Sida acuta, Sida cordifolia, Sida rhombifolia, Etc.

Everything Science and Tradition Knows About the World's Best Herbal Antibiotics, Used by Millions of People Every Day, Top Ayurvedic Herbs, Protein-Rich Survival Plants, Superior Fiber, Grow Them with Your Tomatoes

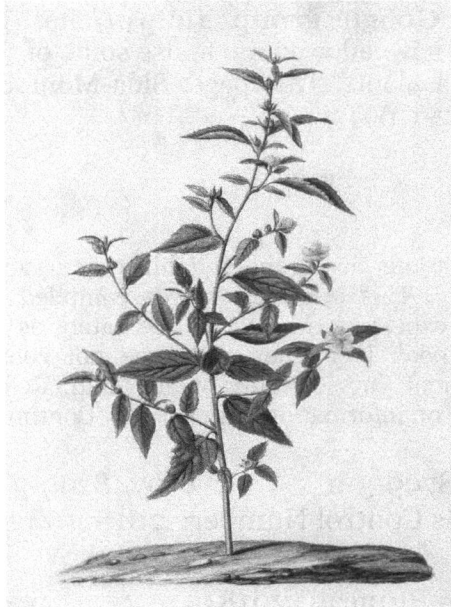

by William Bruneau

WB Publisher, Willits CA

Dedicated to my wife for proof-reading, astute editorial suggestions, and loving support. To friends Brian Ferri-Taylor, Donna D'Terra, and Cynthia Jeavons who have made some excellent suggestions.

I also dedicate this book, in all humility, to the many researchers worldwide who collectively wrote this book.

I am most grateful for essential proof-reading by my friend, and former Ecology Action Garden Manager, Carol Cox. She reviewed certain critical sections of this book, particularly **Cultivation**. More than proof-reading, she made astute observations and asked necessary questions that have added greatly to the accessibility of this book. The information in this book speaks for itself, but reading and understanding this information has become much cleaner and clearer where she has touched it.

Photo credit: Front cover: S. acuta-author. Back cover: S. cordifolia: Prashant Awale & Gurcharan Singh - S. rhombifolia: Dr. Subhasis Panda & Balkar Singh - S. spinosa: Dr. Balkar Singh & Dinesh Valke - S. tiagii; N.S.Dungriyal - S. indica: Satdeep Gill - S. hermaphrodita: Fritz Flohr Reynolds (wikipedia) - S. cordata: J.M.Garg - S. veronicaefolia: Vengolis-wikipedia - S. alba: Marco Schmidt (wikipedia). I am deeply indebted to the **efloraofindia Google group** (https://sites. google.com/site/ efloraofindia/) who have allowed me to use some of their magnificent photographs of Sida plants. Title page: Sida-Moninckx, J., Moninck atlas, vol. 2 t. 1 (1682-1709)

Disclaimer

ISBN: 978-0-9748799-3-2   0-9748799-3-2
Library of Congress Control Number: 2018901425

Title page illustration: Sida-Moninckx, J., Moninckx atlas (1682-1709)
Cover Photos: William Bruneau, The efloraofindia Google group

Contents

....

The leaves of S. acuta possess significant quantities of fat soluble vitamin A precursor, β-Carotene and water soluble vitamins - ascorbic acid, niacin, thiamin and riboflavin. Vitamins are a diverse group of organic molecules required in very small quantities in the diet for health, growth and survival. The absence of vitamin from the diet or an inadequate intake results in characteristics deficiency signs and ultimately death... The composition of calcium, iron, phosphorous, sodium and magnesium in S. acuta leaves as obtained in this study indicates that nutritional benefits would be derived in addition to utilisation of S. acuta leaves for medicinal purposes. **[223]**

Key to the Listings

Most topics in this book are sub-divided by the many species of Sida that have demonstrated that particular quality or benefit. Under each topic each species of Sida has its own paragraph of research. Any listing for a Sida in this book has two parallel tracks: Peer-review research and Ayurvedic/Traditional practice. I personally consider any Ayurvedic use most relevant to the medicinal value of a plant, since herbs have been a core of their medicinal practice for at least 2,000 years. This book is written for herbal practitioners, and in the West peer-review is paramount, so peer-review studies always come first and have their own section clearly marked with the citations in bold.

Peer-review research is clearly separated from Ayurvedic/traditional use. Everything has a citation number that leads you to the research that supports any claim in this book. The peer-review citation number is in **bold** so that it stands out (either in front **145-** or at the end of a listing **[145]**). Ayurvedic and traditional citations are preceded by a bold **Tr** but the citations are not bolded (**Tr** 145-). Look up this number in the **References** section, which gives you the research title, authors, and publishing journal.) Everything with brackets ([??]) is essentially an excerpt or quote from the researchers.

In the three main chapters: (**Composition, Pathogens** and **Benefits**) the individual research citations have a format, but usually the information is incomplete. My ideal listing would be: citation number, what type of research, what part of the plant, what solvent or tea is being used to extract the benefits, and what was learned. You will discover the research is quite incomplete.

In the **Composition** chapter, the actual extract is less important, since most studies are simply looking for its presence. Occasionally the researchers give us the quantity extracted. The extract is more important in the **Benefits** chapter, since the effectiveness might be dependent on that particular extract, perhaps at that concentration. I think the actual extract is most important in the **Pathogens** chapter. One kind of extract, or a certain minimum concentration, affects the pathogen, where other extracts or concentrations from the same source not.

Added benefits come from the synergistic interactions of all the other constituents of the plant. The benefits of Sida are due to its natural defense of itself under tropical conditions. Over millions of years the Sidas have maximized their own internal synergies, marshalling all the constituents they possess. Their performance speaks for itself in these pages.

Who Said What in this Book

- Any comments I make are personal observations and are in this font,
- My comments will not have a citation number.
- The peer-review research is always in this font and will have a citation number at its beginning (**279-**) or end (**[279]**). Traditional and Ayurvedic citations are preceded by a **Tr**, are also bracketed, but are not in bold (**Tr** 279-]. {Short comments I make in the text will be in these brackets}

1

What Sida Does for You

• Sidas are consumed by millions of people every day all over the world, and people have been healing themselves with Sidas for thousands of years.

• Despite being listed as a native plant throughout the Americas, there is no mention of Sida in Western herbals that I can find.

• Nearly everything in this book is from peer-review research, with some expert testimony.

• Sidas control or kill 27 pathogenic bacteria, including many resistant strains, including MRSA.

• Worldwide there have only been 40 studies where Sidas have been tested against cancer. Every one of them has had significant benefits, many were cytotoxic, apoptotic, etc.

• Sidas have shown excellent effect against malaria and other parasites.

• Sidas have tested well against 16 pathogenic fungi, including 15 strains of candida.

• Sidas protect your liver, kidney & brain (and more); are blood cleansing; help to balance your fats/lipids. They are adaptogenic; tonic; aphrodisiac; benefit your digestion; etc.

• This book lists 160 ways that Sida can benefit you.

• Sida acuta can be grown in Zone 8 outdoors. If you can grow tomatoes, you can grow Sida.

For the first time, researchers have found a person in the United States carrying bacteria resistant to antibiotics of last resort, an alarming development that the top U.S. public health official says could mean "the end of the road" for antibiotics. It's the first time this colistin-resistant strain has been found in a person in the United States. In November, public health officials worldwide reacted with alarm when Chinese and British researchers reported finding the colistin-resistant strain in pigs and raw pork and in a small number of people in China. The deadly strain was later discovered in Europe and elsewhere. "It basically shows us that the end of the road isn't very far away for antibiotics — that we may be in a situation where we have patients in our intensive care units, or patients getting urinary-tract infections for which we do not have antibiotics," CDC Director Tom Frieden said in an interview. [723-The Washington Post, May 27, 2016]

Introduction to Sida

This book is the first compilation of known peer-review research and traditional medicinal uses of Sida. This is a reference book and is not to be considered medical advice. Second, this is not a light read! This is an information-dense manual encompassing everything known about the genus Sida.

What I personally add is experience with growing and processing Sida acuta. A smaller book, **User's Guide to Sida acuta and Sida cordifolia**, should be available quite soon. It will cover the two species of Sida currently available to gardeners.

Most, if not all, Sidas originated in Mexico/Central America but they are now ubiquitous in the tropical and sub-tropical worlds: Africa, India, SE Asia, Australia, China, Oceana, American tropics, and the Caribbean among other places. Every day millions of people for thousands of years have gone out and picked Sida leaves (or other parts) to make a tea that will cure many ills. It can be that easy, and it certainly has been for me.

I think everyone is aware that pharmaceutical antibiotics are facing steadily increasing antibiotic resistance from a multitude of pathogens, with few new solutions in sight. Sidas show promise that should be explored. Sidas are non-toxic, benign anti-pathogens that the bugs never figure out. They also augment the potency of many existing pharmaceutical antibiotics, fungicides, etc.

I have successfully grown Sida acuta as an annual for the past four years, outside in our Northern California mountain climate. It is perennial in that it re-seeds profusely. One of the world's great weeds in the tropics, it survives into December in Zone 8, surviving mild freezes. Despite our climate I get a relatively good crop from growing it as an annual outside unprotected. If nothing else Sidas make an excellent protein crop with leaves that can assay at 30% (or better).

To cure the problems caused by infection of such microbes, the current therapy is based on use of synthetic drugs and antibiotics. Although the synthetic drugs have been used in emergency, they possess many side effects. Therefore, it is necessary to introduce an alternative remedial regimen. In the traditional system of India, various indigenous plants are used in the diagnosis, prevention and cure of physical and mental problems of the people. The drugs of herbal origin are used as a medicine in Unani and Ayurveda since ancient times. Medicinal plants are the source of important therapeutic aid for alleviating human and animal ailments. The whole plant or its parts like leaves, stem, bark, root, flower, fruits and seed are used as a source of medicine by the folk healers and local community. Large quantity of this raw drug traded in the market as a raw material for herbal drugs industries. Nowadays, again the people have started using of plants and plant based drugs in order to avoid the toxicity and health hazards associated with indiscriminate use of synthetic drugs and antibiotics. Although, several of plant species have been tested for their antimicrobial properties but the vast majority of plants have not been adequately evaluated. **[639]**

The Pharmaceutical Industry's Response

The pharmaceutical industry has seen incredible growth since 1980. This is due primarily to the industry's strategy to focus efforts towards developing "blockbuster" drugs –those with the potential to generate over $1 billion in sales. However, recent trends indicate that this model may no longer ensure high growth rates for the pharmaceutical industry. One study by Bain Consulting indicates that the average cost of discovering, developing and launching a new drug in June 2004 was $1.7 billion – a 55 % increase over the average cost from 1995 to 2000. This enormous increase is highlighted by the fact that R&D expenses have risen from only $2 billion in 1980 to $39 billion in 2004. Surprisingly, these increases in R&D expenses have not led to a corresponding increase in the number and efficacy of new drug compounds. Comparing 1995-2000 with 1991-1995, the number of New Molecular Entities (NMEs) approvals dropped by nearly 50 percent, to about 40, and the number of New Chemical Entities (NCEs) produced per company declined by 41 percent. **[728-2008]**

Numerous and diverse classes of natural products have been isolated and characterized in the past century. For instance, natural products still remain as major sources of innovative therapeutic agents for infectious diseases, cancer and immunomodulation. Furthermore, natural products and their derivatives still represent more than 30% of the current pharmaceutical market. For example, of the 877 NCEs introduced between 1981 and 2002, 49 % were inspired from natural products in some way or other. So far, **of the estimated 400,000 higher plant species in the world, only about 10% have been characterized chemically to some extent**. Therefore, the unexplored potential of plants as a source of novel bioactive chemicals is enormous. Surprisingly, in the past few years most Big Pharma companies have either terminated or considerably scaled down their natural product operations. This occurs despite a significant number of natural product-derived drugs being ranked in the top 35 worldwide selling ethical drugs in 2000, 2001, and 2002; representing 40% of worldwide drug sales in 2000, 24% in 2001, and 26% in 2002. **[728-2008]**

LONDON, July 7 (Reuters) - At least three people worldwide are infected with totally untreatable "superbug" strains of gonorrhea which they are likely to be spreading to others through sex, the World Health Organization (WHO) said on Friday. Giving details of studies showing **a "very serious situation" with regard to highly drug-resistant forms of the sexually-transmitted disease** (STD), WHO experts said it was "only a matter of time" before last-resort gonorrhea antibiotics would be of no use. "Gonorrhea is a very smart bug," said Teodora Wi, a human reproduction specialist at the Geneva-based U.N. health agency. "Every time you introduce a new type of antibiotic to treat it, this bug develops resistance to it."...(the WHO has) documented three specific cases - of patients with strains of gonorrhea against which no known antibiotic is effective. "These are cases that can infect others. It can be transmitted," she told reporters. "And these cases may just be the tip of the iceberg, since systems to diagnose and report untreatable infections are lacking in lower-income countries where gonorrhea is actually more common."... Manica Balasegaram, director of the Global Antibiotic Research and Development Partnership, **said the situation was "grim" and there was a "pressing need" for new medicines**. The pipeline, however, is very thin, with only three potential new gonorrhea drugs in development and no guarantee any will prove effective in final-stage trials, he said... from 2009 to 2014 there was widespread resistance to the first-line medicine ciprofloxacin, increasing resistance to another antibiotic drug called azithromycin, and the emergence of resistance to last-resort treatments known as extended-spectrum cephalosporins (ESCs). In most countries, it said, ESCs are now the only single antibiotics that remain effective for treating gonorrhea. Yet resistance to them has already been reported in 50 countries... "We urgently need to seize the opportunities we have with existing drugs and candidates in the pipeline," he told reporters. **"Any new treatment developed should be accessible to everyone who needs it, while ensuring it is used appropriately**, so that drug resistance is slowed as much as possible." [742-2017]

Only one peer-review study (ever) has looked into Sida's effectiveness against gonorrhea. A 1995 study found that cryptolepine, an alkaloid extracted from several Sida species, had in vitro activity against gonorrhea (Nekseria gonorrhoeae). I could find no follow-up study, or any other research since then. Nevertheless, for thousands of years Sidas have been prescribed as a specific against gonorrhea around the world, especially as part of Ayurvedic medicine. Again, the one study was positive but never followed up, and Sida has been used to treat gonorrhea in multiple countries since time-out-of-mind.

Stephen Buhner outlined much of the power of Sida in his book, *Herbal Antibiotics,* but more is needed beyond what could be said, however brilliantly, in 18 pages. Herbalists and naturopaths need as much hard data as possible to fashion our health solutions of the future before it is too late.

Sidas in the lab, using concentrated extracts, have worked against something like 65 pathogens including: Staph (18 specific strains of Staph, including several multi-drug resistant strains), Candida (including at least 6 resistant strains), some cancers, gonorrhea, typhoid, Aspergillus mold, E. coli, Herpes simplex, Kebsiella (pneumonia and hospital infections), Malaria, Mycobacterium, Salmonella (both food poisoning and typhoid), Shigella (diarrhea and dysentery), Strep (cavities, pneumonia), and internal worms. Other studies have shown Sida ineffective for about 20 pathogens, including some that have also tested it as effective. You will have to look at the studies and decide who was right. This, of course, is just what has been tested so far, which is not enough.

There are 160 or so other proven benefits from taking Sida including: adaptogenic; anti-oxidant; analgesic; kidney, liver, heart and brain protective; beneficial for human reproduction; and chemoprotective. It is a mineral accumulator; fuel source; and it is a host plant for birds, bees, and butterflies, among other things. The Sidas are excellent fiber plants. The leaves have at least 20% good protein (mine have over 30%); Sida is considered a survival food.

Who Wrote This Book?

I would have preferred to not write this book. I would have much preferred picking up someone else's thorough examination of the genus Sida, including all its traditional and Ayurvedic uses around the world. I waited two years for this book from another author/researcher but it never came. The world desperately needs this book, so I wrote it. It culminates about three years of off-and-on intensive work. Hopefully this will engender future books detailing other known powerful herbal antibiotics. Natural medicinals were our past, and now are our future and our salvation.

Actually, the peer-review researchers themselves wrote this book, because as much as possible I have used the words of the researchers themselves to explain their research, and how Sida benefits humankind. I mostly assembled and edited this book. Assembling a book of this magnitude solo was at moments terrifying, so it was of great comfort to me, knowing that everything in this book leads back to expert research or review. It helps that for the most part, this book is not me. In this first edition I expect mess-ups, for example some material may not have the right citation number (write me and I will correct it for the second edition), but everything in this book is from some peer-review research or expert testimony.

I have been a plant person most of my adult life. My wife and I started Bountiful Gardens Seeds in 1982, which was part of Ecology Action of the Midpeninsula, an organization that has been desperately trying to save the world's soil for the last 45 years, while refining a farming method (Biointensive) that actually creates soil while being very productive. I retired as the third oldest working member of EA after our founder, John Jeavons, and my wife. For years I selected many of the seeds we carried in our catalog, which was not unlike being an Indiana Jones of the plant world. The feedback I have received from farmers all over the world has given me good experience with how plants grow and what plants do. It also helps to be married to a biologist who fills in any blanks.

I consider myself a personal herbalist. I do not have the intimate, extensive knowledge of hundreds of herbs that a professional herbalist needs to know, but rather I know very well the few plants that I need, seeking only my health, and the health of my family. Medicinal herbs have been at the core of my family's health for at least 35 years. I know the plants I use very well, and when I discover a new one that is as good as Sida is, I am completely on board right away, and want to know everything about it. The next step is a thorough and intensive research into its known benefits. So for a year I intensely scoured the world for legitimate research on Sida, and in particular on Sida acuta, the species which I use. The results have exceeded my wildest expectations. Everything known about Sida is pretty much in this book.

I personally believe that the Sidas (the major ones at least) are arguably the most powerful antibiotics known on earth, and Sida acuta the most powerful single herbal antibiotic known. (The discovery of berberine in (only) Sida acuta puts it over the top in my opinion.) Yet the other Sida species, particularly Sida cordifolia, aspire to the crown. The synergies of combining the strengths of several Sida species are largely unknown.

Sidas generally have stronger effects with a stronger dose, and they have a high toxicity limit. Sidas have over 200 known active constituents interlaced in an intricate matrix of effectiveness that "the bugs" never figure out. There has been no evidence of antibiotic resistance to crude Sida extracts no matter how much was taken, or how long they were taken.

I believe from my 35 something years in plants (and especially medicinals) that our anti-pathogenic future is to compound sustainable medications from multiple medicinal herbs. As powerful as any single herbal antibiotic is: there is no single herbal solution that can stop this proliferation of killer pathogens that seventy years of pharmaceutical antibiotics overuse has caused. The next generation of medicinal compounders will have to produce our salvation going forward with herbs like Sida. Again, one herb, even Sida, will ultimately not be enough, but it will be our very best start. And best of all, you can probably grow Sida in your garden just like tomatoes.

Why Write This Book?

Four years ago when I read Stephen Harrod Buhner's classic, *Herbal Antibiotics: Natural Alternatives for Treating Drug-Resistant Bacteria*, it scared the living daylights out of me. He was pronouncing the death of all pharmaceutical antibiotics within 5-10 years (0-5 years now), and his timeline seems right in line with current events. Buhner also proposed that our salvation could come through herbal antibiotics. This was like a key fitting into a locked box that I had to open. I saw a potential cure for a serious health problem I had. I also saw a powerful traditional medicinal that shows immense medicinal promise that begs to be further explored.

7

It took me over a year just to obtain seed. The irony is that several Sidas are considered US natives, and they grow throughout the South. Several Sidas are even considered serious commercial weeds in the South and eradicated, yet ironically the seed is hard to find. I have been actually growing Sida acuta for over three years now and personally benefitting from it all along the way. I have no experience in growing the other Sidas yet, but have acquired some seed. While cultivation of the various Sidas is quite similar (they are all tropical weeds), the next edition of this book will clarify any discrepancies.

This book comprises everything known about the Sidas as of March of 2017, which in actuality is not that much. Consider this: if you go to our National Institute of Health's "Pub Med" website (https://www.ncbi.nlm.nih.gov /pubmed) and look up "folic acid" you will find something like 45,299 peer-review studies. If you look up ascorbic acid, you will get something like 51,292 studies. If you look up the Sida family, most of what you will get as "sida" is the French acronym for HIV/AIDS, so any Sida research is already deeply buried and attenuated under hundreds of French reports on AIDS. Looking up specific varieties we get: Sida acuta = 32 results, Sida cordifolia = 42 results, Sida rhombifolia = 31 results. There is no way this book could have been written with such meager results. Yet I ended up with over 750 references. Everything else came through Google Scholar. I could not have written this book without Google Scholar!

Google Scholar (https://scholar.google.com/) is a freely accessible web search engine that indexes the full text or metadata of scholarly literature across an array of publishing formats and disciplines. This includes journal and conference papers, theses and dissertations, academic books, pre-prints, abstracts, technical reports and other scholarly literature from all broad areas of research. You'll find works from a wide variety of academic publishers, professional societies and university repositories, as well as scholarly articles available anywhere across the web. {bottom line, "We cover academic papers from sensible websites"}....Third-party researchers estimated it to contain roughly 160 million documents as of May 2014 and an earlier statistical estimate...approximately 80-90% coverage of all articles published in English with an estimate of 100 million. [1]

The best single country for Sida research is India. At least five members of the Sida family are primary Ayurvedic herbs, including the renowned "Bala", and many Sidas are considered Rasayana herbs. "Second-world" peer-review research - be it from India, Nigeria, Brazil, Indonesia – was far more useful for me as an herbalist. These studies are far more practical, looking for local solutions to a global health crisis that everyone on earth is facing. India is currently the only country that is looking at rapid replication of Sida. With 1.3 billion people to keep healthy they are aware that there will be a great need for these plants that have traditionally just been harvested from the wild. Many of these "Second-world" peer-review studies also discuss the traditional uses that prompted them to study Sida; this is the basis of much of the research into this book's traditional uses.

An entire section of the Materia Medica of Ayurveda termed Rasayanas is devoted to the enhancement of the body resistance. Interestingly, a somewhat similar role is ascribed to tonics and various herbals in the Chinese and European systems of medicine. [728]   Rasayana drugs are rejuvenating and age-sustaining tonics for promoting vitality and longevity. They are also used for the treatment of asthma and other chest ailments. [464]

How Sidas Stop Pathogens

Nearly every herbalist will tell you that the whole of a plant, as opposed to certain individual constituents, offers additional benefits due to the synergy between the individual elements of the plant. Consider that a plant first and foremost is protecting itself, and that over millennia it has found ways to internally craft great synergies from the natural interactions of its many constituents. Most Western research has been in search of a single compound, a super-star compound, that Western pharmaceutical companies can synthesize, patent, and sell for a ton of money as a sole cure. This compound may or may not be the same as the original.

Unfortunately, pathogens are actually very, very clever and have become quite adept at finding ways to neutralize any single compound that gets in their way. Buhner describes pharma's complete failure in several very clear and thorough chapters in his book, *Herbal Antibiotics*. I highly recommend that everyone read it now! The time grows short. There is now a long list of pathogens that are resistant to all antibiotics except colistin, and colistin's end is quite near.

Colistin is a decades-old drug that fell out of favor in human medicine due to its kidney toxicity... As multi-drug resistant bacteria became more prevalent in the 1990s, colistin started to get a second look as an emergency solution, in spite of toxic effects... It remains one of the last-resort antibiotics for multidrug-resistant bacteria. [1]

When pharmaceutical companies extract individual substances out of the complex that is a plant, and then put them to use killing pathogens, these single compounds are relatively quickly neutralized by those pathogens. So for a short-term gain, the medicinal value from this substance is lessened in the future. This works against its forever value for both the plant and humans. This backwards way of thinking is what got us into this mess to begin with. Creating more single solutions for the bacteria to quickly neutralize just gets us further and further behind in finding a long-term solution, a solution that is sustainable. The only solutions that last are natural complex solutions that the pathogens never figure out.

Most peer-review studies in this book generally use solvents, sometimes exotic, to extract single elements from the plant, because the goal is to find out how much of this element is in the plant, and if this concentrated element kills pathogens by itself. Finding the characteristics of one element is useful, but this ignores any benefits from the synergistic inter-reactions of the many other elements in a Sida plant. We are just beginning to understand how the several hundred elements in a Sida plant interact, but it is already beautiful.

There are very few studies anywhere that look at the benefits of consuming a whole Sida plant together, or all the aerial parts, and they are quite encouraging. Last year I realized that by making the tincture only of the leaves (traditional), I was missing out on additional benefits from the root, stem, bark, seed, fruit, blossom, bud, etc. There is no part of Sida that is not medicinal according to the peer-review research, and the different parts are medicinal in at least somewhat different ways.

The Sidas in this book have been peer-review tested to be essentially non-toxic, anti-inflammatory, and analgesic. They can be considered a tonic and adapto-genic that keeps the body in good health. Sidas are anti-pathogen (antibiotic, anti-malaria, anti-worm, cytoxic, anti-fungal, and somewhat antiviral). The bugs never figure out whole-herb herbal anti-pathogens.

Most of the world takes Sidas by drinking a tea of some leaves or roots. I personally squirt some alcoholic tincture into a glass of water. Sidas are plants that could grow in many temperate gardens. They historically have been easily processed for the health and protection of family, friends, neighbors, etc. Best of all, the Sidas produce these antibiotics for their own preservation, so that these great benefits are constantly "updated" by the plants themselves.

Adaptogens are plant derived biologically active substances that improve your immunity and physical endurance. Many herbal preparations have been evaluated for their adaptogenic activity during exposure to stressful conditions. In response to stressor, a series of behavioral, neurochemical and immunological changes occur that ought to serve in an adaptive capacity.... In conclusion, the above study indicates positive adaptogenic activity of the extract Sida cordata (whole plant). [405]

Sidas are amazing plants. Sida cordifolia is a CNS (central nervous system) sedative and depressant [132], but is also a CNS stimulant [120]. Sida acuta is an abortifacieant [138 et al] and an anti-implantation contraceptive that has no lingering effects [96], but it is also an aphrodisiac [561], uterotonic [313], is essential for post-delivery [305], and has a long history of helping general female problems like vaginal candidiosis [237]. Sida acuta is also aphrodisiac for men [217], improves low or no sperm [201], and is useful for male sexual problems like impotence [526]. I have listed over160 health benefits that the Sidas deliver.

We Know We Need Something Different

CONCLUSION: In general, the mechanisms by which microorganisms survive the action of antimicrobial agents are poorly understood and remain debatable. **[713-2010]**   Increasing risks of infection stemming from antibiotic-resistant microorganisms have made the discovery of new and natural antimicrobial substances the focus of various studies, while the expectations of conscious consumers have encouraged or even forced drug producers and service providers to use natural preservatives. Thus, a need has arisen to investigate and test the efficacy of various plants against microorganisms, and the antibacterial impacts of various plant extracts on microorganisms and, particularly, food pathogens have been reported by several researchers. **[638-2016]**

One of my first thoughts after reading *Herbal Antibiotics* was, "Oh no! I love my community and I would hate to see it decimated." After growing Sida for a few years and trying to convince people of the value of this plant, I made very little progress in terms of raising awareness or growing Sida in my community. The local herbalists want to be on board, but they know nothing about this plant. And after a couple of years the realization came that if I did not write this book, perhaps no one would. The information about the Sida family is very limited and scattered. It took me several years to dig out most of everything known about this plant. All the information in this book is from peer-review research studies, or to a much lesser degree, expert websites.

Since I started this project, there has not been a day passing that I do not feel the urgency to get this information out in a useful form before it is too late. It will take time to spread this information and use Sidas to compound useful herbal antibiotics. I am not sure that we will have enough time to avoid or neutralize the multiple epidemics from pathogens fully resistant to all pharmaceutical antibiotics that are only months away.

This book is specifically written for herbalists and natural healers to give them the Sidas as an additional tool to help preserve life and health. It is mostly based on what little peer-review research has been done to date, with the hope that this will inspire much more research. There is some material taken from expert websites, always with the intention of providing well-researched information from sensible sources. Bottom line: I always cite the name, author, and source for any claims in this book.

The traditional uses are also fully cited, allowing you to easily find the source material. Much of the traditional uses cited in this book come from the peer-review researchers themselves. Not always, but usually these fine "second world" peer-review research studies devote a paragraph or two at the beginning to honor the long-time effective use of Sidas in the traditional healing practices of their country (this is never in "First-world" studies). The best research into the traditional uses of Sida is at institutions and universities in India, Nigeria,

Brazil, and many other countries. The rest of the information on traditional uses comes from international plant websites.

Nearly all this research is easily accessed through Google Scholar. In many cases, there is more than just an abstract summarizing the research, and you can access the whole study! Looking at the actual results can be very edifying! This has been a one-man crusade, and in this first edition mistakes have certainly been made. I am comforted by knowing that no one has to take my word for anything in this book (if you find a misplaced citation, please let me know). I encourage you to always go back to the source and draw your own conclusions. Bottom line: everything in this book comes from some peer-review research even if I got the citation wrong.

Finally, I could not have written this book without the help of Wikipedia. Many, many questions and definitions I was able to answer quickly and authoritatively through Wikipedia. It also has been a very up-to-date source for learning so many new things – it has been my professional oracle. I needed a **Glossary** to keep track of many unfamiliar terms, and most of that comes from Wikipedia. Wikipedia struggles to remain independent. I will be donating a percentage of the proceeds from this book back to Wikipedia in deep gratitude for the essential work they perform, and their role in the creation of this book.

Names, Description, Distribution

Most Sidas, if not all, started in the American tropics. Some varieties like Sida acuta now cover the entire tropical and sub-tropical world. Some are among the world's great weeds. They are incredibly adaptable-their chromosomes are not double-helix, they are multi-helix. As a result diversification within species (and in the genus) is endemic, and identification can be difficult.

Please note: this book is a compilation of known peer-review research and is not to be considered medical advice.

The plants in genus Sida show peculiar features. The plants are herbs or under-shrubs, hairy and with stellate hairs. Leaves toothed; stipules linear, 6-8 mm long. Pedicels auxiliary. Solitary or clustered, disarticulating in fruits at a constriction below the calyx. Involucral bracts o. Sapels 5, valvate, connate with the stamina tube. Stamina tube divided at the top into numerous antheriferous filaments. Ovary of 5-12 cells; ovule 1, in each cell, pendulus; styles as many as carpels; stigmas terminal. Fruit globose, depressed, enclosed by the calyx; carpels separating from each other and from the central axis, beaked or not. Seeds black-chestnut, smooth [88]

The name Sida was validated by Linnaeus in 'Species Plantarum' (1753). The genus comprises about 200 species in tropical and subtropical parts of the World and about 20 species in India... the genus has its main centers of

12

diversity in the New World tropics and in Australia, and hence the genus might be of new World origin. **[555]** "There are 125 or 150 or 200 species of the genus Sida (taxonomy is an exact science). They are distributed throughout the world, mostly in the tropics and subtropics, but some species extend into temperate regions". **[721]**

Sida L. (Malvaceae) has been used for centuries in traditional medicines in different countries for the prevention and treatment of different diseases such as diarrhea, dysentery, gastrointestinal and urinary infections, malarial and other fevers, childbirth and miscarriage problems, skin ailments, cardiac and neural problems, asthma, bronchitis and other respiratory problems, weight loss aid, rheumatic and other inflammations, tuberculosis, etc... A variety of ethnomedicinal uses of Sida species have been found in India, China, African and American countries. Phytochemical investigation of this genus has resulted in identification of about 142 chemical constituents, among which alkaloids, flavonoids and ecdysteroids are the predominant groups. The crude extracts and isolates have exhibited a wide spectrum of in vitro and in vivo pharmacological effects involving antimicrobial, analgesic, anti-inflammatory, abortifacient, neuroprotective, cardiovascular and cardioprotective, antimalarial, antitubercular, antidiabetic and antiobesity, antioxidant and nephroprotective activities among others. Ethnopharmacological preparations containing Sida species as an ingredient in India, African and American countries possess good efficacy in health disorders. From the toxicity perspective, only three Sida species have been assessed and found safe for oral use in rats... Pharmacological results supported some of the uses of Sida species in the traditional medicine. Alkaloids, flavonoids, other phenolics and ecdysteroids were perhaps responsible for the activities of extracts of the plants of this genus. Furthermore, detailed study on quality and safety assurance data on available ethnopharmacological preparations is needed for their commercial exploitation in local and global markets. **[168-2007]** {In this book I have listed 251 constituents}

Medicinal Varieties of Sida

Many Sida species have the same names, and often the same characteristics. Sidas are polyploids, containing more than the normal two paired sets of chromosomes, and thus incredibly adaptive

Sida acuta = var. carpinfolia, broomweed, wireweed, Common Fanpetals, Bala, Brihannagabala, Rajabala

Sida alba = Prickly Sida or Teaweed (usually classified as spinosa)

Sida alnifolia = (a synonym of S. spinosa and S. acuta)

Sida asiatica = Abutilon asiaticum, Sida cordifolia, Sida jamaicensis

Sida cardifolia = Bala, Country Mallow

Sida cordifolia = Abutilon ramosum, Country Mallow, Mahabala

Sida cordata=Long-stalk sida, Heartleaf fanpetals, Nagabala, S. pakistanica

Sida hermaphrodita = River-mallow, Virginia Fanpetals

Sida humilis = var. veronicifolia, a synonym of Sida cordata

Sida indica = Abutilon indicum, Atibala, Monkeybush [English]

Sida javensis = S. veronicaefolia var. javensis, Javanese fanpetals

Sida linfolia = Flaxleaf fanpetals, Balai grand

Sida mysorensis = Sida urticifolia, India Mysore fanpetals

Sida pilosa = S. javensis, Melochia cordata, S. cordata, S. humilis, S. pilosa

Sida rhombifolia = Arrowleaf sida, Cuban jute, Bala, Atibala , Guanxuma

Sida rhomboidea = S. rhombifolia var. rhomboidea, S. retusa

Sida retusa = Sida rhombifolia var. retusa, Cuban jute, Teaweed,

Sida spinosa = S. alba (syn.) , Prickly fanpetals, Indiana mallow, Nagabala

Sida tuberculata = S. tuberculata

Sida tiagii = S. pakistanica, Bal, S. ovata

Sida urens = Tropical fanpetals, Balai-zortie

Sida veronicaefolia = Nagabala, Snake Mallow, Gangeruki

Naming something means its important to you. Sidas have myriad local names all over the world, in particular the tropics and subtropics, because they are used medicinally (as well as for other uses) all over the world. These are very adaptive plants that are constantly causing identification problems for taxonomists. For example, Sida rhomboidea is generally considered to be a variety of Sida rhombifolia, but in India it is considered a variety of Sida spinosa. Sida alba is also considered a synonym. JUSTOR considers Sida spinosa and Sida rhombifolia as synonyms of Sida alba. Fortunately all the major Sidas in this book seem to be generally medicinally equivalent.

All Sidas

General Description: Sida is a genus of flowering plants in the mallow family, Malvaceae. They are distributed in tropical and subtropical regions worldwide, especially in the Americas. Plants of the genus may be known generally as fanpetals or sidas... Sida has historically been a wastebasket taxon, including many plants that simply did not fit into other genera of the Malvaceae. Species have been continually reclassified. The circumscription of Sida is still unclear, with no real agreement regarding how many species belong there. Over 1000 names have been placed in the genus, and many authorities accept about 150 to 250 valid names today. Some sources accept as few as 98 species. There are many plants recognized as Sida that have not yet been described to science [1]   Nine species and varieties of Sida, occurring in wild state, were collected from different localities of West Bengal and regions adjoining it, mostly from the suburbs of Calcutta. S. rhombifolia has a wide occurrence with different varieties adapted to different conditions of the soil and other environmental conditions. Under the present study five distinct forms have been observed.1. S. rhombifolia var. A (typical): Leaves comparatively long rhomboid, narrow, thick, acute and branches green or grayish green.2. S. rhombifolia var. B (rhomboidea): Leaves comparatively large, broad, rhomboid, acute or sub-acute, branches and leaves green.3. S. rhombifolia var. C (obovata): Leaf blades obovate.4. S. rhombifolia var. D: Leaves comparatively short, rhomboid narrow, thin, acute or sub-acute, branches green.5. S. rhombifolia var. E: Leaves comparatively small, short rhomboid, broad, thick, acute or sub-acute; leaves and branches green or light green; distinctly reddish, when young. Forty-eight populations, from different localities, of these varieties were studied. **[216]**

S. acuta can be readily confused with *S. rhombifolia*, and hybridization between the two species has been reported. However, Viarouge et al. (1997) provide a valuable guide to identification of *Sida* species by vegetative characters, in which they point out that *S. rhombifolia* tends to have broader, more rhomboid leaves with dentation restricted to the upper half or two-thirds of the leaf margin, while the leaf margin in *S. acuta* is dentate throughout. The undersides of the leaves of *S. rhombifolia* are also more densely covered in stellate hairs. Other characters suggested by other authors include the stipules, which are uniformly narrow in *S. acuta* but of unequal width in *S. rhombifolia*; also the seeds of *S. rhombifolia* have only one awn; and the flowers are on stalks 1 to 3 cm long, much longer than those of *S. acuta*. **[698]**

Sida species

Sida abutifolia Mill. – accepted – procumbent sida, prostrate sida, spreading fanpetals **Sida acuminata** DC. – not accepted **Sida acuta** Burm. f. – accepted – common wireweed **Sida acuta ssp. carpinifolia** (L. f.) Borss. Waalk. – not accepted **Sida acuta var. carpinifolia** (L. f.) K. Schum. – not accepted **Sida aggregata** C. Presl – accepted – savannah fanpetals **Sida alaba** L. – not accepted **Sida alata** S. Watson – not accepted **Sida alba** L. – not accepted **Sida alcaeoides** Michx. – not accepted **Sida angustifolia** Lam. – not accepted **Sida antillensis** Urb. – accepted – Antilles fanpetals **Sida carpinifolia** L. f. – not accepted **Sida ciliaris** L. – accepted – bracted sida, bracted fanpetals **Sida ciliaris** var. mexicana (Moric. ex Ser.) Shinners – not accepted **Sida cordata** (Burm. f.) Borss. Waalk. – accepted – heartleaf fanpetals **Sida cordifolia** L. – accepted – `ilima **Sida cristata** L. – not **accepted Sida cuneifolia** Roxb. – not accepted **Sida eggersii** Baker f. – not accepted **Sida elliottii** Torr. & A. Gray – accepted – Elliott's fanpetals **Sida elliottii var. parviflora** Chapm. – acc**epted – pineland fanpetals Sida erecta Macfad. – not accepted Sida fallax** Walp. **– accepted – yellow** `ilima **Sida fallax var. kauaiensis** Hochr. – not accepted **Sida filicaulis** Torr. & A. Gray – not accepted **Sida filiformis** Moric. ex Ser. – not accepted **Sida filipes** A. Gray – not accepted **Sida floridana** Siedo – accepted **Sida glabra** Mill. – accepted – smooth fanpetals **Sida glomerata** Cav. – accepted – clustered fanpetals **Sida glutinosa** Comm. ex Cav. – accepted – sticky fanpetals **Sida grayana** Clement – not

15

accepted **Sida hederacea** (Douglas ex Hook.)– not accepted – alkali mallow, alkali sida, dollar weed **Sida helleri** Rose ex A. Heller – not accepted **Sida hermaphrodita** (L.) Rusby – accepted – Virginia mallow, Virginia fanpetals **Sida hispida** Pursh – not accepted **Sida holwayi** Baker f. & Rose – not accepted **Sida humilis sensu** Britton & P. Wilson – not accepted **Sida humilis var. veronicifolia** Lam. – not accepted **Sida inflexa** Fernald – not accepted – pineland fanpetals **Sida jamaicensis** L. – accepted – Jamaican fanpetals **Sida javensis** Cav. – accepted **Sida javensis ssp. expilosa** Borss. Waalk. – not accepted **Sida ledyardii** H. St. John – not accepted **Sida lepidota** A. Gray – not accepted **Sida lepidota var. sagittifolia** A. Gray – not accepted **Sida leprosa** (Ortega) K. Schum. – not accepted **Sida leprosa var. depauperata** (A. Gray) Clement – not accepted Sida leprosa var. hederacea **(Douglas ex Hook.) K. Schum. – not accepted** Sida leprosa var. sagittifolia **(A. Gray) Clement – not accepted** Sida leptophylla **Small – not accepted** Sida lindheimeri **Engelm. & A. Gray – accepted – showy fanpetals** Sida linifolia **Cav. – accepted – flaxleaf fanpetals** Sida longipes A. Gray – accepted – stockflower fanpetals Sida meyeniana **Walp. – not accepted** Sida nelsoni **H. St. John – not accepted** Sida neomexicana **A. Gray – accepted – New Mexico fanpetals** Sida paniculata **L. – not accepted** Sida physaloides **C. Presl – not accepted** Sida physocalyx **A. Gray – not accepted** Sida procumbens **Sw. – not accepted** Sida pyramidata **Cav. – not accepted** Sida repens **Dombey ex Cav. – accepted – Javanese fanpetals** Sida rhombifolia **L. – accepted – arrowleaf sida, Cuban-jute, Cuban jute** Sida rhomboidea **Roxb. ex Fleming is a synonym of Sida rhombifolia L.** Sida rubromarginata **Nash – accepted – red-margin fan**petals Sida sagittifolia (A. Gray) Rydb. – not accepted Sida salviifolia C. Presl – accepted – escoba parade Sida santaremensis Monteiro – accepted – moth fanpetals **Sida setifera** C. Presl – not accepted **Sida spinosa** L. – accepted – prickly sida, prickly fanpetals **Sida stipularis** Cav. – not accepted **Sida stipulata** Cav. – not accepted – stipule fanpetals Sida supina L'Hér. – not accepted **Sida texana** (Torr. & A. Gray) Small – not accepted **Sida tragiifolia** A. Gray – accepted – tuberous sida, catnip noseburn, earleaf fanpetals **Sida ulmifolia** Mill. – accepted – broomweed **Sida urens** L. – accepted – tropical fanpetals **Sida villosa** Mill. – not accepted [720] **Sida garckeana** Pol. (TropicalAfrica) [364] **Sida vogelii** Hook. f. **Sida bodinieri** Gand. **Sida orientalis** DC, Sida scoparia Lour. **[365]**

Species formerly considered Sida but now in other genera include: **Abutilon abutiloides** (Jacq.) Garcke ex Hochr. (as S. abutiloides Jacq. or S. lignosa Cav.) **Abutilon cristata** (L.) Schltdl. (as S. cristata L.) **Abutilon giganteum** (Jacq.) Sweet (as S. gigantea Jacq.) **Abutilon grandifolium** (Willd.) Sweet (as S. grandifolia Willd. or S. mollis Ortega) **Abutilon hirtum** (Lam.) Sweet (as S. graveolens Roxb. ex Hornem.) **Abutilon incanum** (Link) Sweet (as S. incana Link) **Abutilon indicum** (L.) Sweet (as S. indica L.) **Abutilon megapotamicum** (A.Spreng.) A.St.-Hil. & Naudin (as S. megapotamica A.Spreng.) **Abutilon mollissimum** (Cav.) Sweet Sida mollicoma Willd. (as S. mollissima Cav.) **Abutilon pictum**

(Gillies ex Hook. & Arn.) Walp. (as S. picta Gillies ex Hook. & Arn.) **Abutilon reflexum** (Juss. ex Cav.) Sweet (as S. reflexa Juss. ex Cav.) **Abutilon sellowianum** (Klotzsch) Regel (as S. sellowiana Klotzsch) **Abutilon theophrasti** Medik. (as S. abutilon L.)   **Bakeridesia integerrima** (Hook.) D.M.Bates (as S. integerrima Hook.) **Corynabutilon vitifolium** (Cav.) Kearney (as S. vitifolium Cav.) **Malvastrum hispidum** (Pursh) Hochr. (as S. hispida Pursh)   **Malvella leprosa** (Ortega) Krapov. (as S. hederacea (Douglas) Torr. ex A.Gray) **Nototriche compacta** (Gay) A.W.Hill (as S. compacta Gay)   **Pavonia sepium** A. St.-Hil. (as S. malvacea Vell.)   **Sidalcea malviflora** (DC.) A.Gray ex Benth. (as S. malviflora DC.)   **Sidalcea oregana subsp. oregana** (as S. oregana Nutt. ex Torr. & A.Gray)   **Sidastrum micranthum** (A.St.-Hil.) Fryxell (as S. micrantha A.St.-Hil.)   **Sidastrum paniculatum** (L.) Fryxell (as S. paniculata L.)   **Sphaeralcea grossulariifolia** (Hook. & Arn.) Rydb. (as S. grossulariifolia Hook. & Arn.) **Wissadula periplocifolia** (L.) C.Presl ex Thwaites (as S. periplocifolia L.) [1]

Herbal plants used as a remedy against threatened miscarriage... The alkaloid, saponins, resins, flavonoids content of these plants mainly control the miscarriage without any side effects as they are of natural products. So the proper conservation of such precious medicinal plants is required for future use as these are in a verge of extinction due to various environmental constraints. [230]

Sida rhombifolia Linn. is demulcent, diaphoretic, diuretic, emollient, stomachic, tonic, sudorific, appetite and stimulant. Arrowleaf sida has significant medicinal applications for which it is cultivated throughout Bangladesh and India. Leaves and roots are used for piles, gonorrhea, antisoud, diuretic, aphrodisiac. Roots of these herbs are held in great repute in treatment of rheumatism5. Stems abound in mucilage and are employed as demulcents and emollients both for external and internal use. The herb is also useful in calculous troubles and as a febrifuge with pepper. Mucilage is used as an emollient and for scorpion sting. Australian aborigines use the herb to treat diarrhoea. Leaves are smoked in Mexico and a tea is prepared in India for the stimulation it provides. [545]

Sida acuta had very good in vitro antiplasmodial activity (IC50 of 0.05 µg/mL). This may be related to its alkaloid content... Many plants screened for their antimicrobial activities showed interesting results with very low MIC and MBC values. For example, The alkaloids of Sida acuta were also found to exert good in vitro antibacterial activity against several pathogenic bacteria with MIC values ranging from 16 to 400 µg/m.... It is reported that cryptolepine, the main alkaloid of Sida acuta and Cryptrolepis sanguinolenta that is very active in vitro against Plasmodium falciparum failed to cure malaria in vivo and its synthetic analogues such as 2,7-dibromocryptolepine are under investigation. [215]

Individual Sidas

Sida acuta

Sida acuta var. carpinfolia, broomweed, wireweed, Common Fanpetals, Bala, Brihannagabala, Rajabala

Description

Flower Color: pale yellow;.

Attracts Butterflies: y;.

Flower Bloom Period: January;.

Foliage Duration: perennial;.

Habit: sub-shrub

Plant spacing: 12-15" apart;.

Size: 18-24" tall.

Sun Exposure: sun to partial shade.

Temperature Cold Hardiness: 8a. **[360]**

A profusely branching annual herbaceous weed, cosmopolitan in distribution. It is found as a major weed throughout the hotter parts of India and Srilanka. The bark is smooth, greenish, the root is thin, long, cylindrical and very rough; leaves are lanceolate, nearly glabrous, peduncles equal to the petioles, the flowers are yellow, solitary or in pairs; seeds are smooth and black. **[217]** A small, erect, perennial shrub, branching profusely from the base. It usually ranges from 30-150 cm in height, but grows to 3 m in favorable conditions in northern Australia (Lonsdale et al., 1995). The stems are fibrous to almost woody, with a tough stringy bark. There is a deep, tough taproot. The leaves are alternate, lanceolate, acute, tapering towards both ends, and on a short, hairy petiole 3-6 mm long. The leaves have toothed margins, are smooth or have sparse stellate hairs and have prominent veins on the undersurface. The leaves are quite variable in size, from 2-9 cm long and 0.5-4 cm wide. The pair of stipules at the base of each leaf are not equal, with one frequently much narrower than the other. The flowers are yellow, solitary, 1-2 cm in diameter and on a short stalk 0.3-0.8 cm long. There are five petals, joined at the base and with a shallow notch at the apex. The fruit is a hard, brown capsule, 3-5 mm in diameter, breaking into 5-8 triangular segments. Each segment contains one seed and has a pair of sharp awns or 'beaks' 1-1.5 mm long which attach readily to animal fur or clothing. The seeds are small, reddish-brown to black, wedge-shaped, deeply indented on both sides, rounded on the back and about 1.5 mm long. **[698]**

Scientific names - Sida Acuta synonyms

Malvinda carpinifolia (L. fil.) Medic. (synonym)   Sida acuta subsp. carpini-folia (L. fil.) Borss. (syn)   Sida acuta var. carpinifolia K.Schum. (syn) Sida acuta var. intermedia S.Y. Hu (syn)   Sida arrud-iana Monteiro (syn) Sida artensis Montrouz. ex Guillau-min & Beauvis. (syn)   Sida balbisiana DC. (syn)   Sida berlandieri Turcz. (syn) Sida berteriana Spreng. (syn) Sida betulina Lag. ex Spreng. (syn)   Sida brachypetala DC. (syn)   Sida bradei Ulbr. (syn)   Sida brasila Schrank ex Link (syn)   Sida capensis Cav. (syn)   Sida carpinifolia L. fil. (syn)   Sida commixta Gand. (syn) Sida disticha Sessé & Moc. (syn)   Sida foliosa Splitg. ex de Vriese (syn) Sida frutescens Cav. (syn) Sida garckeana Polak. (syn)   Sida glabra Nutt. (syn) Sida jamai- censis Vell. (syn)   Sida lancea Gand. (syn)   Sida lanceolata Retz. (syn)   Sida martinicensis Gand. (syn)   Sida obtusa A.Rich. (syn) Sida orientalis DC. (syn)   Sida ovata G. Don (syn)   Sida planicaulis DC. (syn)   Sida prostrata G. Don (syn)   Sida repanda Roth (syn) Sida rugosa Thunn. (syn)   Sida schrankii DC. (syn)   Sida scoparia Lour. (syn) Sida spiraeifolia Willd. (syn)   Sida stauntoniana DC. (syn)   Sida triv-ialis Macfad. (syn)   Sida vogelii Hook. (syn) **[369]**   syn = synonym

Sida acuta – Some common names:

ENGLISH:Broom weed, broom weed., broomweed, Broomweed, broomweed., Common Fanpetals, common wireweed, Common Wireweed, southern sida, southern sida, Southern Sida, Spiny Head Sida, spiny-head sida, Spiny-Head Sida, spinyhead sida., spiny-head sida., Wire Weed.(English) [362]   CHINESE: Huang hua ren   FRENCH: Balai midi, Balai onze heures, Balai savane, Balyé wonzè (Saint Lucia), Grosse herbe dure, Herbe à panier, Herbe dure   JAPANESE: Hosoba kingojika. LAOTIAN: Khat mon noi   MALAGASY: Tsindahorona   PORTUGUESE: Guaxuma, Relógio-De-Vaqueiro, Tupitixa, Vassoura-Preta, Vassourinha   RUSSIAN: Sida ostraia   SPANISH: Babosilla , Escoba blanca, Escobilla, Huinar, Malva colorado, Malva de castilla   THAI: No-khue-mae, Ya khat bai yao, Ya khat mon, Ya kho, Yung pat. [526]   India - Pilla valatti chedi   Kenya – Mbundugo   Nigeria – Iseketu   Burkina-Faso - Zon-Raaga [220] Indonesia: sidaguri (Javanese), galungang (Sundanese), taghuri (Madurese). Malaysia: bunga telur belangkas, lidah ular, sedeguri (Peninsular). Papua New Guinea: kuriakuria,   Philippines: ualisualisan, takkimbaka (Tagalog), pamalis (Tagalog, Bisaya). Cambodia: kantrang ba sa. Thailand: naa-khui-mee, yaa khat mon (northern), yung kwaat (central). Vietnam: b[as]i ch[oor]i, ch[oor]i d[uwj]c, b[as]i nk[oj]n **[362]**

Sida acuta – Worldwide Distribution

Reported here: Antarctica, Antilles, Argentina, Australia, Austria, Belize, Benin, Bhutan, Bolivia, Brazil, Burkina Faso, Burundi, Cambodia, Cameroon, Central African Republic, China, China: Fujian, China: Guangdong, China: Hainan, China: Yunnan, Christmas Island, Cocos (Keeling) Islands,

Colombia, Comoros, Costa Rica, Cuba, Denmark, Ecuador, El Salvador, Equatorial Guinea, Ethiopia, France, French Guiana, Gabon, Ghana, Guatemala, Guyana, Haiti, Honduras, India, Indonesia, Ireland, Jamaica, Kenya, Laos, Liberia, Madagascar, Malawi, Mali, Mauritius, Mexico, Mexico:Chihuahua, Mexico: Durango, Mexico: Jalisco, Mexico: Michoacan, Mexico: Nuevo Leon, Mexico: Oaxaca, Mexico:Puebla, Mexico: San Luis Potosi, Mexico: Sinaloa, Mexico: Sonora, Mexico: Tamaulipas, Mexico: Veracruz, Micronesia, Nepal, Netherlands, Netherlands Antilles, New Caledonia, Nicaragua, Niger, Nigeria, Norfolk Island, Panama, Papua New Guinea, Paraguay, Peru, Senegal, Seychelles, Solomon Islands, Spain, Sri Lanka, Taiwan, Tanzania, Thailand, Uganda, United Kingdom, United States, Vanuatu, Venezuela, Viet Nam, Zambia, Egypt (Nile Delta), Israel (E-Israel: Rift Valley), Canary Isl. (Gran Canaria, Teneriffa), Cape Verde Isl. (Santo Antao Isl., Ilha de Sao Nicolau, Ilha de Maio, Ilha de Sao Tiago, Fogo Isl., Ilha Brava), Chagos Arch. (Diego Garcia), S-Mali, Sierra Leone, Liberia, Ivory Coast, Ghana, Togo, ?Benin, Nigeria, W-Cameroon, Congo, D.R.Congo (Zaire), Central African Republic, Sudan, Uganda, Rwanda, Burundi, S-Somalia, Kenya, ?Tanzania, Malawi, Mozambique, Zambia, Zimbabwe, Socotra, South Africa (Transvaal, KwaZulu-Natal), Namibia, Swaziland, Bioko Isl. (Fernando Poo), Seychelles, Mauritius, Réunion, Rodrigues, Madagascar, Cook Isl. (Rarotonga), Marquesas Isl., Austral Isl. (Raivavae), Marshall Isl. (Rongelap, Ujelang), Micronesia (Yap, Truk, Moen, Dublon, Tol, Kosrae), Nauru, Niue, Northern Marianas (Pagan, Alamagan, Sarigan, Anatahan), Banaba (Ocean) Isl., Palau Isl. (Angaur), Society Isl. (Tahiti, Moorea, Huahine, Raiatea, Tupai), Southern Marianas (Saipan, Tinian, Rota, Guam), Tonga (Nomuka, Lifuka, Vava'u), Tuamotu Arch. (Makatea Isl.), Western Samoa (Aleipata Isl., Savaii), Bonin Isl. (Chichijima), India, Nepal, Sri Lanka, Andamans, Nicobars, Australia (Western Australia, Northern Territory, Queensland), New Caledonia, Fiji, peninsular Malaysia (common throughout), North Keeling Isl., Christmas Isl. (Austr.), China (Fujian, Guangdong, Yunnan, Guangxi, Hainan), Taiwan, Ryukyu Isl., Laos, Vietnam, Norfolk Isl., Hawaii (introduced) (Kauai (introduced), Oahu (introduced), Maui (introduced), Hawaii Isl. (introduced)), Myanmar [Burma], India (widespread), Bhutan, Sikkim, Pakistan (Sind, Pakistani Punjab), Philippines, Bermuda, Java, USA (Alabama, Florida, Georgia, Louisiana, Mississippi, New Jersey, Pennsylvania, South Carolina, Texas), U.S. Virgin Isl., Puerto Rico, Costa Rica, Bahamas, Turks & Caicos Isl., Nicaragua, Aruba, Curacao, Belize, Panama, Haiti, Dominican Republic, Lesser Antilles (Anguilla, St. Martin, St. Barts, Antigua, Saba, St. Kitts, Montserrat, Guadeloupe, La Desirade, Dominica, Martinique, St. Lucia, St. Vincent, Grenadines, Grenada, Barbados), Mexico (throughout), Cuba, Trinidad, Tobago, N-Brazil (Para, Tocantins), NE-Brazil (Maranhao, Piaui, Ceara, Pernambuco, Bahia), WC-Brazil (Goias), SE-Brazil (Minas Gerais), Venezuela (Amazonas, Anzoategui, Apure, Aragua, Bolivar, Carabobo, Cojedes?, Delta Amacuro, Distrito Federal, Falcon, Lara, Merida, Miranda, Nueva Esparta, Portuguesa, Sucre, Zulia), Ecuador, Galapagos Isl., Jamaica, Peru, Guyana, Surinam, French Guiana [360/369] Japan - Ryukyu Islands, Myanmar, Arizona, Mexico--Campeche, Chiapas, Colima, Guerrero, Jalisco, Morelos, Nayarit, Queretaro, Quintana Roo, Tabasco, Yucatan, Bahamas, Hispaniola, Netherlands Antilles, St. Kitts and Nevis, Suriname, Somalia, Egypt, Mozambique, Zambia, South Africa,

Swaziland, Cote D'Ivoire, Sierra Leone, Togo, Congo, Gabon, Rwanda, Zaire, Western Indian Ocean, Oman, Israel, Jordan, Papuasia, Hawaii, Guam, Marshall Islands, Micronesia, Northern Mariana Islands, Palau, French Polynesia, Fiji, Nauru, Niue, Samoa, Galapagos Islands [366]   Native to Mexico and Central America but has spread throughout the tropics and subtropics. A malvaceous weed that is widely distributed in pan-tropical areas where it is found in bushes, in farms and around habitations, and frequently dominates improved pastures, waste and disturbed places roadsides. S. acuta is widely used as traditional medicine, surveys conducted in indigenous places revealed that the plant had many traditional usages that varied from one region to another. The plant is also used for spiritual practices. [220]

Sida cordifolia

Abutilon ramosum, Country Mallow, Flannel weed, Mahabala

Description

Part Used: seed, leaves, Roots

Stems - stout and strong

Leaves - 2.5-7 cm long and 2.5-5 cm broad, with 7-9 veins.

Flowers - small, yellow or white in color, solitary and axillaries.

Fruits - moong-sized, 6-8 mm in diameter

Seeds - grayish black in color and smooth. [118]

Erect, branched sub-shrubs to 1.5 m tall; stem green, densely tomentose with minute stellate and spreading simple hairs. Leaves 1.5-5.5 x 1-3.5 cm, ovate, rarely suborbicular, base cordate, margins serrate to the base, apex subobtuse or acute, basally 3-5 nerved, densely stellate-tomentose beneath with simple hairs on nerves and soft tomentose above; petiole to 3.5 cm long, pubescent; solitary or aggregated terminally in to congested corymbiform inflorescence; pedicel to 3 mm long in flower, to 1.2 cm in fruits, articulated above the middle. Calyx 6-7 mm long, prominently 10-ribbed, densely tomentose without. Corolla c. 1 cm across, yellow; petals to 8 x 6 mm, obliquely obovate, apex truncate or slightly emarginate. Staminal column c. 3 mm long. Ovary subglobose, pubescent; styles 8-10; stigma capitate, yellow. Schizocarp 6-7 mm diam., pubescent towards apex; mericarps 8-10, to 3 x 2 mm, trigonous with acute angles, apically 2-awned. Seeds brownish or black. [749]

Bloom Characteristics: This plant is attractive to bees, butterflies and/or birds

Water Requirements: Drought-tolerant; suitable for xeriscaping

Height: 18-24 in. (45-60 cm) - 24-36 in. (60-90 cm)

Spacing: 15-18 in. (38-45 cm) - 18-24 in. (45-60 cm)

Hardiness:

USDA Zone 8a: to -12.2 °C (10 °F)

USDA Zone 8b: to -9.4 °C (15 °F)

USDA Zone 9a: to -6.6 °C (20 °F)

USDA Zone 9b: to -3.8 °C (25 °F)

USDA Zone 10a: to -1.1 °C (30 °F)

USDA Zone 10b: to 1.7 °C (35 °F)

USDA Zone 11:   above 4.5 °C (40 °F)

Sun Exposure: Full Sun, Sun to Partial Shade

Propagation Methods: From seed; direct sow after last frost

Self-sows freely; deadhead if you do not want volunteer seedlings next season
[703]

Scientific names - Sida cordifolia synonyms

Abutilon ramosum G. Don (syn)   Malvastrum cordifolium Rojas (syn)
Malvinda cordifolia (L.) Medic. (syn)   Sida althaeifolia Sw. (syn)   Sida
borbonica Cav. (syn)   Sida byssina Schrank (syn)   Sida ciliosa Boj. ex
Baker (syn)   Sida conferta Link (syn)   Sida cordifolia var. althaeifolia
(Sw.) M.Gómez (syn)   Sida cordifolia var. breviaristata Monteiro (syn)
Sida cordifolia var. conferta (Link) Griseb. (syn)   Sida hamulosa Salzm. ex
Griseb. (syn)   Sida herbacea Cav. (syn)   Sida holosericea Willd. ex Spreng.
(syn)   Sida hong-kongensis Gand. (syn)   Sida micans Cav. (syn)   Sida
mollis Herb.Banks ex Griseb. (syn)   Sida multiflora Cav. (syn)   Sida
pellita Kunth (syn)   Sida pungens Kunth (syn) Sida rotundifolia Lam. (syn)
Sida tomentosa Vell. (syn)   Sida truncata Cav. (syn)   Sida velloziana
Steud. (syn)   Sida velutina Willd. ex Spreng. (syn)   Sida vestita Steud.
(syn)   Sida waltheriifolia Boj. ex Baker (syn) **[369]**

Sida cordifolia – Some common names

Gulipas (Sub.)   Country mallow, Flannel weed, Heart-leaf sida, Indian
ephedra, Silky white mallow (Engl.)   ASSAMESE: Bariala   BENGALI:
Berela   CHINESE: Yuan ye jin wu shi hua (Taiwan), Xin ye huang hua ren,
Ke dong   GUJARATI: Jangli methi   FRENCH: Herbe de douze heyres
HINDI: Bariara, Baryal   JAPANESE: Maruba kingojika   KANNADA:
Kadeeru, Hithuthi   KONKANI: Thapkoti   MALAYALAM: Kurumthotti
MARATHI: Chikana, Karaiti   NEPALESE: Balu   ORYA: Bisiripi
PUNJABI: Kharenti   RUSSIAN: Sida serdtselistnaia, Sida kordifolia
SANSKRIT: Bala, Balaa   SPANISH: Escoba negra, Escobilla, llima   TAMIL:
Chitaamuttie   TELUGU: Chirubenda   Mailmanikkam   THAI: Ya khat bai
pom. **[525]**   Hindi- Kungyi   Bengali- Swetberela, Brela, Bala   Gujarati-
Bala baldana, Mahabala, Khapat Telugu- Tella antisa, Tellagorra, Suvarnamu
Tamil- Nila-tutti, Paniar-tuthi   Malyalam- Vellurum, Kathuram   Oriya-
Badianaula, Bisvokopari, suvarna   Punjab- Kowar, Simak   Unani:
Bariyaara, Khirhati, Khireti, Kunayi   English: Bala, Country Sida, Llima
Arabic: الخـبـازة   Bengali: Bedela, Barila   Chinese: Ke dong, 圓葉金午時花
心叶黄花稔   Deutsch: Sandmalve   Gujarati: Kharatee, Baladana,
Janelimethi   Hindi- Bariyaar, Khiratee, Kharantee, Kharenti, Khareti, Barial,

22

Bariar, Bariyara, Kharenti   Japanese: マルバキンゴジカ   Kannada:-Hettuthi, Hettugigada, Kisangi, Chittuharalu   Konkani: Kobirsir-bhaii, Muttava   Marathi.- चिकणा   Mundari.: Marang,Lupaaraba, Huringmindilata

Nepalese: बलु/बरियार   Russian: Бала Bala, Сида сердцелистная Сида кордифолиа   Sindhi: Burrayra   Sinhalese: Hiradona, Valbevila   Thai: หญ้า ขัดใบป้อม   Unani: Bariyaara, Khirhati, Khireti, Kunayi [375]   Brazil: malva branca, malva branca sedosa [66]

Sida cordifolia – Worldwide Distribution

Reported here: USA (Alabama, Florida, Texas), U.S. Virgin Isl., Australia (Western Australia, Northern Territory, Queensland, New South Wales), Galapagos Isl., Jamaica, Peru, Cuba, Nicaragua, Belize, Puerto Rico, Haiti, Dominican Republic, Mexico (widespread), Guatemala, Honduras, Lesser Antilles (St. Martin, St. Barts, Antigua, St. Kitts, Redonda, Montserrat, Guadeloupe, La Desirade, Marie Galante, Dominica, Martinique, St. Lucia, St. Vincent, Barbados), Seychelles, Guyana, Surinam, French Guiana, Ecuador, Bolivia, Argentina (Buenos Aires, Catamarca, Chaco, Corrientes, Formosa, Jujuy, La Rioja, Misiones, Salta, Santiago del Estero, Santa Fe, Tucuman), N-Brazil (Roraima, Para, Amazonas, Tocantins, Rondonia), NE-Brazil (Maranhao, Ceara, Paraiba, Pernambuco, Bahia, Alagoas, Sergipe), WC-Brazil (Mato Grosso, Goias, Distrito Federal, Mato Grosso do Sul), SE-Brazil (Minas Gerais, Espirito Santo, Sao Paulo, Rio de Janeiro), S-Brazil (Parana, Santa Catarina), Paraguay (Alto Paraguay, Amambay, Caaguazu, Caazapa, Central, Cordillera, Guaira, Paraguari, Pres. Hayes), Uruguay (Paysandu, Salto, San Jose), Venezuela (Anzoategui, Bolivar, Carabobo, Delta Amacuro, Distrito Federal, Merida, Miranda, Nueva Esparta, Sucre, Tachira, Trujillo, Zulia), Trinidad, Tobago,?Marshall Isl. (introduced) (?Jaluit (introduced)), Tonga (introduced) (Nomuka (introduced)), Marquesas Isl. (introduced) (Eiao (introduced)), Mauritius, Réunion, Yemen (W-Yemen), Cape Verde Isl. (Santo Antao Isl., Ilha da Boa Vista, Ilha de Sao Tiago, Fogo Isl.), Hawaii (Kauai, Waimea District, East Maui, Kona Coast), Andamans (South Andamans), Nicobars (Car Nicobar Isl., Great Nicobar Isl.), Sri Lanka, Myanmar [Burma] (Bago, Magway, Mandalay, Sagaing, Shan, Yangon), India (widespread), Pakistan (Sind, Swat, Pakistani Punjab, Jhelum), Jammu & Kashmir (Kashmir), Bhutan, Java, peninsular Malaysia (north of Peninsula), Nepal, Philippines, Laos, Vietnam, China (Fujian, Guangdong, Guangxi, Sichuan, Yunnan, Hainan), Taiwan, Antarctica, Argentina, Australia, Benin, Bhutan, Bolivia, Botswana, Brazil, Brazil:Bahia, Burundi, Cameroon, Colombia, Comoros, Côte d'Ivoire, Cuba, Ecuador, El Salvador, French Guiana, Gabon, Ghana, Grenada, Guatemala, Guinea, Guyana, Honduras, Hong Kong, India, Indonesia, Jamaica, Kenya, Liberia, Madagascar, Malawi, Mali, Mayotte, Mexico, Nepal, Nicaragua, Niger, Nigeria, Pakistan, Papua New Guinea, Paraguay, Peru, Philippines, Rwanda, Senegal, South Africa, Sri Lanka, Taiwan, Tanzania, Thailand, United States, Venezuela, Viet Nam, Zambia, Zimbabwe, NW-Angola, Malawi, Mozambique, South Africa (Transvaal, KwaZulu-Natal), Swaziland, Sao Tome [360/369]   Uganda, Middle Atlantic Ocean (St. Helena), Botswana, Namibia, Senegal, Togo,

Central African Republic, Indo-China: Myanmar, Malaysia, Philippines, New Guinea, Argentina - Buenos Aires, Catamarca, Chaco, Corrientes, Formosa, Jujuy, La Rioja, Misiones, Salta, Santa Fe, Santiago del Estero, Tucuman, Paraguay - Alto Paraguay, Amambay, Caaguazu, Caazapa, Central, Cordillera, Guaira, Paraguari, Presidente Hayes, Uruguay, Peru, Ethiopia, Somalia, Yemen, Papua New Guinea, Texas, Georgia, Louisiana, Mississippi, French Polynesia, New Caledonia, Tonga, Cayman Islands, Virgin Islands (British), Virgin Islands (U.S.), El Salvador, Nicaragua [366]

Native of Brazil [171]   A native specie of the Brazilian Northeast [40] native to India [161]   Widely distributed along with other species are common throughout the tropical and sub tropical plains all over India and Srilanka up to an altitude of 1050 m., growing wild along the roadside. It grows as wasteland weed. It is also known as the "Bala" in Hindi and Sanskrit. The plant name Bala is coined on the name of 'Parvati' (goddess of strength and beauty). [118]   Considered an invasive weed in Africa, Australia, the southern United States, Hawaiian Islands, New Guinea, and French Polynesia. [161]

Sida rhombifolia
arrowleaf sida, Cuban jute, Bala, Mahabala, Atibala

S. rhombifolia is one of the most variable species of the genus Sida. As result of this variation it was described by several authors under different names. A satisfactory analysis of this complex is needed. Wild distribution: Almost pan-tropical and extending into the temperate zone. A common weed, growing on roadsides, disturbed places, in urban areas, as well as along streams. [363]

Sida rhombifolia will only continue to play a role locally in the production of fibers. It might be of interest as a local industrial source of the alkaloid ephedrine. However, ephedrine can also be produced synthetically, and its use in medicine is rapidly becoming obsolete. [358] {How wrong they are!}

Description
The stem is erect, branching and covered densely with stellate (star shaped) hairs and is rather twiggy with tough stringy bark. The stem becomes glabrous (without hair or scales) as it approaches the top. The leaves are dull green and lanceolate to linear-oblong sometimes rhombic, alternate and 1.5-8cm long, with serrate margins and finely stellate hairs on the upper surface of the leaf and a dense amount of stellate hairs on the undersurface, making that surface look white. The flowers are small, solitary, pale orange to yellow on slender jointed peduncles (stalks) about 10-30mm long. The peduncles are mostly axillary (formed in the angle between the stems) but sometimes there are clustered of 3 or 4 at the end of branches. The calyx (collectively the sepals of one flower) is a 5-lobed, 10 ribbed ashy green color with stellate (star shaped) hairs. The corolla (the petals collectively) is 7-8mm long and consists of 5 petals that are united at the base. The fruit (schizocarp) is 5-6mm in diameter, glabrous (without hair or scales), a dark brown color, more or less globular and vertically ribbed. It is divided into 9-12 fruitlets

(mericarps) acting as seeds. In the fruit, the mericarps (fruitlets) are hard and often indehiscent (not opening to release the seed) with a wide back and honeycombed or reticulate sides. The mericarps have 2 erect minutely barbed awns. **[748]**

Scientific names - Sida rhombifolia synonyms

Sida canariensis Willd.1800   Sida microphylla Cav. 1785   Sida rhomboidea Roxb. 1810   Sida retusa L. , 1763   Sida orientalis Cav. 1785   Sida pringlei Gandog. 1924   Sida ruderata 1837   Sida riparia   Sida scabrida   Sida blepharoprion   Malva rhombifolia   Napaea rhombifolia   Sida rhombifolia var. rhomboidea   Sida ruderata   Sida ostryaefolia   Sida maderensis   Sida serratifolia   Sida setosa   Sida semicrenata   Sida insularis Hatus   Sida unicornis Marais   Sida ruderata Macfad   Sida cumingii Gand   Sida hondensis Kunth   Sida pringlei Gand   Sida adusta Marais   Sida alnifolia   Sida alba Cav. [370]   Sida rhombifolia var. afrorhomboidea   Sida rhombifolia var. afroscabrida   Sida rhombifolia var. canariensis   Sida rhombifolia var. corynocarpa   Sida rhombifolia var. longipedicellata   Sida rhombifolia var. petherickii   Sida rhombifolia var. scabrida   **[369]**

Sida rhombifolia – Some common names

Alant (Germany)   Mahabala (Ayurveda)   Basbasot (Ilk.)   Elenio (Italy)   Escobilia (Span.)   Eskobang-haba (Tag., Bis., Pamp.)   Eskoba (C. Bis.)   AFRICA: Petoria-bossie   ARABIC: Qinnab el Kûînsland (Egypt)   ASSAMESE: Boriala.   BANGLADESH: Lal berela atibala   BENGALI: Svetbarela   CHINESE: Bai bei huang huo ren, Huang huo, Ya mu tou, Mu wu   FRENCH: Aunee, Balyé wonzè, Chanvre d'Australie, Fausse guimauve, Faux thé, Herbe à balais   GERMAN: Kubajute, Queensland Hanf, Sidafaserpflanze   GUJARATI: Baladana   HINDI: िभयुनी, गुबाटाडा, Baryara, Kharenti, Sahadeva, Swetbarela   INDONESIAN: Sidaguri   JAPANESE: Kingojika   KANNADA: Bolamgadale, Kallangadale   MALAYALAM: Vankuruntotti, Valankuruntotti, Velluram   MARATHI: Baler, Sadeda, Sahadevi   NEPALESE: Saano cilyaa   ORIYA: Bajromuli   PORTUGUESE: Chá-bravo, Erva do chá, Enula campana, Guaxuma, Malva-preta, Relógio, Vassourinha   RUSSIAN: Sida rombolistnaya, Atibala   SANSKRIT: Atibala, Bala, Mahabala   SPANISH: Afata negra, Ancu-sacha, Angosacha, Axpcatzín, Escoba, Escoba blanca, Escobilla, Escobita ceniza, Huinar, Malva de puerco, Malva prieta, Mata-alfalfa, Popotalagua, Tipichaguazu   SRI LANKAN: Chittamadi   TAMIL: Chittamutti, Velaippacai   TELUGU: Guba tada, Mahabala   THAI: Khat mon, Ya khat , Yung pat mae mai   TURKISH: Avsdralia keneviri   URDU: Bala, Baryara   VIETNAMESE: Ké hoa vàng. [524]   ARGENTINA: afata, cañamo crioulo, escoba, tebincha   URUGUAY: afata, malvavisco, mata-alfalfa, tipicha   JAMAICA: broom weed   PERU: limpion   NICARAGUA: escoba amarilla   VENEZUELA: escoba babosa, escoba blanca   PANAMA: hierba de puerco   CUBA: malva de cochino   SOUTH AFRICA: ntswembana, quaquaza **[371]**

Sida rhombifolia – Worldwide Distribution

Reported here: USA (Alabama, Arkansas, Arizona, California, Florida, Georgia, Kansas, Kentucky, Louisiana, Maryland, Mississippi, North Carolina, New Jersey, Oklahoma, Pennsylvania, South Carolina, Tennessee, Texas, Virginia, U.S. Virgin Isl., Portugal (introduced), Spain (introduced), France (introduced), Portugal (introduced), Senegal, Gambia, Guinea-Bissau, Guinea, Sierra Leone, Liberia, Ivory Coast, Ghana, Mali, Burkina Faso, Niger, Togo, Benin, Nigeria, Cameroon, Chad, Central African Republic, Sudan, Ethiopia, Eritrea, Congo, D.R.Congo (Zaire), Uganda, Rwanda, Burundi, Kenya, Tanzania, Angola, Malawi, Mozambique, Zambia, Zimbabwe, South Africa (Transvaal, KwaZulu-Natal, Cape Prov.), Swaziland, Lesotho, Seychelles (introduced), Madagascar, New Caledonia (introduced), Clipperton Isl., Fiji, Lord Howe Isl. (introduced), Norfolk Isl. (introduced), Guyana, Surinam, French Guiana, Ecuador, Bolivia, N-Brazil (Roraima, Amapa, Para, Amazonas, Tocantins, Acre, Rondonia), NE-Brazil (Maranhao, Piaui, Ceara, Rio Grande do Norte, Paraiba, Pernambuco, Bahia, Alagoas, Sergipe), WC-Brazil (Mato Grosso, Goias, Distrito Federal, Mato Grosso do Sul), SE-Brazil (Minas Gerais, Espirito Santo, Sao Paulo, Rio de Janeiro), Argentina (Buenos Aires, Catamarca, Chaco, Cordoba, Corrientes, Entre Rios, Formosa, Jujuy, La Pampa, Misiones, Salta, Santiago del Estero, Santa Fe, San Juan, San Luis, Tucuman), S-Brazil (Parana, Rio Grande do Sul, Santa Catarina), Chile (Coquimbo), Paraguay (Alto Paraguay, Cordillera, Pres. Hayes), Uruguay (Montevideo, Paysandu, Rivera, Salto, Tacuarembo, Treinta y Tres), Venezuela (Amazonas, Bolivar, Delta Amacuro, Distrito Federal, Guarico, Merida, Portuguesa, Sucre, Trujillo, Zulia), Costa Rica, Galapagos Isl., Jamaica, Peru, Nicaragua, Bahamas, Turks & Caicos Isl., Puerto Rico, Belize, Cuba, Panama, Haiti, Dominican Republic, Mexico (widespread), Revillagigedos Isl. (Isla Socorro), Lesser Antilles (St. Martin, Barbuda, Antigua, Saba, St. Kitts, Guadeloupe, Dominica, Martinique, St. Lucia, St. Vincent, Barbados), Trinidad, Tobago, American Samoa (introduced) (Manua Isl. (introduced)), Cook Isl. (introduced) (Rarotonga (introduced)), Mapia Isl. (introduced) (N of Irian Jaya (introduced)), Marquesas Isl. (introduced), Marshall Isl. (introduced) (Jaluit (introduced)), Micronesia (introduced) (Yap (introduced), Ulithi (introduced), Truk (introduced), Moen (introduced), Dublon (introduced), Fefan (introduced), Eten (introduced), Pohnpei (introduced), Kosrae (introduced)), Niue (introduced), N-Line Isl. (introduced) (Washington Isl. (introduced), Christmas Isl. - Kiritimati (introduced)), Northern Marianas (introduced) (Agrihan (introduced), Alamagan (introduced), Sarigan (introduced), Pagan (introduced)), Palau Isl. (introduced) (Babeldaob (introduced), Koror (introduced), Ngarakabesang (introduced), Malakal (introduced), Angaur (introduced)), Society Isl. (introduced) (Mopelia Atoll (introduced), Tahiti (introduced), Huahine (introduced), Raiatea (introduced), Tetiaroa Atoll (introduced), Tupai (introduced), Tahaa (introduced)), Southern Marianas (introduced) (Saipan (introduced), Tinian (introduced), Rota (introduced), Guam (introduced)), Tokelau (introduced) (Swains Isl. (introduced)), Tonga (introduced) (Late Isl. (introduced), Tongatapu (introduced), 'Eua (introduced), Vava'u (introduced), Tafahi (introduced)), Tuamotu Arch. (introduced) (Makatea Isl. (introduced), Rangiroa Atoll (introduced), Takapoto Atoll (introduced), etc.

26

(introduced)), Western Samoa (introduced) (Aleipata Isl. (introduced), Upolu (introduced), Savaii (introduced)), Austral Isl. (introduced) (Tubuai (introduced), Rurutu (introduced), Raivavae (introduced), Rapa Iti (introduced)), Bonin Isl. (Chichijima, Hahajima), Volcano Isl. (Kita-Iwojima, Iwojima), +Mauritius, +Réunion, Oman (Mascat & Oman), Saudi Arabia (NW-Saudi Arabia: Hejaz, SW-Saudi Arabia: Asir), Sinai peninsula (Southern Sinai), Azores (Santa Maria Isl., Sao Miguel Isl., Terceira, Graciosa, Sao Jorge, Pico, Faial, Flores Isl.), Cape Verde Isl. (Santo Antao Isl., Sao Vicente Isl., Ilha de Sao Nicolau, Ilha de Maio, Ilha de Sao Tiago, Fogo Isl., Ilha Brava), Hawaii (introduced) (Midway Isl. (introduced), Kauai (introduced), Oahu (introduced), Molokai (introduced), Lanai (introduced), Maui (introduced), Kahoolawe Isl. (introduced), Hawaii Isl. (introduced), Niihau (introduced)), Andamans (North Andamans, Middle Andamans, South Andamans, Little Andaman Isl.), Nicobars (Car Nicobar Isl., North Nicobars, Central Nicobars, Great Nicobar Isl., Little Nicobar Isl.), Myanmar [Burma], India (widespread), Pakistan (Sind, Baluchistan, Jhelum), Bhutan, China (Fujian, Guangdong, Guangxi, Guizhou, Hainan, Hubei, Sichuan, Yunnan), Taiwan, Laos, Vietnam, Cambodia, Philippines, Caucasus / Transcaucasus, Japan (Yakushima Isl., Tanegashima Isl.), Ryukyu Isl., Nepal, peninsular Malaysia, Sri Lanka, Australia (Northern Territory, Queensland, New South Wales, Victoria Christmas Isl.) **[360/369]** Sida rhombifolia is a plant native to the Americas, occurring extensively in South America. **[189]** Sida rhombifolia: exact native range obscure **[366]** Sida rhombifolia is a plant native to the Americas, occurring extensively in South America and, to a lesser degree, in the southern United States. In Brazil, it is the most common species in the southern region, occurring, however, in all regions. **[516]** A native of Asia. **[671]**

Sida retusa

Sida rhombifolia var. retusa, Cuban jute, Teaweed,
Description – see Sida rhombifolia

Scientific names - Sida retusa synonyms

Sida retusa Linn.   Sida truncatula Blanco   Sida philippica Blanco   Sida rhombifolia Linn. var. retusa [527]   Sida rhombifolia L. (1753)   Sida rhombifolia var. retusa   Sida scabrida   Sida alnifolia L.   Sida blepharoprion   Sida riparia   Sida canariensis Cav. (1801)   Sida angustifolia   Sida rhombifolia var. surinamensis   Sida rhombifolia var. obovata   Sida rhombifolia var. canescens **[364]**

Sida retusa – Some common names

Basbasot (Ilk.)   Eskoba (Tag., C. Bis.)   Eskobang-bilog, Sasaang-parang (Tag.)   Jelly leaf (Engl.)   JAPANESE: Yahazu kingojika   RUSSIAN: Sida retuza, Sida prituplennaia. [527]   English: Arrow-Leaf Sida, Cuban Jute, Paddy´s Lucerne, Queensland Hemp, Teaweed   French: Faux Thé   German: Kubajute   Portuguese: Chá-Bravo   Portuguese (Brazil): Malva Preta,

Relógio, Vassourinha, Vassourinha Relógio   Spanish: Axpcatzín, Escoba, Escobilla, Escobita Ceniza, Huinar, Malva Prieta, Popotalagua   **[360]**

Sida retusa – Worldwide Distribution

Distribution of Sida retusa-In open grasslands, on paddy banks, at low and medium altitudes - Also reported from India to Malaysia. **[527]**

Sida cordata

Long-stalk sida, heartleaf fanpetals, Nagabala,

Description

Sub-shrubs procumbent, to 1 m. Stems slender, with simple pilose hairs, stiffly stellate hairs, and sometimes small simple multicellular hairs. Stipule filiform, 2-3 mm, sparsely pilose; petiole 1-3 cm, with conspicuous long simple hairs; leaf blade broadly ovate, (1-)2-5 × 1.8-4.5 cm, both surfaces stellate puberulent and ± apressed pilose, base cordate, margin crenate or dentate, apex acuminate. Flowers usually solitary, axillary, often on leafy, racemelike, axillary shoots. Pedicel slender, 1.5-4 cm, articulate on distal part, sparsely stellate and with long hairs. Calyx cup-shaped, 4-6 mm, sparsely pilose with long hairs, lobes 2-3 mm, acute. Corolla yellow, 8-9 mm in diam. Filament tube ca. 2 mm, glabrous or sparsely pilose. Schizocarp nearly globose, ca. 3 mm in diam.; mericarps 5, ovoid-tetrahedral, ca. 2.5 mm, smooth, glabrous or sparsely minutely hairy at apex, apex not beaked, not awned. **[747]**

Scientific names - Sida cordata synonyms

Sida cordata   Melochia cordata   Sida humilis   Sida multicaulis   Sida veronicifolia

Sida cordata – Some common names

English: heartleaf fanpetals   Assamese: Bor Sonborial   Bengali: Berela
Hindi: भुइनी bhuinii   Kannada: ಬೆಕ್ಕಿನ ಥಳೆ ಗಿಡ bekkinathale gida   Malayalam: kuruntotti, nela-vaga, വള്ളിക്കുറുന്തൊട്ടി vallikkurgunthotti   Sanskrit: भूमिबल bhumibala, नागबल nagabala   Tamil: kurunthotti, mayirmanikkam Telugu: Paavani, Chitta muta, Bedara, Beedara, Gadda chettu [375]   India: Farid buti, Rajbala, Bhumibala, and Shaktibala in India and Simak in Pakistan   Parkiston: Simak [496]   Transcribed Chinese   chang geng huang hua ren [F ChinaEng]   long-stalk sida [Herbs Commerce ed2]

Sida cordata – Worldwide Distribution

Reported here: China: (Fujian, Guangdong, Guangxi, Hainan, Yunnan), Taiwan, Bhutan, India, Pakistan, Sri Lanka, Indo-China, Myanmar, Thailand,

Philippines, Dominican Republic, Puerto Rico, Virgin Islands (British), Virgin Islands (U.S.), Suriname [366] USA (District of Columbia, Indiana, Kentucky, Massachusetts (introduced), Maryland, Michigan, New Jersey (introduced), New York (introduced), Ohio, Pennsylvania, +Tennessee, Virginia, West Virginia), Canada-Ontario [369] Alaska, Greenland, Hawaii, VI St. Pierre and Miquelon [724] Exact native range obscure. **[366]**

Sida indica

Abutilon indicum, Atibala, monkeybush [English]

Description

A perennial, half-woody, branched, erect shrub, 0.5 to 3 meters high. Leaves are green and toothed, orbicular-ovate to broadly ovate, 5 to 12 centimeters long and nearly as wide, with a prominently heart-shaped base and pointed apex, the margins entire or irregularly toothed. Flowers are yellow, 2 to 2.5 centimeters, solitary, borne in the axils of the leaves, and opens in the evening. Fruits is a rounded capsule, 1.5 to 2 centimeters in diameter, with 15 to 20 somewhat hairy, shortly awned carpels. **[729]**

Scientific names - Sida indica synonyms

Abutilon grandiflorum (S Africa)   Abutilon grantii A (S Africa)   Abutilon mauritianum (S Africa)   Abutilon grandiflorum (Trop. Africa)   Abutilon grantii (Trop. Africa)   Sida asiatica   Abutilon taiwanensis (China) Abutilon muticum var. parvifolia   Sida guineensis   Sida beloere L'Hér. Sida populifolia   Sida indica   Abutilon populifolium   **[367]**

Sida indica – Some common names

Bengali: Jhampi, Jhumka, Petari, Potari   Cutch: Balbij   Goa & Konkani: Petari, Tupkadi   Gujarati: Dabali, Kansaki   Hindi: Jhampi, Kandhi, Kanghani, Kanghi, Potari, Tepar, काधी   Kannada: Srimndrigida   Konkani: Voddlipettari   Malayalam: Jhoukaped, Katturam, Katturan, Pitikkapattu, Uram   Marathi: Akakai, Chakrabhenda, Kansuli, Karandi, Madmi, Mudra Mumbai: Chakrabenda, Etari, Kangoi, Kangori, Madmi   Punjabi & Sind: Atikhirate, Khapate, Peelee-bootee   Sanskrit: Atibala, Balika, Balya, Bhuribala, Ghanta, Kankati, Kotibala, Rishiprokta, Shita, Shitapushpa, Vikankata, Vatyapushpika, Vrishyagandha, Vrishyagandhika   Tamil: Nallatutti, Paniyarattutti, Perundutti, Ponnaithuthi, Tutti   Telugu: Adavibenda, Botlabenda, Dudi, Kammalaku, Papidlakaya, Thuthurbenda, Tutti   Uriya: Nakochono   English: Country Mallow **[437]**   Arabic: أبو طيلون هندي   Chinese: 冬葵子   English: Country mallow, Indian Abutilon, Monkey bush, Monkeybush   French: Guimauve, Herbe de douze heures, Mauve du pays   Greek: Avutilon to indikon   Italian: Abutilone   Japanese: Takasago ichibi   Malayalam: ഊരം   Marathi (Marāṭhī): पेटारी   Oriya: ପେଡ଼ିପେଡ଼ିକା Portuguese: Abutilo   Spanish: Boton de oro   Tamil: துத்திக்கீரை   Telugu: దువ్వెన బెండ   Thai: Khrop chak krawaan   Vietnamese: Cây cối xay **[360]**

Sida indica – Worldwide Distribution

Reported here: Saudi Arabia (NW-Saudi Arabia: Hejaz), Iraq (SE-Iraq: Mesopotamia), Israel (E-Israel: Rift Valley, Negev Desert, SC-Israel: Judean Desert), Oman (Mascat & Oman, Dhofar), Yemen (N-Inner Yemen, Tihama, W-Yemen), Afghanistan, Andamans (North Andamans, Middle Andamans, South Andamans, Little Andaman Isl.), Nicobars (Car Nicobar Isl., North Nicobars, Central Nicobars, Great Nicobar Isl., Little Nicobar Isl.), Myanmar [Burma], Bhutan, India (widespread), Pakistan (Karachi, Sind, Baluchistan, Pakistani Punjab, Lahore, Rawalpindi), Jammu & Kashmir (Kashmir), Thailand, Java, Malesia, Nepal, Ryukyu Isl., peninsular Malaysia (common throughout), Singapore (introduced), Cambodia, Laos, Vietnam, Philippines, China (Fujian, Guangdong, Guangxi, Guizhou, Sichuan, Yunnan, Hainan), Taiwan, New Caledonia (Loyalty Isl.), Australia (Northern Territory), Jamaica (introduced), Peru (introduced), Haiti (introduced), Dominican Republic (introduced), Cuba (introduced), Puerto Rico (introduced), Mona Isl. (introduced), Lesser Antilles (introduced) (Anguilla (introduced), St. Martin (introduced), St. Barts (introduced), Antigua (introduced), St. Kitts (introduced), Montserrat (introduced), Guadeloupe (introduced), Marie Galante (introduced), Dominica (introduced), Martinique (introduced), Grenada (introduced), Barbados (introduced)), Trinidad (introduced), Turks & Caicos Isl. (introduced), Virgin Isl. (introduced), Brazil (introduced), Seychelles (introduced), New Caledonia, Fiji, Guyana (introduced), Surinam (introduced), Colombia (introduced), Banaba (Ocean) Isl., Chagos Arch. (Diego Garcia), Gilbert Isl. (Tarawa), Micronesia (Yap), Nauru, Niue, Northern Marianas (Sarigan), Palau Isl. (Sonsorol), Southern Marianas (Saipan, Tinian, Rota, Guam), Marquesas Isl. (introduced) (Hiva Oa (introduced), Ua Huka (introduced), Nuku Hiva (introduced)), Tuamotu Arch. (introduced), Austral Isl. (Tubuai), Bonin Isl. (Keetaajima, Nakohdojima, Chichijima, Hahajima, Hirashima), Volcano Isl. (Kita-Iwojima, Iwojima, Minami-Iwojima), Mauritius, Réunion, Rodrigues, Madagascar (introduced), Hawaii (introduced) (Oahu (introduced) (Honolulu (introduced)), Algeria (introduced), Morocco (introduced) [369]   China: (Jiangsu, Jiangxi), Antarctica, Australia: (Queensland, Western Australia), Comoros, French Polynesia, Germany, Indonesia, Mayotte, Mexico, Morocco, Netherlands, New Zealand, Papua New Guinea, Spain, Sri Lanka, Thailand, United States, Viet Nam, Yemen. [360]   Japan-Ryukyu Islands, Afghanistan, Israel, Jordan, Bhutan, India, Nepal, Pakistan, Sri Lanka, Myanmar, Thailand, Indonesia, Malaysia, Australia: (Queensland, Western Australia, Northern Territory) [366]   Alaska, Canada, Greenland, St. Pierre and Miquelon, U.S. Virgin Islands [724]

....

It is concluded that alcoholic extract of S. cordifolia at a dose of 400 mg/kg have potency to act as anti diabetic, hypoglycemic and anti oxidant properties and also helps to check muscle wasting. Further it also protects from LPO that damages the cell membrane. [148]

30

Sida rhomboidea

Sida rhombifolia var. rhomboidea

Description

An under-shrub with a height of 1 to 2 feet with stellate hairs. Stem is circular; leaves ovate, toothed in the distal half; flowers solitary cyme, pedicels fused at the base; stamens filamentous and numerous; fruits capsule; carpels numbering 6-10 are without awns. It is a variety of S. rhombifolia which is found as a weed of marshy places throughout India. [217]   Erect, much branched sub-shrubs to 1.2 m tall; stem usually purplish. Leaves 1.5-5 x 1-3 cm, obovate, rhomboid to lanceolate, base rounded, margins coarsely serrate to crenate, entire towards base, apex subobtuse or acute, 3-nerved from base, sparsely pubescent above and densely stellate-tomentose beneath; petiole to 8 mm long; stipules c. 6 mm long, linear, caducous. Flowers axillary, solitary; pedicels c. 5 mm in flowers, to 3 cm in fruits, filiform, articulated at about the middle. Calyx c.7 mm across, campanulate, 5-lobed; lobes c. 3 mm long, triangular, tomentose without. Petals yellow, 6-7 x 4-5 mm, obliquely obovate, retuse or emarginate at apex. Staminal column to 3 mm long, stellate-pubescent, antheriferous at apex. Ovary c. 1.5 mm across, depressed globose; styles 8-10; stigmas capitate. Schizocarp 3-4 mm long; mericarps 8-10, c. 3 x 2 mm, trigonous, apex beaked, completely included. Seeds c. 2 mm long, brownish-black. [749]

Scientific names - Sida rhomboidea synonyms

Sida rhomboidea   Sida rhombifolia L. subsp. rhombifolia   Sida rhombifolia subsp. retusa   Sida retusa L.   Sida scabrida   Sida alnifolia L.   Sida blepharoprion Ulbr.   Sida riparia   Sida canariensis   Sida angustifolia   Sida rhombifolia var.   Sida rhombifolia var. obovata   Sida rhombifolia var. canescens [364]   Sida unicornis   Sida microphylla   Sida retusa L.   Sida orientalis Cav.   Sida pringlei   Sida hondoensis   Sida ruderata   Sida adusta [363]   Sida spinosa L. (accepted name)   Malva   Malvinda alba Medic   Malvinda alnifolia Medic   Malvinda spinosa   Sida affinis   Sida alba L   Sida betonicifolia   Sida bicolor   Sida bicuspidata   Sida bicuspidate   Sida boriara   Sida emarginata   Sida glandulosa   Sida heterocarpa   Sida milleri   Sida minor   Sida obliqua   Sida orientalis   Sida pimpinellifolia   Sida pusilla   Sida scabra   Sida spinosa var. kazmii   Sida spinosa var. sennaarensis   Sida tenuicaulis   Sida truncata L'Herit. (synonym) [369]

Sida rhomboidea – Some common names

Balai blanc   Balai savane   Balai-onze-heures   Escoba   Escoba espinosa (Puerto Rico)   Escobilla (Dominican Republic)   Fe teck teck (Haiti)   Fi tectec   Malva caballo   Malva de caballo (Cuba)   Prickly fanpetals (English)   False mallow (Bahamas)   White broomweed (Lesser Antilles)   [369]

Sida rhomboidea – Worldwide Distribution

Reported here: Africa, East Tropical Africa, Kenya, Tanzania, Uganda , Macaronesia, Azores, Canary Is, Cape Verde, Madeira , Northeast Tropical Africa, Chad, Ethiopia, Socotra, Somalia, Sudan , South Tropical Africa, Angola, Malawi, Mozambique, Zambia , Southern Africa, Botswana, Cape Province, Natal, Swaziland, Transvaal , West Tropical Africa, Ghana, Guinea, Liberia, Mali, Niger, Nigeria, Sierre Leone, The Gambia, Togo , West-Central Tropical Africa, Burundi, Cameroon, Congo, Equatorial Guinea, Rwanda, Sao Tome, Zaire , Western Indian Ocean, Madagascar, Mauritius, Seychelles Asia-Temperate, Arabian Peninsula, North Yemen, Oman, Saudi Arabia , China, Fujian, Guangdong, Hong Kong, Yunnan , Eastern Asia, Japan, Taiwan , Western Asia, Sinai Asia-Tropical, Indian Subcontinent, Assam, Bangladesh, Bihar, Maharashtra, Manipur, Orissa, Pakistan, Punjab, Sikkim, Sri Lanka, Tamil Nadu, Uttar Pradesh, West Bengal , Indo-China, Burma, Thailand, Vietnam , Malesia, Christmas I, Jawa, Lesser Sunda Is s.l., Moluccas, Papua New Guinea, Peninsular Malaysia, Philippines, Sabah, Sarawak, Sulawesi, Sumatera , North Indian Ocean, Maldives Europe, Southwestern Europe, Spain Northern America, Northern Mexico, Baja California Sur, Hawaii , Northwestern Pacific, Guam , South-Central Pacific, Cook Is, Marquesas, Society Is , Southwestern Pacific, Fiji, New Caledonia, Niue, North Solomons, South Solomons, Tonga, Vanuatu, Western Samoa Southern America, Brazil, Bahia, Brazilia Distrito Federal, Goias, Maranhao, Minas Gerais, Para, Parana, Pernambuco, Rio Grande do Sul, Santa Catarina, Sao Paulo , Caribbean, Cuba, Dominica, Guadeloupe, Haiti, Jamaica, Montserrat, Puerto Rico, Trinidad-Tobago , Mesoamerica, Belize, Chiapas, Costa Rica, El Salvador, Honduras, Nicaragua, Panama , Northern South America, French Guiana, Guyana, Surinam, Venezuela , Southern South America, Paraguay, Uruguay , Western South America, Bolivia, Colombia, Ecuador, Galapagos, Peru [361] USA (Alabama, Arkansas, Arizona, California, Connecticut, District of Columbia, Delaware, Florida, Georgia, Iowa, Illinois, Indiana, Kansas, Kentucky, Louisiana, Massachusetts, Maryland, Maine, Michigan, Missouri, Mississippi, North Carolina, Nebraska, New Jersey, New York, Ohio, Oklahoma, Pennsylvania, South Carolina, Tennessee, Texas, Virginia, West Virginia), Canada (Ontario), Bahamas, Turks & Caicos Isl., Cayman Isl., Cuba, Hispaniola, Jamaica, Puerto Rico, Virgin Isl. (St. Croix, St. John, St. Thomas, Virgin Gorda), Lesser Antilles (Anguilla, Antigua, Barbados, Barbuda, Grenada, Grenadines, Guadeloupe, Martinique, St. Barthelemy, St. Lucia, St. Martin), Aruba, Bonaire, Curacao, Isla Margarita, Tobago (introduced), Galapagos Isl., Peru, Mexico (Campeche, Chiapas, Chihuahua, Coahuila, Colima, Durango, Guanajuato, Guerrero, Hidalgo, Jalisco, Mexico State, Michoacan, Morelos, Nayarit, Nuevo Leon, Oaxaca, Puebla, Queretaro, Quintana Roo, San Luis Potosi, Sinaloa, Sonora, Tamaulipas, Veracruz, Yucatan, Zacatecas), Guyana, French Guiana, Ecuador, Argentina (Buenos Aires, Catamarca, Chaco, Cordoba, Corrientes, Distrito Federal, Entre Rios, Formosa, Jujuy, La Rioja, Mendoza, Misiones, Salta, Santiago del Estero, San Juan, San Luis, Tucuman), S-Brazil (Parana, Rio Grande do Sul), Chile (Tarapaca, Atacama), Paraguay (Alto Paraguay, Cordillera, Guaira, Pres. Hayes), Uruguay (Canelones, Montevideo), Belize, Costa Rica, Bolivia (Beni, Chuquisaca, Cochabamba, La Paz, Santa Cruz, Tarija), NE-Brazil (Ceara, Rio

Grande do Norte, Paraiba, Pernambuco, Bahia), WC-Brazil (Mato Grosso do Sul), SE-Brazil (Minas Gerais, Rio de Janeiro), Venezuela (Anzoategui?, Aragua?, Carabobo, Cojedes?, Distrito Federal?, Falcon?, Guarico, Lara, Merida, Miranda?, Nueva Esparta, Portuguesa, Sucre?, Tachira, Zulia?), Panama, Nicaragua, Colombia (Antioquia, Cauca, Cesar, Cundinamarca, Huila, Magdalena, Norte de Santander, Santander, Tolima, Valle), Egypt (Desert Oases, Great Southwestern Desert, Nile Delta, Nile Valley, NW-coastal Egypt), Oman (Mascat & Oman), Saudi Arabia (NW-Saudi Arabia: Hejaz, SW-Saudi Arabia: Asir), Yemen (Tihama, W-Yemen), Namibia, Swaziland, Botswana, Mauritania, Mali, Senegal, Gambia, Sierra Leone, Ghana, Togo, Niger, Burkina Faso, N-Benin, Nigeria, Chad, Bioko Isl. (Fernando Poo), Annobon Isl., Sudan, South Sudan, Congo (Brazzaville), D.R.Congo (Zaire), Angola, Mozambique, Zambia, Zimbabwe, ?Kenya, ?Tanzania, Uganda, Rwanda, ?Burundi, Ethiopia, Eritrea, Somalia, South Africa (Transvaal, Free State, KwaZulu-Natal), Madagascar (introduced), +Mauritius, Réunion, Rodrigues (introduced), Cape Verde Isl. (Santo Antao Isl., Sao Vicente Isl., Ilha de Sao Nicolau, Sal Isl., Ilha da Boa Vista, Ilha de Maio, Ilha de Sao Tiago), Spain (introduced), France (introduced), Caucasus, Transcaucasus, Russian Far East, Japan (Honshu, Shikoku, Kyushu), Ryukyu Isl., Taiwan, China (S-Yunnan, Zhejiang), Korea (introduced), Java, Australia (Western Australia, Northern Territory, Queensland, New South Wales, Ashmoore Reef), India (widespread), Pakistan (Karachi, Sind, Hazara, Pakistani Punjab, Rawalpindi), Jammu & Kashmir (Kashmir), Sri Lanka, Bhutan, Philippines, Myanmar [Burma], Chagos Arch. (introduced) (Diego Garcia (introduced)), Micronesia (introduced) (Pohnpei (introduced)), Northern Marianas (introduced) (Alamagan (introduced)), Palau Isl. (introduced) (Angaur (introduced)), Society Isl. (introduced) (Tahiti (introduced)), Tonga (introduced) (Tongatapu (introduced)), Hawaii (introduced) (Kauai (introduced), Oahu (introduced), Lanai (introduced), West Maui (introduced), Hawaii Isl. (introduced)) **[369]**

Sida spinosa

Prickly fanpetals, Indiana mallow,Nagabala (S. alba is a synonym)

Description

A summer annual with yellow flowers and very small spines at the base of each leaf and branch. This weed is one of the ten most common and troublesome weeds in peanuts, cotton, and soybeans in most of the southern states. Prickly sida is primarily a weed of agronomic crops, but can also be found in horticultural crops, landscapes, pastures, hay fields, and gardens.

Seedlings: Both cotyledons are generally heart-shaped with a small indentation at the cotyledon apexes. The cotyledons and the stems below the cotyledons (hypocotyls) are covered with short hairs.

Leaves: Arranged alternately along the stem, approximately 3/4 to 2 inches long, and inconspicuously hairy. Leaves are oval to lanceolate in outline with toothed margins. Leaves occur on petioles that are 1/2 to 1 1/4 inches long and have small spines (stipules) that are 5 to 8 mm long at the base of each leaf petiole.

Stems: Erect, branched, ranging from 8 to 20 inches in height. Stems also have hairs.

Roots: A taproot and a fibrous root system.

Flowers: Occur singly or in clusters on flower stalks (peduncles) that arise from the area between the stems and leaf petioles. Flowers consist of 5 yellow petals that are 4 to 6 mm long.

Identifying Characteristics: The seedlings with 2 heart-shaped cotyledons, and the small spines that occur at the base of each leaf petiole are both features that help in the identification of prickly sida.   Velvetleaf (Abutilon thophrasti), Spurred Anoda (Anoda cristata), and Arrowleaf Sida (Sida rhombifolia) seedlings are very similar to those of prickly sida. However, prickly and arrowleaf sida have 2 heart-shaped cotyledons unlike the round and heart-shaped cotyledons of velvetleaf. Spurred anoda also has two heart-shaped cotyledons like prickly and arrowleaf sida, however the first true leaf of spurred anoda is not as coarsely toothed as that of prickly or arrowleaf sida. The cotyledons of arrowleaf sida are essentially identical to those of prickly sida, however the first true leaf of arrowleaf sida is rhombic in outline and tapers to the base unlike the first true leaf of prickly sida. [751]

Scientific names - Sida spinosa synonyms

Sida spinosa   Sida alba   Malva spinosa   Malvinda alba Medic   Malvinda alnifolia Medic   Malvinda spinosa (L.) Medic   Sida affinis   Sida angustifolia   Sida betonicifolia   Sida bicolor   Sida bicuspidata   Sida boriara   Sida emarginata   Sida glandulosa   Sida heterocarpa   Sida linearis   Sida milleri   Sida minor   Sida obliqua   Sida orientalis   Sida pimpinellifolia   Sida pusilla   Sida retusa   Sida scabra   Sida spinosa var. sennaarensis   Sida subdistans   Sida truncata L'Herit [369]

Sida spinosa – Some common names

English: prickly sida, prickly-mallow, guanchuma   Portuguese (Brazil): guaxima, relógio, vassourinha-de-relógio   Spanish: popotalagua, quesillo [366]   Puerto Rico: Balai blanc, Balai-onze-heures, Escoba, Escoba espinosa   Dominican Republic: Escobilla   Haiti: Fe teck teck   Cuba: Fi tec-tec, Malva caballo, Malva de caballo   English: Prickly fanpetals   Bahamas: False mallow   Lesser Antilles: White broomweed [369]

Sida spinosa – Worldwide Distribution

Reported here: USA   (Alabama,   Arkansas,   Arizona,   California, Connecticut, District of Columbia, Delaware, Florida, Georgia, Iowa, Illinois, Indiana, Kansas, Kentucky, Louisiana, Massachusetts, Maryland, Maine, Michigan, Missouri, Mississippi, North Carolina, Nebraska, New Jersey, New York, Ohio, Oklahoma, Pennsylvania, South Carolina, Tennessee, Texas, Virginia, West Virginia), U.S. Virgin Isl., Canada (Ontario), Galapagos Isl., Jamaica, Peru, Aruba, Bonaire, Curacao, Puerto Rico, Haiti, Dominican Republic, Mexico (widespread), Guyana, French Guiana, Ecuador, Argentina

(Buenos Aires, Catamarca, Chaco, Cordoba, Corrientes, Distrito Federal, Entre Rios, Formosa, Jujuy, La Rioja, Mendoza, Misiones, Salta, Santiago del Estero, San Juan, San Luis, Tucuman), S-Brazil (Parana, Rio Grande do Sul), Chile (Tarapaca, Atacama), Paraguay (Alto Paraguay, Cordillera, Guaira, Pres. Hayes), Uruguay (Canelones, Montevideo), Belize, Costa Rica, Bolivia, NE-Brazil (Ceara, Rio Grande do Norte, Paraiba, Pernambuco, Bahia), WC-Brazil (Mato Grosso do Sul), SE-Brazil (Minas Gerais, Rio de Janeiro), Venezuela (Anzoategui?, Aragua?, Carabobo, Cojedes?, Distrito Federal?, Falcon?, Guarico, Lara, Merida, Miranda?, Nueva Esparta, Portuguesa, Sucre?, Tachira, Zulia?), Panama, Lesser Antilles (Anguilla, St. Martin, St. Barts, Barbuda, Antigua, Guadeloupe, La Desirade, Martinique, St. Lucia, Grenadines, Grenada, Barbados), Tobago, Nicaragua, Jamaica, Puerto Rico, Virgin Gorda, Bahamas, Turks & Caicos Isl., Cuba, Egypt (Desert Oases, Great Southwestern Desert, Nile Delta, Nile Valley, NW-coastal Egypt), Oman (Mascat & Oman), Saudi Arabia (NW-Saudi Arabia: Hejaz, SW-Saudi Arabia: Asir), Yemen (Tihama, W-Yemen), Namibia, Swaziland, Botswana, Mauritania, Mali, Senegal, Gambia, Sierra Leone, Ghana, Togo, Niger, Burkina Faso, N-Benin, Nigeria, Chad, Sudan, Congo, D.R.Congo (Zaire), Angola, Mozambique, Zambia, Zimbabwe, ?Kenya, ?Tanzania, Uganda, Rwanda, ?Burundi, Ethiopia, Eritrea, Somalia, South Africa (Transvaal, Free State, KwaZulu-Natal), Madagascar (introduced), +Mauritius, Réunion, Rodrigues (introduced), Cape Verde Isl. (Santo Antao Isl., Sao Vicente Isl., Ilha de Sao Nicolau, Sal Isl., Ilha da Boa Vista, Ilha de Maio, Ilha de Sao Tiago), Spain (introduced), France (introduced), Caucasus / Transcaucasus, Russian Far East, Zhejiang, Japan (Honshu, Shikoku, Kyushu), Ryukyu Isl., Taiwan, China (S-Yunnan), Java, Australia (Western Australia, Northern Territory, Queensland, New South Wales, Ashmoore Reef), India (widespread), Pakistan (Karachi, Sind, Hazara, Pakistani Punjab, Rawalpindi), Jammu & Kashmir (Kashmir), Sri Lanka, Bhutan, Philippines, Myanmar [Burma], Chagos Arch. (introduced) (Diego Garcia (introduced)), Micronesia (introduced) (Pohnpei (introduced)), Northern Marianas (introduced) (Alamagan (introduced)), Palau Isl. (introduced) (Angaur (introduced)), Society Isl. (introduced) (Tahiti (introduced)), Tonga (introduced) (Tongatapu (introduced)), Hawaii (introduced) (Kauai (introduced), Oahu (introduced), Lanai (introduced), West Maui (introduced), Hawaii Isl. (introduced)) [369] Burundi, Congo, Equatorial Guinea, Zaire, Anguilla, Antigua and Barbuda, Bahamas, Barbados, Cayman Islands, Cuba, Grenada, Hispaniola, Jamaica, Martinique, Puerto Rico, St. Lucia, Virgin Islands (British), Virgin Islands (U.S.), El Salvador, Guatemala, Honduras, Panama, French Guiana, Guyana **[366]**

Sida hermaphrodita

River-mallow, Virginia Fanpetals

Description

The branching stem of Sida hermaphrodita is 1 to 4 meters tall, and up to 3 centimeters in diameter. The leaves are 10 to 20 centimeters long and borne on petioles. The leaves are simple, but palmately cleft into 3 to 7 lanceolate lobes. The flowers are borne in terminal clusters. Each flower has 5 petals, which are about a centimeter long. The fruit is a schizocarp that splits into segments when ripe. [1]

Scientific names - Sida hermaphrodita synonyms

Accepted scientific name: Sida hermaphrodita   Napaea hermaphrodita L. [369]

Sida hermaphrodita – Some common names

English: river-mallow, Virginia-mallow, alkali sida, Virginia Fanpetals   [366] French: mauve de Virginie · sida hermaphrodite   Polish: Ślazowiec pensylwański [360]

Sida hermaphrodita – Worldwide Distribution

Reported here: Southern parts of USA.   **[363]**   USA (District of Columbia, Indiana, Kentucky, Massachusetts (introduced), Maryland, Michigan, New Jersey (introduced), New York (introduced), Ohio, Pennsylvania, Tennessee, Virginia, West Virginia), Canada: (Ontario (introduced)) **[366, 369]**   Alaska, Greenland, Hawaii, Puerto Rico, Virgin Islands: St. Pierre and Miquelon, Delaware **[724]**   Native range thought to center on 4 disjunct areas: Potomac and Susquehanna watersheds in Pennsylvania, Maryland, District of Columbia, and Virginia; southeastern Indiana, extreme southern Ohio, western West Virginia, and adjacent northeastern Kentucky; (formerly) northeastern corner of Tennessee; and the Great Lakes region (northeastern Indiana, northwestern Ohio, Michigan, and southeastern Ontario). The native status of some occurrences in the Great Lakes region is uncertain (some are currently thought to have been introduced), but at least the Ontario occurrences are considered native, and at least one source (Spooner et al. 1985) argues that this region is part of the native distribution. **[725]**

Sida urens

Description

Perennial herb up to c. 60 cm tall, branching from the base. Stems and branches covered with stiff hairs both appressed and spreading. Leaves ovate, up to 7 × 4 cm, usually with a long drawn-out pointed apex and a distinctly cordate base, covered with more or less stiff appressed hairs on both surfaces; margin regularly serrate; petiole almost a long as the leaf blade, covered with stiff appressed and spreading hairs. Flowers in axillary clusters. Calyx 5-7 mm long, angular, with stiff appressed and spreading hairs, lobed to just beyond the middle; lobes triangular with a bristle-like tip; petals c. 9 mm long, more or less notched, pale yellow to buff, sometimes reddish in the centre. Mericarps 5, c. 2.5 mm long, shortly beaked. **[750]**

Scientific names - Sida urens synonyms

Sida sessiliflora   Sida breviflora   Sida pseudo-urens   Sida debilis   Sida congensis   Sida verticillata   Sida conferta   Sida boivini   Sida densiflora   Sida rufescens [363]

Sida urens – Some common names

English: balai-zortie, ortie long, malva montés   Spanish: ortie-razier, tomoztla, tunillo [366]

Sida Javensis

Sida veronicaefolia var. javensis (Cav.) Baker f, Javanese fanpetals

Description

Herbs procumbent, 50-70 cm tall, rooting at nodes. Stems, petiole, and pedicels subglabrous or sparsely stellate strigose, sometimes sparsely pilose. Stipule subulate, ca. 2 mm; petiole 1-3 cm; leaf blade ovate or subcordate, sometimes obscurely 3-lobed, 1-3 × 1-2 cm, abaxially stellate strigose, adaxially sparsely strigose, base subcordate, margin dentate, apex obtuse. Flower solitary, axillary, mostly subterminal. Pedicel 2-2.5(-3.5) cm. Calyx 4-5 mm, sparsely pilose with long hairs. Corolla yellow; petals slightly longer than sepals. Filament tube glabrous. Schizocarp globose, ca. 3 mm in diam.; mericarps 5, segmentiform with sharp angles, ca. 2.5 mm, smooth, minutely hairy apically, with 2 tightly convergent awns to 1.5 mm, side walls thin, partly disintegrating. [747]   An annual, procumbent herb up to 70 cm (28 inches) tall, rooting at the nodes. Leaves are ovate or subcordate, up to 30cm (1.2 inches) long. Flowers are yellow, solitary, forming in the axils of the leaves. Fruit is spherical, about 3 mm in diameter. The species is closely related to S. cordata, differing by having fewer hairs along the stems, roots forming at the nodes, a glabrous filament tube, and 2 awns on the mericarp. [1]

Scientific names - Sida javensis synonyms

Sida javensis Cav, Sida veronicaefolia var. javensis (Cav.) Baker f. [528]

Sida javensis – Some common names

Tagalog: Hapuang-niknik, Igat-igat   Ilk.: Marmaraipus, Padapadakpusa English: Javanese fanpetals   CHINESE: Zhao wa huang hua ren   FRENCH: Sida de Java. [528]

....

We demonstrated for the first time that Cryptolepine induces cell cycle arrest through p21WAF1/CIP1 expression, indicating that Cryptolepine might be an attractive compound for molecular-targeting chemotherapy or chemoprevension. [400]

Sida Veronicaefolia

Nagabala, Snake Mallow, Gangeruki. It is also known as Rajbala, Bhumibala, Farid buti, Shaktibala, etc.

Description

A straggling way side herb found very often growing in shady places. It grows mainly in clearing in the forest and as weeds in the over grown grass of public parks and gardens. [347]   A hairy herb with coarsely gray, brown colored hairy branches. Leaves are cordate, ovate and sparingly hispid with 6-14 cm length and 2-3.5 cm in width. Flowers are axillary, solitary, or borne in pairs or in small cymes. Color of fower is white, which gradually turns yellow and brown when they are fully grown. Fruits are small sized and also yellow in color. Seeds are of brown color. Herbs bear the fruits and flower throughout the year. **[807]**

Sida acuta – An Introduction

When I started growing Sida acuta I was very cognizant of and concerned by its status as a world-class weed, but that is in the tropics/sub-tropics. In our Zone 8 it is one of my hardier annuals. In 2016 I finally pulled up the last Sida acuta plants in early December, weeks after the tomatoes, squash, basil, etc. had gone. In 2017 I still have some residual plants doing well in January. Yet in four growing seasons there has been no re-growth from any roots left in the soil (such a waste of root anyhow), but it most vigorously re-sprouts from hundreds of hardy seeds when the soil warms up.

Sida's problem is that when it is perennial, it grows woody and prickly and legendarily entrenched in the soil. The solution is to not let it get entrenched. First-year Sida acuta has a root system that can be pulled out of the soil intact; basically weeding it out at the end of the season. With luck the plant will re-sprout the next Spring from seed left in the same bed. It is absurdly easy to transplant.

So I grow it as an annual. Harvest the leaves and seeds throughout the growing season, and then take the whole plant at the end. This gives me a good supply of the root, considered the most medicinal part by some, as well as the rest of the plant. This also maximizes the length and amount of fiber from the stalk.

There is absolutely no data on whether a Sida acuta plant gets stronger medicinally over multiple growing seasons, or even during a single year's growth. My experience so far is that Sida acuta leaves, even when harvested at three months, are already medicinally potent.

One immediate result of my research was to expand the base of my tinctures from containing just leaves to containing everything but the fiber. All parts of

Sida are similarly medicinal, and they all have their own strengths, so why not put them all together? In support of this I find a tea made of "branch sida," made from a small handful of freshly harvested aerial parts steeped for ten minutes is very healthy.

Up to this year I was making 40% vodka tinctures of just the leaves and it was working well. I would add 50% more to the dose, presumably making up for the superior ethanol content of the commercial tincture I used to buy. I am now putting up several 70% extracts: roots, aerial parts, and everything but fiber.

Sida acuta is a good bee plant in the tropics, and our bees seem to like it, especially when it is still flowering in November. I find a lot of worms around its roots. Birds do not bother it – the sharp points on the seeds are a deterrent {viz 358}. Needless to say deer love it, rodents love it. You have to protect its nutritious tastiness from the wildlife until it can survive serious browsing. Our dog hangs out in the garden a lot, so I have been fortunate to have had no losses to predation so far.

There are only two species of Sida that are commercially available: Sida acuta and Sida cordifolia. Generally they are medicinally equivalent (Sida acuta is the only Sida that contains berberine). While cordifolia is the "official" Bala of Ayurvedic medicine, Sida acuta is a functional alternate. Many Sida species are considered Rasayana herbs. I am trying hard to make more Sidas available ASAP, contact me if this is important to you.

There is controversy over possible toxicity of Sida acuta. Sida acuta is the only species that has been implicated with toxicity, but it also is the most beneficial. Sida carpinfolia (a variety of Sida acuta that occurs only in one area of South America) has several studies finding it toxic to grazing animals, while at least one other study found no toxicity. There are some studies that concluded that Sida acuta affected human kidneys of humans consuming it long term above 100 mg/kg. On the other hand I have been using my extract at 240-700 drops a day for over five years with no ill effects, and my blood tests show no problems with my kidneys, quite the opposite.

Growing Sida

Commercial Sida grower: We recommend using 10 lb. 10-10-10 fertilizer per 1,000 sq. ft. at planting and then side dressing with that much or more every year in May. The protein level and digestibility increase dramatically with fertilization and commonly analyses come back at around 40% crude protein! Incidentally, it is also higher in calcium and phosphorus (critical for antler development) than iron clay peas, soybeans or alfalfa. [699]

In early May of 2017 I was worried. I had hypothesized that my Sida would re-sprout from fallen seed but there were no sprouts. I planted several flats of Sida seed to assure myself of a crop. In late May my wife came in and said, "You have got to look at your Sida bed!" As she was removing the Winter ground cover she discovered hundreds of sprouts! More like 400 sprouts in a 50-square-foot bed. That is wonderful news! That could allow us to multiply Sida out for my whole county in two years if enthusiastically embraced. At the same time all the Sidas came up in the flats!

These Sidas had sprouted despite having completely exhausted the nitrogen from both beds in the previous growing season. So I dug up all the Sida sprouts, and replaced a foot of soil with good quality manufactured organic soil. Still far from ideal, but closer to good garden soil. I added a generous dose of organic 12-12-12 with a liberal dose of kelp meal. Then replanted the best 100 plants to one foot centers (or four to a five gallon can). I put the remaining starts in any available container I could find, flats, quart containers, sixpacs, even a cardboard box.

The remaining 200+ starts got jammed into the end of a bed, which I called the jungle. I wanted to observe the dynamics of really close planting. I have not noticed any dead plants in the jungle. Months later all the plants are still there, many with their growth retarded, but all still reaching for the sky, all healthy. They were much smaller in size, with very few side branches due to the crowding, resulting in a completely vertical Sida acuta.

When these vertical Sidas got to be 4-5' tall they were harvested for fiber along with the taller plants in pots. These unbranched "verticals" have fiber lengths of up to four feet or more! They have good stiffness and strength once dried. My hope is that first-year fibers, even from young plants, are comparable in fiber quality to older plants and certainly will have longer fibers. So far these fibers have demonstrated very good strength. The harvest was about the same - there is at least as much net leaf and roots as in the rest of the garden. Harvesting will be more laborious.

These are hardy weeds. More than once I have discovered to my dismay yet another six pack of grossly overgrown Sidas. Pulling them out of the chambers reveals what appears to be a mass of roots with a little soil. At this point I rip off the bottom inch of root hairs and save it for tinctures. Then I dig a hole that allows me to hang the remaining roots freely and fill dirt under and around them and water them down, and they all survive! Five-foot Sidas in a gallon tub happily trade the trauma of being ripped out and root hairs ripped off, to be able to be in real soil. Have never lost a plant – these are strong weeds in the wrong climate.

Starting From Seed

The best way to have plants next year is to let them go to seed and they will re-sprout in the same bed when the soil gets warm enough. Even if you are vigorously collecting seed, the plant will find ways to drop seed. The only other thing you need is ground cover. The seed has to be in very shallow soil, or right on top, to germinate. This leaves it exposed to things that would like a tasty nutritious seed. Last year the bed that did not have ground cover, but was the

40

better soil, had virtually no sprouts; while the other bed, with worse soil but ground cover, had perhaps four hundred sprouts! We're in zone 8b (down to 15-20 degrees); those in a colder zone let me know how this works for you.

If you are starting from saved seed, immerse the seed in boiling water for 20 seconds, and then plant immediately, very shallowly, barely covering the seed. I had 100 per cent germination doing this with last year's seed. Plants started from seed will pause after emergence for a period of weeks before continuing on their growth, so don't fret. Seed that was 2-3 years old was very very slow to develop, still struggling to get bigger than a few inches in late September.

Maintenance and Growth

After preparing the soil, I have not added subsequent fertilizer. Betsy faithfully waters once a day. I left Sidas in a six pack for five days in the office without watering and they were fine.

The leaves are a known treat for deer, which in the wild browse it heavily. Once established this plant can survive a lot of harvesting. I harvest leaves and seeds every week or two once established.

Fertilization

An herb like rosemary I would stress for better medicinal production. Sidas are much more complex. The general attitude is feed them well for medicinal production. There is evidence of improved growth with fertilization, but equal evidence that fertilization makes no difference in growth! I found that applying 12-12-12 fertilizer to Sida acuta made no difference in growth or lushness. There is ample evidence that they are essentially indifferent to fertilizer in terms of growth. Sidas do like nitrogen and that does seem to improve size; yet early this year it sprouted and was growing in a bed that had been stripped of nitrogen the growing season before. There is no knowing what maximizes its medicinals yet, but commercial growers stress feeding well for the best protein and nutrients, so I assume medicinal value as well. Despite not very good soils and varied amounts of fertilizer used over the years, all my Sida acuta crops have produced an adequate medicinal crop for my needs.

Harvesting Sida acuta

I like to let my Sidas get to the branching stage before picking leaves; then I harvest leaves and seeds every week or two throughout the growing season. When they start to produce seed, they also produce some very large leaves; I call them the "come browse me" leaves because they are right next to seed pods. I think Sida produces these leaves to get the deer to browse the plant, disturb the seed pods, get seed in its fur, and spread the seed. I prefer to pick those big leaves, since that replicates browsing, and they do not seem to last long anyhow. So I harvest the big leaves weekly and then thin the remaining leaves. I probably take only about 10% of the leaves at a time, but could probably take much more. I find it efficient to harvest the seeds separately.

Collecting seed

The fruit is like a tiny naval orange, but where the navel is, it begins to open up and peel back as it matures. When the fruit dries out it turns brown and finally almost black. Once brown the seed pod will generally be open enough to harvest the seeds. When black it will drop seed with the lightest touch (unless moist). To harvest seed I position my fingers over the seed pod and grab it with my thumb and forefinger. If it is truly ripe it will crumble to my touch and I have the seeds pinched between my fingers. If it does not crumble under a strong pinch, then it is not ripe enough no matter how it looks. If you do not pinch the seeds firmly, they will crumble and scatter and you will lose seeds. The seeds do have a sharp short point which you generally avoid by pinching it this way, but if you have sensitive fingers, it is best to wear gloves.

Another method is to carry a wide-mouth jar in one hand, and with the other hand dip a seed cluster into the jar, and roughly rub the cluster of ripe and unripe seed pods. The ripe seed clusters will break apart, and you will get most of the seeds. The unripe pods will resist your efforts; they are hard to break up.

This is a tropical plant, so just keep the seeds cool and dry. Seed saved at room temperature should be good for two years. Research has shown that properly saved seed can be viable for many years.

Processing Sida

Here is how I process Sida plants. Loosen the soil and carefully dig them up to preserve as much root as possible. I then separate the roots from the aerial parts for later processing since they are hard to clean (use wire cutters; scissors do not work).

The aerial parts have a whole variety of forms from single unbranched stem to a tangled multi-branched plant. Since I now value all the aerial parts, harvesting has become easier. I put on old nitrile gloves – as they age they harden which is better for stripping stalks. I pinch the stem firmly between my thumb and forefinger at the top and strip everything downwards. If I get some bark, that is great; bark has its own special benefits. Sometimes I can just strip a straight plant once straight down. Tangled multi-branched plants are too large, so I cut off all the side branches for individual processing (use wire cutters; scissors do not work). With all that done there will still be tufts of goodies along the stem and at the top for harvesting. Each plant demands particular attention.

Like everything Sida there is a great variation in roots. Bare roots with few root hairs are easy to clean in a bucket of water. Roots with whole tangles of root hairs are a real pain. They grab onto everything, so if your soil is rocky you will be peeling off a lot of pebbles. If your soil has clay, you will have resistant blobs of clay/root hairs that wetting only makes worse – **so I recommend that you**

avoid clay. Once the roots are dry, crush the soil blobs away, and then wash in water. The main roots should be a creamy yellow/brown with brown filaments.

N.B.: If you are processing dried Sida parts, I would recommend a mask and maybe even eye protection, and process with a wind current or a fan. The dry dust can be very irritating.

Medicinal benefits of Sida acuta

Elsewhere in this book are listings of pathogens that Sida has shown action against. Beyond direct action, Sida acuta is a great supporter of pharmaceuticals. There is no incidence of Sida interfering with any pharmaceutical, rather a lot of instances in the literature of Sida augmenting their effects. There are a few examples in the chapter **Sida Benefits Narrative.**

There is also Sida's particular ability to create silver, gold, or zinc nanoparticles in a water solution which greatly augments its power. This process seems relatively simple, primitive and potentially useful to all herbalists.

Sida acuta – leaves -- hot distilled water extract -- 20g of ground leaves added to 200mL of distilled water -- boiled for 15 minutes -- Aqueous solution of $AgNO_3$ (0.1 M) was prepared and used for the synthesis of silver nanoparticles. 5mL of aqueous extract of Sida acuta was added to 95mL of 0.1M aqueous solution of silver nitrate in 250mL Erlenmeyer flask, mixed thoroughly by manual shaking and placed under sunlight for reduction into silver nanoparticles (AgNPs). [77]   Silver nanoparticles possess unique properties which find myriad applications such as antimicrobial, anticancer, larvicidal, catalytic, and wound-healing activities. Biogenic syntheses of silver nanoparticles using plants and their pharmacological and other potential applications are gaining momentum owing to its assured rewards. [58] Biosynthesized silver nanoparticles (are a) novel biolarvicidal agent and can be used along with traditional insecticides as approach of Integrated Pest Management (IPM). This is the first report on the mosquito larvicidal activity of the plant aqueous extract and synthesized silver nanoparticles. [768] The biomolecules present in plants mediate the synthesis of nanoparticles and also stabilize the nanoparticles formed with desired size and shape as well play a role in reducing the ions to the nanosize, and in the capping of nanoparticles. [683]   Silver nanoparticles (AgNps) were formed within 10-15 minutes by sunlight irradiation of aqueous solution (0.1M) of silver nitrate ($AgNO_3$) with leaves extract of Sida acuta [364]

What else does Sida do?

Sida acuta is a valuable food plant

"Oh, Sida acuta! That poor people food." – Ecology Action intern from Haiti

Sida acuta is one of the food plants of the Luo of Siaya district, Kenya. [258]

Sida acuta Protein Score Card

Leaf	18% [274]	22% [230]	33.7% [546]	30-40% [699]
Root	5.7% [538]	9.4% [52]		
Seed	12.6% [352]	23.2% [359]	22% [158]	

Sida acuta is a valuable animal forage plant

Fertile Plant Parts: seeds, primates; flower buds, primates. Aerial Parts: leaves, sheep, forage; stems, game mammals, grazing; stems, camels, fodder; stems, horses, browse; goats, forage. Seeds: flower buds, primates: Baboons eat the seeds and flower buds. [361]

Sida acuta has been a sole feed for rabbits with improved weight gains. [229]   Also reported as a supplement for rabbits [694]
Goats - forage-SE Nigeria   [643]
Goats - forage-Philippines   [776]
Goats - forage-Nigeria   [780]
Goats - forage-Nigeria   [781]
Goats - forage-Nigeria   [782]
Animal feed - NE Brazil   [783]

Why I grow it as an Annual

Until last summer my mantra was, "I want this in every greenhouse in the county." I live in the Emerald Triangle and there are a number of 'commercial greenhouses' right in my neighborhood growing marijuana, and hundreds in our county. So I was still thinking, "Sida is tropical, so it must be grown in a greenhouse." Then I realized that I had already been successfully harvesting my first-year beds for years with adequate results.

Sida is perennial, in that it re-sprouts every year from its perennial roots, but that does not happen in Willits. My experience in four years of over-wintering is that the roots cannot survive Mendocino's combination of a cold and wet winter. In four growing seasons there has been no re-growth from the old roots. But I got hundreds of Sida sprouts in my main Sida beds because of all the dropped seeds from the previous season.

After selectively harvesting the aerial parts throughout the growing season, you can get a good final harvest as well (mine was in December). By harvesting the plant at the end of the year (just like tomatoes, but hardier) you get all the first year roots, rather than struggling to cut second- and later-year roots out of an incredibly resisting mass. The real payoff is the following Spring - you should have hundreds of high-protein micro-greens begging for your attention. Do be sure to cover the seedlings since the seeds are surface sown and need to be hidden from things that would gleefully eat them.

It will be interested to know the experience of gardeners in the North closer to Canada. Sida alba is considered "an herbal waif" in Boston. It is amazing that any tropical Sida could in any way survive Boston, but occasionally it does. So where on the scale are you? If you are fully Boston with your Winters, then germination from seeds overwintering outside might be scant. In Willits it gets down into the 20s every winter but that does not appear to affect the seeds. Success will depend on the cold-hardiness of some very tough seeds, and enough soil temperature in the next Spring to get them to sprout.

After the first year or so Sida matures, it becomes a woody, prickly shrub that will deny you passage. It is called "wireweed" because it is so hard to dig up. So I see no benefit so far in letting it get more than one year old. My fiber friend is wildly enthusiastic over the strength and quality of the first-year bark fibers, further indication of the maturity of first-year plants.

If your climate is too cold for seed re-sprouting, and you have a greenhouse and have some room in it, you could grow Sida with an extended season. Two greenhouses in my area that have tried to grow Sida were ultimately not successful. I am sure that it can be done, but why bother unless you are unable to grow it outdoors?

Pathogens and Sida

Pathogen = an infectious agent such as a virus, bacterium, protozoa, prion, a fungus, or other micro-organism [1]

Sida L. (Malvaceae) has been used for centuries in traditional medicines in different countries for the prevention and treatment of different diseases such as diarrhea, dysentery, gastrointestinal and urinary infections, malarial and other fevers, childbirth and miscarriage problems, skin ailments, cardiac and neural problems, asthma, bronchitis and other respiratory problems, weight loss aid, rheumatic and other inflammations, tuberculosis, etc. [609]

MIC = minimum inhibitory concentration. [609]   It was considered that if the extracts displayed an MIC less than 100 μg/ml, the antimicrobial activity was good ; from 100 to 500 μg/ml the antimicrobial activity was moderate; from 500 to 1000 μg/ml the antimicrobial activity was weak; over 1000 μg/ml, the extract was considered inactive. It was also considered that if the extracts displayed an MIC of 8 mg/ml or below against any of the yeast tested, the antimicrobial activity was good. [106]

The use of plants for healing is as ancient and universal as medicine itself. Plants act generally to stimulate and supplement the body's healing forces, they are the natural food for human beings. Many infectious diseases are known to be treated with herbal remedies throughout the history of man kind. Even today, plant materials continue to play a major role in primary health care as therapeutic remedies in many developing countries. [83]

Pathogen Listings

Pathogen Description: In the header in large bold is the name of the pathogen, and what type of pathogen it is in smaller bold type. Following this there might be some text describing what this pathogen does. At the beginning or end of any header or listing, there is a citation number in bold (143- or [143]). This number leads you to the original research in **the References**. (Any special sub-species of this pathogen that were tested appear just below the pathogen name).

This book is a compilation of peer-review research, and is not meant to be used as medical advice. Under each pathogen listed are the Sidas tested against it. Sida acuta and Sida cordifolia dominate the listings, but realize that most listings might only have one entry for one type of Sida tested against one pathogen. There is ample evidence in this book that the top ten Sidas all have about the same awesome medicinal properties (see **Traditional Use/Ayurveda/Bala Controversy**), so if one Sida is listed as successful, the other Sidas might be as well. The section that follows this one (**Pathogen Narratives**) covers some pathogen related topics in greater detail.

I have an ideal listing format that frequently does not happen. I am talking about the specific pathogen listings under each species of Sida. Often there is not enough information presented in the research, or I only have access to an abstract of the research. My ideal listing would go thus: Pathogen, type of research, part(s) of the plant studied, what extract used, results. The information in this book is way too incomplete and hopefully by the time of the next edition the information will be more complete.

Sample Listing

Bacillus spp.   **Gram positive bacteria**

B. cereus - B. cereus LMG 13569 - B. licheniformis - B. megaterium - Bacillus subtilis - B. subtilis(MTCC441) - B. subtilis (NCM 2439) - NCIM 2063

Bacillus species are common microbes found in most natural environments including soil, water, plant and animal tissues. While most *Bacillus* species are regarded as having little pathogenic potential, both *Bacillus cereus* and *Bacillus subtilis* have been known to act as primary invaders or secondary infectious agents in a number of diseases and have been implicated in some cases of food poisoning. **[450]**

Sida acuta

Bacillus cereus   7-invitro-aerial parts-chloroform extract-MIC=400 µg/ml--MBC=240 µg/ml-microbiostactic-Bacillus cereus LMG 13569,

----

1: **Pathogen species**   Bacillus spp. (spp.= several species covered)

The header in bold is the pathogen species tested: Bacillus subtilis If several sub-species were tested, they will be listed immediately below.

2.   **Type of Pathogen:** Gram positive bacteria

This could be bacteria, microbes, worms, fungi, etc. Grouped by type of pathogen, sub-listed under this alphabetically.

3.   **Pathogen varieties in this section (if specified):**

B. cereus - B. cereus LMG 13569 - B. licheniformis - B. megaterium - Bacillus subtilis - B. subtilis (MTCC441) - B. subtitlis (NCM 2439) - B. subtilis NCIM 2063

Codes with the pathogen usually denote either a standard lab strain or a pharmaceutically resistant variety.

4. **Pathogen information (not always):**

Bacillus species are common microbes found in most natural environments including soil, water, plant and animal tissues. While most *Bacillus* species are regarded as having little pathogenic potential, both *Bacillus cereus* and *Bacillus subtilis* have been known to act as primary invaders or secondary infectious agents in a number of diseases and have been implicated in some cases of food poisoning.

Additional information about this particular pathogen, usually in the words of the researchers themselves. Also refer to the next chapter, **Pathogen Narratives**, covers some pathogen related topics in greater detail

5. **Citation Number** = 102.

Just about everything in this book has a citation number, which leads you to the original peer-review research (sometimes expert testimonty). Match this number in the References section to find the study's title, the author's names, and the journal in which it was published. It is particularly easy to find this study by its exact title in Google Scholar (https://scholar.google.com/) Many of the citations lead you to the complete studies - which gives you the complete source of the information.

6. **Species of Sida tested:** Sida acuta. Each species has its own paragraph

7.   **Pathogen tested:**   Bacillus cereus. Every pathogen has its own entry under the species of Sida tested.

8. **Citation numbers:** 7, 106 (look them up in the References section)

9.   **Type of test:** invitro

"invitro" means it happened in the lab in test tubes and petri dishes. If animals are involved in the research they are named here instead. Things like "field study" means an expert observational study in the field. "Review" means research cited in other peer-review studies not otherwise available.

10. Parts of the plant tested: Leaf

Every part of Sidas are medicinal to varying degrees, and often have their own strengths and weaknesses. For example, comparing results for root can be different than results for leaf. Whole plant, aerial parts are other options.

11. Method of extraction: chloroform extract

Several methods of extraction may be attempted in one study. Sometimes two methods are done together, such as various concentrations of ethanol and water. If two or more different methods of extraction are employed seperately, they will be seperated by commas. Any sequential extraction or subsequent fractionizations would be noted with >. For example: ethanol> ether would be an ethanol extraction with a secondary extraction with ether.

12. How outcome measured: MIC=240 µg/ml--MBC=400 µg/ml

MIC=Minimum inhibitory concentration. The concentration that inhibits the growth or multiplication of microbiota; MBC=Minimum bactericidal concentration. Lowest concentration of an antibacterial agent required to kill a particular bacterium. Other ways of expressing an outcome: ZI (Zone of inhibition) the size of this zone shows how effective the antibiotic is at stopping the growth of the pathogen. LC90 = death of 90% of a pathogen.

13. Measure of success: MIC, MBC

In this case, death (MBC) or inhibition (MIC) of the pathogen. ZI would express in mm. how far the pathogen is inhibited.

14. Concentration of extract: 240 µg/ml, 400 µg/ml

How much Sida was needed for this outcome? 240 µg/ml stops the pathogen from growing further. 400 µg/ml kills the pathogen outright. Often, but not always, Sida's effectiveness is dependent on the size of the dose.

15. Notes: (microbiostactic-Gentamicin Zone of Inhibition=18mm)

If there is some additional information that could be helpful, it is included here. First reaffirming that the 240 µg/ml is microbiostactic-another way of expressing MIC. Second, a particular strain was tested: Bacillus cereus LMG 13569.

The next chapter, **Pathogen Narratives**, combines some excellent narrative from the researchers on some basic concepts of disease and pathogen resistance. I begin with my opinion on our situation vis-à-vis pathogens, and close with product longevity and how to make the perfect cup of tea.

···

In earlier studies, selected pathogens have been proved to be the major causal organisms of various human infections viz. Eschirichia coli and Proteus mirabilis are the culprits of human urinary tract infections 11 and most of the human intestinal infections are due to E. coli. S. aureus causes a variety of suppurative, wound infections and food poisoning in human beings. S. aureus is a major causative agent of nosocomial infections. **[221]**

Pathogens covered (by class)

A listing by pathogen class, alphabetically within the section:

Bacteria

Bacillus spp.
Bordetella bronchiseptica
Campylobacter spp.
Citrobacter freundii
Corynebacteriun diphtheriae
Enterobacter spp.
Escherichia coli (E. coli)
Helicobacter pylori (H. pylori)
Kebsiella spp.
Listeria innocua
Micrococcus luteus (Sarcina lutea)
Moraxella catarrhalis
Morganella morganii
Mycobacterium spp.
Neisseria gonorrhoeae
Nocardia asteroids
Pantoea agglomerans
Pasturella multocida
Proteus spp
Pseudomonas spp.
Salmonella spp.
Sarcina lutea (Micrococcus luteus)
Shigella spp.
Staphylococcus spp.
Streptococcus spp.
Vibrio spp.
Xanthonomonas axonopodies pv. Malvacearum
Six Pathogens

Cancer

Cancer, In General
Cancer Treatment
Adenocarcinoma
Blood cancer
Breast cancer
Liver cancer
Colon cancer
Hepatoma
Leukemia
Cancer, Liver
Lung cancer

Lung fibroblast cells
Hepatoma
Osteosarcoma (Bone cancer)
Ovarian cancer
Preneoplastic lesions
Cancer, Other Cancer
Cancer, Cytoxic

Insects

Bean Weevil
Earias vittella
Mosquito - Aedes aegypti
Mosquito - Anopheles stephensi
Mosquito-Culex quinquefasciatus
Plasmodium berghei
Plasmodium falciparum

Fungi

Alterneria Alternata
Aspergillus spp.
Candida spp.
Cryptococcus neoformans
Cunninghamella elegans
Dreschlera turcica
Fusarium oxysporum
Fusarium verticillioides
Microsporum gypseum
Rhizopus oryzae
Saccharomyces cerevisiae
Scpulariopsis candida
Trichoderma spp.
Trichophyton spp.
Trichosporon inkin
Ustilago maydis

Virus

Herpes-simplex virus
Polio virus
Sindbis virus

....

S. hermaphrodita is harvested in the winter and consists of dry leafless stems which are used in small combustion units. Energy contents of pellets made from its stems are comparable to those of pine wood chips with calorific values ranging from 16 to 18 MJ per kg dry mass (Borkowska and Molas, 2012)... the agronomic value of S. hermaphrodita has not yet been realized in Northern America, probably because it is nowadays a rare species. [475]

Bacteria

Bacillus spp.   Gram positive bacteria

B. cereus - B. cereus LMG 13569 - B. licheniformis - B. megaterium - Bacillus subtilis - B. subtilis(MTCC441) - B. subtitlis (NCM 2439) - B. subtilis NCIM 2063

Bacillus species are common microbes found in most natural environments including soil, water, plant and animal tissues. While most *Bacillus* species are regarded as having little pathogenic potential, both *Bacillus cereus* and *Bacillus subtilis* have been known to act as primary invaders or secondary infectious agents in a number of diseases and have been implicated in some cases of food poisoning. [450]

Sida acuta

Bacillus cereus   7-invitro-microbiostactic-Bacillus cereus LMG 13569, **106**-invitro-Methanol Zone of inhibition=9 mm-Methanol & Water (1/1)Zone of inhibition=11 mm--Ethanol Zone of inhibition=10 mm—Ethanol & Water(1/1)/ Ethyl acetate/Water extracts-no Zone of Inhibition,

Bacillus megaterium   83-invitro-plant oils-no effect,

Bacillus subtilis 5-invitro-methanol extract-susceptible,   6-invitro-leaf-95% ethanol extracts-Inhibition zone 17mm-activity index=.53-Gentamycin 10 mcg-Inhibition zone 34-also chloroform extract--similar results for Bacillus subtilis NCIM 2063,   55-in vitro,   83-invitro-plant oils-Hydro distillation in the ratio of 3:1-not antimicrobial in tests-no effect,   101-invitro-MIC 10 mm/ml-ZI=16mm (25 mg/ml)--ZI Ciprofloxacin=19.8mm (5 µg/ml)--ZI Amoxycillin 18mm (25 µg/ml),   102-invitro-leaf-1000 mg/ml-100% ethanolic extract-zone of inhibition=22mm---gentamicin-zone of inhibition=18mm--cold water extract-zone of inhibition=12mm--gentamicin-zone of inhibition=18mm,   168-invitro-aerial parts-90 % ethanol extract-Zone of inhibition (25 mg/ml)-16 mm-MIC (10 mg/ml),   179-invitro-seed-showed relatively large inhibition zones,   168-invitro-aerial parts-ethanolic extract,   238-invitro-stems with leaves and reproductive structures-100% methanol extract-zone of inhibition=0,   362-review-seed-The untreated seeds in dung heaps show antibacterial activities on Bacillus subtilis,   523-invitro-leaves-MIC=4 ug/well-zone of inhibition (40ug/well)- 90% ethanol 28mm - methanol 20mm - ethyl acetate 17mm - aqueous extract 15mm,

Sida cordifolia

Bacillus cereus 143-invitro-chloroform and methanol extracts of leaves and roots exhibited significant activity against,

Bacillus subtilis 143-invitro-chloroform and methanol extracts of leaves and roots exhibited significant activity against,   173-invitro-leaf and root-methanol extract-Zone of Inhibition (mm)-root=16--leaf=18--same effect as Streptomycin sulfate.

Sida indica

Bacillus cereus **446**-invitro-acqueous and methanol extracts-nothing detected, **450**-invitro-fruit,root,leaf-dichloromethane:methanol (1:1, v/v) extract-no effect-Bacillus cereus var. mycoides (ATCC 11778), **52**-brine shrimp-carbon tetrachloride zone of inhibition 8.0 -(chloroform extract, n-hexane extract, aqueous soluble partitionate of methanolic extract) none had an effect, **713**-invitro-leaves-methanol extract>dissolved in 10% aqueous methanol>n-hexane extract>carbon tetrachloride extract ZI 8.0 ± 0.44 mm--kanamycin ZI 30.4 ± 0.10 mm—chloroform/n-hexane/aqueous fraction of methanol extracts ZI=none,

Bacillus subtilis **689**-invitro-root, bark and fresh leaves methanol extract-root ZI= 15@90μg/ml-leaf ZI=16 @90μg/ml, **704**--n-hexane/methanol extraction—re-dissolved in distilled water—leaf MIC=604μg/ml—stem MIC=2333μg/ml—root MIC=254 μg/ml, **713**-invitro-leaves-methanol extract>dissolved in 10% aqueous methanol>n-hexane extract>carbon tetrachloride extract ZI 7.1 ± 0.66 mm--kanamycin ZI 33.0 ± 1.10 mm—chloroform/ n-hexane/ aqueous fraction of methanol extracts ZI=none, **718**-invitro-leaf-chloroform extract ZI 13mm—ethanol extract ZI 14mm--water extract ZI 0mm--Chloramphenicol (Control) ZI 27mm,

Other Bacillus **704**-Bacillus licheniformis-n-hexane/methanol extraction—re-dissolved in distilled water—leaf MIC=160μg/ml—stem MIC= 852μg/ml—root MIC=225 μg/ml, **713**-**Bacillus megaterium**-invitro-leaves-methanol extract>dissolved in 10% aqueous methanol>n-hexane extract>carbon tetrachloride extract ZI 8.2 ± 0.55 mm--kanamycin ZI 33.3 ± 1.20 mm—chloroform/ n-hexane/ aqueous fraction of methanol extracts ZI=none,

Cryptolepine (found in S. acuta, cordifolia, rhombifolia, alba, at least)
Bacillus cereus **390**- -invitro-acid alcoholic extract-MIC <7.8 /mi-MBC 15.75 pg/mi,

Bordetella bronchiseptica
Infectious bronchitis in dogs [1]   **Gram negative bacteria**

Sida indica
450--(ATCC 4617)--invitro--fruit, root, leaf--dichloromethane: methanol (1:1, v/v) extract--no effect,

Campylobacter spp.   Gram negative bacteria
Campylobacter spp. - C. coli - C. jejuni

Bacterial food borne disease, blood infections in individuals with AIDS, recurrent diarrhea in children, opportunistic pathogen in humans. Periodontitis. [1]

Cryptolepine (found in S. acuta, cordifolia, rhombifolia, alba, at least)
392-invivo?-MIC90%=12.5 µg/ml-41 strains-the ethanol extract activity against Campylobacter strains (MIC 90%=25µg/ml) is higher than that of co-trimoxazole and sulfamethoxazole and Campylobacter strains susceptibility for cryptolepine is equal to ampicillin,

Citrobacter freundii   Gram negative bacteria

As an opportunistic pathogen, C. freundii is responsible for a number of significant infections. It is known to be the cause of nosocomial infections of the respiratory tract, urinary tract, blood, and many other normally sterile sites in patients. C. freundii represents about 29% of all opportunistic infections. [1]

Sida acuta

106-invitro-Methanol/Methanol&Water (1/1)/Ethanol/Ethanol&Water (1/1) / Ethyl acetate/Water/Water extracts-no Zone of Inhibition.

Corynebacteriun diphtheriae
Gram positive bacteria

Diphtheria causes a thick covering in the back of the throat. It can lead to difficulty breathing, heart failure, paralysis, and even death. The pathogenic bacterium that produces diphtheria toxin.... is sensitive to the majority of antibiotics [1]

Sida cordifolia   **38**-invitro-leaf-extract- showed a maximum zone (20 mm) against Corynebacteriun diphtheriae.

Sida retusa   **436**-Sida retusa-invitro-seed-ethanolic extract-exhibited potent inhibitory effects against Diptheriae spp. with inhibitory zone something like 18-26 mm.

Sida rhombifolia-invitro-root-petroleum ether/chloroform/methanol extracts -Though their antibacterial activities were relatively lower than that of the reference compound (ciprofloxacin), the three crude extracts showed significant activities against all the bacterial species-antibacterial activities were comparable. **[150]**

Enterobacter spp.   Gram positive bacteria

E. aerogenes - E. aeruginosa - E. agglomerans - E. cloacae - E. faecalis Opportunistic infections in immunocompromised hosts-commonly urinary and respiratory tract infections. **[1]**

Sida acuta

Enterobacter agglomerans, Enterobacter cloacae

106-invitro-Methanol/Methanol&Water(1/1)/Ethanol/Ethanol&Water(1/1)/Ethyl acetate/Water extracts-no Zone of Inhibition.

Enterobacter faecalis **238**-invitro-whole plant-methanolic extract-no effect.

Sida alba (Sida spinosa)

Enterobacter aeruginosa **11**-invitro-leaves?-aqueous acetone (80%, v/v) washed with hexane-Inhibition zone= 22.00 ± 2.65 mm-MIC (25 µg/ml) - MBC (100 µg/ml)-net effect bacteriostatic--Inhibition zone Co-trimoxazol= none -when combined with Co-trimoxazol killed all bacteria (both gram positive and negative) within 5 hours-combined-Zone inhibition 14.66 ± 1.53 mm-MIC 100 (µg/ml)-MBC 400 (µg/ml)-net effect bacteriostatic.

Sida indica

Enterobacter faecalis **238**-invitro-methanolic extract-no effect

Cryptolepine (found in S. acuta, cordifolia, rhombifolia, alba, at least)

Enterobacter aerogenes **390**-invitro-acid alcoholic extract-MIC 125 /mi-MBC 250 pg/mi.

Enterococcus spp.   Gram positive bacteria

Enterococcus spp. - E. faecalis CIP 103907 (Enterobacter faecalis) - E. faecalis   Urinary tract infections, bacteremia, bacterial endocarditis, diverticulitis, and meningitis [1]

Sida acuta

Enterococcus faecalis **7**-(CIP 103907)-invitro-microbiostactic, **11**-invitro-leaves?-aqueous acetone (80%, v/v) washed with hexane- All test bacteria were susceptible to the polyphenol-rich fractions-the effect was faster on Enterococcus faecalis, **101**-invitro-aerial parts-90% ethanol extract--aerial parts--ZI=14@25 mg/ml, **238**-(CIP 103907)-invitro-stems with leaves and reproductive structures-100% methanol extract-zone of inhibition=0, **523**-invitro-leaves-clinical isolates-- zone of inhibition (40ug/well)- 90% ethanol 25mm - methanol 15mm - ethyl acetate none - aqueous extract none.

Sida cordifolia

Enterococcus faecalis **125**-review-leaf-methanol extract ZI=0mm (2 mg/disc)—water extract ZI=14mm (2 mg/disc)—Ciprofloxlacin ZI=24mm (5 ug/disc),

Sida alba (Sida spinosa)

Enterococcus faecalis **11**-invitro-leaves?-aqueous acetone (80%, v/v) washed with hexane-Inhibition zone=50 mm-MIC 50 (µg/ml) -MBC 200

(µg/ml)-net effect bacteriostatic--Inhibition zone Co-trimoxazol= 25 mm-when combined with Co-trimoxazol killed all bacteria (both gram positive and negative) within 5 hours-combined-Zone inhibition 29.66 ± 2.89 mm-MIC 12.5 (µg/ml)-MBC 25 (µg/ml)-net effect bacteriocidal.

Sida indica

Enterococcus spp. **639**-stem-methanol extract-ZI (100 µg /ml) 4.3 mm.

Enterococcus faecalis (CIP 10390) **450**-Sida indica-invitro-fruit, root, leaf-dichloromethane: methanol (1:1, v/v) extract-no effect--Streptococcus faecalis (MTCC 8043)

Escherichia coli   Gram negative bacteria

Escherichia coli (E. coli) - Escherichia coli ATCC25722 -- Escherichia coli (MTCC 40) -- Escherichia coli CIP 105182 -- Eschorichia coli NCIM 2065 -- Escherichia coli NCM 2965 -- Escherichia coli NCTC 10418 -- Escherichia coli NCTC 11560

Harmless strains are part of the normal flora of the gut, virulent strains can cause gastroenteritis, urinary tract infections, neonatal meningitis, hemorrhagic colitis, and Crohn's disease [1]   Infection due to ESBL-producing E. coli and Klebsiella species continue to increase in frequency and severity... a recent single-center study showed that blood stream infection due to an ESBL-producing organism was an independent predictor of mortality, prolonged length of stay, delay in initiation of appropriate antimicrobial therapy, and increased hospitalization costs. In a meta-analysis of 16 studies reported for 1996–2003, ESBL-producing BSI was significantly associated with delayed initiation of effective therapy and increased crude mortality [456]

Sida acuta

Escherichia coli spp. **5**-invitro-methanol extract-susceptible-UVA only, **6**-invitro-leaf-95% ethanol extract-100mg/disc-Inhibition zone 42mm-activity index=.98--Gentamycin 10 mcg-Inhibition zone 43--also chloroform extract- similar results-did about as well as Gentamycin 10 mcg/Nystatin 100 units, **7**-(CIP 105182)-invitro-microbicide, **77**-invitro-leaves-boiled distilled water extract-used immediately after-**ZI=nil**--with silver nanoparticles 13mm--silver nitrate alone 10mm--Gentamycin 38mm, **83**-invitro-plant oils-Hydro distillation in the ratio of 3:1-not antimicrobial in tests-no effect, **89**-invitro-whole plant- aqueous acetone extract-ZI=0--also CIP 105182 no effect, **101**-invitro-MIC (no activity)-ZI=(no activity)--ZI Ciprofloxacin=26.5mm (5 µg/ml)--ZI Amoxycillin 16.5mm (25 µg/ml), **102**-invitro-leaf-1000 mg/ml-100% ethanolic extract-zone of inhibition=26mm--gentamicin-zone of inhibition=35mm--cold water extract-zone of inhibition=18mm--gentamicin-zone of inhibition=35mm, **106**-invitro-Methanol/ Methanol&Water (1/1)/Ethanol/Ethanol&Water (1/1)/ Ethyl acetate/Water extracts-no ZI, **113**-invitro-whole plant?- ethanolic and aqueous extracts- quite susceptible, **168**-invitro-aerial parts-90% ethanol extract-no effect, **179**-invitro-seed-showed relatively large inhibition zones,

214-invitro-whole plant?-70% aqueous methanol extracts-at 20+g/ml-zone of inhibition 13.4±0.26--MIC 0.248±0.02, **221**-invitro-roots/stems/leaves/buds-10% acetic acid in ethanol extract-all inactive against E. coli, **224**-invitro-all methods of extraction were effective, **238**-invitro-stems with leaves and reproductive structures-100% methanol extract-zone of inhibition=0, **271**-invitro-water extract (distilled water)-80% methanol extract-MIC-root/stem/bud-0.625 mg/ml-MBC-root/bud-1.25 mg/ml-stem-.625 mg/ml-leaf-0 mg/ml, **362**-review-seed-The untreated seeds in dung heaps show antibacterial activities on Escherichia coli, **523**-invitro-leaves-MIC=5 ug/well - zone of inhibition (40ug/well)-90% ethanol 29mm - methanol 20mm - ethyl acetate 18mm - aqueous extract none, **645**-invitro-leaf-cold water extract-ZI 10mm@50 ug-ZI 15mm@600 ug, **645**-invitro-leaf-acetone extract-ZI 10mm@50 ug-ZI 16mm@600 ug,

Sida cordifolia

Escherichia coli spp. **152**-invitro-seed oil-petroleum ether (40-600C) extract-ZI 22-26mm (300 µg)-ZI 0-10mm at 100 µg -- chloroform extract ZI 0-26mm (300 µg)-ZI 0-10mm at 100 µg--Norfloxacin ZI 23mm (50µg/ml), **173**-invitro-leaf and root-methanol extract-Zone of Inhibition (mm)-root=12--leaf=15--same effect as Streptomycin sulfate, **664**-invitro-whole plant-95% ethanolic extract-ZI 10.66±1.15mm-100µl, **667**-(MTCC 1303)-invitro-roots-ethyl acetate ZI=18mm @100µg/ml-ethanol extract ZI=11mm @100µg/ml,

Sida rhombifolia

Escherichia coli spp. **47**-invitro-whole plant?-aqueous methanol extract (1v:4v)- Diameter of inhibition 11.80 ± 1.04 mm-200 (µg/disc)-Gentamycin-Diameter of inhibition 23.00 ± 0.06 (133 µg/disc), **51**-invitro-fruit-methanol (CH3OH) extract-MIC=300 µg/ml-Zone Inhibition-21 mm(200 µg/ml)- Ciprofloxacin zone of inhibition=24 mm (200 µg/ml)-also included Petroleum ether (C2H5-O- C2H5), chloroform (CHCl3) extracts-less effective-Escherichia coli (MTCC 40), **126**-invitro-ethanolic extract-50 to 500 ug-leaves, stalk, root had no effect, **150**-invitro-root-50 mg/ml-petroleum ether extract ZI=16 mm, chloroform extract ZI=17 mm and methanol extracts ZI=20 mm-Ciprofloxacin ZI=35 mm, **278**-invitro-root-50 mg/ml-petroleum ether extract ZI=16.1 mm, chloroform extract ZI=17 mm and methanol extracts ZI=20 mm-Ciprofloxacin ZI=35 mm-Escherichia coli ATCC25722, **282**-invitro-roots-petroleum ether, chloroform and methanol-100 mg/ml solution-Escherichia coli ATCC25722, **353**-fruit- Escherichia coli (KL2DSM 498) - "n-hexacosa-11-enoic acid"-50 µg/ml-zone inhibition 11mm,

Sida alba

Escherichia coli spp. **11**-invitro-leaves?-aqueous acetone (80%, v/v) washed with hexane-Inhibition zone=29 mm-MIC 50 (µg/ml) -MBC 200 (µg/ml)-net effect bacteriostatic--Inhibition zone Co-trimoxazol=none-when combined with Co-trimoxazol killed all bacteria (both gram positive and negative) within 5 hours-combined-Zone inhibition 12.33 ± 3.22 mm-MIC 100 (µg/ml)-MBC 400 (µg/ml)-net effect bacteriostatic, **55**-invitro-leaf-ethanolic extract-500 µg/ disc-zone of inhibition 15 mm-Ciprofloxacin-5 µg /

disc- zone of inhibition 37 mm, 99-(NCM 2965)-invitro-whole plant-hot 60-80% ethanolic extract- showed antimicrobial activity-Zone of inhibition 21 mm at 500 μg/ disc, **633**-invitro-methanolic extract-whole plant?-ZI 7mm, **667**-(MTCC 1303)-invitro-roots-ethyl acetate ZI=16mm @75μg/ml-ethanol extract ZI=10mm @25μg/ml,

Sida indica

Escherichia coli spp. **450**-invitro-fruit,root,leaf-dichloromethane:methanol (1:1, v/v) extract-no effect-Escherichia coli (ATCC 10536), **452**-brine shrimp-carbon tetrachloride zone of inhibition 9.2mm-Neither chloroform, n-hexane extract nor aqueous soluble partitionate of methanolic extract had an effect, **453**-whole plant-100mg/kg bw-zone of inhibition (mm)-Acqueous extract 16 mm-ethanolic extract 20.2 mm, Hexane extract 12 mm, chloroform extract 0 mm, streptomycin (1.mg/ml) 29.2 mm, **639**- stem-methanol extract-ZI (100 μg /ml) 2 mm, **675**-invitro-leaves-80% methanol extract using distilled water no ZI-distilled cold water extract no ZI, **689**-invitro-root, bark and fresh leaves-methanol extract-root ZI= 11@90μg/ml-leaf ZI=12@90μg/ml, **704**-leaf/stem/root--n-hexane/methanol extraction-redissolved in distilled water--MIC 239 to 1250 μg/ml, **713**-invitro-leaves-methanol extract>dissolved in 10% aqueous methanol>n-hexane extract>carbon tetrachloride extract ZI 9.2 ± 0.72 mm--kanamycin ZI 33.0 ± 0.49 mm—chloroform/n-hexane/aqueous fraction of methanol extracts ZI=none, **718**-invitro-leaf-chloroform extract ZI 15mm—ethanol extract ZI 17mm--water extract ZI 0mm--Chloramphenicol (Control) ZI 22mm.

Cryptolepine (found in S. acuta, cordifolia, rhombifolia, alba, at least)

Escherichia coli spp. **108**-invitro-showed activity against, **385**-cryptolepine-invitro-MIC-80 to 160 μg ml– Candida albicans ATCC 10231-Biocidal effects were noted at concentrations 2–4 times those of the MIC of the alkaloid, **390**-invitro-acid alcoholic extract-MIC 62.5 pg/mi-MBC 500 pg/mi,

Helicobacter pylori (H. pylori)

Gram negative bacteria

Chronic gastritis and gastric ulcers, duodenal ulcers and stomach cancer. [1]

Sida indica **639**-Sida indica-stem-methanol extract-ZI (100 μg /ml) 3 mm.

Kebsiella spp. Gram negative bacteria

Klebsiella spp. - K. aerogenes (Enterobacter aerogenes) - K. oxytoca - K. ozenae - K. Pneumonia Urinary tract infections, septicemia, meningitis, diarrhea, soft tissue infections, and spondyloarthropathies [1]

Sida acuta

Klebsiella oxytoca 89-invitro-whole plant- aqueous acetone extract-no effect,

Kebsiella ozenae 89-invitro-whole plant- aqueous acetone extract-Freshly prepared extracts ZI=0--Stored extracts for 21 days ZI=18mm--Microbiostatic activity

Kebsiella pneumonia 5-invitro-methanol extract-no effect, 83-invitro-plant oils-Hydro distillation in the ratio of 3:1-not antimicrobial in tests-no effect, 86-invitro (weak), 89-invitro-whole plant- aqueous acetone extract-no effect, 101-invitro-aerial parts-ethanol extract- MIC (no activity)-ZI=(no activity)--ZI Ciprofloxacin=27mm (5 µg/ml)--ZI Amoxycillin (no activity),neither the concentrated extract nor its dilutions inhibited-no effect, 106-invitro-Methanol Zone of inhibition=11mm-Methanol&Water (1/1)Zone of inhibition=10mm-Ethyl Acetate extract Zone of inhibition=9.5mm--Ethanol/ Ethanol&Water(1/1) /Water-no Zone of Inhibition, 113-invitro-whole plant?- ethanolic and aqueous extracts-somewhat susceptible, 168-invitro-aerial parts-90 % ethanol extract-no effect, 224-invitro-no method of extraction worked-no effect, 523-invitro-leaves-MIC=none - ZI none-90% ethanol none - methanol none - ethyl acetate none - aqueous extract none.

Sida cordifolia

Kebsiella pneumonia 664-invitro-whole plant-95% ethanolic extract-ZI 11±1 mm, 667-(MTCC 1303)-invitro-roots-ethyl acetate ZI=20mm @100µg/ml-ethanol extract ZI=12mm @100µg/ml,

Sida rhombifolia

Klebsiella spp. 48-in vitro-stem-methanol extract>ethyl acetate-ZI=14@ 500 µg/disc. **Kebsiella pneumonia** 47-invitro-whole plant?-aqueous methanol extract (1v:4v)- Diameter if inhibition 19.50 ± 0.50 mm (200 µg/disc)-MIC 50 (µg/ml)-Gentamycin-Diameter of inhibition 26 mm (133 µg/disc)-MIC 16.66 ± 3.33 (µg/ml), 202-invitro-extract-marked antibacterial activity,

Sida alba

Klebsiella aerogenes (Enterobacter aerogenes) 11-invitro-leaves-aqueous acetone (80% v/v)-washed with hexane-Inhibition zone=14 mm-MIC 100 (µg/ml) -MBC 400 (µg/ml)-net effect bacteriostatic--Inhibition zone Co-trimoxazol=none-when combined with Co-trimoxazol killed all bacteria (both gram positive and negative) within 5 hours-combined-Zone inhibition 12.66 ± 3.79 mm-MIC 100 (µg/ml)-MBC 400 (µg/ml)-net effect bacteriostatic,.

Kebsiella pneumonia 11-invitro-leaves?-aqueous acetone (80%, v/v) washed with hexane-Inhibition zone=29.66 mm-MIC (100µg/ml) -MBC (400 µg/ml)-net effect bacteriostatic--Inhibition zone Co-trimoxazol=none-when combined with Co-trimoxazol killed all bacteria (both gram positive and negative) within 5 hours-combined-Zone inhibition 13.33 mm-MIC (100 µg/ml)-MBC (400µg/ml)-net effect bacteriostatic, **667**-(MTCC 1303)-invitro-roots-ethyl acetate ZI=20mm @100µg/ml-ethanol extract ZI=12mm @100µg/ml,

Sida indica

Kebsiella pneumonia (ATCC 10031) **450**-invitro-fruit,root,leaf-dichloro-methane:methanol (1:1, v/v) extract-no effect, **718**-invitro-leaf-chloroform extract ZI 8mm—ethanol extract ZI 14mm--water extract ZI 0mm--Chloramphenicol (Control) ZI 30mm,

Cryptolepine (found in S. acuta, cordifolia, rhombifolia, alba, at least)

Kebsiella pneumonia **390**-invitro-acid alcoholic extract-MIC 500 pg/mi-MBC 500 pg/mi,

Listeria innocua Gram positive bacteria

Non-pathogenic bacteria [1]

Sida acuta 7-(LMG 13568)-invitro-aerial parts-chloroform extract-MIC=400 µg/ml--MBC=240 µg/ml-microbiostactic,

Micrococcus luteus Gram variable bacteria

(Sarcina lutea) Although of low virulence, the germ may become pathogenic in patients with impaired resistance, colonizing the surface of heart valves **[https://www.ncbi.nlm.nih.gov/pubmed/1862670]**

Sida cordifolia

24-mice-roots-ethanol extract-no effect, **72**-(ATCC 9341)-invitro-distillation?-leaf essential oil (2%)-ZI=12mm (50 uL)—Chloramphenicol ZI=20mm (30 ug/ml).

Sida rhombifolia **48**-in vitro--stems—methanol extract> ether/ chloroform/ ethyl acetate --MIC=64mm,

Sida indica

450- fruit/root/leaf-dichloromethane and methanol extract (1:1, v/v)-no antimicrobial or antifungal effect,-Micrococcus luteus (ATCC 9341), **453**-whole plant-100mg/kg bw-zone of inhibition (mm)-Acqueous extract 0mm-ethanolic extract 21mm,Hexane extract 13.8 mm, chloroform extract 12.8 mm, streptomycin (1mg/ml) 22.6mm, **704**--n-hexane/methanol extraction--redissolved in distilled water—leaf MIC=795µg/ml—stem MIC=547µg/ml—root MIC=274 µg/ml, **713**-invitro-leaves-methanol extract>dissolved in 10% aqueous methanol>n-hexane extract>carbon tetrachloride extract>chloroform extract ZI 8.4 ± 0.49mm--carbon tetrachloride extract ZI 10.4 ± 0.15mm—chloroform/n-hexane/aqueous fraction of methanol extracts ZI=none,

Moraxella catarrhalis   Gram negative bacteria

Infections of the respiratory system, middle ear, eye, central nervous system, and joints of humans [1]

Sida urens

499- rats-aerial parts-80% acetone extract-ZI 16.66 ± 1.15mm-MIC (250µg/ml)-MBC (1000 µg/ml)-net effect bacteriostatic--Gentamicin-ZI 23.66 ± 1.53mm-MIC (625µg/ml),

Morganella morganii   Gram negative bacteria

Causes sepsis, ecthyma, endophthalmitis, and chorioamnionitis, and more commonly urinary tract infections, soft tissue infections, septic arthritis, meningitis, and bacteremia, often with fatal consequences. **[1]**

Sida acuta

106-invitro-Methanol/Methanol&Water (1/1)/Ethanol/Ethanol&Water(1/1)/ Ethyl acetate/Water extracts-**no Zone of Inhibition,**

Sida rhombifolia

47-invitro-whole plant?-aqueous methanol extract (1v:4v)- Diameter of inhibition 11.50 ± 0.28 mm (200 µg/disc)-Gentamycin-Diameter of inhibition 19 (133 µg/disc),

Mycobacterium spp.   acid fast gram positive bacteria

M. abcessus −M. aurum −M. bovis BCG − M. fortuitum − M. phlei − M. smegmatis − M. tuberculosis   This genus includes pathogens known to cause serious diseases in mammals, including tuberculosis and leprosy. Mycobacterial infections are notoriously difficult to treat. **[1]**

Sida acuta

Mycobacterium phlei 5-invitro-methanol extract-susceptible, **238**-invitro-stems with leaves and reproductive structures-100% methanol extract-zone of inhibition=14.0−17.9mm.

Mycobacterium smegmatis 7-invitro-aerial parts-chloroform extract-MIC=400 µg/ml--MBC=240 µg/ml-microbiostactic, **585**-leaf-chloroform extract.

Tr 361-tuberculosis, 561-Ayurveda-root-tuberculosis, 609-India-tuberculosis,

Sida cordifolia

Tr 71-Ayurveda-root-pulmonary tuberculosis, 118-Ayurveda-bark-tuberculosis, 217-Ayurveda-pulmonary tuberculosis, 167-Ayurveda-root-pulmonary tuberculosis or a similar progressive systemic disease, 548-Ayurveda-pulmonary tuberculosis, 561-Ayurveda-root-tuberculosis,

Sida rhombifolia

Mycobacterium tuberculosis **544**—invitro--leaves (roots less effective)--Ethyl acetate extract--The anti-mycobacterial screening showed that the ethyl acetate extract of Sida rhombifolia L. leaves has the potential to cure tuberculosis (and M. tuberculosis resistant to S, H, R & E).....The maximum inhibitory activity was seen in the Ethyl acetate extract of the leaves which is 83.61 % inhibition at 500 µg/ml concentration. This is even more significant as this activity was noted against a clinical strain which was resistant to S, H, R and E....For the roots, the ethyl acetate extract showed 29.02 % and 62.37 % inhibition at the concentration of 100 µg/ml and 500 µg/ml,

Tr 47-India-tuberculosis, 51-India-whole plant?-tuberculosis, 136-Ayurveda-root and leaves-tuberculosis, 361-Malaysia-whole plant?-tuberculosis, 362-review-Malaysia-whole plant?-tuberculosis, 522-India-decoction of root-orally-pulmonary tuberculosis, 561-Ayurveda-root-tuberculosis,

Sida cordata
Tr 496-Pakistan-Siddha and Ayurveda-tuberculosis, 549-Ayurveda-tuberculosis,

Sida indica
Tr 448-Ayurveda-pulmonary tuberculosis, 452-Bangladesh-tuberculosis, 684-India-pulmonary tuberculosis,

Other Sida

436-Sida retusa-Mycobacterium tuberculosis-invitro-seed-methanol extract-potent cytotoxic, antibacterial, antitubercular and antimycotic activities, **471-Sida hermaphrodita**-review-caused decrease of viability and deformation of *Mycobacterium smegmatis* cells.

Tr 561- Sida alba (Sida spinosa)-Ayurveda-root-tuberculosis,

Cryptolepine (found in S. acuta, cordifolia, rhombifolia, alba, at least)

Mycobacterium fortuitum, M. phlei, M. aurum, M. smegmatis, M. bovis BCG, M. abcessus **384**-invitro- cryptolepine hydrochloride- dose (16 µg/mL)-antitubercular drugs-MICs ranged over 2–32 µg/mL.

Neisseria gonorrhoeae   Gram negative bacteria
Gonorrhea [1]

Cryptolepine (found in S. acuta, cordifolia, rhombifolia, alba, at least)
108-invitro-showed activity against.

....

An ethnobotanical investigation in the central region of Burkina Faso has shown that many species are traditionally used to treat various kinds of pain diseases. Among such plants, S. acuta Burn f. and S. cordifolia L. (Malvaceae) are the most frequently and widely used. [75]

Nocardia asteroids Gram positive bacteria

nocardiosis, a severe pulmonary infection in immunocompromised hosts [1]

Sida indica

704--n-hexane/methanol extraction--redissolved in distilled water—leaf MIC=512µg/ml—stem MIC=815µg/ml—root MIC=379µg/ml,

Pantoea agglomerans Gram negative bacteria

Occasionally reported to be an opportunistic pathogen in immunocompromised patients, causing wound, blood, and urinary-tract infections [1]

Sida acuta

106-invitro-methyl/ethyl/water/acetone extracts-none worked,

Pasturella multocida Gram negative bacteria

Infection from bites or scratches from domestic pets [1]

Sida acuta **224**-invitro-leaves-all but water extraction worked.

All the flavonoid extracts showed varying degrees of antifungal activity on *C. albicans*. Some of these extracts were more effective than traditional antibiotic terbinafine to combat the pathogenic fungi. **[98]**

Proteus spp. Gram negative bacteria

P. mirabilis - P. vulgaris - P. vulgaris MTCC 426

Opportunistic pathogens, often causing urinary and septic infections **[1]**

Sida acuta

Proteus mirabilis 83-invitro-plant oils-Hydro distillation in the ratio of 3:1-not antimicrobial in tests-no effect, **106**-invitro-Ethanol Zone of inhibition=10mm-Ethanol&Water(1/1) Zone of inhibition=12 mm--Methanol/Methanol&Water (1/1)/Ethyl acetate/Water extracts-no Zone of Inhibition, **125**-invitro-methanolic extract slightly better than acqueous, **214**-invitro-whole plant?-70% aqueous methanol extracts-at 20 +g/ml-zone of inhibition 11±0.21 --MIC 0.178±0.01, **221**-invitro-leaves>stems>roots>buds-10% acetic acid in ethanol extract-all the tested alkaloid extracts of S. acuta have potent antibacterial activity, **271**-invitro-water extract (distilled water)-80% methanol extract-MIC-bud/stem-0.625 mg/ml-leaf-0.312 mg/ml-root-0.156 mg/ml-MBC-bud/stem-0.156mg/ml-leaf-0.625mg/ml-root-0.312 mg/ml.

Proteus vulgaris 106-invitro-Methanol Zone of inhibition=14mm-Methanol&Water (1/1)Zone of inhibition=9mm--Ethanol/Ethanol &Water(1/1)/ Ethyl acetate/Water extracts-no Zone of Inhibition, **761**-invitro-whole plant-The major alkaloid of Sida acuta was shown to be cryptolepine which has antimicrobial activity against Proteus vulgaris, **523**-invitro-leaves-MIC=4 ug/well - zone of inhibition (40ug/well)- 90% ethanol 30mm - methanol 22mm - ethyl acetate 17mm - aqueous extract none.

Sida cordifolia

Proteus mirabilis **38**-invitro-leaf-extract-slightly inhibitory, **72**-invitro, **125**-review-leaf-methanol extract ZI=15mm (2 mg/disc)—water extract ZI=12mm (2 mg/disc)—Ciprofloxlacin ZI=29mm (5 ug/disc),

Proteus vulgaris **143**-invitro-chloroform and methanol extracts of leaves and roots exhibited moderate activity against,

Sida rhombifolia

Proteus vulgaris **47**-invitro-whole plant?-aqueous methanol extract (1v:4v)- Diameter of inhibition 16.20 ± 0.57 mm-200 (µg/disc)-MIC 78.30 ± 0.10 (µg/ml)-Gentamycin-Diameter of inhibition 26 (133 µg/disc)-MIC 10.16 ± 0.16 (µg/ml), **51**-invitro-fruit-methanol (CH3OH) extract-MIC=300 µg/ml-Zone Inhibition- 21 mm(200 µg/ml)- Ciprofloxacin zone of inhibition=23 mm (200 µg/ml)-also included Petroleum ether (C2H5-O-C2H5), chloroform (CHCl3) extracts-less effective-Proteus vulgaris MTCC 426,

Sida alba

Proteus mirabilis **11**-invitro-leaves?-aqueous acetone (80%, v/v) washed with hexane-Inhibition zone= 24.66 ± 1.53 mm-MIC (25 µg/ml) -MBC (50 µg/ml)-net effect bacteriocidal--Inhibition zone Co-trimoxazol= 20.66 ± 1.53 mm-when combined with Co-trimoxazol killed all bacteria (both gram positive and negative) within 5 hours-combined-Zone inhibition 27.00 ± 1.00 mm-MIC 12.5 (µg/ml)-MBC 25 (µg/ml)-net effect bacteriocidal.

Proteus vulgaris **11**-invitro-aerial parts?-aqueous acetone (80%, v/v) washed with hexane-All test bacteria were susceptible to the polyphenol-rich fractions, **51**-invitro-fruit- methanol (CH3OH) extract-MIC=300 µg/ml-Zone Inhibition- 21 mm(200 µg/ml)- Ciprofloxacin zone of inhibition=23mm (200 µg/ml)-also included Petroleum ether (C2H5-O- C2H5), chloroform (CHCl3) extracts-less effective.

Sida indica

446--**Proteus vulgaris**-invitro-acqueous and methanol extract had a 1 mm zone of inhibition-acqueous extract had no effect, **704-Proteus mirablis**--n-hexane/methanol extraction--redissolved in distilled water—leaf MIC=642µg/ml—stem MIC=235µg/ml—root MIC=446µg/ml/

Cryptolepine (found in S. acuta, cordifolia, rhombifolia, alba, at least)

Proteus vulgaris **108**-invitro-showed activity against, **320**-invitro-has antimicrobial activity, **390**-invitro-acid alcoholic extract-MIC 250/mi-MBC 250 pg/mi.

Pseudomonas spp. Gram negative bacteria

P. aeruginosa - P. aeruginosa ATCC 27853 - P. aeruginosa DSMZ1117 - P. aeruginosa MTCC 424 - P. aeruginosa NCM 2036 - P. cichorii - P. fluorescence   Second-most common infection in hospitalized patients [1]

Sida acuta

Pseudomonas aeruginosa 5-invitro-whole plant?-methanol extract-no effect,   6-(NCM 2036)invitro-leaf-ethanolic extract-ZI=20--AI=.54,   55-invitro-leaf-ethanolic extract-*500 µg/ disc*-zone of inhibition 20 mm-*Ciprofloxacin – 5 µg / disc*- zone of inhibition 41 mm,   83-invitro-plant oils-Hydro distillation in the ratio of 3:1-not antimicrobial in tests-no effect,   86-whole plant?-implied somewhat effective,   101-invitro-aerial parts-90% ethanol-MIC (no activity)-ZI=(no activity)--ZI Ciprofloxacin=19.5mm (5 µg/ml)--ZI Amoxycillin (no activity),   102-invitro-leaf-1000 mg/ml-100% ethanolic extract-zone of inhibition=10mm--gentamicin-zone of inhibition=28mm--cold water extract-zone of inhibition=4mm--gentamicin-zone of inhibition=26mm,   106-invitro-Methanol/Methanol &Water (1/1)/Ethanol/Ethanol&Water(1/1)/ Ethyl acetate/Water extracts-ZI=0, 113-invitro-whole plant?-ethanolic and aqueous extracts-susceptible,   125-invitro-leaf-both methanolic and acqueous extracts effective,   168-invitro-aerial parts-ethanolic extract-25 mg/ml-no effect,   214-invitro-whole plant?-70% aqueous methanol extracts-at 20+g/ml-zone of inhibition 8.9±0.16--MIC 0.178±0.01,   238-(H187)-invitro-methanolic extract-no effect,   645-invitro-leaf-cold water extract-ZI 10mm@50 ug-ZI 15mm@600 ug,   645-invitro-leaf-acetone extract-ZI 9mm@50 ug-ZI 16mm@600 ug,

Pseudomonas cichorii   179-invitro-seed-showed relatively large inhibition zones,

Sida cordifolia

Pseudomonas aeruginosa 24-mice-roots-95% ethanol extract (distilled water)- ZI=0@500µg/disc,   72-(ATCC 27853)-invitro-leaf essential oil (100%)-ZI=no effect (50 uL)—Chloramphenicol ZI=10mm (30 ug/ml),   125-review-leaf-methanol extract ZI=15mm (2 mg/disc)—water extract ZI=16mm (2 mg/disc)—Ciprofloxlacin ZI=20mm (5 ug/disc),   238-invitro-stems with leaves and reproductive structures-100% methanol extract-Pseudomonas aeruginosa H187-zone of inhibition=0,   667-(MTCC 1303)-invitro-roots-ethyl acetate ZI=16mm @100µg/ml-ethanol extract ZI=0mm @25µg/ml,

Pseudomonas fluorescence   173-invitro-leaf and root-methanol extract-ZI root=14mm@100 µg ml —ZI leaf=16mm@100 µg ml -- Streptomycin sulfate ZI=14@10 µg ml.

Sida rhombifolia

Pseudomonas aeruginosa 51-(MTCC 424)-invitro-fruit-Petroleum ether (C2H5-O- C2H5), chloroform (CHCl3) and methanol (CH3OH) fruit extracts-MIC 50-200 (µg/ml)-Zone Inhibition-200 (µg/ml)-18 mm,   126-invitro-Ethanol extracts-MIC-leaves 50ug=7mm-stem 50ug=6mm-root 50ug=9mm--ethyl acetate and chloroform fractions   150-invitro-root-50 mg/ml-petroleum ether extract ZI=10 mm, chloroform extract ZI=13.8 mm and methanol extracts ZI=16 mm-Ciprofloxacin ZI=28 mm, **278**-(DSMZ1117)-invitro-root-50 mg/ml-petroleum ether extract ZI=10 mm, chloroform extract ZI=13.8mm and methanol extracts ZI= 16 mm-Ciprofloxacin ZI=28 mm, **282**-(DSMZ1117)-invitro-roots-petroleum ether, chloroform and methanol-100 mg/ml solution, **353**-fruit-Pseudomonas aeruginosa–"n-hexacosa-11-enoic acid"-50μg/ml-zone inhibition=10mm-half the effect of Gentamicine-"1, 3-dilinoleoyl-2-oleine"-zone of inhibition=9, **362**-review-whole plant?-methanolic plant extract-activity against.

Sida alba

Pseudomonas aeruginosa **55**-invitro-leaf-ethanolic extract-500 μg/ disc-zone of inhibition 20 mm-Ciprofloxacin-5 μg / disc- zone of inhibition 41 mm, **99**-(NCM 2036)-invitro-whole plant-hot 60-80% ethanolic extract-showed antimicrobial activity-Zone of inhibition 22 mm at 500 μg/disc, **667**-(MTCC 1303)-invitro-roots-ethyl acetate ZI=18mm @100μg/ml-ethanol extract ZI=0mm @25μg/ml,

Sida indica

Pseudomonas aeruginosa **450**-(ATCC 9027)-invitro-fruit, root, leaf-dichloromethane: methanol (1:1, v/v) extract-no effect, **452**-brine shrimp-carbon tetrachloride zone of inhibition 6.2mm-Neither chloroform, n-hexane extract nor aqueous soluble partitionate of methanolic extract had an effect, **453**-whole plant-100mg/kg bw-zone of inhibition (mm)-Acqueous extract 16.8 mm-ethanolic extract 21.6 mm-Hexane extract 0 mm-chloroform extract 18.8 mm-streptomycin (1.mg/ml) 24.8 mm, **713**-invitro-leaves-methanol extract> dissolved in 10% aqueous methanol>n-hexane extract>carbon tetrachloride extract ZI 6.2 ± 0.15 mm--kanamycin ZI 34.4 ± 0.40 mm—chloroform/n-hexane/aqueous fraction of methanol extracts ZI=none, **718**-invitro-leaf-chloroform extract ZI 15mm—ethanol extract ZI 25mm--water extract ZI 0mm--Chloramphenicol (Control) ZI 23mm,

Pseudomonas fluorescence **689**-invitro-root, bark and fresh leaves-methanol extract-root ZI= 13@90μg/ml-leaf ZI=17@90μg/ml,

Sida Urens

499-**Pseudomonas aeruginosa**-rats-aerial parts-80% acetone extract-ZI=0 -MIC no effect-MBC no activity--Gentamicin-ZI 23.67 ± 1.00mm-MIC 31.25 (μg/ml),

Cryptolepine (found in S. acuta, cordifolia, rhombifolia, alba, at least)
390-**Pseudomonas aeruginosa**-invitro-acid alcoholic extract-MIC 250 pg/mi - MBC 250 pg/mi.

Salmonella spp. Gram negative bacteria

S. boydi - S. enterica (S. choleraesuis) - S. enteritidis - S. parathyphi - S. typhi (S. enterica typhi) - S. typhimurium (typhoid) - S. thyphimurium ATCC13311

Typhoid fever, paratyphoid fever, and food poisoning (salmonellosis) [1]

Sida acuta

Salmonella parathyphi   7-(parathyphi B)-invitro-aerial parts-chloroform extract-ZI nil-MIC nil-MBC nil,   **89**-(parathyphi B)-invitro-whole plant-aqueous acetone extract-fresh leaf extract ZI=0--Stored extracts for 21 days ZI=16mm,

Salmonella typhi (Salmonella enterica typhi)   7-aerial parts-cold chloroform extract-invitro-ZI=nil,   **89**-invitro-whole plant-aqueous acetone extract-no effect,   **106**-invitro-Methanol-ZI =15mm-MIC=(100 µg/ml)-MBC=(400µg/ml)/ Methanol&Water (1/1)-Zone of inhibition= 17mm—Ethanol/Ethanol&Water (1/1)/ Ethyl acetate/ Water extracts-no Zone of Inhibition,   **224**-invitro-methanol, hexane, chloroform and aqueous extracts-none worked

Salmonella typhimurium (typhoid)   5-invitro-methanol extract-no effect,   **179**-invitro-seed-showed relatively large inhibition zones-"active against"69%,   **224**-invitro-leaves-Water extract-ZI=6.5mm@20gm/100ml-only water extract had effect at fairly high dosage,   **362**-review-seed-The untreated seeds in dung heaps show antibacterial activities against.

Sida rhombifolia

Salmonella enteritidis   47-invitro-whole plant?-methanolic extract ZI 14.1mm@500µg/disc--aqueous   methanol   extract   (1v:4v)-ZI 8.50mm@500µg/ disc-ZI 8mm@100 µg/disc--water /MeOH extract (1v:1v)-ZI none--water/MeOH   (3v:2v)-ZI   15.6mm@500µg/disc--Gentamycin-Diameter of inhibition 22.2mm@(133 µg/disc).

Salmonella typhi (Salmonella enterica typhi)   47-MeOH ZI 12.5mm@500 µg/disc--water/MeOH (1v:4v) ZI 15.8mm@500 µg/disc--water /MeOH   (1v:1v)   ZI   13.3mm@500   µg/disc--water/MeOH   (3v:2v)   ZI 10.3mm@500 µg/disc--Gentamycin ZI 26.5mm@133 µg/disc,

Sida alba

Salmonella enterica (Salmonella choleraesuis)   **633**-invitro-methanolic extract-whole plant?-Salmonella spp.-ZI nil,

Salmonella typhi (Salmonella enterica typhi)   11-invitro-leaves?-aqueous acetone (80%, v/v) washed with hexane-Inhibition zone=24.33 mm-MIC 100 (µg/ml)-MBC (400µg/ml)-net effect=bacteriostatic--Inhibition zone Co-trimoxazol=none-when combined with Co-trimoxazol killed all bacteria (both gram positive and negative) within 5 hours-combined-Zone inhibition 12.33 mm-MIC 25 (µg/ml)-MBC 200 (µg/ml)-net effect=bacteriostatic.

Sida indica

Salmonella boydi

713-invitro-leaves-methanol extract>dissolved in 10% aqueous methanol>n-hexane extract>carbon tetrachloride extract ZI 8.4 ± 0.20 mm--kanamycin ZI 35.0 ± 1.00 mm—chloroform/n-hexane/aqueous fraction of methanol extracts ZI=none,

Salmonella enterica (Salmonella choleraesuis)

453-whole plant-100mg/kg bw-zone of inhibition (mm)-Acqueous extract 15.6 mm-ethanolic extract 17.6 mm, Hexane extract 0 mm, chloroform extract 0 mm, streptomycin (1.mg/ml) 21.8 mm,

Salmonella parathyphi

452-brine shrimp-carbon tetrachloride zone of inhibition 8.4mm-Neither chloroform, n-hexane extract nor aqueous soluble partitionate of methanolic extract had an effect, 713-invitro-leaves-methanol extract>dissolved in 10% aqueous methanol>n-hexane extract>carbon tetrachloride extract ZI 8.4 ± 0.49 mm--kanamycin ZI 29.8 ± 0.90 mm—chloroform/n-hexane/aqueous fraction of methanol extracts ZI=none,

Salmonella typhi (Salmonella enterica typhi)

452-brine shrimp-carbon tetrachloride zone of inhibition 6.9mm-Neither chloroform, n-hexane extract nor aqueous soluble partitionate of methanolic extract had an effect, 639-Sida indica-stem-methanol extract-ZI (100 μg /ml) 11 mm, 713-invitro-leaves-methanol extract>dissolved in 10% aqueous methanol>n-hexane extract>carbon tetrachloride extract ZI 6.9 ± 0.51 mm--kanamycin ZI 35.0 ± 1.00 mm—chloroform/n-hexane/aqueous fraction of methanol extracts ZI=none,

Salmonella typhimurium (typhoid)

446-invitro-acqueous and methanol extracts-nothing detected, 704--n-hexane/methanol extraction--redissolved in distilled water—leaf MIC=336μg/ml —stem MIC=610μg/ml—root had no activity,

Cryptolepine   (found in S. acuta, cordifolia, rhombifolia, alba, at least)
Salmonella typhi (Salmonella enterica typhi) 390-invitro-acid alcoholic extract-MIC 62.5 /mi-MBC 125 pg/mi,

Sarcina lutea   gram positive bacteria
(Micrococcus luteus)   Human flora found in the skin and large intestine [1]

Sida indica

452- brine shrimp-carbon tetrachloride zone of inhibition 10.4mm-chloroform zone of inhibition 8.4 mm -Neither n-hexane extract nor aqueous soluble partitionate of methanolic extract had an effect.

Shigella spp.   Gram negative bacteria

S. boydii – S. dysentariae – S. dysenteriae CIP 54051 – S. flexneri – S. flexneri MTCC 1457 – S. shiga – S. sonnei

The causative agent of human shigellosis. One of leading bacterial causes of diarrhea. may cause dysentery. Reactive arthritis. **[1]**

Sida acuta

Shigella boydii 7-invitro-aerial parts-chloroform extract-ZI=17--MIC=80 µg/ml--MBC=240 µg/ml-microbiostactic, **89**-invitro-whole plant- aqueous acetone extract-no effect,

Shigella dysentariae 7-invitro-aerial parts-chloroform extract-ZI=18--MIC=400 µg/ml--MBC=240 µg/ml-microbiostactic—also CIP 54051, **89**-invitro-whole plant- aqueous acetone extract-fresh leaves extract-ZI 15mm-Stored extracts for 21 days-ZI 25mm, **89**-(CIP 54051)-invitro-whole plant-aqueous acetone extract-no effect, **106**-invitro-Methanol Zone of inhibition=10mm-Methanol&Water (1/1) Zone of inhibition=10mm-Ethanol Zone of inhibition=10mm--Ethanol&Water(1/1)/ Ethyl acetate/Water extracts-no Zone of Inhibition.

Shigella flexneri 7-invitro-aerial parts-chloroform extract-ZI=18--MIC=80 µg/ml--MBC=186 µg/ml-microbiostactic, **89**-invitro-whole plant-aqueous acetone extract- no effect, **106**-invitro-whole plant?-Methanol extract ZI=10mm—Methanol &Water extract (1/1) ZI=12mm--Ethanol/ Ethanol&Water extract (1/1)/ Ethyl acetate/ Water extracts-no Zone of Inhibition.

Sida rhombifolia

Shigella boydii, Shigella shiga, Shigella sonnei

48-in vitro-stem-phenyl ethyl B-D-glucopyranoside via exotic extracts,

Shigella dysentariae

47-invitro-whole plant?-aqueous methanol extract (1v:4v)- Diameter if inhibition 24.10±0.50 mm-(200 µg/disc)-MIC 49.40 ±0.30 (µg/ml)-Gentamycin-Diameter of inhibition 22.50 mm (133 µg/disc)-MIC 10.16±0.16 (µg/ml), **48**-in vitro-stems-chloroform-ZI=20 @500µg/disc,

Shigella flexneri

51-invitro-fruit- Petroleum ether (C2H5-O- C2H5), chloroform (CHCl3) and methanol (CH3OH) fruit extracts-MIC 200 (µg/ml)-Zone Inhibition-200 (µg/ml)-21-22 mm--also MTCC 1457,

Sida alba

Shigella boydii, Shigella dysentariae, Shigella flexneri

11-invitro-leaves?-aqueous acetone (80%, v/v) washed with hexane-Inhibition zone=24.66 mm-MIC (100µg/ml) -MBC (200 µg/ml)-net effect=bacteriostatic--Inhibition zone Co-trimoxazol=19 mm-when combined with Co-trimoxazol killed all bacteria (both gram positive and negative) within 5 hours-combined-Zone inhibition 29 mm-MIC (25µg/ml)-MBC (50 µg/ml)-net effect=bacteriocidal,

Sida indica

Shigella boydii

52-brine shrimp-carbon tetrachloride zone of inhibition 8.4mm-Neither chloroform, n-hexane extract nor aqueous soluble partitionate of methanolic extract had an effect, **713**-invitro-leaves-methanol extract>dissolved in 10% aqueous methanol>n-hexane extract>carbon tetrachloride extract ZI 8.4 ± 0.20 mm--kanamycin ZI 35.0 ± 1.00 mm—chloroform/n-hexane/aqueous fraction of methanol extracts ZI=none,

Shigella dysentariae

452-brine shrimp-carbon tetrachloride ZI=10.7mm-Neither chloroform, n-hexane extract nor aqueous soluble partitionate of methanolic extract had an effect, **713**-invitro-leaves-methanol extract>carbon tetrachloride extract-ZI 10.7±0.15mm--kanamycin ZI 34.5 ± 0.50 mm—chloroform/n-hexane/aqueous fraction of methanol extracts ZI=none,

Staphylococcus spp.   gram positive bacteria

S. aureus - S. aureus (MRSA) - (NCM 2010) - ATCC25903 - ATCC 25923 - S. aureus ATCC 53154 - MTCC 87 - NCIM 2079 - NCTC 10788 (MRSA) - NCTC 11561 (MRSA) - SS-1VC - SS-2VM - SS-3SW - SS-4OM - SS-5BC - SS-6AF - SS-7DS -- S. carmonum carmonum LMG 13567 -- S. epidermidis - S. epidermidis ATCC 12228 - S. epidermidis MTCC 2639

Can cause a wide variety of diseases in humans and animals through either toxin production or penetration [1]

Sida acuta

Staphylococcus aureus

5-invitro-methanol extract-susceptible, **6**-invitro-both chloroform and ethanolic extracts-did about as well as Gentamycin 10 mcg/Nystatin 100 units, **7**—invitro--aerial parts--chloroform extract--resistant penicillin-MIC=240µg/ml-MBC=240µg/ml--susceptible penicillin-MIC=80µg/ml-MBC=80µg/ml--ATCC 25923-MIC=400 µg/ml-MBC=>400 µg/ml—ATCC 53154-MIC=400 µg/ml-MBC=>400 µg/ml. **55**-in vitro-leaf-ethanolic extract-ZI=17 @500 µg/ disc, **77**-invitro-leaves-hot distilled water extract-20g of ground leaves added to 200mL of distilled water-boiled for 15 minutes-used immediately after-Zones of inhibition-just leaves 15mm-with silver nanoparticles 10mm-silver nitrate alone (no activity)-Gentamycin 35mm, **86**-implied somewhat effective, **89**-invitro-whole plant- aqueous acetone extract--Freshly prepared extracts ZI=0--Stored extracts for 21 days ZI=15mm—also ATCC 25923-no effect, **101**-invitro-MIC 5 mg/ml-ZI=21.3mm (25 mg/ml)--ZI Ciprofloxacin=26mm (5 µg/ml)--ZI Amoxycillin 15.3mm (25 µg/ml), **102**-invitro-leaf-100% ethanolic extract-1000 mg/ml-works against 4 bacteria and 3 fungi-has better ZI (zone of inhibition) (22) than gentamicin (18) against B. subtilis-has better ZI (44) than gentamicin (34) against Staph aureus-skin disease--cold water extract-ZI=28mm-gentamicin ZI=35mm, **106**-invitro-Methanol Zone of inhibition= 17mm - Ethanol Zone of inhibition= 13mm--Methanol&Water (1/1)/Ethanol &Water (1/1) / Ethyl acetate/Water extracts-no Zone of Inhibition, **113**-invitro-whole plant?- ethanolic and aqueous extracts-susceptible, **125**-invitro-both acqueous and methanolic effective, **168**-invitro-aerial parts-90 % ethanol extract-Zone of inhibition (25 mg/ml)-21.3 mm-MIC (5 mg/ml), **214**-

invitro-whole plant?-70% aqueous methanol extracts-at 20 +g/ml-zone of inhibition 11±0.21--MIC 0.220±0.01, **219**-invitro-leaf-hot water and ethanol extract-ethanol extracts produced the highest antimicrobial activity against S. aureus (86%), followed by hot water (61%), and cold water extracts (48%)-where lincomycin (control) only killed 80%-The result of killing rate studies showed that the test organisms were killed within 0-10 minutes for ethanol and hot water extracts and 5-60 minutes for cold water extracts-The activity was concentration dependent, **221**-invitro-buds>leaves>stems>roots-All the strains were inhibited by the aqueous extract=10% acetic acid in ethanol extract-all the tested alkaloid extracts of S. acuta have potent antibacterial activity, **226**-invitro-had activity against the Gram positive microorganism Staphylococcus aureus including methicillin-resistant Staphylococcus aureus (MRSA). **238**-invitro-ethanolic extract>Lyncomycia>hot water>cold water-also had photo enhanced activity, **271**-invitro-(bud/leaf/root/stem tested)-root methanol> ethyl acetate-ZI=20 (bound flavenoids)—ZI=13 (free flavenoids)--@1 mg/disc, **273**-invitro-leaf-45 clinical isolates isolated from nasal cavity of HIV/AIDS patients of S aureus-ethanol extract antimicrobial activity 86%-MIC .96-1.8 ug/mL—hot water extract-100degC-stand for 5 hours with occasional shaking--antimicrobial activity 61%-MIC 7.8-31.2 ug/mL—cold water extract-soaked for 48 hours-antimicrobial activity 48%-MIC 15-35 ug/mL, **523**-invitro-leaves-MIC=6 ug/well - zone of inhibition (40ug/well)- 90% ethanol 30mm - methanol 20mm - ethyl acetate 10mm - aqueous extract none, **523**-(clinical isolate)-invitro-leaves-clinical isolates-MIC=6 ug/well - zone of inhibition (40ug/well)- 90% ethanol 30mm - methanol 17mm - ethyl acetate none - aqueous extract none, **645**-invitro-leaf-cold water extract-ZI 8mm@50 ug-ZI 14mm@600 ug, **645**-invitro-leaf-acetone extract-ZI 11mm@50 ug-ZI 15mm@600 ug,

Staphylococcus aureus (MRSA)

226-invitro-had activity against the Gram positive microorganism Staphylococcus aureus including methicillin-resistant Staphylococcus aureus (MRSA), **273**-invitro-leaf-45 clinical isolates isolated from nasal cavity of HIV/AIDS patients of S aureus-ethanol extract antimicrobial activity 86%-MIC .96-1.8 ug/mL—hot water extract-100degC-stand for 5 hours with occasional shaking--antimicrobial activity 61%-MIC 7.8-31.2 ug/mL—cold water extract-soaked for 48 hours-antimicrobial activity 48%-MIC 15-35 ug/mL,

Sida cordifolia

Staphylococcus aureus

72-(ATCC 25923)-invitro-leaf essential oil (2%)-ZI=16mm (50 uL)- 80% inhib-itory activity—Chloramphenicol-ZI=16mm (30 ug/ml), **125**-review-leaf-methanol extract ZI=17 mm (2 mg/disc)—water extract ZI=13mm (2 mg/disc)—Ciprofloxlacin ZI=29 mm (5 ug/disc), **143**-invitro-chloroform and methanol extracts of leaves and roots exhibited significant activity against, **152**-invitro-seed oil-petroleum ether (40-600C) extract-ZI 10-12mm (300 µg)- resistant at 100 µg -- chloroform extract ZI 14-16mm (300 µg)-resistant at 100 µg--Norfloxacin ZI 18mm (50µg/ml), **173**-invitro-leaf and root-methanol extract-Zone of Inhibition (mm)-root=16--leaf=18--same effect as Streptomycin sulfate, **664**-invitro-whole plant-95% ethanolic extract-ZI 13±1mm, **667**-(MTCC 1303)-invitro-roots-ethyl acetate ZI=25mm @100µg/ml-ethanol extract ZI=0mm @25µg/ml,

Sida rhombifolia

Staphylococcus aureus

48-in vitro-stem-phenyl ethyl B-D-glucopyranoside via exotic extracts, **51**-(MTCC 87)-invitro-fruit-methanol (CH3OH) extract-MIC=300 µg/ml-Zone Inhibition- 21 mm(200 µg/ml)- Ciprofloxacin zone of inhibition=24 mm (200 µg/ml)-also included Petroleum ether (C2H5-O- C2H5), chloroform (CHCl3) extracts-less effective, **126**-invitro-ethanol/ethyl acetate/chloroform extracts-all had activity against-leaves—ethanolic extract- - 50ug=8mm--stem 50ug= 8mm—root 50ug=11mm, **150**-invitro-root-50 mg/ml-petroleum ether extract ZI=16 mm, chloroform extract ZI=18 mm and methanol extracts ZI=15 mm-Ciprofloxacin ZI=32 mm, **202**-invitro-whole plant?-some extract-marked antibacterial activity, **278**-(ATCC25903)-invitro-root-50 mg/ml-petroleum ether extract ZI=16.2 mm, chloroform extract ZI=18 ± 1 mm and methanol extracts ZI=15 ± 2 mm-Ciprofloxacin ZI=32 mm, **282**-(ATCC25903)-invitro-roots-petroleum ether, chloroform and methanol-100 mg/ml solution, **353**-(DSMZ346)-fruit-"n-hexacosa-11-enoic acid" -50 µg/ml-zone inhibition 14mm- about 80% of the effect of Gentamicine - "1, 3-dilinoleoyl-2-oleine" - zone of inhibition=8mm, **362**-review-whole plant?-methanolic plant extract-activity against, **436**-invitro-seed-ethanolic extract-exhibited potent inhibitory effects against Staphylococcus aureus with inhibitory zone something like 18-26 mm,

Staphylococcus epidermidis MTCC 2639

51-invitro-fruit-methanol (CH3OH) extract-MIC=300 µg/ml-Zone Inhibition 21mm(200µg/ml)- Ciprofloxacin zone of inhibition=22 mm (200 µg/ml)-also included Petroleum ether (C2H5-O- C2H5), chloroform (CHCl3) extracts-less effective,

Sida alba

Staphylococcus aureus

55-invitro-leaf-ethanolic extract-500 µg/ disc-zone of inhibition 17 mm-Ciprofloxacin-5 µg / disc- zone of inhibition 37 mm, **99**-(NCM 2079)-invitro-whole plant-hot 60-80% ethanolic extract- showed antimicrobial activity-Zone of inhibition 19mm at 500 µg/disc , **99**-(NCM 2010)-invitro-whole plant-ethanolic extract-bacteriostatic, **667**-(MTCC 1303)-invitro-roots-ethyl acetate ZI=23mm @100µg/ml-ethanol extract ZI=0mm @25µg/ml,

Sida retusa

Staphylococcus aureus **436**-invitro-seed-ethanolic extract-exhibited potent inhibitory effects with inhibitory zones something like 18-26 mm.

Sida indica

Staphylococcus aureus

450--(ATCC 29737)--invitro--fruit, root, leaf--dichloro-methane/methanol extract (1:1,v/v)--no effect--Staphylococcus aureus,   **452**-brine shrimp-carbon tetrachloride zone of inhibition 6.2mm -Neither chloroform extract, n-hexane extract, nor aqueous soluble partitionate of methanolic extract had an effect,   **453**-invitro-whole plant-100mg/kg bw-zone of inhibition (mm)-Acqueous extract 15.4 mm-ethanolic extract 19.2 mm, Hexane extract 13.8 mm, chloroform extract 12.8 mm, streptomycin (1.mg/ml) 22.6mm,   **633**-invitro-methanolic extract-whole plant?-ZI 5mm,   **639**-Sida indica-stem-methanol extract-ZI (100 µg /ml) 6 mm,   **675**-Sida indica-invitro-leaves-80% methanol extract using distilled water ZI 23mm-distilled cold water extract no ZI,   **689**-invitro-root, bark and fresh leaves-methanol extract-root ZI= 15@90µg/ml -leaf ZI=18@90µg/ml,   **713**-invitro-leaves-methanol extract>dissolved in 10% aqueous methanol>n-hexane extract>carbon tetrachloride extract ZI 6.2 ± 0.25 mm--kanamycin ZI 29.6 ± 0.49 mm—chloroform/n-hexane/aqueous fraction of methanol extracts ZI=none, **718**-invitro-leaf-chloroform extract ZI 17mm—ethanol extract ZI 25mm--water extract ZI 0mm--Chloramphenicol (Control) ZI 25mm,

Staphylococcus epidermidis

446-(ATCC 12228)-invitro-acqueous and methanol extracts-nothing detected,   **450**-(ATCC 12228)-invitro-fruit, root, leaf--dichloromethane: methanol (1:1, v/v) extract-no effect,   **638**-invitro-methanol extract-no effect,

Cryptolepine   (found in S. acuta, cordifolia, rhombifolia, alba, at least)

Staphylococcus aureus

108-invitro-showed activity against,   **249**-invitro-at 10, 20 or 40 µg ml)1 produced killing effects on S. aureus NCTC 11561 (>3 log reductions in viable counts) within 6 h and these levels of kill were maintained at 24 h. For S. aureus NCTC 10788, 20 µg ml)1 cryptolepine produced a 2 log reduction in viable count within 5 h. However, there was an apparent re-growth at 24 h where 0Æ5 log recovery was noted. Inhibitory effects recorded for 5 or 10 µg ml)1 within the first 6 h were small--Scanning electron micrograph of S. aureus NCTC 10788 after exposure to 20 µg ml)1 of cryptolepine for 24 h. Cells 'bursting' and starting to lose contents.-The lytic effect appears more extensive in strain NCTC 11561-At 24 h, extensive lysis was taking place with the cells leaching their contents and/or almost all the cells bore very rough and distorted outer surfaces. Cells thus affected represented approx. 75% of the treated population,   **383**-invitro- Cryptolepine possesses bacteriostatic and bactericidal actions-the bactericidal action predominates in subsequent stages-action was linear in the entire concentration range and... resulted in a kill or lysis of the cells,   **387**-(NCTC11561 MRSA)-invitro-10, 20 or 40 µg ml)1 produced killing effects on S. aureus NCTC 11561 (>3 log reductions in viable counts) within 6 h and these levels of kill were maintained at 24 h-Lysis to staphylococcal cells was observed following exposure to cryptolepine and this coincided with sharp falls in viable counts of the bacteria. There was the formation of deformed cells as depicted in the SEM photomicrographs of S. aureus cells after 3, 6 or 24 h exposure to inhibitory concentrations of cryptolepine. **390**-invitro-acid alcoholic extract-MIC <7.8 pg/mi-MBC 125 pg/ml.

Streptococcus spp.   **gram positive bacteria**

S. faecalis – S. mutans – S. mutans (ATCC 700610-resistant strain) – S. mutans (w7,w11,w13) – S. pneumoniae – S. pyogenes – S. salivarius – S. sanguis (ATCC 10556) – S. sanguis w14,w18,w20) – S. viridans (group name)

Certain species cause pink eye, meningitis, bacterial pneumonia, endocarditis, erysipelas, and necrotizing fasciitis (the 'flesh-eating' bacterial infections) [1]

Sida acuta

Streptococcus faecalis

77-invitro-leaves-boiled distilled water extract-ZI=nil--imbrued with silver nanoparticles-ZI 12mm--Gentamycin ZI 40mm,   **86**-invitro- ethanolic and aqueous extracts-quite susceptible,   **101**-invitro-MIC 10 mm/ml-ZI=14mm (25 mg/ml)--ZI Ciprofloxacin=19mm (5 µg/ml)--ZI Amoxycillin 16mm (25 µg/ml),   **106**-invitro-Methanol Zone of inhibition=8.5 mm-Ethyl acetate Zone of inhibition=12 mm--Methanol&Water (1/1)/Ethanol/Ethanol&Water(1/1)/Water extracts-no Zone of Inhibition, **113**-invitro-whole plant?- ethanolic and aqueous extracts-quite susceptible, **168**-invitro-aerial parts-90 % ethanol extract-Zone of inhibition (25 mg/ml)-14 mm-MIC (10 mg/ml).

Streptococcus jecalis   5-invitro-methanol extract-**no effect**,

Streptococcus mutans

234-(w7,w11,w13)-invitro-ethanolic extract-leaves-Ghana strains-inhibition zone was greater than penicillin and gentamicin (positive control)-aqueous and ethanolic extract effective from 50mg/ml,

Streptococcus pneumoniae   **224**-invitro-no extraction method worked,

Streptococcus pyogenes

224-invitro-leaf and bud-methanol extract ZI=9mm (1000mg)-hexane extract ZI=16mm (900mg)-chloroform extract ZI=12mm (1000mg)-aqueous extract ZI=nil,   **645**-invitro-leaf-cold water extract-ZI 9mm@50 ug-ZI 14mm@600 ug,   **645**-invitro-leaf-acetone extract-ZI 11mm@50 ug-ZI 16mm@600 ug,

Streptococcus sanguis

234-(ATCC 10556, w14,w18,w20 clinical strains)-invitro-leaf- aqueous and ethanolic extracts-effective from 50mg/ml -aqueous extract showed a maximum zone of inhibition against the standard strain- greater than the positive controls Penicillin and Gentamicin,

Tr   361-roots-pneumonia,   507-Sida acuta-roots-Plant powder administered orally for pneumonia,

Sida rhombifolia

202- Streptococcus mutans-invitro-extract-marked antibacterial activity,

Tr   358-Senegal, the Central African Republic and Madagascar-leaves and roots.

Sida urens

Streptococcus mutans

499- invitro-aqueous acetone extract (80%, v/v)-Inhibition Zone=18.67-MIC=125 ug/ml-MBC=500 ug/ml-net effect bacteriostatic--Gentamicin-ZI none-MIC no effect,

Streptococcus salivarius

499- invitro-aqueous acetone extract (80%, v/v)-Inhibition Zone=20.33-MIC=65 ug/ml-MBC=125 ug/ml-net effect bacteriocidal--Gentamicin-ZI 19.00 ± 0.58mm-MIC 125(µg/ml).

Streptococcus viridans

499- invitro-aqueous acetone extract (80%, v/v)-Inhibition Zone=19-MIC=125 ug/ml-MBC=250 ug/ml-net effect bacteriocidal--Gentamicin-ZI no effect-MIC none(µg/ml),

Sida indica

638-Streptococcus pyogenes -invitro-methanol extract-weak.

Cryptolepine   (found in S. acuta, cordifolia, rhombifolia, alba, at least)
Streptococcus pyogenes   390-invitro-acid alcoholic extract-MIC <7.8/ml /MBC <7.8 pg/ml.

Vibrio spp.   **gram negative bacteria**
V. cholerae – V. mimicus – V. parahemolyticus

Disease-causing strains are associated with gastroenteritis, but can also infect open wounds and cause septicemia, or cholera. [1]

Sida cordifolia

Vibrio cholerae   **664**-invitro-whole plant-95% ethanolic extract-ZI 30±1mm,

Sida indica

Vibrio mimicus

452-brine shrimp-carbon tetrachloride zone of inhibition 8.4mm-Neither chloroform, n-hexane extract nor aqueous soluble partitionate of methanolic extract had an effect,   **713**-invitro-leaves-methanol extract>dissolved in 10% aqueous methanol>n-hexane extract>carbon tetrachloride extract   ZI 8.4 ± 0.46 mm--kanamycin ZI 30.7 ± 0.60 mm—chloroform/n-hexane/aqueous fraction of methanol extracts ZI=none.

Vibrio parahemolyticus

452-brine shrimp-carbon tetrachloride zone of inhibition 7.6mm-Neither chloroform, n-hexane extract nor aqueous soluble partitionate of methanolic extract had an effect, **713**-invitro-leaves-methanol extract>dissolved in 10% aqueous methanol>n-hexane extract>carbon tetrachloride extract ZI 7.6 ± 0.15 mm--kanamycin ZI 32.3 ± 0.30 mm—chloroform/n-hexane/aqueous fraction of methanol extracts ZI=none.

Cryptolepine   (found in S. acuta, cordifolia, rhombifolia, alba, at least)
Vibrio cholerae   **392**-invitro-some activity against 86 Vibrio cholerae strains-activities are lower than that of tetracycline.

Xanthonomonas axonopodies pv. Malvacearum

Xanthomonas species can cause bacterial spots and blights of leaves, stems, and fruits on a wide variety of plant species. Pathogenic species show high degrees of specificity [1]   **gram negative bacteria**

Sida cordifolia   **173**-invitro-leaf and root-methanol extract-Zone of Inhibition (mm)-root=13--leaf=16--same effect as Streptomycin sulfate,

Sida indica   **689**-invitro-root, bark and fresh leaves-methanol extract-root ZI= 13@90µg/ml-leaf ZI=15@90µg/ml.

Cancer, In General

The rate of increase of cancer incidence and the lack of anticancer drugs has forced scientists to pharmacological and chemical investigations in the area of medicinal plants to search for anticancer agents... The strong association between the increasing of the consumption of these natural products and human diseases prevention has been explained by the content of the phytonutrients... The results of the screening of plant extracts for antiproliferative activity have shown that higher plants are a potential source of antioncogenic agents which can compete favorably with chemotherapy and hormonal treatments. In vitro studies have provided evidence that chemotherapeutic agents such as extracts may induce apoptotic tumor cell death in vivo. [141]   Screenings of medicinal plants used as anticancer drugs has provided modern medicine with effective cytotoxic pharmaceuticals. More than 60% of the approved anticancer drugs in United States of America (from 1983 to 1994) were from natural origin. In this last decade, investigations on natural compounds have been particularly successful in the field of anticancer drug research. [64-2010]

Adenocarcinoma is a type of cancer that forms in mucus-secreting glands throughout the body. It can occur in many different places in the body, and is most prevalent in the following cancer types: Lung cancer: Non-small cell lung cancer accounts for 80 percent of lung cancers, and adenocarcinoma is the most common type. Prostate cancer: Cancer that forms in the prostate gland is typically an adenocarcinoma, which makes up 99 percent of all prostate cancers. Pancreatic cancer: Exocrine pancreatic cancer tumors are called adenocar-cinomas. They form in the pancreas ducts. Esophageal cancer: Cancer that forms in the glandular cells of the esophagus is known as adenocarcinoma. This is the most common type of esophageal cancer. Colorectal cancer: Cancer that develops in the intestinal gland cells that line the inside of the colon and/or rectum is an adenocarcinoma. It makes up 95 percent of colon and rectal cancers. [398]

Cancer Treatment

Plants that are used as traditional medicine represent a relevant pool for selecting plant candidates that may have anticancer properties... Sida acuta-invitro-leaves, seeds, stems and bark-methanol extract- promising cytotoxic activity against 7 of 8 human carcinoma cell lines. [95]

Sida acuta

95-invitro-leaves, seeds, stems and bark-methanol extract- promising cytotoxic activity against 7 of 8 human carcinoma cell lines,   460-rats-whole plant-70% ethanol extract-400mg/kg bw-induced hepatocellular cancers-significantly quenched the free radical damage-The treatment with the ethanolic extract of Sida acuta at both dose levels 200mg/kg and 400mg/kg showed a prominent anticancer activity by restoring the altered parameters to near normal levels due to the presence of alkaloids, flavonoids, tannins and phenolic compounds which contributes to antioxidant activity inhibiting the free radical mechanism.

Tr 64-Camaroon,   580-India-whole plant-ethanol extract-anticancer,

Sida cordifolia   Tr 64-Camaroon,   358-Benin-whole plant-used
as a cure for cancer and leukemia,

Sida rhombifolia   Tr 13-Zaire-leaves, 64-Camaroon,   522-
Madagascar-leaf- The leaves are pounded and applied to tumors,   522-
Peru-leaf-tumors,

Sida retusa

464- mice/rats-seed-80% methanol extract-treatment with seed extract significantly inhibited the increase in DEN/CCl4 induced activities of pre-cancerous marker enzymes,

Adenocarcinoma   Cancer of mucus-secreting glands

Adenocarcinoma is a type of cancer that forms in mucus-secreting glands throughout the body. It can occur in many different places in the body, and is most prevalent in the following cancer types: Lung cancer: Non-small cell lung cancer accounts for 80 percent of lung cancers, and adenocarcinoma is the most common type. Prostate cancer: Cancer that forms in the prostate gland is typically an adenocarcinoma, which makes up 99 percent of all prostate cancers. Pancreatic cancer: Exocrine pancreatic cancer tumors are called adenocarcinomas. They form in the pancreas ducts. Esophageal cancer: Cancer that forms in the glandular cells of the esophagus is known as adenocarcinoma. This is the most common type of esophageal cancer. Colorectal cancer: Cancer that develops in the intestinal gland cells that line the inside of the colon and/or rectum is an adenocarcinoma. It makes up 95 percent of colon and rectal cancers. **[398]**

Sida Veronicaefolia

348-mice-leaves-acetone and ethanol extracts-doses of 500 mg/kg body weight per day for 14 days after 24 h of tumor inoculation-significantly decreased the tumor volume, tumor weight, tumor cell count, body weight, and brought back the haematological parameters to more or less normal levels- Ehrlich Ascites Carcinoma.

Cryptolepine (found in S. acuta, cordifolia, rhombifolia, alba, at least)
Adenocarcinoma 17-invitro- Cryptolepine, isolated from Sida acuta, sensitizes human gastric adenocarcinoma cells to TRAIL-induced apoptosis, **62**-invitro-whole plant- showed strong activity in overcoming TRAIL-resistance in human gastric adenocarcinoma (AGS) cells at 1.25, 2.5 and 5 μm. Combined treatment of 1 and TRAIL sensitized AGS cells to TRAIL-induced apoptosis at the aforementioned concentrations, **397**-invitro-Cryptolepine induced G1 phase block at 1.25-2.5 μM, S phase and G2/M phase block at 2.5-5 μM, and cell death at 10 μM. The dead cells displayed condensed and fragmented nuclei, features of apoptosis.

Blood cancer

Blood cancers affect the production and function of your blood cells. Most of these cancers start in your bone marrow where blood is produced **[http://www.hematology.org/Patients/Cancers/]**

Cryptolepine (found in S. acuta, cordifolia, rhombifolia, alba, at least)
399-invitro-Among patient solid tumour samples, those from breast cancer were the most sensitive and essentially as sensitive as haematological malignancies. Cryptolepine activity was essentially unaffected by established mechanisms of drug resistance. In conclusion, cryptolepine shows interesting in vitro cytotoxic properties and its further evaluation as an anti-cancer drug seems warranted.

....

S. spinosa leaves are bruised in water and the filtrate is administered. Root is used as a tonic and diaphoretic: given in mild cases of debility and fever. **[99]**

Breast cancer

Cancer that develops from breast tissue [1]   The demonstration of a broad-spectrum activity {by cryptolepine} on a variety of cancer cell lines, apoptotic cell death, and apparently low genotoxicity suggest that these agents may have potential as candidates for cancer chemotherapy. very cytotoxic and may be weak mammalian mutagens and/or clastogens. The poor genotoxicity of CSE and CLP coupled with their potent cytotoxic action support their anticancer potential. [297]

Sida acuta

human breast adenocarcinoma   95- stems and leaves-methanol extract-human breast adenocarcinoma BT-20 (ATCC No. HTB-19)-percentage of inhibition-20 µg/ml 25 ± 5.03%-200 µg/ml 97 ± 0.57%--IC50 cytoxicity (41.1 ± 1.05µg/mL),   **297**-invitro-MCF7 human breast adenocarcinoma cell line-IC50 genotoxicity 1 +-.04(uM),

Cryptolepine   (found in S. acuta, cordifolia, rhombifolia, alba, at least)
399-invitro-Among patient solid tumour samples, those from breast cancer were the most sensitive and essentially as sensitive as haematological malignancies. Cryptolepine activity was essentially unaffected by established mechanisms of drug resistance. In conclusion, cryptolepine shows interesting in vitro cytotoxic properties and its further evaluation as an anti-cancer drug seems warranted.

Colon cancer   Cancer of the colon or rectum

Sida indica

705-leaf-aqueous extract-showed a dose dependant anti-proliferative effect against COLO 205 (human colon cancer) and MDCK (normal) cells with an IC50 of 3 and 4µg/mL and 100 and 75µg/mL, respectively after 24 and 48h-The mode of action through the induction apoptosis by AIAgNPs in COLO 205 cells is exciting with promising application of nano-materials in biomedical research,   **707**-leaf-aqueous extract-showed a dose dependant anti-proliferative effect against COLO 205 (human colon cancer) and MDCK (normal) cells with an IC50 of 3 and 4µg/mL and 100 and 75µg/mL, respectively after 24 and 48h- The mode of action through the induction apoptosis by AIAgNPs in COLO 205 cells is exciting with promising application of nano-materials in biomedical research,

Cryptolepine   (found in S. acuta, cordifolia, rhombifolia, alba, at least)
HCT116 human colon adenocarcinoma cell line   **297**-invitro-HCT116 human colon adenocarcinoma cell line-IC50 genotoxicity (.7+-.02uM),

78

Hepatoma
A cancer of the cells of the liver

Cryptolepine   (found in S. acuta, cordifolia, rhombifolia, alba, at least)
394-invitro- HepG2, a human hepatoma cell line showed morphology that was more like necrosis after treatment with Cryptolepine,

Cancer, Leukemia
Bone/Blood cancer
A group of cancers that usually begin in the bone marrow [1]

Sida acuta
acute T cell leukemia Jurkat (ATCC No. TIB-152)   **95**-stems and leaves-methanol extract-acute T cell leukemia Jurkat (ATCC No. TIB-152)-IC50 cytoxicity (42.3 ± 0.79µg/mL),

Cancer, Liver
Tr   no reported use
Cancer which has spread from elsewhere to the liver, known as liver metastasis, is more common than that which starts in the liver. [1]   Sida rhombifolia ssp. retusa is a well established drug in the Ayurveda system of medicine used for antirheumatism and antiasthmatism... The chemopreventive and hepatoprotect-ive potentials of seed extract are due to free radical scavenging activity and restoration of dhalwal cellular structural integrity. **[464]**

Sida acuta
79- Scopoletin was found to exert a dual action on tumoral lymphocytes exhibiting both a cytostatic and a cytotoxic effect. These results indicate that scopoletin could be a potential antitumoral compound to be used for cancer treatment... Scopoletin was also isolated from Sida acuta and constitutes an active compound that inhibits proliferation of Hepa 1c1c7 mouse hepatoma cells-These effects varied with the concentrations analysed,   **92**-invitro-HepG-2 cells,**141**-invitro-methanolic extract-viability of HepG-2 liver cancer cells about 30% after 72 hours-(461.53±0.23 gmL–1) cytotoxic concentration (CC50),   **232**-invitro-overcomes TRAIL resistance-It sensitized AGS cells to TRAIL induced apoptosis by the activation of caspase-3/7,   **460**-rats-whole plant-70% ethanol extract-200&400mg/kg bw-28 days-at both dose levels showed a prominent anticancer activity by restoring the altered parameters to near normal levels-400mg/kg bw-significantly quenched the free radical damage-showed a significant increase in activities of antioxidant enzymes that reduces the oxidative stress induced damage exhibiting a potent antioxidant and anticancer activity,

Sida cordifolia   **141**-whole plant?-methanol extract-was the less active among the five extracts tested,

Sida rhombifolia

92-invitro—methanol extract-HepG-2 cells—IC50-475 gmL–1, **141**-whole plant?-methanol extract-cytotoxic concentration (CC50) 475.33±0.65_gmL–1), **436**-invitro-seed-ethanolic extract-marked cytotoxic activity at GI50 ≤ 20 µg/ml- Carcinoma (Hep G2), **464**-the chemopreventive and hepatoprotective potentials of seed extract are due to free radical scavenging activity and restoration of dhalwal cellular structural integrity,

Sida retusa
436-invitro-seed-methanol extract-marked cytotoxic activity against HOP 62, Hep G2 cells at GI50 ≤ 20 µg/ml, **464**-mice/rats,invitro-80% methanol extract-It exhibited marked reduction in incidence of preneoplastic lesions

Cryptolepine (found in S. acuta, cordifolia, rhombifolia, alba, at least)
394-invitro-HepG2, a human hepatoma cell line showed morphology that was more like necrosis after treatment with CLP-the CLP-mediated demise of HepG2 cells is not apoptotic.

Lung Cancer   Non-Small-Cell Lung Cancer

Human Non-Small-Cell Lung Cancer accounts for about 85% of all lung cancers. NSCLCs are relatively insensitive to chemotherapy, compared to small cell carcinoma. When possible, they are primarily treated by surgical resection with curative intent. [1]

Sida rhombifolia
Human Non-Small-Cell Lung Cancer (HOP 62) **436**-invitro-seed-ethanolic extract-marked cytotoxic activity at GI50 ≤ 20 µg/ml,

Sida retusa
Human Non-Small-Cell Lung Cancer (HOP 62) **436**-Sida retusa-invitro-seed-methanol extract-marked cytotoxic activity against HOP 62, Hep G2 cells at GI50 ≤ 20 µg/ml.

Lung fibroblast cells   DNA damage

V-79 A Chinese hamster fibroblast cell line commonly used in genetic toxicity studies has been widely used in studies of DNA damage and DNA repair. [1] **MCL-5** Commonly utilized in vaccine development, as a transfection host in virology research, and for in vitro cytotoxicity testing [https://micro.magnet.fsu.edu/primer/techniques/fluorescence/gallery/cells/mrc5/mrc5cells.html]

Cryptolepine (found in S. acuta, cordifolia, rhombifolia, alba, at least)
V79 cells **297**-invitro-V79 MZ Chinese hamster lung fibroblast cell line-IC50 genotoxicity (2.1 +-.11uM), **394**-invitro-apoptosis as the mode of cell

death in CLP-treated MCL-5 cells, but the CLP-mediated demise of HepG2 cells is not apoptotic-morphology consistent with apoptosis after treatment with CLP, **396**-invitro-DNA damage-treatment of mammalian cells with cryptolepine can lead to DNA damage- cryptolepine did not appear to be mutagenic in the dosage range used (up to 2.5 μM, equivalent to 1.1 μg/ml)- after 24 h treatment of V79 cells cryptolepine induced a dose-dependent increase in micronuclei.

Osteosarcoma (Bone cancer)

An osteosarcoma is a cancerous tumor in a bone. [1]

Cryptolepine (found in S. acuta, cordifolia, rhombifolia, alba, at least)
35-invitro—cryptolepine-p53-mutated human osteosarcoma MG63 cells- induces p21WAF1/CIP1 and cell cycle arrest- in a dose-dependent manner, **164**-invitro-human osteosarcoma MG63 cells- induces the expression of p21WAF1/CIP1 with growth arrest-completely inhibited the growth and caused G2/M-phase arrest, **400**-invitro-cryptolepine inhibits the growth of human osteosarcoma MG63 cells. A dose-dependent inhibition of the cell growth was observed at concentrations of ≥0.5 μM. Seventy-two hours after the addition of CLP, the growth of cells was inhibited to 77.6, 31.6, 10.3, 4.7, and 2.1% of the control level by 0.5, 1, 2, 3 and 4 μM CLP, respectively - In this study, we demonstrated for the first time that CLP induces cell cycle arrest through p21WAF1/CIP1 expression, indicating that CLP might be an attractive compound for molecular-targeting chemotherapy or chemoprevention. These results raise a possibility that treatment with CLP is promising for the chemotherapy of osteosarcoma.

Ovarian cancer

Cryptolepine (found in S. acuta, cordifolia, rhombifolia, alba, at least)
297-invitro-SKOV3 human ovary adenocarcinoma cell line-IC50 genotoxicity (.9 +-.04uM).

Preneoplastic lesions
Before the formation of a tumor

The development of primary tumors is often preceded, both in humans and experimental animals (mainly rodents), by the appearance of lesions referred to as preneoplastic. These consist of genetically and phenotypically altered cells exhibiting a higher risk of malignant evolution than normal cells. **[https://link.springer.com/referenceworkentry/10.1007%2F978-3-642-16483-5_4724#page-1]**

Sida acuta

7,12-dimethylbenz[a]anthracene-induced preneoplastic lesions **253**-invitro-whole plant-EtOAc-soluble extract-cryptolepine-10 microg/mL-

83.3% inhibition of 7,12-dimethylbenz[a]anthracene-induced preneoplastic lesions,

Cancer, Other Cancer

The evaluation of anticancer and anti-HIV activities of extracts from nine medicinal plants collected in Zaire was carried out against the National Cancer Institute (NCI) panel of human tumor cell lines provided for the preliminary screening of natural products. The leaves of Sida rhombifolia, exhibited cytotoxic activity against the 60 human cell lines tested. [282] Cryptolepine-has been found to bind to DNA in a formerly unknown intercalation mode- a basis for the design of new anticancer drugs. [244] Cryptolepine inhibits the growth of human osteosarcoma MG63 cells. A dose-dependent inhibition of the cell growth was observed at concentrations of ≥0.5 µM. [400]

Sida acuta

17-invitro- Cryptolepine, isolated from Sida acuta, sensitizes human gastric adenocarcinoma cells to TRAIL-induced apoptosis,   62-invitro-whole plant- showed strong activity in overcoming TRAIL-resistance in human gastric adenocarcinoma (AGS) cells at 1.25, 2.5 and 5 µm. Combined treatment of 1 and TRAIL sensitized AGS cells to TRAIL-induced apoptosis at the aforementioned concentrations,   64-review-widely used in cancer treatment was recently screened for cytoxicity against Hep G2 hepatocarcinoma cells-showed moderate anti-proliferative effects,   95-breast cancer-stems and leaves-methanol extract-human breast adenocarcinoma BT-20--percentage of inhibition-20 µg/ml 27 ± 2.20%--200 µg/ml 97 ± 1.80%,

Tr   64-Camaroon,   219-Nigeria-leaf usually used-breast cancer following inflammation,   220-Nigeria-breast cancer,   221-India-leaf-breast cancer, 224-Nigeria-breast cancer,   273-Nigeria-breast cancer following inflammation,   580-India-whole plant-ethanol extract-anticancer,

Sida cordifolia

64-review-widely used in cancer treatment was recently screened for cytoxicity against Hep G2 hepatocarcinoma cells-showed moderate anti-proliferative effects.   Tr   64-Camaroon,   358-Benin-whole plant-used as a cure for cancer and leukemia,

Sida rhombifolia

13-rhombifolia-exhibited cytotoxic activity against the National Cancer Institute (NCI) panel of 60 human tumor cell lines,   64-review-widely used in cancer treatment was recently screened for cytoxicity against Hep G2 hepatocarcinoma cells-showed moderate anti-proliferative effects,

Tr   13-Zaire-leaves,   64-Camaroon,   522-Madagascar-leaf-pounded and applied to tumors,   522-Peru-leaf-tumors,

82

Sida cordata
282-leaves- brine shrimp-methanol extract-lethality concentration LC50 for crude extract was 263.02 µg/ml,

Sida indica
13-invitro-leaves-methanolic extract-cellular sensitivity against-3 NCI cell lines, 674- invitro-leaf-boiling distilled water extract- polyphenol stabilized gold nanoparticles had potential cytotoxic effects in HT-29 human colon cancer cell line, 683-invitro-leaves-cold distilled water extract- The Zn nanoparticles synthesized using (Sida indica), showed positive results for cytotoxic activity with an IC50 value of 45.82 µg/ml. These positive results confirmed the cytotoxic potential of the Zn nanoparticles against cervical cancer. Thus Zn nanoparticles can be used as a potent drug in alternative therapy for treating the cervical cancer patients in the near future,

Cryptolepine
(S. acuta, cordifolia, rhombifolia, alba, and ?)
17-invitro- Cryptolepine, isolated from Sida acuta, sensitizes human gastric adenocarcinoma cells to TRAIL-induced apoptosis, 35-invitro—cryptolepine-p53-mutated human osteosarcoma MG63 cells-induces p21WAF1/CIP1 and cell cycle arrest- in a dose-dependent manner, 62-invitro-whole plant- showed strong activity in overcoming TRAIL-resistance in human gastric adenocar-cinoma (AGS) cells at 1.25, 2.5 and 5 µm. Combined treatment of 1 and TRAIL sensitized AGS cells to TRAIL-induced apoptosis at the aforementioned concentrations, 164-invitro-human osteosarcoma MG63 cells- induces the expression of p21WAF1/CIP1 with growth arrest-completely inhibited the growth and caused G2/M-phase arrest, might be a suitable chemotherapeutic agent for treatment of osteosarcoma, 244-has been found to bind to DNA in a formerly unknown intercalation mode- a basis for the design of new anticancer drugs, 380-invitro- Cryptolepine easily crosses the cell membranes and accumulates selectively into the nuclei rather than in the cytoplasm of B16 melanoma cells, 396-invitro-DNA damage-treatment of mammalian cells with cryptolepine can lead to DNA damage- cryptolepine did not appear to be mutagenic in the dosage range used (up to 2.5 µM, equivalent to 1.1 µg/ml)-after 24 h treatment of V79 cells cryptolepine induced a dose-dependent increase in micronuclei, 397-invitro-This study using human lung adenocarcinoma A549 cells as a model demonstrated that cryptolepine selects different molecular pathways to cell cycle checkpoint activation in a dose specific manner and evokes a wortmannin sensitive anti-apoptosis response, 400-invitro-CLP induces the expression of p21WAF1/CIP1 with growth arrest in p53-mutated human osteosarcoma MG63 cells, 592-crypotlepine-invitro-p53-mutated human osteosarcoma MG63 cells- These findings suggest that CLP arrests the growth of MG63 cells- might be a suitable chemotherapeutic agent for treatment of osteosarcoma,

Cancer, Cytoxic
The results of the screening of plant extracts for antiproliferative activity have shown that higher plants are a potential source of antioncogenic agents which

can compete favorably with chemotherapy and hormonal treatments. In vitro studies have provided evidence that chemotherapeutic agents such as extracts may induce apoptotic tumor cell death in vivo. **[92]** Our observations revealed that the crude extract of Sida cordata show significant antioxidant and cytotoxic properties... it can be inferred that Sida cordata may be a good source for the further investigation to discover a new drug for cancer treatment. **[282]**

Sida acuta

5-sida acuta-invitro-methanol extract-1,000 pg/ml dried plant material and 1% methanol-cytoxicity 500 (WgIml)- Cellular changes 250 (pg/ml)- cells become rounded but remain attached; g, granules evident in cytoplasm, **64**-review-widely used in cancer treatment was recently screened for cytoxicity against Hep G2 hepatocarcinoma cells-showed moderate anti-proliferative effects, **79**-invitro-isolated from Sida acuta-Scopoletin was found to exert a dual action on tumoral lymphocytes exhibiting both a cytostatic and a cytotoxic effect- associated to the induction of apoptosis-These results indicate that scopoletin could be a potential antitumoral compound to be used for cancer treatment... Scopoletin constitutes an active compound that inhibits proliferation of Hepa 1c1c7 mouse hepatoma cells-These effects varied with the concentrations analyzed, **92**-invitro-whole plant?-methanol extract-cytotoxic concentration (CC50) value=(461.53±0.23_ gmL−1)- it seems that the extracts of S. acuta utilize their antioxidant properties by increasing SOD activity to nearly 1.8−2.2 its normal level in order to protect cells against negative effects of stress produced by the proliferation of HepG-2 cells, **93**-invitro-leaves-70% methanol extract(v/v)-acidified to pH 2- demonstrated a cytotoxic activity on murine and human cancer cell lines- showed a cytotoxic activity of metabolites from plant extract in cancer cells, which after treatment reduced significantly cellular growth and survival-CHP100 (human neuroblastoma), **95**-Sida acuta-invitro-leaves, seeds, stems and bark-methanol extract-promising cytotoxic activity against 7 of 8 human carcinoma cell lines, **141**-an effective anti-cancer agent, whereas S. cordifolia and S. rhombifolia were marginal in this. Acuta has antiproliferative activity against HepG-2 liver cancer cells and reduced their viability to about 30% after 72 hours, **174**-rats-whole plant-ethanol extract-300 mg/kg wt-cytoprotective (protects cell against harmful agents), **232**-invitro-showed strong activity to overcome TRAIL resistance-It sensitized AGS cells to TRAIL induced apoptosis by the activation of caspase-3/7, **253**-invitro-human neuroblastoma-cytoprotective (protects cell against harmful agents), **460**-rats-whole plant-70% ethanol extract-200 and 400mg/kg bw-NDEA and CCl4 induced hepatocellular cancers-at both dose levels showed a prominent anticancer activity by restoring the altered parameters to near normal levels, **647**-invitro/invivo-aerial parts-hot petroleum ether, toluene, chloroform, acetone, ethyl acetate and hydroalcoholic extracts-the results of the DPPH scavenging assay demonstrated a moderate scavenging activity for the toluene, chloroform and ethyl acetate extracts. Furthermore, the cytotoxicity test (CTC50) on DLA and EAC cells helped in identifying the chloroform and toluene extracts to be highly potent and therefore, the eligible candidates for in vivo evaluation...By employing the DLA model of cancer development, we were able to establish the in vivo efficacy of the chloroform and toluene extracts. A significant increase in life span was observed in the mice treated with the higher dose of both extracts with negligible changes in the body weights,   **649**- brine shrimp-dried flowers-95% methanol extract-The fraction showed potential cytotoxic activity with LC50 value of 67.5μg/ml. Vincristin sulphate served as the positive control for this brine shrimp lethality assay and its LC50 value was 14.55μg/ml...the extremely significant effect of Sida acuta demonstrates it to be the best cytotoxic component for further processing-80μg/ml = 70% mortality.

Tr   82-India-cytoprotective (protects cell against harmful agents),   95-Nigeria,   221-India,

Sida cordifolia

64-review-widely used in cancer treatment was recently screened for cytoxicity against Hep G2 hepatocarcinoma cells-showed moderate anti-proliferative effects,   **92**-invitro-HepG-2 cells-weaker than the other two, **176**-invitro-whole plant?- The results of cytotoxic activity on hela cells treated with Sida cordifolia extracts showed cells with uncontrolled growth has been arrested and there is decline level of cancerous cells,   **590**-Medicinally important S. cordifolia leaf extract was successfully used to synthesize stable AgNPs in the presence of sunlight... The effect of nanoparticles on cancer cell growth inhibition allows us to predict their anti-cancer potential. The anticancer effect of AgNPs of the present study might be due to the presence of bioactive compounds that are incorporated from the aqueous leaf extract of S. cordifolia with AgNPs... the nanoparticles synthesized from S. cordifolia, also recorded impressive anticancer effect against two different types of cancer cells... the biofunctionalized AgNPs displayed remarkable antioxidant and anticancer activities.   **591**-invitro-whole plant-70% ethanol extract-it was concluded that the herbal extract of EESC at both dose levels (250 & 500mg/kg body weight) has a prominent role in showing anticancer activity and in a dose dependent manner,   **662**-invitro-leaves-cold distilled water extract- silver nanoparticles (AgNPs) in presence of sunlight recorded impressive anticancer effect against two different types of cancer cells-In vitro cytotoxic activity of AgNPs was evaluated at different concentrations and it showed a dose dependent activity against EAC and HT-29 cell lines with IC50 value of 204.7and129.3 mg/ml, respectively,

Tr   152-India-anticancer,   358-Benin-whole plant-used as a cure for cancer and leukemia,

Sida rhombifolia

13-invitro-leaves exhibited cytotoxic activity against the   National Cancer Institute (NCI) panel of 60 human tumor cell lines,   **54**-review-anticancer activity,   **64**-review-widely used in cancer treatment was recently screened for cytoxicity against Hep G2 hepatocarcinoma cells-showed moderate anti-proliferative effects,   **126**-invitro-leaves-ethanol and acqueous extract-Ethanol extracts presented important genotoxicity (CL50 35 ppm); it is worth pointing out that the leaves' aqueous extracts displayed low genotoxicity (CL50 900 ppm), **129**-invitro-ethyl acetate extract showed potent cytotoxicity with LC50 values (5.41 ppm) comparable to the reference standard, gallic acid, **176**-invitro-whole plant?-detected-decline in cancer cells, **522**-review-The pharmacological activities reported include anticancer activity, **545**-invitro-aerial parts-80% ethanol extract-brine shrimp lethality bioassay indicates cytotoxicity-mortality LC50 = 40 µg/ml; LC90= 80 µg/ml)-The cytotoxic activity of the ethanol extract of dried aerial part of Sida rhombifolia Linn. was tested by using brine shrimp lethality bioassay. The extract was found to show potent activity against the brine shrimp nauplii. Therefore the positive response obtained in this assay suggests that the extract may contain antitumor, antibacterial or pesticidal compounds. **619**-whole plant--n-hexane extract-cytoxic-human cancer cells, SNU-1 and Hep G2 inhibition was 68.52% and 47.82%, **744**-invitro-leaf- ethyl acetate extract-showed potent cytotoxicity with LC50 values (5.41 ppm) comparable to the reference standard, gallic acid,

Tr 13-Zaire-leaves, 54-India,

Sida retusa

49-rats-seed-80% methanol extract-DEN induced murine hepatic-Treatment with seed extract significantly inhibited the increase in DEN/CCl(4) induced activities of pre-cancerous marker enzymes, **407**-rats-seed-80% methanol extract-The results of the present study indicates significant inhibitory effects of seed extract on the development of preneoplastic foci, **436**- invitro-seed-methanol extract- potent cytotoxic effect-marked cytotoxic activity against HOP 62, Hep G2 cells at GI50 ≤ 20 µg/ml, **464**-mice/rats-seed-80% methanol extract-treatment with seed extract significantly inhibited the increase in DEN/CCl4 induced activities of pre-cancerous marker enzymes.

Sida indica

452-invivo-brine shrimp-chloroform extracts showed strongly significant cytotoxicity-LC50 (µg/ml)=1.51, **684**-invitro-leaf--hydro-methanolic extract—phytol-AP1 was found to induce chromatin condensation and apoptosis. This is the first report of an apoptosis inducing compound identified from the hydromethanolic extract of S. indica leaves. Hence the phytol isolated from S. indica leaves not only decreased the viability (42%), but also showed DNA degradation and different phases of programmed cell death (ROS mediated) in AO–EtBr stained S. pombe cells as well as in DAPI staining, **705**-leaf-aqueous extract-the biological properties of AIAgNPs were free radical scavenging activity, antibacterial effect and anti-proliferative activity- showed a dose dependant anti-proliferative effect against COLO 205 (human colon cancer) and MDCK (normal) cells with an IC50 of 3 and 4µg/mL and 100 and 75µg/mL, respectively after 24 and 48h., **707**-leaf-aqueous extract-silver nanoparticles (AIAgNPs) using aqueous leaf extract (AILE)- the biological properties of AIAgNPs were free radical scavenging activity, antibacterial effect and anti-proliferative activity-AIAgNPs showed a dose dependant anti-proliferative effect against COLO 205 (human colon cancer) and MDCK (normal) cells with an IC50 of 3 and 4µg/mL and 100 and 75µg/mL, respectively after 24 and 48h., **713**-invitro-leaves-methanol extract>dissolved in 10% aqueous methanol>n-hexane extract> carbon tetrachloride/ chloroform extract-Cytotoxic activity-From the results of the brine shrimp lethality bioassay it can be well predicted that the crude extracts have considerable cytotoxic potency. Among the four fractions, chloroform extracts showed strongly significant cytotoxicity. The degree of lethality was directly proportional to the concentration of the extracts from the lowest concentration (0.781µg/ml) to highly significant with the highest concentration (400µg/ml)-mortality increased gradually with the increase in concentration of the test samples,

Sida cordata

282-invitro-leaf-methanol extract- LC50 for crude extract was 263.02 µg/ml -Our observations revealed that the crude extract shows significant antioxidant and cytotoxic properties. According the discussion above on introduction paragraph and on the basis of the results of the research it can be inferred that Sida cordata may be a good source for the further investigation to discover a new drug for cancer treatment.

Cryptolepine (S. acuta, cordifolia, rhombifolia, alba, and ?)

17-invitro-Cryptolepine, isolated from Sida acuta, sensitizes human gastric adenocarcinoma cells to TRAIL-induced apoptosis **35**-invitro—cryptolepine-p53-mutated human osteosarcoma MG63 cells-induces p21WAF1/CIP1 and cell cycle arrest- in a dose-dependent manner, **73**-invitro- strongly cytotoxic to tumour cells, **164**-invitro-human osteosarcoma MG63 cells- induces the expression of p21WAF1/CIP1 with growth arrest-completely inhibited the growth and caused G2/M-phase arrest, might be a suitable chemotherapeutic agent for treatment of osteosarcoma, **165**-invitro-HL-60 human leukemia cells-treatment with cryptolepine leads to the appearance of a hypo-diploid DNA content peak (sub-G1) characteristic of the apoptotic cell population, **166**-invitro-a potent topoisomerase II inhibitor and a promising antitumor agent, **172**-invitro-cryptolepine-displays potent cytotoxic activities against tumour cells-cryptolepine, but not neocryptolepine, induces cleavage of poly(ADP-ribose) polymerase but both alkaloids induce the release of cytochrome c from the mitochondria, **232**-invitro-showed strong activity to overcome TRAIL resistance, **244**-invitro-cryptolepine-has been found to bind to DNA in a formerly unknown intercalation mode- a basis for the design of new anticancer drugs, **249**-invitro-Lysis to staphylococcal cells was observed following exposure to cryptolepine and this coincided with sharp falls in viable counts of the bacteria. There was the formation of deformed cells as depicted in the SEM photomicrographs of S. aureus cells after 3, 6 or 24 h exposure to inhibitory concentrations of cryptolepine, **297**—invitro--IC50- --MDA MB 361 human breast adenocarcinoma cell line-IC50 genotoxicity 4.7+-.48(uM)--The demon-stration of a broad-spectrum activity on a variety of cancer cell lines, apoptotic cell death, and apparently low genotoxicity suggest that these agents may have potential as candidates for cancer chemotherapy. very cytotoxic and may be weak mammalian mutagens and/or clastogens. The poor genotoxicity of CSE and CLP coupled with their potent cytotoxic action support their anticancer potential. **298**-invitro-is a direct cytotoxin that readily generates damaging ROS (reactive oxygen species), **308**-invitro-bind tightly to DNA and behave as typical intercalating agent-The poisoning effect is more pronounced with cryptolepine-Cryptolepine-treated cells probably die via necrosis rather than via apoptosis, **309**-review-Neocryptolepine-DNA-binding and inhibition of the enzyme topoisomerase II, **380**-invitro-This study has also led to the discovery that cryptolepine is a potent topoisomerase II inhibitor and a promising antitumor agent, **382**-invitro- The poisoning effect is more pronounced with cryptolepine-cytotoxic toward B16 melanoma cells, **393**-invitro-quindoline and cryptolepine-quite cytotoxic in the antiviral test system down to a concentration of 1 µg/ml, **394**-invitro-apoptosis as the mode of cell death in CLP-treated MCL-5 cells, but the CLP-mediated demise of HepG2 cells is not apoptotic, **397**-invitro-This study using human lung adenocarcinoma A549 cells as a model demonstrated that cryptolepine selects different molecular pathways to cell cycle checkpoint activation in a dose specific manner and evokes a wortmannin sensitive anti-apoptosis response, **399**-invitro-cryptolepine shows interesting in vitro cytotoxic properties and its further evaluation as an anti-cancer drug seems warranted- In the cell lines cryptolepine activity was essentially unaffected by established mechanisms of drug resistance, **400**-invitro-cryptolepine-induces the expression of p21WAF1/CIP1 with growth arrest in p53-mutated human osteosarcoma MG63 cells/human colon cancer HCT116 cells, **592**-invitro-p53-mutated human osteosarcoma MG63 cells- These findings suggest that CLP arrests the growth of MG63 cells- might be a suitable chemotherapeutic agent for treatment of osteosarcoma.

Insects

Bean Weevil   Crop damage
Acanthoscelides obtectus feeds on vetches, beans and other leguminous plants. A significant pest in some parts of the world, damages crops both in-situ and when stored in warehouses, and can potentially reduce crop yields by 60% as the larvae develop at the expense of the seeds. [1]

Sida acuta
265-leaf-80% ethanol extract-4% solution-1.5 hours-mortality 48%+--this study suggested that S. acuta possesses insecticidal properties and can be used to control variety of insect pests and vectors, **516**-invivo-leaf-One of the least effective was S. acuta.

Earias vittella   Insect, cotton predator
Spiny bollworm. Attacks cotton and okra crops. [http://www.plantwise.org/ KnowledgeBank/Datasheet.aspx?dsid =20306]

Sida acuta

362-review-leaf-extract-strong feeding deterrence and toxicity against the larvae, **422**-invivo-leaf-solvent ether and ethyl alcohol-extracts exhibited strong feeding deterrence and toxicity against the larva.

Mosquito - Aedes aegypti   Yellow fever

Can spread dengue fever, chikungunya, Zika fever, Mayaro and yellow fever viruses, and other diseases. [1]

Sida acuta

4-invitro-larvacidal-LC 50 values 38 to 48 mg/L,   **4**-invivo-repellant-150 minutes,   **354**-invivo-acqueous extract-leaf-119.32 µg/mL and LC90, 213.84 µg/mL- silver nanoparticles synthesized using Sida acuta plant leaf extract- LC50 23.96and LC90 44.05 µg/mL

Sida indica   **441**-invivo-β-sitosterol-LC50 11.49.

Mosquito - Anopheles stephensi   Malaria

Important vector for the human malaria species Plasmodium falciparum. [1]

Sida acuta

4-invitro-larvacidal-LC 50 values 38 to 48 mg/L--repellant-120 minutes-it can be concluded the crude extract of Sida acuta was an excellent potential for controlling Culex quinquefasciatus, Aedes aegypti and Anopleles stephensi mosquitoes,   **354**-invivo-acqueous extract-leaf-LC50, 109.94 µg/mL and LC90, 202.42 µg/mL- silver nanoparticles synthesized using Sida acuta plant leaf extract- LC50 21.92 and LC90 41.07 µg/mL,   **463**-leaf and root extract-methanol extract-showed higher mortality against mosquito larvae, lethal dose (Lc50),

Sida indica   **441**- invivo-β-sitosterol-LC50 value of 3.58.

Mosquito-Culex quinquefasciatus   Malaria

Southern House Mosquito, the vector of Wuchereria bancrofti, avian malaria, and arboviruses, including St. Louis encephalitis virus, Western equine encephalitis virus, zika virus, and West Nile virus. [1]

Sida acuta

4-invitro-larvacidal-LC 50 values 38 to 48 mg/L,   **4**-invivo-repellant-120 minutes,   **354**-invivo-acqueous extract-leaf-kills mosquito larvae-LC50, 130.30 µg/mL and LC90, 228.20 µg/mL- silver nanoparticles synthesized using Sida acuta plant leaf extract- LC50 26.13 and LC90 47.52 µg/mL,   **586**-invivo-whole plant?-acetone extract-significant juvenile hormone analogue activity against.

Sida rhombifolia

587-invivo-stem-methanolic extract-It was concluded that the isolated compound (phenyl ethyl B-D-glucopyranoside) from Sida rhombifolia offers a significant potential as new control agent against Culex quinquefasciatus larvae,

Sida indica

441-invivo-β-sitosterol as a potential new mosquito larvicidal compound with LC50 value of 26.67 against Culex quinquefasciatus Say (Diptera: Culicidae)

Plasmodium berghei　　　　　mice malaria

A protozoan parasite that causes malaria in certain rodents. [1]

Sida acuta

463-leaf and root extract-methanol extract-both extracts showed significant antiplasmodial activity-showed markedly significant antimalarial activity and antivectorial activity effects even at low concentrations,

Cryptolepine (found in S. acuta, cordifolia, rhombifolia, alba, at least)
245-mice/invitro-orally-50 mg/kg/day-parasitemia was suppressed by 80%,

Plasmodium falciparum
parasitic protozoa, malaria

A protozoan parasite, one of the species of Plasmodium that cause malaria in humans. It is transmitted by the female Anopheles mosquito. This species causes the disease's most dangerous form, malignant or falciparum malaria. It has the highest complication rates and mortality. [1]

Sida acuta

12-invitro-whole plant?-extract?-IC50<5 µg/ml- was related to its alkaloid contents,　**19**-invivo-lwhole plant?-water decoction/ethanol extract-IC50 values obtained for these extracts ranged from 3.9 to -5.4 microg/ml,　**20**-20-invitro- its alkaloid contents-IC50 < 5 microg/ml,　**108**-invitro-multidrug resistant (K1) strain-highly active with an IC50 value of 0.031±0.0085 (SE) µg/mL, equivalent to 0.134±0.037 µM (n = 3),　**252**-invivo-acqueous extract+ethanolic extract- FcM29-Cameroon (chloroquine-resistant strain) and a Nigerian chloroquine-sensitive strain-antiplasmodial-IC50 values 3.9 to −5.4 µg/ml,　**294**-review,　**459**-invitro-whole plant-acqueous, ethanolic extracts-IC50 3.9 to −5.4 µg/ml-two chloroquine-resistant strains of Plasmodium falciparum from Cameroon and Nigeria.

Cryptolepine (found in S. acuta, cordifolia, rhombifolia, alba, at least)
245-mice-50 mg/kg bw/day-parasitaemia was suppressed by 80.5% of that of the untreated control animals. However, with chloroquine diphosphate at 5

90

mg/kg/day parasitaemia was suppressed by 93.5%, **251**-invitro-multidrug resistant (K1) strain -IC50 0.134±0.037 µM- this compound appears to intercalate with DNA and this may explain the high degree of antimalarial activity demonstrated in vitro,

Fungi, Anti-fungal (antimycotic)

In the last three decades, pathogenic resistant fungi particularly candida strains, have caused major health problems throughout the world in women although the pharmacological industries produced quantities of antibiotics. Unfortunately, the resistance of fungi to these drugs is increasingly important. The search for plants with antifungal activity has gained increasing importance in recent years due to the development of resistance. **[211]**   The emergence of pathogens resistant to antibiotics as a result of their excessive use in clinical and veterinary applications represents a serious public health concern. In the last three decades, pathogenic resistant fungi particularly candida strains, have caused major health problems throughout the world in women although the pharmacological industries produced quantities of antibiotics. Unfortunately, the resistance of fungi to these drugs is increasingly important. The search for plants with antifungal activity has gained increasing importance in recent years due to the development of resistance. **[27]**

Alterneria Alternata   opportunistic fungus

An opportunistic pathogen on numerous hosts causing leaf spots, rots and blights on many plant parts. It can also cause upper respiratory tract infections and asthma in humans with compromised immunity. **[1]**

Sida alba   **633**-invitro-methanolic extract-whole plant?-ZI 20 mm.

Aspergillus spp.   toxic fungus
A. flavus - A. fumigates - A. niger - A. niger NCIM 1054 - A. ochraceus

A fungus best known for its colonization of cereal grains, legumes, and tree nuts. Many strains produce significant quantities of toxic compounds known as aflatoxins, which are poisonous and cancer-causing chemicals.... Children are particularly affected. Adults are also at risk. No animal species is immune. Aflatoxins are among the most carcinogenic substances known. **[1]**

Sida acuta

Aspergillus flavus

83-invitro-plant oils-Hydro distillation in the ratio of 3:1-as effective as control (Streptomycin?),   **271**-invitro-root, stem, leaf and buds-water extract (distilled water)-80% methanol extract-no effect against Aspergillus flavus and Aspergillus niger-Previously, antibacterial and antifungal activities of crude extracts of S. acuta have been reported.

Aspergillus fumigates

102-invitro-leaf-1000 mg/ml-100% ethanolic extract-ZI=2mm--cold distilled water extract-ZI=1mm--griseofulvin-ZI=5mm--Unlike the root of the plant which has been reported to exhibit antifungal activity, the extracts from the leaves has been shown to be less active against fungi.

Aspergillus niger

6-(NCIM 1054)-invitro-leaf-chlorofom/95% ethanol extracts-ZI 11mm--activity index=.5—(Gentamycin 10 mcg//Nystatin 100 units)-ZI 22mm,   **55**-in vitro,   **83**-invitro-plant oils-Hydro distillation in the ratio of 3:1-not antimicrobial in tests-good effect-Aspergillus niger,   **102**-invitro-leaf-1000 mg/ml-100% ethanolic extract-ZI=3mm--cold distilled water extract-ZI=1mm--griseofulvin-ZI=8mm-Unlike the root of the plant which has been reported to exhibit antifungal activity, the extracts from the leaves has been shown to be less active against fungi,   **271**-invitro-water extract (distilled water)-80% methanol extract-MIC-none-MBC-none,   **523**-invitro-leaves-MIC=4 ug/well - zone of inhibition (40ug/well)- 90% ethanol 30mm - methanol 22mm - ethyl acetate none - aqueous extract none,

Sida cordifolia

Aspergillus flavus   **173**-invitro-leaf and root-methanol extract-Zone of Inhibition (mm)-root=8--leaf=8-100 µg ml.

Aspergillus fumigates 143-invitro-chloroform and methanol extracts of leaves and roots exhibited moderate activity against.

Aspergillus niger

143-invitro-chloroform and methanol extracts of leaves and roots exhibited moderate activity against,   **152**-invitro-seed oil-petroleum ether (40-600C) extract-ZI 22-28mm (300 µg)-ZI 12-14mm at 100 µg -- chloroform extract ZI 28-30mm (300 µg)-ZI 12mm at 100 µg--Griseofulvin ZI 18mm (50 µg/ml), **202**- ethyl acetate and aqueous fractions-exhibited significant antifungal activity,

Sida rhombifolia

Aspergillus niger   202-invitro-extract-significant antibacterial activity,

Aspergillus ochraceus   **362**-review-whole plant?-methanolic plant extract-activity against,

Sida alba (Sida spinosa)

Aspergillus niger   **55**-invitro-leaf-ethanolic extract-500 µg/disc-zone of inhibition 22 mm-Amphotericin B-30 µg / disc- zone of inhibition 40 mm, **99**-(NCM 105)-invitro-whole plant-hot 60-80% ethanolic extract-had no effect.

Sida retusa

Aspergillus flavus   436-invitro-seed- ethanolic extract-exhibited potent inhib-itory effects with inhibitory zones something like 18-26 mm.

Sida indica

Aspergillus flavus   689-Sida indica-invitro-root, bark and fresh leaves-methanol extract-root ZI= 9@90µg/ml--leaf ZI=13@90µg/ml,

Aspergillus niger

450-invitro-fruit,root,leaf-dichloromethane:methanol (1:1, v/v) extract-no effect-Aspergillus niger (MTCC 1344),   **452**-Sida indica-brine shrimp-carbon tetrachloride zone of inhibition 8.7mm-Neither chloroform, n-hexane extract nor aqueous soluble partitionate of methanolic extract had an effect, **704**--n-hexane/methanol extraction--redissolved in distilled water—leaf MIC=none µg/ml—stem MIC=581µg/ml—root MIC=255 µg/ml,   ZI 8.7 ± 0.20 mm--kanamycin ZI 36.7 ± 1.50 mm—chloroform/n-hexane/aqueous fraction of methanol extracts ZI=none,   **713**-invitro-leaves-methanol extract>dissolved in 10% aqueous methanol>n-hexane extract>carbon tetrachloride extract ZI 8.7 ± 0.20 mm--kanamycin ZI 36.7 ± 1.50 mm—chloroform/n-hexane/aqueous fraction of methanol extracts ZI=none,

Multiple Aspergillus   717-invitro-new steroidal compound-100% effective at 5000 ppm in controlling the mycelial growth of Aspergillus parasiticus var. globosus and Aspergillus terreus var. aureus using the poison food technique. For other fungi like Aspergillus flavus, A. versicolor and A. fischeri, it was fungistatic,

Candida spp.   Fungal infections

Candida albicans -- Candida albicans (MTCC No. 183) -- Candida albicans ATCC 10231 -- Candida albicans ATCC 2091 -- Candida albicans ATCC 9002 -- Candida albicans ATCC 90028 -- Candida albicans NCIM 3102 -- Candida albicans NCPF 3242 -- Candida albicans NCPF 3262 -- Candida glabrata -- Candida guilliermondii - Candida guilliermondii LM 28 -- Candida intermedia -- Candida krusei -- Candida krusei ATCC 6258 -- Candida krusei LM 07 -- Candida parapsilosis -- Candida parapsilosis ATCC 22019 -- Candida tropicalis -- Candida tropicalis ATCC 750 -- Candida tropicalis LM 25 -- Candida tropicalis NCPF --Candida tropicalis NCPF -- Candida tropicalis NCPF 3242 -- Candida tropicalis NCPF 3262   A genus of yeasts that is the most common cause of fungal infections worldwide [1]

Sida acuta

Candida albicans

5-invitro-methanol extract-no effect,   6-(NCIM 3102)-invitro-leaf-chlorofom/95% ethanol extracts-ZI 24mm--activity index=.92—(Gentamycin 10 mcg//Nystatin 100 units)-ZI 26mm,   77-invitro-leaves-hot distilled water extract-20g of ground leaves added to 200mL of distilled water-boiled for 15 minutes-used immediately after-Zones of inhibition-just leaves (no activity)-with silver nanoparticles 21mm-silver nitrate alone 10mm,   **98**-(MTCC No. 183)-invitro-root, stem, leaves and buds-80% methanol extract>petroleum ether, ethyl ether and ethyl acetate extraction- In the present study total 8 extracts of different parts of the plant were tested for their bioactivity against C. albicans (MTCC No. 183), among which 7 extracts showed significant activity against test fungi-order of activity-stem>root>leaf> terbinafine>bud, **101**-invitro-aerial parts-ethanol extract-neither the concentrated extract nor its dilutions inhibited-MIC (no activity)-ZI=(no activity)--ZI Ciprofloxacin=(no activity)--ZI Amoxycillin (no activity)-ZI Fluconazole 35mm (20 µg/ml), **106**-invitro-Methanol Zone of inhibition=10 mm--Methanol& Water (1/1)/Ethanol/ Ethanol&Water(1/1)/ Ethyl acetate/Water extracts-no Zone of Inhibition, **168**-invitro-aerial parts-90% ethanolic extract-no inhibition, **184**-invitro-root, stem, leaves and buds-80% ethanol extract>petroleum ether, ethyl ether and ethyl acetate extracts- All the flavonoid extracts showed varying degrees of antifungal activity on C. albicans. Some of these extracts were more effective than traditional antibiotic terbinafine to combat the pathogenic fungi, **238**-invitro-100% methanolic extract-no effect, **523**-invitro-leaves-MIC=2 ug/well - zone of inhibition (40ug/well)- 90% ethanol 21mm - methanol 27mm - ethyl acetate 20mm - aqueous extract none.

Candida glabrata **106**-invitro-Methanol/Methanol&Water (1/1)/Ethanol /Ethanol&Water(1/1)/ Ethyl acetate/Water extracts-no ZI-no extract worked,

Sida cordifolia

Candida albicans

27-(ATCC 2091)-invitro-whole plant?-80% acetone extract>chloroform extract for alkaloid compounds-MIC 8.33±3.61 (µg/ml)-MFC 29.17±19.09 (µg/ml)--Nystatin MIC=4.17±1.80 (µg/ml)-MFC 12.5±0.00 (µg/ml)--Clotrimazole MIC= 6.25±0.00 (µg/ml)-MFC 12.5±0.00 (µg/ml)--S. cordifolia+Nystatin-MIC 1.04±0.45 (µg/ml)--S. cordifolia+Clotrimazole-MIC 1.30±0.45 (µg/ml), **27**-(ATCC 9002)-invitro- aerial parts?- 80% acetone extract (400 ml acetone + 100 ml water) for 24 h under mechanic agitation at room temperature-MIC 10.42±3.61 (µg/ml)-MIC Nystatin 4.17±1.80 (µg/ml)-MIC Clotrimazole 4.17±1.80 (µg/ml), **72**-(ATCC 90028)-invitro-steam distilled leaf essential oil (100%)-ZI=14mm (50 uL)—Ketoconazole ZI=10mm (50 ug/ml), **125**-leaf-water extract-exhibited high antifungal activity at a concentration of 2mg/disc--methanolic extract-did not show any antifungal activity, 100µg/ml concentration, whereas the same extracts at 300µg/ml concentration showed promising activity and comparable to standard drug griseofulvin, **143**-invitro-leaf and root-chloroform and methanol extracts-significant activity against Candida albicans, **152**-invitro-seed oil-petroleum ether (40-600C) extract-ZI 26-28mm (300 µg)-ZI no activity at 100 µg -- chloroform extract ZI 22-26mm (300 µg)-ZI no activity at 100 µg-- Griseofulvin ZI 25mm (50 µg/ml)- Against C. albicans seed extracts were resistant at 100µg/ml concentration, whereas the same extracts at 300µg/ml concentration showed promising activity and comparable to standard drug griseofulvin, **202**- ethyl acetate and aqueous fractions-exhibited significant antifungal activity, **211**-invitro- aerial parts?- 80% acetone extract (400 ml acetone + 100 ml water) for 24 h under mechanic agitation at room temperature- alkaloid compounds in combination with antifungal references (Nystatin and Clotrimazole) exhibited antimicrobial effects against candida strains tested-MIC 10.42±3.61 (µg/ml)-MIC Nystatin 4.17±1.80 (µg/ml)-MIC Clotrimazole 4.17±1.80 (µg/ml),

Candida guilliermondii 72-invitro-steam distilled leaf essential oil (2%)-80% inhibitory activity, 72-(LM 28)-invitro-steam distilled leaf essential oil (100%)-ZI=20mm (50 uL)—Ketoconazole ZI=12mm (50 ug/ml),

Candida krusei
27-(ATCC 6258)-invitro-whole plant?-80% acetone extract>chloroform extract for alkaloid compounds-MIC 8.33±3.61 (μg/ml)-MFC 29.17±19.09 (μg/ml)--Nystatin MIC=4.17±1.80 (μg/ml)-MFC 12.5±0.00 (μg/ml)--Clotrimazole MIC= 4.17±1.80 (μg/ml)-MFC 14.58±9.55 (μg/ml)--S. cordifolia+Nystatin-MIC 1.04±0.45 (μg/ml)--S. cordifolia+Clotrimazole-MIC 1.30±0.45 (μg/ml), 72-(LM 07)-invitro-steam distilled leaf essential oil (100%)-ZI=12mm (50 uL)—Ketoconazole ZI=no effect (50 ug/ml).

Candida parapsilosis 27-(ATCC 22019)-invitro-whole plant?-80% acetone extract>chloroform extract for alkaloid compounds-MIC 12.5±0.00 (μg/ml)-MFC 41.67±14.43 (μg/ml)--Nystatin MIC=6.25±0.00 (μg/ml)-MFC 14.58±9.55 (μg/ml)--Clotrimazole MIC= 6.25±0.00 (μg/ml)-MFC 16.67±7.22 (μg/ml)--S. cordifolia+Nystatin-MIC 1.30±0.45 (μg/ml)--S. cordifolia+Clotrimazole-MIC 1.56±0.00 (μg/ml),

Candida stellatoidea (LM 96) 72-invitro-steam distilled leaf essential oil (100%)-ZI=no effect (50 uL)—Ketoconazole ZI=14mm (50 ug/ml),

Candida tropicalis
27-(ATCC 750)-invitro-whole plant?-80% acetone extract>chloroform extract for alkaloid compounds-MIC 10.42±3.61 (μg/ml)-MFC 29.17±19.09 (μg/ml)--Nystatin MIC=4.17±1.80 (μg/ml)-MFC 12.5±0.00 (μg/ml)--Clotrimazole MIC= 6.25±0.00 (μg/ml)-MFC 14.58±9.55 (μg/ml)--S. cordifolia+Nystatin-MIC 1.04±0.45 (μg/ml)--S. cordifolia+Clotrimazole-MIC 1.56±0.00 (μg/ml), 72-(LM 25)-invitro-steam distilled leaf essential oil (100%)-ZI=14mm (50 uL)—Ketoconazole ZI=12mm (50 ug/ml),

Sida rhombifolia
Candida albicans 202-invitro-significant antifungal activity, 362-review-whole plant?-methanolic plant extract-activity against.

Candida intermedia 362-review-whole plant?-methanolic plant extract-activity against,

Sida retusa
Candida krusei 436-invitro-seed-ethanolic extract-exhibited potent inhibitory effects against Candida krusei with inhibitory zone something like 18-26 mm,

Sida tuberculata
490-invitro- leaves, roots-acqueous extract-ethanolic extract three ethanol con-centrations were tested on extraction: 20, 30 and 40% (v/v) for leaves and 50, 70 and 90% (v/v) for roots, 613-leaves and roots-hot water infusion-biofilm removal efficiency in contaminated central venous catheter (CVC) coupons-removed biofilm after 90 min of exposure-MIC 3.90 to 62.50 μg/ml,

Sida alba

Candida albicans   55-(NCM 3102)-invitro-leaf-ethanolic extract-500 µg/ disc-zone of inhibition 23 mm-Amphotericin B-30 µg / disc- zone of inhibition 43 mm,   99-(NCIM 3102)-invitro-whole plant-ethanolic extract-bacteriostatic-ZI 21mm (500 µg/ disc)-Ciprofloxacin ZI 32mm (5 µg / disc).

Sida indica

Candida albicans   450-(MTCC 10231)-invitro-fruit, root, leaf-dichloromethane: methanol (1:1, v/v) extract-no effect,   452-brine shrimp-carbon tetrachloride zone of inhibition 6.1mm-Neither chloroform, n-hexane extract nor aqueous soluble partitionate of methanolic extract had an effect,   713-invitro-leaves-methanol extract>dissolved in 10% aqueous methanol>n-hexane extract>carbon tetrachloride extract ZI 6.1 ± 0.62 mm--kanamycin ZI 36.0 ± 1.00 mm—chloroform/n-hexane/aqueous fraction of methanol extracts ZI=none.

Cryptolepine   (found in S. acuta, cordifolia, rhombifolia, alba, at least)

Candida albicans

108-invitro-showed activity against,   **301**-invitro-neocryptolepine inhibited the growth of the yeast C. albicans,   **385**-(ATCC 10231)- cryptolepine-invitro-MIC-40–80 µg ml–1-extreme disturbance of surface structure, including partial and total collapse, followed by lysis--Time-kill studies showed a reduction in viable count from 106 to < 10 cfu ml–1 in 4 h to 320 µg ml–1 of the agent-Biocidal effects were noted at concentrations 2–4 times those of the MIC of the alkaloid,   **385**-invitro--MIC µg ml–1= 40-80,   **385**-(NCPF 3242)-cryptolepine-invitro-MIC-80 to 160 µg ml–Biocidal effects were noted at concentrations 2–4 times those of the MIC of the alkaloid,   **385**-(NCPF 3262)-invitro-MIC-80–160 µg ml–1--Biocidal effects were noted at concentrations 2–4 times those of the MIC of the alkaloid following challenge with 106 cfu ml–1 of micro-organisms.   **388**-invitro-liposome size of 400 nm-negatively charged cryptolepine liposomes were at least 2-4 times more active than free cryptolepine or positively charged liposomes- none of the liposome preparations were superior to amphotericin B in their antifungal activity,   **390**-invitro-acid alcoholic extract-MIC 31.25/mi-MBC 250 pg/mi,

Candida tropicalis   **385**-(NCPF)-invitro--MIC µg ml–1= 40-80--Biocidal effects were noted at concentrations 2–4 times those of the MIC of the alkaloid following challenge with 106 cfu ml–1 of micro-organisms,   **385**-(NCPF 3242, NCPF 3262)-invitro--MIC µg ml–1= 80-100--Biocidal effects were noted at concentrations 2–4 times those of the MIC of the alkaloid following challenge with 106 cfu ml–1 of micro-organisms.

Cryptococcus neoformans   Infectious yeast

Most infections occur in the lungs. However, fungal meningitis and encephalitis, especially as a secondary infection for AIDS patients, are often caused, making it a particularly dangerous fungus. [1]

Sida cordifolia

125-review-leaf-methanol extract ZI=0mm (2 mg/disc)—water extract ZI=20mm (2 mg/disc)—Fluconazole ZI=20mm (25 ug/disc),

Cunninghamella elegans   non-pathogenic fungus

Able to degrade xenobiotics, pesticides, and synthetic phenolytics-has uses in biotechnology. [1]

Sida rhombifolia   **362**-review-whole plant?-methanolic plant extract-activity against.

Dreschlera turcica   Corn fungus

A serious fungal disease prevalent in cooler climates and tropical highlands wherever corn is grown. [1]

Sida cordifolia   **173**-invitro-leaf and root-methanol extract-Zone of Inhibition (mm)-root=8--leaf=9,

Sida indica   **689**-invitro-root, bark and fresh leaves-methanol extract-root ZI= 11@90µg/ml-leaf ZI=14@90µg/ml,

Fusarium oxysporum   Fungus, plant pathogen

Some of the most abundant and widespread microbes of the global soil microflora...many strains are pathogenic to plants, especially in agricultural settings. [1]

Sida cordifolia

120-leaves and inflorescences-water, methanol, methanol-water (95:5), ethanol-water (95:5) and ethanol (1 g:10 mL plant/solvent) extracts-No activity against,

Sida alba   **633**-invitro-methanolic extract-whole plant?-ZI 2 mm-100 µl,

Fusarium verticillioides   Pathogenic corn fungus

This infection of maize can result in highly variable disease symptoms ranging from asymptomatic plants to severe rotting and wilting. [745]

Sida cordifolia   **173**-invitro-leaf and root-methanol extract-ZI (mm)-root=10--leaf=12.

Sida indica   **689**- invitro-root, bark and fresh leaves-methanol extract-root ZI= 12@90µg/ml-leaf ZI=14@90µg/ml,

Microsporum gypseum
Fungi, ringworm

Known for causing diseases on human skin. Contains a number of pathogens to both humans and animals. Causes Tinea or ringworm. [1]

Sida rhombifolia

202-invitro-significant antifungal activity -MIC value of 62.5 µg/ml, **545**-extract-significant antibacterial activity.

Penicillium (FCF 281)
fungi

Ascomycetous fungi of major importance in the natural environment as well as food and drug production. [1]

Sida cordifolia
72-invitro-steam distilled leaf essential oil (100%)-ZI=no effect (50 uL)—Ketoconazole ZI=no effect (50 ug/ml),

Rhizopus oryzae
fungus, causes mucormycosis

An opportunistic human pathogen, it is one causative agent of zygomycosis, These rare yet serious and potentially life-threatening fungal infections usually affect the face or oropharyngeal (nose and mouth) cavity. [1]

Sida cordifolia

120-invitro-leaves and inflorescences-water, methanol, methanol-water (95:5), ethanol-water (95:5) and ethanol (1 g:10 mL plant/solvent) extracts-No activity against,

Sida indica

704—(Rhizopus microsporus)--n-hexane/methanol extraction--redissolved in distilled water—leaf MIC= 512µg/ml—stem MIC=815µg/ml—root MIC=379µg/ml,

Saccharomyces cerevisiae
Non-infective yeast

Saccharomyces cerevisiae -- Saccharomyces cerevisiae NCPF 3139 -- Saccharomyces cerevisiae NCPF 3178

Sida indica

450-(ATCC9763)-invitro-fruit, root, leaf-dichloromethane: methanol (1:1, v/v) extract-**no effect**, **452**-brine shrimp-carbon tetrachloride zone of inhibition 7.6mm-Neither chloroform, n-hexane extract nor aqueous soluble partitionate of methanolic extract had an effect-no effect, **713**-invitro-leaves-methanol extract>dissolved in 10% aqueous methanol>n-hexane extract>carbon tetrachloride extract ZI 7.6 ± 0.21 mm--kanamycin ZI 35.5 ± 0.50 mm—chloroform/n-hexane/aqueous fraction of methanol extracts ZI=none.

Cryptolepine   (found in S. acuta, cordifolia, rhombifolia, alba, at least)

385-(NCPF 3139)-invitro-MIC-5 to 10 µg ml−1 --extreme disturbance of surface structure, including partial and total collapse, followed by lysis-- Biocidal effects were noted at concentrations 2−4 times those of the MIC of the alkaloid following challenge with 106 cfu ml−1 of micro-organisms--3 log cycle reductions were recorded for the 6 h counts of S. cerevisiae NCPF 3139 exposed to 40µg ml−1 and 160 µg ml−1 of the alkaloid respectively,   **385**-(NCPF 3178)-invitro-MIC-20−40 µg ml−1--Biocidal effects were noted at concentrations 2−4 times those of the MIC of the alkaloid following challenge with 106 cfu ml−1 of micro-organisms,   **388**-invitro-liposome size of 400 nm-negatively charged cryptolepine liposomes were at least 2-4 times more active than free cryptolepine or positively charged liposomes- none of the liposome preparations were superior to amphotericin B in their antifungal activity.

Scpulariopsis candida   opportunistic mold

Anamorphic fungi that are saprobic and pathogenic to animals. [1] Commonly isolated from soil, air, plant debris, paper, and moist indoor environments. Some species are known to be opportunistic pathogens, mainly causing superficial tissue infections...have also been involved in deep tissue infections, mainly in immunocompromised and occasionally in immunocompetent patients, causing, for example, pneumonia, endophthalmitis, subcutaneous and brain abscesses, invasive sinusitis, peritonitis, and endocarditis. **[744]**

Sida acuta

102-invitro-leaf-1000 mg/ml-100% ethanolic extract-ZI=6mm-- cold distilled water extract-ZI=2mm--griseofulvin-ZI=5mm--Unlike the root of the plant which has been reported to exhibit antifungal activity, the extracts from the leaves has been shown to be less active against fungi,

Trichoderma spp.   Toxic fungi

Ubiquitous in soil, causes toxic house mold, highly resistant to heat and antimicrobials making primary prevention the only management option. Certain species cause green mold, a disease of cultivated button mushrooms and onions. **[1]**

Sida acuta   **83**-invitro-plant oils-Hydro distillation in the ratio of 3:1-- 24 hrs ZI = 30mm--48 hours ZI = 34mm—72 hrs ZI= 82mm.

Sida indica

704--n-hexane/methanol extraction--redissolved in distilled water—leaf MIC=642µg/ml—stem MIC=235µg/ml—root MIC=446µg/ml-- Trichoderma viride   ,

Trichophyton spp.   **Athlete's foot fungi**

Sida cordifolia
72-invitro-steam distilled leaf essential oil (100%)-ZI=12mm (50 uL)—Ketoconazole ZI=12mm (50 ug/ml) –(Trichophyton mentagrophytes LM103),

Sida indica
736-leaves-methanolic extract-remarkable antifungal activity against Trichophyton rubrum,

Trichosporon inkin   **opportunistic fungi**

Sida cordifolia
72-invitro-steam distilled leaf essential oil (100%)-ZI=24mm (50 uL)—Ketoconazole ZI=no effect (50 ug/ml).

Ustilago maydis   **corn smut fungi**

Cryptolepine   (found in S. acuta, cordifolia, rhombifolia, alba, at least)
388-invitro-liposome size of 400 nm-negatively charged cryptolepine liposomes were at least 2-4 times more active than free cryptolepine or positively charged liposomes- none of the liposome preparations were superior to amphotericin B in their antifungal activity.

Virus

A virus is a small infectious agent that replicates only inside the living cells of other organisms. Viruses can infect all types of life forms, from animals and plants to microorganisms....   A virus is a biological agent that reproduces inside the cells of living hosts. When infected by a virus, a host cell is forced to produce many thousands of identical copies of the original virus at an extraordinary rate. Unlike most living things, viruses do not have cells that divide; new viruses are assembled in the infected host cell. But unlike still simpler infectious agents, viruses contain genes, which gives them the ability to mutate and evolve. [1]   Widespread usage of antiviral agents has led to drug resistant varieties of viruses, especially in immunocompramised patients. Resistance of virus to synthetic nucleoside analogues has been reported to develop in vitro and in vivo (Field, 2001). It is therefore necessary to find new and effective antiviral agents to treat the viral infections and to counter the resistant varieties of viruses. In view of a significant number of plant extracts that have yielded positive results, it can be concluded that a rich source of antiviral agents are still present in natural products, which are yet to be explored. [795]

Herpes-simplex   Face or mouth infection

Oral herpes involves the face or mouth and may result in small blisters called cold sores or a sore throat. Genital herpes may in small ulcers. Other disorders include: herpetic whitlow with the fingers, herpes of the eye, herpes infection of the brain, and neonatal herpes when it affects a newborn. Worldwide rates of either HSV-1 or HSV-2 are between 60% and 95% in adults. [1]

Sida acuta

5-Antiviral activity measured as complete or partial alleviation of viral cpe (cytopathic effects) at minimum concentration of 250 pg/ml.

Cryptolepine   (found in S. acuta, cordifolia, rhombifolia, alba, at least)

393-invitro-cryptolepine HCl-possess an antiherpetic activity.

Sida cordifolia

Herpes simplex virus, type 1   **795**-At 100 TCID50 of HSV-I challenge dose, Toluene, Hydro-alcoholic and methanolic extracts of Sida cordifolia showed promising cell protection with IC50 values 37µg/ml, 12µg/ml and 22µg/ml when challenged with 50µg/ml treated dose. Those values were compared with acyclovir, standard drug used for the study which showed 98.33% protection with IC50= 7µg/ml.

Influenza   virus type A H1N1

Sida cordifolia

795-the antiviral activity was performed with two strains of influenza A i.e., PR-8/34 and IFV-296. The maximum cell protection was offered by HA extract of Sida cordifolia against both the viral strains. hydroalcohol extract offered highest selectivity index of 41 and 13.66 against IFV-296 and PR-8 strains. The results were compared with the standard drug oseltamivir which showed maximum virus inhibition at 10µg/ml it offered 94% protection with IC50= 7µg/ml.

Polio   human enterovirus

Sida acuta   5-invitro-methanol extract-no antiviral activity measured as complete or partial alleviation of virus (cytopathic effects).

Sida cordifolia

Poliovirus type I   **795**-All the extracts of Sida cordifolia offered 100% protection - Pe extract at 50µg/ml it offered 90% protection with IC50= 18µg/ml followed by HA and Tol extracts at 50 µg/ml showed 89.33% and

88.66% virus inhibition with IC50= 19µg/ml. The results were compared with standard Guanidine hydrochloride which showed 99.00% protection at 12.5µg/ml with IC50= 8µg/ml. all other extracts showed moderate activity.

Sindbis alphavirus

Sida acuta 5-invitro-methanol extract-1,000 pg/ml dried plant material and 1% methanol-cytoxicity (500 WgIml)- Cellular changes (250 pg/ml)- cells become rounded but remain attached; g, granules evident in cytoplasm.

Virus, General Antiviral

Sida acuta 5-invitro-methanol extract-250 pg/ml-Antiviral activity measured as complete or partial alleviation of viral cpe (cytopathic effects)-active against herpes simplex-no effect against Virus targets Sindbis or Polio.

Tr 6-Ayurveda-cold, 7-Central America, 93-Italy/Burkina Faso-leaves-colds, 220-Nicaragua/Guatemala, 223-India, 358-hepatitis (viral), 653-Ayurveda-by cold perhaps they mean this.

Sida cordifolia **Tr** 32-Ayurveda-cold and flu, 88-Ayurveda-root bark, 118-Ayurveda-cold and flu, 161-Ayurveda-cold and flu, 312-USA-Ayurveda-root bark, 312-Brazil,

Sida rhombifolia **Tr** 522-Mexico-entire plant-decoction-treats head cold when applied externally, 522-Nicaragua-leaf-decoction-taken orally for colds,

Sida indica

704--n-hexane/methanol extraction--redissolved in distilled water—leaf MIC=512µg/ml—stem MIC=815µg/ml—root MIC=379µg/ml,

Tr 445-Sida indica-India and China, 448-Ayurveda-mumps, 452-Bangladesh-colds-mumps, 684-India-mumps,

Other Sidas **Tr** 11-Sida spinosa--Burkina-Faso, 631-Sida schimperiana-Ethiopia-influenza-Leaf juice is used against cough and influenza,

Cryptolepine (found in S. acuta, cordifolia, rhombifolia, alba, and ?) **393**-invitro-cryptolepine HCl-possess an antiherpetic activity.

Multiple Pathogens

705-Sida indica-leaf-aqueous extract-the intense zone of inhibition displayed by them in six different pathogenic species indicate the potential antibacterial effect,   **707-Sida indica**-leaf-aqueous extract-the intense zone of inhibition displayed by them in six different pathogenic species indicate the potential antibacterial effect,   **129-Sida rhombifolia**-invitro-leaf-all extracts showed weak antibacterial activity against both Gram-positive and Gram-negative test organisms,

Sida indica

704--excellent activity against three Gram-negative bacteria, four Gram-positive rods, and three fungi--n-hexane/methanol extraction--redissolved in distilled   water—leaf   MIC=512µg/ml—stem   MIC=815µg/ml—root MIC=379µg/ml,

Disease, Miscellaneous   No peer review

{Traditional solutions not otherwise noted}

Sida acuta   **Tr**   76-W Africa-smallpox,   124-India-roots orally with sugar-sun stroke,   428-India-sun stroke,   593-Burkina Faso-hepatitis B, **Elephantiasis   Tr**   88-Ayurveda-juice,   107-juice of the leaves is boiled in oil,   109-juice of the leaves is boiled in oil,   217-Ayurveda,   270-India-boiled in gingelly oil,   361-India-leaves-are boiled in oil and applied to elephantiasis,   362-review-India-leaves-boiled in oil and applied to elephantiasis.

Sida cordifolia

Tr   76-W Africa-smallpox,   203-Burkina-Faso-children-smallpox,   358-review-The powdered whole plant is applied to open wounds of horses in Niger,   378-medical website-the juice of the whole plant has been pounded with a little water, made into paste with the juice of the palmyra tree, and applied to the affected area- elephantiasis,   593-Burkina Faso-hepatitis B,

Sida rhombifolia

Tr   51-India-whole plant?-herpes,   51-India-skin application in chicken pox,   150-Ethiopia-fruit- chicken pox,   150-Ethiopia-leaf-rabies,   524-Phillipines-whole plant?-poultice- chicken pox,   524-Phillipines-whole plant?-poultice-herpes,   593-Burkina Faso-hepatitis B.

Sida spinosa   **Tr**   593-Burkina Faso-hepatitis B,

Other Sidas   **Tr**   593- Sida urens-Burkina Faso-hepatitis B,   593-Cienfuegosia digitata Cav -Burkina Faso-hepatitis B.

Pathogen Narratives

This narrative part of the Pathogens section was an afterthought of my research, where I collected interesting paragraphs from the peer-reviewers themselves. Putting the book together I found that the researchers themselves could describe or explain a topic better than I could. There has not been enough research to cover all topics.

The first thing this chapter provides is my thoughts on where we stand with pathogens. The second part contains some narrative from the researchers themselves that define some basic concepts of disease and how it affects us.

Each peer-review entry should have a bracketed number **[79]**. You can then use this number to look up the web page of the actual research in the **References**. I sometimes add the date of the research if applicable ([1-2017]). Additionally, this is the font that is used for expert testimony, while any comments that are mine should be in this font. If I interject personal comments in the text, they will be bracketed thus: {just to be clear about this}. My words offer not expert testimony but experienced herbalist user testimony.

About The Research

Research Topics

About The Research

This chapter starts with my studied evaluation of the quality and productivity of the peer-review studies in this book. The researchers then weigh in on the current situation, and clarify some basic concepts of pathogenesis.

We should consider some severe limitations on these studies, and on the value of such studies in general:

- There are not enough of them.
- How peer-review research is designed
- How the studies were carried out
- The conclusions they arrived at

There are not enough of them

This book demonstrates that many Sidas are everywhere in the tropics and sub-tropics, with some species being world-wide. Everywhere they grow, they are used for medicinal purposes (See **Traditional Use**).

When I started to research this book, I went to Pub Med. This website run by our National Institutes for Health claims to cover all medical research in the world since the 1970s. It currently has over 15 million studies! But not much on Sida. The first problem in searching for Sida is that the French acronym for AIDS is SIDA, as well as being a term for "Stable Isotope Dilution Assay". So searching for "sida" was futile. So I had to search for individual Sidas: Sida acuta 30 studies. Sida cordifolia 42 studies, Sida rhombifolia 30 studies, other Sidas much less. I could not have written this book with only those studies. Fortunately there is another source for peer-review research that allowed me to collect most of the nearly 800 cited studies in this book, and that source is Google Scholar.

What was the difference? Google Scholar (https://scholar.google.com/) includes peer-review research done in India, Nigeria, Brazil, and many other "second world" universities and institutions. I have found this research to be adequate to excellent, but don't take my word for it - I have provided you with a path to all the source material in this book. Every claim made in this book is backed by peer-review research or other expert testimony.

"Google Scholar provides a simple way to broadly search for scholarly literature. From one place, you can search across many disciplines and sources: articles, theses, books, abstracts and court opinions, from academic publishers, professional societies, online repositories, universities and other web sites. Google Scholar helps you find relevant work across the world of scholarly research." Google scholar was implemented soon after Google was incorporated in 2004. **[google.com]**

Even with Google Scholar, nearly 800 citations is not that much for medicinal plants that have been used as medicinals everywhere in the tropics and sub-tropics from time-out-of-mind. Today Sidas are currently being used daily by millions (if not billions) of people. Sidas are five of the top Ayurvedic herbs, including the legendary "Bala". Many sidas are Ayurvedic rasayanas, the rejuvenating, adaptogenic herbs that restore strength. 800 studies is not nearly enough to fully validate all of this.

Almost all peer-review studies that demonstrate Sida's prowess against pathogens have occurred since 2000. We are trying to find replacements for pharmaceutical antibiotics, but are we too late? And are we really looking for any solution that works?

How peer-review research is designed

The pharmaceutical industry is trying, belatedly, to come up with new anti-pathogens. (antibiotics, anti-malarials, antifungals, etc.) Unfortunately most of the research is to find a particular super single compound, that can then be synthesized, patented, and then sold to the public for a lot of money. This has become a failed process in my opinion; any one compound will inevitably be figured out by the pathogens and one way or another neutralized, thus forever made useless.

The real search should be to identify the synergistic effects of the whole plant which the pathogens never figure out. We can then compound several powerful medicinal plants into effective and affordable medicine that stops all pathogens; medicine that the pathogens never figure out. Unfortunately most of the peer-review research is searching for the next big "bullet".

How the studies were carried out

Lab studies have limited validity. They are usually performed on rats (also mice, guinea pigs, rabbits, etc), because a rat's metabolism is close to ours (but not the same). These studies are also largely based on supra-normal concentrations of a single compound. The pathologic conditions that are studied in rats are often induced into healthy rats by other toxic substances, which is not the real condition, and so there is possible error there as well. This leaves some doubt about the applicability of these lab studies to humans. That is why in this book peer-review research is placed next to traditional practice. Correspondence of traditional uses (used successfully for thousands of years) to peer-review research on any given pathogen would alleviate much of my doubt.

Most of the studies have some structural flaws. First and foremost, most studies appear to have used distilled water in their experiments. Some of the most profound medical effects of Sidas come from the alkaloids. Acidic water best extracts alkaloids, so the results may not be as robust as they could be in those studies. Acidic water should always be used to maximally extract the alkaloids.

Second flaw, choice of extracts. Researchers have typically used the solvent that extracts the most of the single element they want to study. This can be methanol, acetone, chloroform, n-hexane, and other high tech methods. While this provides valuable information, these solvents are beyond community use, and are toxic. Most researchers in these studies use methanol, which extracts the most of a given compound; but methanol is toxic to ingest and cannot be consumed. So methanol is a poor choice for those who actually need to use Sida as a medicine, and there are better alternatives.

After being immersed in Sida research for the last four years I personally think the ethanol and hot water extracts are often are as effective, or at least in the same ball park, as any and all of the exotic extraction methods. The public, and especially natural healers, want results from either water or alcohol extraction - results which can be easily replicated. This would allow us to make our own Sida extracts. I have been making ethanolic Sida acuta extracts for three years now. The studies in this book and my experience say they compete well with the other extracts.

It is ultimately up to you dear reader to decide – I have provided you with all the available data. I would settle for less yield or strength for a non-toxic extraction. Most of the world simply uses a hot water extract – a tea. There are some excellent whole herb studies that are part of this book.

The conclusions they arrived at

By extracting and concentrating a single compound, and then testing it against pathogens, researchers get results based upon higher than natural concentrations, which might be difficult to replicate in everyday use by natural healers. The conclusions are absent any benefits from other plant constituents. The results from a single compound is actually a small part of what the plant can presumably offer.

A single compound's success is inherently limited by how fast pathogens can neutralize its effects. Ultimately any single compound has quite limited use. I refer you to the first two chapters of Buhner's pioneering book, *Herbal Antibiotics: Natural Alternatives for Treating Drug-Resistant Bacteria* : "The End of Antibiotics", and "The Resistant Organisms, the Diseases They Cause, and How to Treat Them." These two chapters present a terrifying case for all pharmaceutical antibiotics (which are essentially single ingredients) becoming essentially useless in the next few years. Using multiple pharmaceutical antibiotics at once has bought us a bit more time but the outcome seems to be the same.

Despite these limitations, I am grateful to have access to so many full research papers, and you should be as well. They do give me as an herbalist useful information that I need (although very spotty): parts of the plant tested, what solvents and other compounds are employed in this process, and what the quantitative and qualitative results are. There is often a toxicity study. Some studies look to find an effectiveness in natural concentrations, and a section in

Sida Actions is dedicated to the effectiveness of Sida compounds compared to standard pharmaceuticals (**Sida actions/Relations with pharmaceutical medicines**). There may be caveats about the process of these studies, and some reservations about the results, but in the end there is a lot of very useful information in these studies.

A World Desperate for Antibiotics

Even though pharmacological industries have produced a number of new antibiotics in the last three decades, resistance to these drugs in microorganisms has gradually increased. In general, bacteria have the genetic ability to transmit and acquire resistance to drugs, which are utilized frequently as therapeutic agents. This fact is the cause for concern, as numbers of patients are not responding positively towards existing antibiotics. Further emerging new multi-resistant bacterial strains, aggravate the problem. The problem of microbial resistance is continuously growing hence the use of existing antimicrobial drugs in future is still uncertain. Therefore, immediate action is required to combat the problem, by encouraging research to develop new drugs; more so of herbal origin as synthetic drugs are known to cause side effects. **[221-2012]**

July 7, 2017 WHO warns of imminent spread of untreatable superbug gonorrhoea: Manica Balasegaram, director of the Global Antibiotic Research and Development Partnership, said the situation was "grim" and there was a "pressing need" for new medicines. The pipeline, however, is very thin, with only three potential new gonorrhoea drugs in development and no guarantee any will prove effective in final-stage trials, he said... from 2009 to 2014 there was widespread resistance to the first-line medicine ciprofloxacin, increasing resistance to another antibiotic drugs called azithromycin, and the emergence of resistance to last-resort treatments known as extended-spectrum cephalosporins (ESCs). In most countries, it said, ESCs are now the only single antibiotics that remain effective for treating gonorrhoea. Yet resistance to them has already been reported in 50 countries... "We urgently need to seize the opportunities we have with existing drugs and candidates in the pipeline," he told reporters. "Any new treatment developed should be accessible to everyone who needs it, while ensuring it is used appropriately, so that drug resistance is slowed as much as possible." {Ayurveda medicine has used Sidas to treat gonorrhea and other venereal diseases for thousands of years.} **[742-2017]**

To date, MCR-1 has been detected in five human isolates in the United States. The US Centers for Disease Control and Prevention says it has increased surveillance for the gene in healthcare settings. Two studies today in The Lancet Infectious Diseases indicate that a gene that can confer resistance to the last-resort antibiotic colistin has spread widely in clinical settings in China. The gene, known as MCR-1, was first identified in China in November 2015 in Escherichia coli samples from pigs, pork products, and a handful of human cases. It has since been detected in more than 30 countries, including the United States. The emergence of the resistance gene was believed to be connected to widespread use of colistin in Chinese agriculture. China banned use of the drug in animal feed in 2016, based in part on the findings of that study. Though there have been few cases so far of human infections involving the gene—which has mostly been found in animals—MCR-1 has become a significant public health concern because colistin is one of the few antibiotics left that can be used to treat multidrug-resistant infections. And because the gene is carried on mobile pieces of DNA called plasmids, it can be passed not only to different strains within a single family of bacteria—such as E coli—but also to different types of bacteria. Among the most worrisome scenarios is the emergence of bacteria that harbors the MCR-1 gene along with other antibiotic-resistance genes. If the superbug carbapenem-resistant Enterobacteriaceae (CRE) were to acquire the gene, for example, it could present clinicians with infections that are nearly impossible to treat with current antibiotics." **"Therefore, at this stage we can conclude that the doomsday scenario of convergence of carbapenem resistance and colistin resistance (via MCR-1) has not yet occurred to any great extent in China."** [618-2017]

Infection due to ESBL-producing E. coli and Klebsiella species continue to increase in frequency and severity... a recent single-center study showed that blood stream infection due to an ESBL-producing organism was an independent predictor of mortality, prolonged length of stay, delay in initiation of appropriate antimicrobial therapy, and increased hospitalization costs. In a meta-analysis of 16 studies reported for 1996–2003, ESBL-producing BSI was significantly associated with delayed initiation of effective therapy and increased crude mortality. **[456-2009]**

There is a wide range of medicinal plant parts possessing a variety of pharmacological activities, such as flowers, leaves, barks, stems, fruits and roots extracts which are used as powerful raw drug. Recently there is a widespread interest of plants derived drugs which reflect its recognition of the validity of many traditional claims regarding the value of natural products in health care. For the quality control of traditional medicine phytochemical screening is mainly applied. Nowadays, secondary plant metabolites previously with unknown pharmacological activities have been extensively investigated as a source of medicinal agents. Thus it is anticipated that phytochemicals with enough antibacterial efficacy will be used for the treatment of the bacterial infections. According to WHO, to obtain a variety of new herbal drugs, medicinal plants are the best sources. Therefore, in order to determine the potential use of herbal medicine, it is important to emphasize the study of medicinal plants that (are) found in folklore. **[106-2011]**

Numerous and diverse classes of natural products have been isolated and characterized in the past century... of the 877 New Chemical Entities introduced between 1981 and 2002, 49 % were inspired from natural products in some way or other. So far, of the estimated 400,000 higher plant species in the world, only about 10% have been characterized chemically to some extent. Therefore, the unexplored potential of plants as a source of novel bioactive chemicals is enormous... **Surprisingly, in the past few years most Big Pharma companies have either terminated or**

considerably scaled down their natural product operations. This occurs despite a significant number of natural product-derived drugs being ranked in the top 35 worldwide selling ethical drugs in 2000, 2001, and 2002; representing 40% of worldwide drug sales in 2000, 24% in 2001, and 26% in 2002. **[728-2008]**

Infectious diseases caused by fungi are still a major threat to public health, despite numerous efforts by researchers. Their impact is particularly large in developing countries due to the relative unavailability of medicines and the emergence of widespread drug resistance. Use of ethnopharmacological knowledge is one attractive way to reduce empiricism and enhance the probability of success in new drug-finding efforts. **[211-2012]**

The Solution

A considerable number of plant extracts and isolated compounds possess significant antimicrobial, anti-parasitic including antimalarial, anti-proliferative, anti-inflammatory, anti-diabetes, and antioxidant effects. Most of the biologically active compounds belong to terpenoids, phenolics, and alkaloids. **[64]**

In conclusion, the alkaloids displayed good antimicrobial activity against several test microorganisms. The GC-MS analysis of the same alkaloid extract revealed the presence of two major alkaloids; cryptolepine and quindoline. The results of the present study support the traditional medicinal use of S. acuta and suggest that a great attention should be paid to this plant which is found to have many pharmacological properties. **[7]**

The ethanol extract of Sida acuta exhibited a broad spectrum of antimicrobial activity ranging from gram positive to a few gram negative bacteria and common fungi. The water extract only worked against Bacillus subtilis. The other organic extracts (methanol, ethyl acetate,) exhibited moderate inhibitory activity against: Bacillus subtilis NCIM 2063, Staphylococcus aureus NCIM 3021, Escherichia coli NCIM 2066, Kebsiella pneumoniae NCIM 2957, Proteus vulgaris NCIM 2027, Candida albicans NCIM 3557, Aspergillus niger NCIM 1054, Strep faecalis. **[523]**

Research Topics

110

Polyphenolic compounds

Some previous studies showed that polyphenolic compounds cause inhibition of a wide range of microorganisms. Phenol is well known as a chemical antiseptic. In addition, Phenolic and terpenic antimicrobial activities are well documented. Polyphenols, such as tannins and flavonoids, are important antibacterial activity. The antimicrobial activity of flavonoids is due to their ability to complex with extracellular and soluble protein and to complex with bacterial cell wall while that of tannins may be related to their ability to inactivate microbial adhesions, enzymes and cell envelop proteins. [11]

The presence of flavonoids, phenolics in plants has been shown to be responsible for antimicrobial activity in plants. Their role is to protect plants against microbial or insect damage. [499]

Antibiotic Resistance

Antibiotic resistance is the ability of a microorganism to withstand the effects of an antibiotic. It is a specific type of drug resistance. Antibiotic resistance evolves naturally via natural selection through random mutation, but it could also be engineered by applying an evolutionary stress on a population. Once such a gene is generated, bacteria can then transfer the genetic information in a horizontal fashion (between individuals) by plasmid exchange. The patterns of antibiotic usage greatly affect the number of resistant organisms which develop. Overuse of broad spectrum antibiotics, such as second and third generation greatly hastens the development of resistance. [556]

The problem of microbial resistance is continuously growing hence the use of existing antimicrobial drugs in future is still uncertain. Therefore, immediate action is required to combat the problem, by encouraging research to develop new drugs; more so of herbal origin as synthetic drugs are known to cause side effects. The ultimate goal is to offer appropriate and efficient antimicrobial and present study is an effort in this direction. [221-2012]

The resistance problem demands that a renewed effort be made to seek antibacterial agents effective against pathogenic bacteria resistant to current antibiotics... One of the possible strategies towards this objective is the rational localization of bioactive phytochemicals. Plants have a limitless ability to synthesize aromatic substances, most of which are phenols or their oxygen substituted derivatives such as tannins. Many of the herbs and spices used by humans to season food yield have useful medicinal compounds including those having antibacterial activity. [499-2013]

Gram Negative Bacteria

Generally therefore, Gram-negative bacteria are more resistant than Gram-positive bacteria because of the complexity of the cell wall of Gram negative bacteria...(there is an) extra outer membrane in their cell wall acting as a barrier for the compound(s) to diffuse into the bacterial cells [499-2013]

111

Since 2002, the Infectious Diseases Society of America (IDSA) has voiced concern with the absence of progress in developing novel therapeutics to treat multidrug-resistant (MDR) infections, including those caused by gram negative bacteria. In our 2009 report, no antibacterial agent in development with a purely gram-negative spectrum had reached phase 2 of clinical study. The need for new agents to treat infections caused by gram negative bacteria resistant to currently available agents is even more urgent than at the time of our 2009 report. Furthermore, the withdrawal of several large pharmaceutical companies from antibacterial research and development (R&D) has compromised the infrastructure for discovering and developing new antimicrobials, especially in the United States. [617-2013]

Several highly resistant gram-negative pathogens—namely Acinetobacter species, multidrug-resistant (MDR) P. aeruginosa, and carbapenem-resistant Klebsiella species and Escherichia coli—are emerging as significant pathogens in both the United States and other parts of the world. Our thera-peutic options for these pathogens are so extremely limited that clinicians are forced to use older, previously discarded drugs, such as colistin, that are associated with significant toxicity and for which there is a lack of robust data to guide selection of dosage regimen or duration of therapy. The growing number of elderly patients and patients undergoing surgery, transplantation, and chemotherapy and dramatic increases in population in neonatal intensive care units will produce an even greater number of immunocompromised individuals at risk of these infections... None of these agents addresses the growing need created by the emergence of carbapenemases. We found no antibacterial drugs with a pure gram-negative spectrum that have reached phase 2 development. [456-2009]

The plant antibiotic substances appear to be more inhibitory to Gram-positive organisms than to the Gram-negative type. It may be remembered that penicillin and some of the other prominent antibiotic agents of fungal origin are also rather selective in their inhibitory action, most of them being inhibitory to Gram-positive organisms. Unlike Gram-positive bacteria, the lipopolysaccharide layer along with proteins and phosholipids are the major components in the outer surface of Gram-negative bacteria. Access of most compounds to the peptidoglycan layer of the cell wall is hindered by the outer lipopolysaccharide layer. This explains the resistance of Gram negative strains to the lytic action of most extracts exhibiting activity. [450-2006]

Sida cordifolia zones of inhibition

pathogen	methanolic	acqueous	Ciprofloxacin
Staphylococcus aureus	17	13	29
Enterococcus faecalis	0	14	24
Proteus mirabilis	15	12	29
Pseudomonas aeruginosa	15	16	20
Candida albicans	0	20	25
Cryptococcus neoformans	0	20	20
(2 mg extract- Ciprofloxacin 5mcg)	[125]		

Cytotoxicity

Cytotoxicity is the nature of being harmful to cells. Cells presented to a cytotoxic compound can react in various ways. The cells may undergo necrosis, in which they lose membrane integrity and die rapidly as a result of cell lysis; they can stop growing and dividing; or they can activate a genetic program of controlled cell death, termed apoptosis...Cytotoxicity assays are used widely in drug discovery research to help predict which lead compounds might have safety concerns in humans before significant time and expense are incurred in their development. Other researchers study mechanisms of cytotoxicity as a way to gain a better understanding of the normal and abnormal biological processes that control cell growth, division, and death. **[649]**

Sida rhombifolia-invitro-aerial parts-80% ethanol extract- In brine shrimp lethality bioassay, the extract showed lethality against the brine shrimp nauplii. It showed different mortality rate at different concentrations. From the plot of percent mortality versus log concentration on the graph paper LC50 and LC90 were deduced (LC50 = 40 µg/ml; LC90 = 80 µg/ml). **[545]**

Sida acuta-invitro-leaves, seeds, stems and bark-methanol extract-promising cytotoxic activity against 5 of 6 human carcinoma cell lines--against one cancer cell line (BT-549), Sida acuta showed between 83% - 91% at 20 µg/ml. **[95]** ..... Five medicinal plants widely used in cancer treatment, Sida acuta, Sida cordifolia, Sida rhombifolia, Urena lobata, Viscum album, were recently screened for their cytoxicity against Hep G2 hepatocarcinoma cells rather showed moderate anti-proliferative effects. **[64]** Sida indica-invitro-leaves-cold distilled water extract- The Zn nanoparticles synthesized using *Sida indica*, showed positive results for cytotoxic activity with an IC50 value of 45.82 µg/ml. These positive results confirmed the cytotoxic potential of the Zn nanoparticles against cervical cancer. Thus Zn nanoparticles can be used as a potent drug in alternative therapy for treating the cervical cancer patients in the near future. **[683]**

Medical Nanoparticles

Nanoparticles can be synthesized by chemical processes like pyrolysis, hydrothermal method, chemical precipitation etc. But these chemical processes cause pollution and are costly practices...However using "green" methods in the synthesis of Zinc nanoparticles has increasingly become a topic of interest. Nanoparticles in recent days have revolutionized the modern medicinal practices because of their potential activities in treatment of various diseases. Plants have been used from centuries to treat various human diseases. Herbal drugs as compared to synthetic drugs have no or lesser side effects and are less expensive. Since plant mediated synthesis is easy and safe with one-step protocol and don't involve the use of harsh solvents or surfactant as the reducing agents, studies have suggested their use to be more ideal and compatible for their use in nanomedicine because of their stability in various biological media. The biomolecules present in plants mediates the synthesis of nanoparticles and also stabilize the nanoparticles formed with desired size and shape as well play a role in reducing the ions to the nanosize, and in the capping of nanoparticles. **[683-2016]**

The metallic nanoparticles whose synthesis involves natural products derived from plants are found to be biocompatible. Thus such metallic nanoparticles could be suitable candidates for safe delivery of drugs, molecular imaging and biomedical diagnostics. Among the available varieties of nano-materials, gold nanoparticles possess some unique characteristics: small size, good biocompatibility, low toxicity, simple surface chemistry and easy surface modification. These characteristic features of the gold nanoparticles make them promising candidates for biomedical use and such gold nanoparticles have been used for various biological applications such as biosensors and as drug delivery vectors for cancer chemotherapy and radiotherapy. **[674-2016]**

Inflammation

Inflammation is a pathophysiological response of living tissue to injury that leads to local accumulation of plasmatic fluid and blood cells. Although it is a defense mechanism that helps body to protect itself against infection, burns, toxic chemicals, allergens or other noxious stimuli. The complex events and mediators involved in the inflammatory reaction can induce, maintain or aggravate many diseases... Anti-inflammatory agents have been traditionally evaluated by studying their effects on inflammation produced in animals by injecting foreign or noxious agents. **[537]**

Inflammation (Latin, inflammare, to set on fire) is part of the complex biological response of vascular tissues to harmful stimuli, such as pathogens, damaged cells, or irritants. Inflammation is a protective attempt by the organism to remove the injurious stimuli and to initiate the healing process. Inflammation is one of the responses of the organism to the pathogen as infection is caused by various microorganisms. Inflammation is some of the most common manifestations of many diseases afflicting millions of people worldwide. Although there are number treatment available for inflammation, but yet is not satisfying the need of patients suffering from disease. Recently there is vast prevalence of the disease due to the continuous change in life style of people.... Despite the progress made in medical research during the past decades, the treatment of many serious diseases is still problematic. Inflammatory diseases remain one of the world's major health problems. It involves a complex array of enzyme activation, mediator release, and extravasations of fluid, cell migration, tissue breakdown and repair. **Inflammation has become the focus of global scientific research because of its implication in virtually all human and animal diseases.** The efficacy of plant-based drugs used in the traditional medicine have been paid great attention because they are cheap, have little side effects and according to WHO still about 80% of the world population rely mainly on plant-based drugs. **[551]**

Inflammation is a local response of living mammalian tissues to injury. It is a body defense reaction in order to eliminate or limit the spread of injurious agent. There are various components to an inflammatory reaction that can

114

contribute to the associated symptoms and tissue injury... **Aging is also considered to be inflammatory response**.... Currently available anti-inflammatory agents are associated with unwanted side effects and have their own limitations. About 34-46% of the users of NSAIDs usually sustain some gastrointestinal damage due to the inhibition of the protective cyclo-oxygenase enzyme in gastric mucosa. Therefore, new anti-inflammatory and analgesic drugs lacking these side effects are being researched as alternatives to NSAID and opiates. Attention is being focused on the investigation of the efficacy of plant based drugs used in the traditional medicine because they are cheap, have little side effects and according to WHO, about 80% of world population still rely mainly on herbal remedies. [186]

The present study revealed that *Sida cordifolia* has mild to moderate antiinflammatory activity. The activity of the ethyl acetate (EA) extract of root at a dose of 600 mg/kg is equivalent to that of indomethacin and exhibited no ulcerogenicity indicating its safety on the gastrointestinal tract (data not shown). A drug having good anti-inflammatory activity with lesser or negligible ulcerogenicity is preferable for treating chronic disease related to inflammation. Interestingly the extracts showed very good peripheral and central analgesic activity as evident from the writhing and hot plate tests. [285]

Oxidative stress

In a healthy body prooxidants and antioxidants maintain a ratio and a shift in this ratio towards prooxidants gives rise to oxidative stress. This oxidative stress may be either mild or severe depending on the extent of shift. This causes several diseases such as cardiovascular diseases, neurological diseases, renal diseases, diabetes, skin diseases, ageing, respiratory diseases and inflammatory problems. Over 70 degenerative diseases are due to oxidative stress. These free radicals are produced from two important sources, cellular metabolism and environmental sources. [200-2015]

It is reported that many diseases such as brain dysfunction, cancer, heart diseases and immune decline could be the result of free radicals... In physiological conditions, the human body can compensate for a mild degree of oxidant stress and remove oxydatively damaged molecules by activating antioxidant enzymes like super oxide dismutase, catalase, gluthation peroxidase etc. Oxidative stress is a state of imbalance between the level of antioxidant defense system and the production of oxygen-derivatives. Thus antioxidants have been of interest to pharmacologists, biochemists and other health professionals because they are supposed to reduce oxidative damages. Antioxidants are compounds that can delay or inhibit lipid oxidation or oxidation chain reaction propagation. Nowadays, there is a great interest in replacing synthetic antioxidants with natural ingredients because of the concern over the possible carcinogenic effects of synthetic antioxidants in foods... Except for a few examples, the majority of studies always stop after the active compound is identified or the crude extract shown to be active. [215-2007]

There is a linear correlation between antioxidant capacities and reducing power of plant extracts. The reducing properties are generally related to the presence of reductones, which have been shown to exert antioxidant action by breaking the free radical chain through donating a hydrogen atom and may have great relevance in the prevention and treatment of diseases associated with oxidants or free radicals. [24]

Free radical stress leads to tissue injury and progression of disease conditions such as arthritis, hemorrhagic shock, atherosclerosis, diabetes, hepatic injury, aging and ischemia, reperfusion injury of many tissues, gastritis, tumor promotion, neurodegenerative diseases and carcinogenesis. Safer anti-oxidants suitable for long term use are needed to prevent or stop the progression of free radical mediated disorders. [127]

In the defense against oxidative stress, the antioxidant enzyme system of cells plays an important role. The primary antioxidative enzyme, superoxide dismutase (SOD) is among the most important antioxidative system parameters of the organism. [141]

Free radicals and other reactive oxygen species are considered to be important causative factors in the development of diseases of aging such as neurodegenerative diseases, cancer and cardiovascular diseases. Free radicals play a crucial role in a complex interplay of different mechanisms in both normal aging and neurodegenerative diseases... Free radicals and other reactive oxygen species, collectively known as ROS, are generated continuously via normal physiological processes, more so in pathological conditions. They are simultaneously degraded to non-reactive forms by enzymatic and non-enzymatic antioxidant defense mechanisms. [123]

Reactive oxygen species (ROS), such as superoxide radicals, hydroxyl (OH) radicals and peroxyl radicals, are natural byproducts of the normal metabolism of oxygen in living organisms with important roles in cell signaling. However, excessive amounts of ROS may be a primary cause of biomolecular oxidation and may result in significant damage to cell structure, contributing to various diseases, such as cancer, stroke, diabetes and degenerative processes associated with ageing. Thus, antioxidants are important inhibitors of lipid peroxidation not only for food protection but also as a defense mechanism of living cells against oxidative damage... Plant polyphenols with antioxidant capacity could scavenge reactive chemical species as well as minimize oxidative damage resulting from excessive light exposure. Some plant polyphenols are important components of both human and animal diets and they are safe to be consumed... Natural antioxidants are known to exhibit a wide range of biological effects including antibacterial, antiviral, antiinflammatory, anti-allergic, antithrombotic and vasodilatory activities. [195]

Even though almost all organisms possess antioxidants and several enzyme systems like superoxide dismutase, catalase, glutathione peroxidase and glutathione reductase to protect them from oxidative damage, these systems are inadequate to prevent the damage entirely. Hence antioxidant supplements or foods containing high concentrations of antioxidants are needed which may help scavenge free radicals and reduce oxidative damage. Currently available synthetic antioxidants including Butylated hydroxytoluene (BHT), Butylated hydroxyanisole (BHA), Gallic acid, etc., have been found to cause negative health effects. Hence, their application has been restricted and there is a trend to substitute them with naturally occurring antioxidants. Since several methods exist for the in vitro determination of antioxidant capacity, it becomes necessary to select the right method that can give accurate results for the antioxidants in study. The three spectrophotometric methods selected were (1, 1-diphenyl-2-picrylhydrazyl) free radical scavenging activity assay (DPPH), [2,2'-azinobis(3-ethylbenzothiazoline-6-sulphonic acid)] free radical scavenging activity assay (ABTS) and Ferric ion Reducing Antioxidant Power assay (FRAP).

Comparison between Antioxidant Assays

All the three methods used (DPPH, ABTS, FRAP) for the evaluation of antioxidant activity of aqueous extract of the three mushroom species were spectrophotometric methods.

1) DPPH Assay: DPPH is one of the few stable and commercially available organic nitrogen radicals. It is one of the most widely reported methods for the determination of antioxidant activity. DPPH is not a very tedious assay in terms of preparation of chemicals and also in terms of performing the assay and hence can be used for its operational simplicity. In the present study, the antioxidant activity of each sample was measured three times to test the reproducibility of the assay. DPPH showed high reproducibility. The only disadvantage of this assay is that it is not very cost effective and is not suitable for measuring the antioxidant capacity of plasma, because proteins are precipitated in the alcoholic reaction medium.

2) ABTS Assay: The ABTS assay uses ABTS radicals preformed by oxidation of ABTS with potassium persulphate. Thus, this assay becomes time consuming in terms of waiting for the ABTS radicals to be generated as it takes around 12-16 hours for the reaction of ABTS with potassium persulphate, unlike the DPPH assay where one does not have to wait for it to be generated. However, once the radicals are generated, it is a very simple assay in terms of performing the assay. The ABTS radical is soluble in water and organic solvents, enabling the determination of antioxidant capacity of both hydrophilic and lipophilic compounds/samples. One major drawback of this assay is that the radicals formed are not very stable and the results are not reproducible. Nevertheless, this assay is also widely reported for the measurement of antioxidant activity.

3) FRAP Assay: The FRAP assay is more tedious and time consuming in terms of preparing the chemicals of the working solution. It is a simple and inexpensive method and does not require the use of any exclusive chemicals. The results obtained in FRAP are found to be reproducible for all the concentrations. Hence, FRAP is a suitable method for the determination of antioxidant activity. In one study done by Katalinic et al., in 2006, they suggested that from the methodological point of view, the DPPH method is easy and accurate with regard to measuring the antioxidant activity of the extracts and also the results are highly reproducible and comparable to other antioxidant methods such as ABTS. In another study done by Thaipong et al.,

in 2006 for estimating antioxidant activity from guava fruit extracts, they concluded that the FRAP assay showed high reproducibility, was simple and could be rapidly performed. **[760]**

Antioxidant

An antioxidant causes prevention or slowing the oxidation reactions of other molecules. An oxidation reaction produces free radicals which start chain reactions that damage cells. Antioxidants being oxidized themselves, causes termination of these chain reactions by removing free radical intermediates. As a result, antioxidants are often reducing agents such as thiols, ascorbic acid or polyphenols. **[677]**

Medicinal plants are largely used either for the prevention, or for the curative treatment of several diseases. **Among the properties behind these virtues, the antioxidant activity holds the first place. [27]**

A lot of research is are going on worldwide directed towards finding natural antioxidants of plants origins... Active research has been driven in recent years on plant components due to their biologically beneficial effects emanating from antioxidant activities of phenolic phytochemicals. The antioxidant activity is mainly due to the presence of phytochemicals such as phenolics, flavonoids and anthocyanins.... It is well known that plant produce these metabolites to protect itself but recent research demonstrates that different phytochemicals have various protective and therapeutic effects which are essential to prevent diseases and maintain a state of well being... Phenolic compounds are naturally occurring secondary metabolites that are of great pharmacological interest.... Researchers and food manufacturers have become more interested in polyphenols due to their potent antioxidant properties, their abundance in the diet, and their credible effects in the prevention of various oxidative stress associated diseases. **[200]**

However, the use of synthetic antioxidants has been debated due to their toxic and carcinogenic effects, which can result in liver damage, so the discovery of new, reliable and harmless antioxidants from natural resources has become a prominent research topic. **[686]**

An antioxidant causes prevention or slowing the oxidation reactions of other molecules. An oxidation reaction produces free radicals which start chain reactions that damage cells. Antioxidants being oxidized themselves, causes termination of these chain reactions by removing free radical intermediates. As a result, antioxidants are often reducing agents such as thiols, ascorbic acid or polyphenols. Natural antioxidants in plants like vitamin C, vitamin E and polyphenols scavenges free radicals which can cause several diseases including diabetes, cancer, cataracts, cardiovascular diseases, arthritis, atherosclerosis and ageing. **[677]**

Although aerobic metabolism is efficient, the presence of oxygen in cellular environment possesses a constant oxidative threat to cellular structures and processes. In fact, the evolution of oxygen dependent metabolic processes such as aerobic respiration, photosynthesis and photorespiration unavoid-

118

ably leads to the production of reactive oxygen species (ROS) in mitochondria... with the resultant generation of highly toxic ROS... In a normal plant cell the generation of prooxidants in the form of ROS is delicately balanced by antioxidative defense systems. Exposure of plant cells to prooxidants results in oxidative stresses that shifts the balance in favor of prooxidants. The reactive oxygen species capable of causing oxidative damage include superoxide... The manifestation of this state of cell that leads to the generation and subsequent accumulation of ROS ranges from membrane damage, metabolic impairment to genomic lesions, associated with ageing that senescence of plant cells... Lipid peroxidation is commonly used as an indicator of oxidative damage by free radical accumulation in plants... **[Reactive Oxygen Species and Antioxidants in Higher Plants (book), S. Dutta Gupta, CRC Press, Sep 15, 2010 - 384 pages]**

Free radicals

Natural antioxidants present in the plants scavenge harmful free radicals from our body. Free radical is any species capable of independent existence that contains one or more unpaired electrons which reacts with other molecule by taking or giving electrons and involved in many pathological conditions. It is possible to reduce the risk of chronic diseases and prevent disease progression by either enhancing the body's natural antioxidant defenses or by supplementing with proven dietary antioxidants.... Most sources of natural antioxidants originate from plant materials. **[433]**

Free radicals are fundamental to any biochemical process and represent an essential part of aerobic life and metabolism. Various metabolic processes, UV radiations, smoke etc, trigger the production of free radicals.... excessive production of free radicals leads to oxidative stress... Recent evidences suggested that involvement of oxidative stress in the pathogenesis of various diseases and had attracted much attention of scientists and general public on the role of antioxidants in the maintenance of human health and prevention and treatment of diseases. Free radical reactions have been implicated in the pathology of many human diseases like atherosclerosis, ischemic heart disease, diabetes and neurodegenerative disease etc., and disease conditions like ageing process, inflammation, immunosuppresion, etc. A number of plants and plant isolates have been reported to protect free radical induced damage in various experimental models. **[653-2016]**

Many forms of cancer are thought to be the result of reactions between free radicals and DNA, resulting in mutations that can adversely affect the cell cycle and potentially lead to malignancy. Some of the symptoms of aging such as atherosclerosis are also attributed to free-radical induced oxidation of many of the chemicals making up the body. In addition free radicals contribute to alcohol-induced liver damage, perhaps more than alcohol itself. **[115]**

The aim of this research is to determine DPPH, nitric oxide, hydroxyl and hydrogen peroxide scavenging activity. The Gallic acid was used as standard. In all tests inhibition percentages increased with increasing concentrations of the extracts. The chloroform extract was somewhat stronger than the alcoholic extract in all tests. Sida acuta shows good activity in all the tested methods at 100µg/ml concentration...Phenolic content shows good scavenging of all the tested methods at 100µg/ml concentration, when compared to that of whole extracts...The results of free radical scavenging activity showed that the leaves have significant antioxidant activity... had comparably more nitric oxide scavenging activity, and hydrogen peroxide scavenging activity, than Gallic acid... The leaf extract had strong hydroxyl scavenging activity. [653]

Free radical stress leads to tissue injury and progression of disease conditions such as arthritis, hemorrhagic shock, atherosclerosis, diabetes, hepatic injury, aging and ischemia, reperfusion injury of many tissues, gastritis, tumor promotion, neurodegenerative diseases and carcinogenesis. Safer anti-oxidants suitable for long term use are needed to prevent or stop the progression of free radical mediated disorders. [46-2012]

Reactive oxygen species (ROS) such as superoxide (O_2 -), hydroxyl radicals (OH-) and hydrogen peroxide (H_2O_2-) form an important factor in the etiology of several pathological conditions such as Alzheimer's disease. Parkinsons's disease, arthritis, hemorrhoids, rheumatism, heart attack, AIDS, immune system and disorders, cataract, stroke, cancer stress, varicose veins, hepatitis, diabetes and several degenerative diseases including aging. ROS are degraded to non-reactive forms by enzymatic and non-enzymatic antioxidant defense mechanisms. [461]

Superoxide is biologically quite toxic and is deployed by the immune system to kill invading microorganisms... Superoxide is also deleterious when produced as a byproduct of mitochondrial respiration... Because superoxide is toxic, nearly all organisms living in the presence of oxygen contain isoforms of the superoxide-scavenging enzyme superoxide dismutase, or SOD. SOD is an extremely efficient enzyme; it catalyzes the neutralization of superoxide nearly as quickly as the two can diffuse together spontaneously in solution... Absence of cytosolic SOD causes a dramatic increase in muta-genesis and genomic instability... Superoxide may contribute to the patho-genesis of many diseases (the evidence is particularly strong for radiation poisoning and hyperoxic injury), and perhaps also to aging via the oxidative damage that it inflicts on cells. [1]

Increasing evidence has implicated free radical mechanism in the initiation of carcinogenesis... Reactive oxygen species (ROS) have damaging effects upon the cells due to peroxidation of unsaturated lipids in biological membranes, interactions with DNA, or attack on enzymes and proteins. Cell and tissue destruction leads to more lipid peroxidation because antioxidants are diluted out and transition metal ions that stimulate the peroxidation process are released from the disrupted cells. This increase in lipid conjugated dienes and hydroperoxides was counteracted significantly on treatment with seed extract administration. [464]

(Research title: Anti-inflammatory and anti-oxidant proprties of Sida rhom-bifolia stems and roots in adjuvant induced arthritic rats) Free radicals prime the immune response and recruit inflammatory cells and are innately bactericidal. Some of these free radicals play positive roles in vivo such as energy production, phagocytosis, regulation of cell growth and intercellular signaling or synthesis of biologically important compounds.... The most commonly prescribed medication for rheumatoid arthritis treatment is steroidal, non-steroidal anti-inflammatory, disease modifying anti-rheumatic and immunosuppressant drugs. Though the goal of these drugs has been to relieve pain and to decrease joint inflammation, to prevent joint destruction and to restore function of disabled joints, these drugs are known to produce various side effects including gastrointestinal disorders, immunodeficiency and humoral disturbances. Accordingly, reducing side effects should be considered while designing improved therapeutics for rheumatoid arthritis, besides enhancing medicinal effectiveness. [127]

Cryptolepine

Cryptolepine is but one of the indoloquinoline alkaloids in the Sidas, but it has been relatively well researched. The results below are probably indicative of what the other indoloquinoline alkaloids can do. The other known indoloquinoline alkaloids include: cryptolepinone, berberine (Sida acuta), quindoline, vascicine, and many others less studied, for a total of 13 found in the Sidas so far. This does not include other types of alkaloids such as ephedrine. See the **Constituents** section for a listing of all known constituents in the Sida family.

Phytochemicals exert their antimicrobial activity through different mechanisms, tannins for example act by iron deprivation, hydrogen bounding or non specific interactions with vital proteins such as enzymes. In the case of indoloquinoline alkaloids the mechanism remains unclear. Sawer et al. (2005) demonstrated that the main indoloquinoline alkaloid, cryptolepine, causes cell lysis and morphological changes of *S. aureus*, but the antimicrobial effects of the alkaloid may be through another mechanism, since the compound is known to be a DNA intercalator and an inhibitor of DNA synthesis through topoisomerase inhibition. [7]

Considerable interest in this family (indoloquinoline alkaloids) has been shown by several teams throughout the world due to their various and important biological properties such as: antimuscarinic, antibacterial, antiviral, antiplasmodial, and antihyperglycemic activities. Recently, two reports mentioned the cytotoxicity of cryptolepine and analogues toward B16 melanoma cells20 and M109 Madison lung carcinoma. Bonjean et al. also showed that cryptolepine interferes with topoisomerase II and primarily inhibits DNA synthesis. Moreover, some quindoline derivatives have been described as potent antitumor-active compounds. [295]

Cryptolepine presents a large spectrum of biological properties. [582]   The activity of cryptolepine hydrochloride... was assessed against the fast growing mycobacterial species Mycobacterium fortuitum, which has recently been shown to be of use in the evaluation of antitubercular drugs. The low minimum inhibitory concentration (MIC) of this compound (16 µg/mL) prompted further evaluation against other fast growing mycobacteria namely, M. phlei, M. aurum, M. smegmatis, M. bovis BCG and M. abcessus and the MICs ranged over 2–32 µg/mL for these species. The strong activity of this agent, the need for new antibiotics with activity against Mycobacterium tuberculosis, coupled with the ethnobotanical use of C. sanguinolenta extracts to treat infections, highlight the potential of the cryptolepine template for development of antimycobacterial agents. **[383]**

Cryptolepine possesses bacteriostatic and bactericidal actions. Both phenomena occur in the initial stages of drug-bacteria reaction, but the bactericidal action predominates in subsequent stages. **[383]** Lysis to staphylococcal cells was observed following exposure to cryptolepine and this coincided with sharp falls in viable counts of the bacteria. There was the formation of deformed cells as depicted in the SEM photomicrographs of S. aureus cells after 3, 6 or 24 h exposure to inhibitory concentrations of cryptolepine. **[240]** These results were consistent with findings using scanning electron microscopy. Exposure of cells to biocidal concentrations of cryptolepine produced filamentation prior to lysis in E. coli NCTC 10418 and extreme disturbance of surface structure, including partial and total collapse, followed by lysis in C. albicans ATCC 10231 and S. cerevisiae NCPF 3139. **[385]**

Cryptolepine, a naturally occurring indoloquinoline alkaloid used as an antimalarial drug in Central and Western Africa, has been found to bind to DNA in a formerly unknown intercalation mode...a basis for the design of new anticancer drugs. **[244]** **Cryptolepine activity was essentially unaffected by established mechanisms of drug resistance**. In conclusion, cryptolepine shows interesting in vitro cytotoxic properties and its further evaluation as an anti-cancer drug seems warranted. **[399]** The poisoning effect (of) B16 melanoma cells is more pronounced with cryptolepine than its analogues. Cryptolepine-treated cells probably die via necrosis rather than via apoptosis. **[308]** This study has also led to the discovery that cryptolepine is a potent topoisomerase II inhibitor and a promising antitumor agent. Altogether, the results provide direct evidence that DNA is the primary target of cryptolepine and suggest that this alkaloid is a valid candidate for the development of tumor-active compounds. Cryptolepine easily crosses the cell membranes and accumulates selectively into the nuclei rather than in the cytoplasm of B16 melanoma cells. **[380]**

The Perfect Cup of Tea

Many thanks to Indigo Herbs of Glastonbury [379] for this information. They have a delightful website in England, carrying many things you wouldn't expect.

How to make a perfect herbal tea infusion.

The word 'tea' here is a bit of a misnomer. Tea in this context refers, not to camellia sinensis (who's various leaves are used to make black tea, green tea and white tea) but to what a herbalist would call an infusion, tisane or ptisan.

Making a herbal tea is effectively a method of extracting the active ingredients of a herb into an easy to digest form.

To make a perfect cup of herbal tea for one person, you will need a teapot or cafetiere, 750 ml of spring water (or filtered water will do) and enough top quality cut, dried herb depending on your herb of choice and how strong you want your tea to be.

1. Bring all the water to the boil

2. Add roughly a third of the water to your empty, clean teapot or cafetiere, replace the lid and allow the vessel to warm for a few moments.

3. Empty the teapot of its warming water and add the herbs. The amount you add will depend on which herbal tea you are making and how strong you want it but a good amount is usually about 2 heaped teaspoons.

4. Immediately pour over the remaining boiling water (make sure it is still boiling) and quickly and calmly put the lid on the teapot and cover with a tea cosy or other insulating cover.

5. Leave the tea for between 5 and 15 minutes allowing the herbs to infuse into the water.

6. Pour your delicious herbal tea into a clean cup, through a tea strainer and drink.

Larger volumes of herbal tea infusions can be stored for up to 3 days if kept covered and refrigerated. **[379]**

Product Longevity

Q. How long will my product last?

All of our products will have a best before date on the back of the pack when it is sent out. How long is on the product varies on the batch of the product. We do however guarantee the products will have the following time before they expire at a minimum when we send them to you:

Tinctures – 12 months minimum

Powders- 6 months minimum

Whole foods – 3 months minimum

Raw Chocolates – 3 weeks minimum

Tea Blends and loose teas – 6 months minimum

Oils blends and rollers – 6 months minimum

Essential Oils – 12 months minimum

In our experience however lots of our products have a much longer before they expire than these minimums. **[379]**

Prelude Medicinal Plants Database [370]

Royal Museum of Central Africa

http://www.africamuseum.be/collections/external/prelude/

The Royal Museum for Central Africa (RMCA) is known for being one of the world's most beautiful and impressive museums devoted to Africa. Since its founding in 1898, its task has been to preserve and manage collections, carry out scientific research, and disseminate knowledge to a wide audience through its scientific, educational, and museological activities.

Their Prelude database contains hundreds of references to the medical application of herbs. They have categorized nearly all human ailments into a table, and this is the reference for every herb in the database. From the home page Choose "Collections" from the top menu. Choose "External online collection" on the left, once there near the bottom is a hyperlink, "Consult the database Prelude." For example, Sida acuta has medicinal action in over 50 categories, with multiple entries for some.

The medical effects are in code like abbreviations, in another part of this website. The table that decodes these is accessed through their Practical Guide. Once there scroll to near the bottom for, "a list of abbreviations accessible by hyperlinks" Or jump to: Shttp://www.africamuseum.be/collections/external/prelude/browse_symptoms **[370]**

Sida Actions and Benefits

Methanolic root extracts (10% w/v) of Sida species, viz., S. acuta, S. cordata, S. cordifolia, S. indica, S. mysorensis, S. retusa, S. rhombifolia, and S. spinosa were analyzed... The high contents of phenolic compounds in the root extracts of selected Sida species have direct correlation with their antioxidant properties. Conclusively, roots of S. cordifolia can be considered as the potential source of polyphenols and antioxidants. **[15]**

In tropical Africa Sida species are used and traded at the local level only, for medicinal purposes. Chinese and Ayurvedic herbalists stock Sida rhombifolia plants and trade them through Internet. **[358]**

Sida plants have so much to offer! Certainly the anti-pathogen, anti-fungal, and anti-many-bad-things action is foremost. The 25%+ protein content in the leaves is important. They are also excellent fiber plants with extremely long fibers. There is literally no waste at harvest – every part has great value.

This chapter covers the many actions and benefits that are not directly linked to a pathogen. This chapter, like the whole book, is a compilation of known peer-review research and is not to be considered medical advice.

Personally, I value any documented Ayurvedic use most, because they have been using Sida medicinally for something like 2,000 years. Then I value peer-review, and a close third is (other than Ayurveda) traditional. Remember the scientific research is very incomplete; often only one substance from one species has been tested. My personal priority for the likelihood that a reported Sida benefit might benefit me: First would be Ayurvedic use or strong peer-review, second would be some peer-review and traditional use. I am merely presenting what valid information there is about the genus Sida, and you must decide its applicability to your life.

There is good evidence that the main medicinal species of Sida are generally interchangeable in their medicinal properties, even though they all have their specialties (Heck, each part of each species has its own specialties). The "major" Sidas have their own headings in the following listings. The occasional study of other species of Sida is usually lumped into Other Sidas.

Sida Benefits By Category

Trying to combine the actions and benefits from peer review, traditional, and Ayurvedic into one table was quite a challenge! Each approaches medicine in slightly different ways. My choice of category might very well not be yours, so check out other similar categories if you do not immediately find what you are looking for.

There are surprisingly few complete entries. Sometimes I can only work from the abstract of a research study which often is devoid of useful information. Full studies often omit important details like what part of the plant, or the working concentration. This hopefully will be corrected with future editions filling in many of the blanks. For now, much of this book is a general guide, a departure point crying for further experimentation, and most importantly, a validator of the many known actions and benefits of Sida.

Traditional benefits are nearly all positive. The number of studies for a given topic are less meaningful than for peer-review because I stopped counting traditional uses if I already had a bunch of them on a particular condition. If marked "India" the study may very well be an Ayurvedic benefit, but without some clear indication otherwise I always defaulted to a generic India. Many benefits that are marked "no traditional use" may actually be treated by Ayurveda, which as a holistic system that effectively treats a condition indirectly. It is too complicated for a non-practitioner to fully understand its benefits, but Ayurveda is an herb-based medical system that has been successful for 6,000 years. I personally consider Ayurveda to be equal to Western medicine in its results. The book chapter on **Traditional Use** has a whole section devoted to Ayurveda.

Each entry from peer-review research or other expert source should have a bold number in one of two forms (**139-** or **[139]**). This is the citation number for that research study. You can use this number to look up the name of the study, its authors, and the journal publishing the results in the **References**. Nearly all of these studies can be accessed through Google Scholar. I sometimes add the date of the research if it seems time sensitive (**[139-2017]**). Sometimes two studies have the same results (**[139,272]**). Traditional and Ayurvedic uses have a bold **Tr** preceding an un-bolded citation number (**Tr** 139-).

Additionally, this is the font that is used for expert testimony, while any comments that are mine should be in this font. I may interject personal comments in the text as well {just to be clear about this}. For my part, I do not offer expert testimony, rather experienced herbalist user testimony.

Who Said What in this Book

- Any comments I make are in this font,
- My comments will not have a citation number.

  - The peer-review research is always in this font and will have a citation number at its beginning (**279-**) or end (**[279]**). Traditional and Ayurvedic citations are preceded by a **Tr**, are also bracketed, but are not in bold (**Tr** 279-]. {Short comments I make in the text will be in these brackets}

-

Sample Listing Explained

Blood, Hypoglycemic

Hypoglycemia (low blood sugar) is when blood sugar decreases to below normal levels. This may result in a variety of symptoms including clumsiness, trouble talking, confusion, loss of consciousness, seizures, or death. **[1]**

Sida acuta

103--rats—leaf--ethanolic and methanolic extracts--200 mg/kg bw--the hypoglycemic effects were comparable to that of glibenclamide, EESA exhibiting greater antioxidant activity.

• **Blood, Hypoglycemic** = This is the benefit that Sida brings.

Next to the Benefit at the top of the listing might be these statements:

No peer review – There are no peer-review studies in this category.

Tr no reported use -- No traditional uses reported in this category.

(blank) -- There are both peer-review and traditional benefits.

• *Hypoglycemia* **(low blood sugar) is when blood sugar decreases to below normal levels. This may result in a variety of symptoms including clumsiness, trouble talking, confusion, loss of consciousness, seizures, or death. [1]** = This describes the benefit.

[1] = citation number for this passage. You can look up this number in the **References** to find the name of the study, its authors, and the publishing journal.

• **Sida acuta** = the species of Sida studied. (**K**=cryptolepine alkaloid)

• **103** = citation number for this benefit. Look it up as described above.

• **rats** = type of study: invitro=lab research, animal name=research was performed on this animal, field=field study, observing what happens out in nature, review=summation of the state of research.

• **leaf** = part of Sida studied. There can be more than one part studied. Aerial parts and whole plant are options as well.

• **ethanolic and methanolic extracts** = how was the medicinal benefit extracted? Look to the Appendix for a full listing of extracts. There may have been more than one extract used. If several were tried separately (A, L, E). If they were used together then they are joined (LS). If they were sequential or derivative (M>E). If the cited method is one of several options-it is in **bold**.

• **200 mg/kg bw** = how much of the medicinal was used. Usually expressed as the amount of the extract given per kilogram of body weight of the animal studied.

• **the hypoglycemic effects were comparable to that of gliben-clamide, EESA exhibiting greater antioxidant activity.** = Outcomes and notes. In this case comparing the effectiveness against a standard pharmaceutical, glibenclamide, in two different ways. There may be additional information here as well.

Full Listing of Benefits

Adaptogenic - Nerves, Stress, Anxiety
Allergy, Antihistamine
Animals, Disease
Arteries, Atherosclerosis
Arteries – Thrombosis
Arteries, Vasorelaxation
Ayurveda – aromatic
Ayurveda – atitikta (bitter)
Ayurveda – Daha (burning sensation)

Ayurveda – Hima – Cold
Ayurveda – svadu-sweet in taste
Ayurveda – Tridoshanut
Ayurveda – vata–pitta diseases
Other Ayurveda
Bladder, Cystitis
Bladder, Diuretic
Bladder, Hematuria
Bladder, Problems
Bladder, Stones (calculus)
Bladder, Urinary disease
Bladder, Urinary disorders
Blood, Anti-diabetic
Blood Cleaner
Blood disorders
Blood, Diabetes mellitus
Blood, Haemolysis
Blood, Hypoglycemic
Blood pressure depressant
Blood, Stops bleeding,
Blood, Thrombolytic activity
Body, Adaptogenic
Body, Alertness
Body, Anti-convulsant
Body, Antioxidant
Body, Arthritis and Osteoarthritis
Body, Chemoprotective
Body, Chills
Body, Depression
Body, Detoxification
Body, Edema
Body, Fever (Antipyretic)
Body, Gout
Body, Immuno-stimulant
Body, Immuno-supportive
Body, Inflammation
Body, Jaundice
Body, Leprosy
Body, Muscles
Body, Obesity
Body, Rheumatism
Body, Stimulant
Body, Strength
Body, Thirst
Body, Tonic
Body, Weight Change
Body, Wound healing
Brain, Myocardial injury (MI)
Brain, Neurodamage
Brain, Neurotoxicity

Brain, Other conditions
Children, Child's remedy
Companion/Catch Plant
Disease, Miscellaneous
Disease, Virus, Antiviral
Ear and Nose Problems
Eye Problems
Fat/lipids - Increases HDL
Fat/lipids – Inhibit lipid peroxidation
Fat/lipids – Lowers cholesterol
Fat/lipids – Lowers LDL
Fat/lipids – Lowers Triglycerides
Fiber
Fiberglass
Food, Food storage protection
Food, For humans
Food, Other than human   See also, Insects, Food and Sustenance
Food, Tea
Fuel, Heat production
Fungi, Anti-fungal (antimycotic)
GI tract, Abdominal pains
GI tract, Colic
GI tract, Constipation
GI tract, Diarrhea
GI tract, Digestive Problems
GI tract, Dysentery
GI tract, Flatulence   (farts)
GI tract, Gastric disorders
GI tract, Haemorrhoids
GI tract, Laxative/Enema
GI tract, Stomach, Disorders
GI tract, Stomach, Ulcer
GI tract, Stomachic
GI tract, Tenesmus
Hair
Head, Headache
Heart, Aarhythmia
Heart, Bradycardia
Heart, Cardioprotective
Heart, myocardial infraction
Heart, Heart disease
HIV/AIDS
Insect, Anti-sida
Insects, Beneficial
Insects, Defense against
Insects, Food and Sustenance
Kidney, Nephroprotective
Kidney, Stones
Liver, Bile disorders
Liver Disorders

Liver, Hepatoprotective
Lungs, Asthma
Lungs, Bronchitis
Lungs, Cough and wheezing
Lungs, Expectorant
Lungs, Pneumonia
Lungs, Tuberculosis
Metal, Anti-corrosion
Minerals, Mineral accumulator, Chelator
Minerals, Nanoparticles
Mollusks, Molluscicide
Mouth, Demulcent
Mouth, Dental hygiene
Mouth, Inflamed (stomatitis)
Mouth, Toothache
Nausea, Antiemetic
Nerves, CNS central nervous system depressant
Nerves, Nervous disorders
Nerves, Neurodegenerative diseases
Nerves, Paralysis
Nerves, Sciatica
Nerves, Sedative
Noise Reduction
Pain, Analgesic
Pain, Antinociceptive
Parasites, Anthelmintic
Parasitic protozoa, Malaria
Parasitic protozoa, Other
Poison, Alexertic
Poison, Neutralizes poison
Reproduction, Abortifacient
Reproduction, Anti-fertility
Reproduction, Aphrodisiac
Reproduction, Contraceptive, anti-implantation
Reproduction, During labor
Reproduction, estrogenic activity
Reproduction, Female sexual problems
Reproduction, Leucorrhoea
Reproduction, Low or no sperm
Reproduction, Male sexual problems
Reproduction, Pregnancy
Reproduction, Uterine disorders
Sanity, Delerium
Skin, Abscess
Skin, Astringent
Skin, Boils
Skin, Cooling
Skin, Diaphoretic/Sudorfic
Skin, Emollient
Skin, Rashes and Inflammation

Skin, Skin beauty
Skin, Skin disease
Skin, Sores
Skin, Lessen Perspiration
Skin, Wound healing
Sleep, Sleeping time
Soap, For Washing
Soil, Rejuvenates degraded soil
Toxicity, Low/no toxicity
Toxicity, Protection from toxic metals
Toxicity, Toxic to living things
Veneral Disease, Gonorrhea
Veneral disease
Worms, Earthworm friendly
Other Uses

Adaptogenic - Nerves, Stress, Anxiety

Adaptogens have even been described as "medicine[sic] for healthy people; administration results in stabilization of physiological processes and promotion of homeostasis, for example, decreased cellular sensitivity to stress. [1]   Stressors are external, environmental demands placed on us to feel stressed, whereas an Adaptogen increases the power of resistance against physical, chemical or biological noxious agents. [32]   The mode of action of Adaptogens is basically associated with stress system. Adaptogen increase the capacity of stress to respond to the external signals of activating and deactivating mediators of stress response subsequently. [32]   Ayurveda has a special class of botanicals known as Rasayana with immunomodulatory and adaptogenic activities. [728]

Sida acuta

186-invitro-whole plant-methanol extract-the extract prolonged the stress tolerance capacity of the mice, indicating the possible involvement of a higher center,   **275**-mice-leaves and stems-100% ethanolic extract-500 and 1000 mg/kg-for anxiety.

Sida cordifolia

32-mice-root-40% ethanol extract-possess antistress, and adaptogenic activity, hence can be categorized as plant adaptogen.-The stress induced increase in total white blood cell count is decreased indicating antistress, adaptogenic activity-Plant adaptogen are smooth prostressors which reduce the reactivity of host defense system. The mode of action of adaptogens is basically associated with stress system. Adaptogen increase the capacity of stress to respond to the external signals of activating and deactivating mediators of stress response subsequently. The stress induced increase in total WBC count is decreased by SCE, indicating antistress, adaptogenic activity,   **289**-invitro-root-Both sitoindoside IX and X (extracted from Sida cordifolia) exhibited significant adaptogenic effects in the battery of tests accepted for this purpose. The phagocytotic index determined for the two compounds in vitro and the dose-dependent blastogenic response produced in thymocytes and splenic lymphocytes suggest their strong potential as immunostimulatory agents. Sitoindoside X significantly inhibited the production of oxygen metabolites by activated PMN. These findings validate the use of the two plant drugs as health promotive agents in Ayurvedic medicine,

Tr   118-Ayurveda-relief from anxiety,   127-Ayurveda,   664-Ayurveda-whole plant?,

Sida rhombifolia

543-mice-whole plant-petroleum ether (60-80°C), chloroform, ethanol and water extracts-It was concluded from the present study that ethanolic extract of Sida rhombifolia Linn exhibited good anti-anxiety activity at the dose of 300 mg/kg in mice using elevated plus maze model of anxiety.

Other Sidas

205-Sida tiagii-invitro-mice -fruit-ethanolic extract-100-200 mg/kg bw-anxiolytic,   405-Sida cordata-whole plant-adaptogens are the plant derived biologically active substances that improves the immunity and physical endurance. Many herbals preparations have been evaluated for their adaptogenic activity during exposure to stressful conditions. In response to stressor, a series of behavioral, neurochemical and immunological changes occur that ought to serve in an adaptive capacity.... In conclusion, the above study indicates positive adaptogenic activity of the extract Sida cordata (whole plant), by forced swim test and resultant biochemical studies.

Tr   358-Sida linfolia-Benin- Twig sap is drunk as a remedy for anxiety, 552-SIDA TIAGII-India,

Allergy, Antihistamine

Antihistamines are drugs which treat allergies... Antihistamines can give relief when a person has nasal congestion, sneezing, or hives because of pollen, dust mites, or animal allergy. Although typical people use the word "antihistamine" to describe drugs for treating allergies, doctors and scientists use the term to describe a class of drug that opposes the activity of histamine receptors in the body. [1]

Sida rhombifolia

194-mice-whole plant?-80% acetone/water extract-The antihistamine property of extract could be due to the neutralization of histamine and serotonin,   201-rats-aerial parts-methanolic extract- showed inhibitory effects on the release of histamine like substances,   324-rats-aerial parts-water extract- inhibitory effects on the release of histamine like substances,

Other Sida   Tr   270-Sida acuta-India-extract-hay fever,   596-Sida cordifolia-Nigeria-leaf/root/seed-hay fever,

132

Cryptolepine 583- isolated guinea pig ileum-antagonized histamine,

Animals, Disease   **No peer review**

Sida indica   Hemorrhagic septicemia
Tr 708-Ayurveda-fruit-decoction mixed with ammonium chloride is given orally to treat hemorrhagic septicemia,   712 India-fruit and/or seeds-Hemorrhagic septicemia,

Other Sida
Tr 209-Sida acuta-Ethiopia-livestock diseases,   358-Sida cordifolia-review-The powdered whole plant is applied to open wounds of horses in Niger

Arteries, Atherosclerosis   **Tr   no reported use**
A specific form of arteriosclerosis in which an artery wall thickens as a result of invasion and accumulation of white blood cells (foam cells) and proliferation of intimal-smooth-muscle cell creating an atheromatous (fibrofatty) plaque. [1]

Sida rhomboidea
321-rats+invitro-leaves-acqueous extract-has the potency of controlling experimental atherosclerosis and can be used as promising herbal supplement in combating atherosclerosis,   **323**-invitro-leaf-?extract-This scientific report is the first detailed investigation that establishes anti-atherosclerotic potential of SR extract.   **547**-invitro-leaf-extract-Results clearly indicated that SR was capable of reducing LDL oxidation and formation of intermediary oxidation products. Also, SR successfully attenuated peroxyl radical formation, mitochondrial dysfunction, nuclear condensation, and apoptosis in Ox-LDL-exposed HMDMs. This scientific report is the first detailed investigation that establishes anti-atherosclerotic potential of SR extract.

Arteries, Thrombosis   **Tr   no reported use**
Demonstration of inhibition of CaCl2-induced human platelet aggregation in vitro with ethanol extract of *Sida acuta* leaves suggest anti-platelet properties [655]

Sida acuta
115-invitro-leaf-water extract-human blood clots reduced 24.786 % by 100 ul of aqueous extract-extract has notable Thrombolytic activity-clot lysis increased with increase in concentration---reducing activity and absorption both increase with concentration but no mention of lysis at 500 ul tested, **649**-invtro- dried flowers-95% methanol extract-The thrombolytic potency of

Sida acuta is found 48.87% and the standard have 80.22%. It seems good result or may be said significant as the extract was the mixture of many phytochemical, it shows nearby percent of clot lysis. The cytotoxic result obtained 67.5µg/ml (LC50) it so good, but proper isolation can make it more potent and useful, **655**-invitro-leaves-absolute ethanol extract-Demonstration of inhibition of CaCl2-induced human platelet aggregation in vitro with ethanol extract of Sida acuta leaves suggest anti-platelet properties -The extract inhibits prostaglandin activity, phospholipase A2 activity and positive effect on platelet aggregation, membrane stabilization which showed a significant inhibition of in-vitro haemolysis and could have a potential therapeutic effect on disease processes causing destabilization of biological membranes.

Cryptolepine   (S. acuta, cordifolia, rhombifolia, spinosa, and ?)

391-mouse-cryptolepine- mouse model of arterial thrombosis- cryptolepine produced 25% maximal protection at 1 mg/kg while dipyridamole produced a 20% maximal effect at 2 mg/kg- The use of 20% ethanol as a dosage vehicle enhanced the protective effects of all drugs tested and the ethanol vehicle alone provided 45% protection,   **401**-invitro-exhibited antiplatelet effects in vitro in human, rabbit and rat-it exhibited an indirect fibrinolytic action in the rat.

Arteries, Vasorelaxation

The aqueous fraction of the hydroalcoholic extract of the Sida cordifolia leaves induced relaxation of phenylephrine-induced contractions in the rat superior mesenteric artery. **[39]**

Sida acuta

160-vasicine produces hypotension and bradycardia, which appears to be due to a direct and indirect stimulation of cardiac muscarinic receptors, and by a decrease of the total peripheral resistances.   **Tr**   148-India,

Sida cordifolia

39-rats-leaf- hydroalcoholic extract- vasorelaxation induced in the rat superior mesenteric artery,   **160**-vasicine produces hypotension and bradycardia, which appears to be due to a direct and indirect stimulation of cardiac muscarinic receptors, and by a decrease of the total peripheral resistances. **162**-rats-leaf- hydroalcoholic extract- the vasorelaxation induced in the rat superior mesenteric artery.

Tr   148-India-aerial parts,   161-Ayurveda-rejuvenating action,   664-Ayurveda-crushed leaves-poultice-anti-plaque,

Sida rhombifolia

59-rat-whole plant?-the vasorelaxant activity of cryptolepinone in rat mesenteric artery rings is reported herein for the first time, vasorelaxant activity in rat cranial mesenteric artery with and without functional vascular endothelium,   **160**-vasicine produces hypotension and bradycardia, which appears to be due to a direct and indirect stimulation of cardiac muscarinic receptors, and by a decrease of the total peripheral resistances. **622**-invitro-aerial parts-?extract-quindolinone (6) and the salt of cryptolepine (9) induced vasorelaxation dependent on the vascular endothelium,

Tr   524-Phillipines,

Ayurveda – aromatic   No peer review
Ayurveda makes use of aromatics to prevent and treat various health conditions. Inhalation of the aroma of plants and the essential oils extracted from those plants is trusted to enhance the sense of smell and directly contributes to mental health and treats hormonal imbalances. **[http://ayurvedicoils.com/tag/relationship-between-ayurveda-and-aromatherapy]**

Sida acuta   **Tr**   88-root bark,   118 -root bark,

Sida cordifolia   **Tr**   312-USA-root bark

Ayurveda -- atitikta (bitter)   No peer review
{bitter herbs are beneficial in deranged pitta}

Sida acuta   **Tr**   88-root bark,   118-root bark,   377-root,

Sida cordifolia   **Tr**   161-Ayurveda-extremely bitter,   312-Ayurveda-USA-root bark,   377-root,

Other Sida   **Tr**   293-Sida cordata-roots,   377-Sida rhombifolia-roots,   377-Sida indica-root,

Ayurveda – Daha (burning sensation)
{Burning sensation of the body is a characteristic feature in many diseases, mainly influenced by increase of Pitta Dosha.}   **No peer review**

Sida cordata   **Tr**   293-flower and ripe fruits,

Sida rhomboidea   **Tr**   288-Ayurveda?-burning sensation,   320-Sri Lanka,   520-India,

Ayurveda – Hima – Cold   No peer review
{Hima or cold infusion is usually used for treating disorders due to the pitta imbalance}

Sida acuta   **Tr**   6- Ayurveda,   653-Ayurveda,

Sida cordifolia   Tr   444-Ayurveda-Bala,

Ayurveda – svadu-sweet in taste

{The taste in the mouth is called svadu-applies not only to the perception of taste buds located on the tongue, but to the final reaction of food in the acid medium of the stomach}   **No peer review**

Sida cordifolia Tr   444-Ayurveda-Bala-svadu,   561-Ayurveda -root,

Other Sida   Tr   293-Sida cordata-roots,   561-Sida acuta-Ayurveda-root,   561-Ayurveda-Sida rhombifolia and Sida spinosa-root,

Ayurveda – Tridoshanut   No peer review
{Balances Tridosha – vata, Pitta and kapha}

Sida cordifolia   Tr   437-Ayurveda-bark-remove vata,   444-Ayurveda Bala-balances Tridosha-vata, Pitta and kapha

Sida rhombifolia   Tr   437-Ayurveda-bark-remove tridosha,   522-roots and leaves-removes tridosha,

Other Sida   Tr   437 -Sida cordata-Ayurveda-bark-remove tridosha, 437-Sida indica-Ayurveda-bark-remove tridosha,   710-Sida indica-Ayurvedic-bark-removes "Vatta and tridosha",

Ayurveda – vata–pitta diseases

{The dry, nervous qualities of the Vata type or the hot, dynamic qualities of the Pitta type, the Vata person is the most innovative and creative and the Pitta person is the most practical and dynamic}   **No peer review**

Sida cordifolia   Tr   161-Ayurveda-beneficial in deranged pitta, 437-Ayurveda -roots-vata–pitta diseases,

Sida rhombifolia   Tr   161-Ayurveda-beneficial in deranged pitta., 437-Ayurveda -roots-vata–pitta diseases,

Sida cordata   Tr   437-Ayurveda -roots-vata–pitta diseases,   496-Pakistan-Siddha and Ayurveda-seeds,

Sida indica   Tr   437-Ayurveda -roots-vata–pitta diseases,   710-Ayurveda-Sida indica-bark-removes "Vatta and tridosha",

....
Alkaloids are capable of reducing headache associated with hypertension. It has been reported that alkaloids can be used in the management of cold, fever and chronic catarrh. **[223]**

136

Other Ayurveda

Sida cordifolia
Tr 118-Ayurveda-balances all the doshas-vata, pitta, kapha-has more effect on vata dosha, 444-Ayurveda -Snigdha (unctuous, oilyness), 444-Ayurveda -Grahi-absorbant

Sida cordata
Tr 293-India-roots-sour, 405-Ayurveda-Kayakarpam-imparting immunity to diseases.

Sida indica
449-mice-leaves (flowering stage)- petroleum ether (60-800)>petroleum ether (60-800)/distilled water and chloroform (9:1)-significantly high phagocytic index-indicates stimulation of the reticulo-endothelial system-validates the traditional use of S. indica as a 'Rasayana' in Ayurveda system of medicine,

Tr 443-India-rakttapitta-simply means bleeding-can be both internal as well as external, 443-India-dosha-each of three energies believed to circulate in the body and govern physiological activity. 449-Ayurveda-L-R-validates the traditional use of S. indica as a 'Rasayana' in Ayurveda system of medicine, 678-Ayurveda-root-haemorrhagic diseases,

Bladder, Cystitis No peer review
Inflammation of the urinary bladder. It is often caused by infection and is usually accompanied by frequent, painful urination. **[738]**

Sida cordifolia
Tr 161-Ayurveda 167-Ayurveda-root, seeds, 312-USA-Ayurveda-seeds-cystitis, 358-DR Congo, 362-review-Malaysia-seeds, 437-Ayurveda-seeds,

Sida rhombifolia
Tr 407-Ayurveda-seeds, 437-Ayurveda-seeds,

Sida spinosa
Tr 55-Ayurveda-root-decoction-irritability of bladder, 99-India-root-decoction as a demulcent in irritability of bladder,

Sida indica
Tr 238-Sri Lanka-leaf-bladder infection, 437-Ayurveda-seeds- chronic cystitis, 451-Thailand-leaf extract-inflammation of the bladder, 678—Ayurveda-India-leaves-decoction-inflammation of the bladder, 684-Ayurveda-leaf juice-inflammation of the bladder, 708-Ayurveda-seed-in treatment chronic cystitis, 708-Ayurveda-leaves-internally for inflammation of bladder, 735-Ayurveda-review-seeds-chronic cystitis, 737-India-seeds-infusion in water-chronic cystitis,

Sida cordata
Tr 437-Ayurveda-seeds, 496-Sida cordata-Pakistan-Siddha and Ayurveda-seeds or roots.

Bladder, Diuretic

A substance that promotes *diuresis*, that is, the increased production of urine. [1]

Sida acuta

Tr 3-India-leaves, 6-Ayurveda, 21-Siddha (Tamil)-leaves, 21-Ayurveda-root, 29-Ayurveda, 52-India-hot water extract of the dried entire plant, 82-India, 88-Portuguese, 101-India, 107-Ayurveda-leaves, 107-Ayurveda-in rheumatic conditions, 109-Siddah, 137-leaf-Guatemala, 138-India-whole plant-hot water extract, 168-India-dried entire plant-hot water extract, 174-India, 186-India, 223-Ayurveda, 270-India-leaves, 271-India-hot water extract of the dried entire plant-taken orally, 358-review-leaves, 571-India, 653-Ayurveda,

Sida cordifolia

132-mice?-roots-[citing Rastogi, R.P., Malhotra, B.N., 1985. Compendium of Indian Medical Plants 4, 674]. **142**-rats-chloroform, ethyl acetate and methanol extract of roots of Sida cordifolia exhibited dose dependent diuretic property,-The onset of diuretic action was extremely prompt (within 1h), **412**-rats-roots- significant diuretic activity-petroleum ether, chloroform, ethyl acetate or methanol extract-250, 500 mg/kg- onset of diuretic action was extremely prompt (within 1h) and lasted through out the studied period (up to 5 h).

Tr 29-Ayurveda, 40-Brazil, 88-Cambodia, 88-Ayurveda-root bark, 118-Ayurveda-root bark, 125-Ayurveda, 312-Ayurveda-invitro-root?, 138-India, 148-India-aerial parts, 152-India, 161-Ayurveda, 161-Ayurveda, 162-Brazil, 180-Ayurveda, 312-USA-Ayurveda-root bark, 312-Brazil, 358-Mauritius-leaf decoction, 437-Ayurveda-bark,

Sida rhombifolia

Tr 47-India-leaf-infusion, 51-India-leaf, 57-Ayurveda, 75-India, 136-India- root and leaves, 377-Ayurveda, 437-Ayurveda-bark, 522-Peru-leaf, 524-Phillipines, 524-Ayurveda, 545- Bangladesh-leaves and roots,

Sida indica

Tr 238-Sri Lanka-roots, 285-Ayurveda-root, 377-Ayurveda-root, 437-Ayurveda-bark-diuretic, 443-Ayurveda-leaves-is a stronger diuretic, 445-Thailand, 448-Ayurveda, 451-Thailand-root, 452-Bangladesh, 454- India-bark, 678-India-root, 678-India-bark or root and bark, 708-Ayurveda-root, 708-Ayurveda-bark, 711-Ayurveda-root and bark, 711-Chinese-bark and root, 711-India-root, 712-India-stem bark, 735-Ayurveda-review-roots, 735-Ayurveda-review-bark,

Sida retusa

Tr   75-India,   131-Sida retusa-Ayurveda-widely used in Ayurveda as a diuretic,   435-Sida retusa-Japan,   529-Ayurveda-used in calculus troubles as a diuretic.

Sida cordata

Tr   437-Ayurveda-bark,   496-Pakistan-Siddha and Ayurveda-roots.

Bladder, Hematuria   No peer review

The presence of blood in urine. [738]

Sida acuta   **Tr**   71-Ayurveda-roots,   217-Ayurveda,

Sida cordifolia   **Tr**   71-Ayurveda-root,   437-Ayurveda-roots,
548-Ayurveda-roots

Sida rhombifolia   **Tr**   437-Ayurveda-roots,   522-Peru-leaf,

Sida indica   **Tr**   437-Ayurveda-roots-haematuria, 451-Thailand-root-can be taken for the relief of hematuria,   678-Ayurveda-root infusion,   711-India-root,   712-India-roots,

Sida cordata   **Tr**   437-Ayurveda-roots,

Bladder, Problems   No peer review

Sida acuta   **Tr**   358-Sida acuta-gall bladder-roots,

Sida cordifolia   **Tr**   437- Ayurveda-Sida cordifolia-leucoderma-India-roots,

Sida rhombifolia   **Tr**   437- Ayurveda-Sida rhombifolia-leucoderma-India-roots,

Sida cordata   **Tr**   437-Ayurveda-Sida cordata-leucoderma-India-roots,

Sida indica

Tr   437-Ayurveda-roots-in strangury,   710-Ayurveda-leaves-decoction-inflammation of the bladder,   711-Ayurveda-seed-used in urinary disorders, 711-India-leaf extract-inflammation of the bladder,   711-India-seed-urinary disorders,   712-India-roots-strangury, polyuria, urinary discharge, or uretyhritis,   735-Ayurveda-review-decoction of the leaves-bladder inflammation,   737-India-root-infusion-strangury and hematuria,

139

Bladder, Stones

Bladder stones are caused by a buildup of minerals. They can occur if the bladder is not completely emptied after urination. Eventually, the leftover urine becomes concentrated and minerals within the liquid turn into crystals. [738] Deposition of calcium oxalate microcrystal in human body can be a significant problem and it is recognized that 70 - 80 % of kidney stones contain calcium oxalate. [90]

Sida acuta 90-invitro-methanolic and aqueous extracts,

Sida rhombifolia Tr 437-Ayurveda-roots, 522-Ayurveda-whole plant?-fresh juice-to dissolve stones in urinary tract,

Sida retusa Tr 435-Sida retusa-Japan, 529-Sida retusa-Ayurveda,

Other Sida Tr 437-Sida cordata- Ayurveda-roots, 437-Sida cordifolia-Ayurveda-roots, 437-Sida indica-Ayurveda-roots-bladder stones, 526-Sida spinosa-Togo-leaves-kidney stones,

Bladder, Urinary disease

Urinary tract infection (UTI) is one of the major widespread infections standing next to upper respiratory infection with an rising conflict to antimicrobial agents. These sicknesses affect patients in all age of groups and sexes. Majority of UTIs are not life aggressive and do not cause any permanent damage. Multiple anti-microbial resistances among gram negative and gram positive organism have been a long term and well documented trouble with urinary tract infection. [645]

Sida acuta 645-leaf-aqueous and acetone extracts-it was concluded that aqueous and acetone extracts has antibacterial activity against ESBL producing E. coli from UTI.
Tr 6-Ayurveda, 18-India, 63-India, 88-Ayurveda, 90-India-root, 186-Inida, 223-India, 264-Nigeria-urinary infections, 275-Brazil-leaves and stems-100% ethanolic extract, 561-Ayurveda-roots, 571-India, 653-Ayurveda,

Sida cordifolia Tr 32-Ayurveda-root infusion, 71-Ayurveda-roots, 118-Ayurveda, 358-Benin-roots-urinary tract problems, 548-Ayurveda-roots, 561-Ayurveda-root, 664-Ayurveda-bark,

Sida rhombifolia Tr 47-India-urogenital diseases, 51-India, 522-India-entire plant-hot aqueous extract-orally-in treatment of urinary diseases, 524-India-Hindus, 561-Ayurveda-root,

Other Sidas Tr 445-Sida indica-India and China, 561-Sida veronicaefolia-Ayurveda-roots, 561-Sida spinosa-Ayurveda-roots,

Bladder, Urinary disorders No peer review

Sida acuta

Tr 3-India-whole plant, 82-India, 88-Ayurveda-urinary discharges-leaf, 111-India, 174-India, 186-India, 217-Ayurveda, 270-India-tonic-root, 358-roots-gall bladder Genitourinary System Disorders, 609-India, 644-Ayurveda-root,

Sida cordifolia

Tr 118-Ayurveda-bark, 118-Ayurveda-Powder of the root and bark together, is given with milk and sugar for frequent urination, 124-India-paste of flowers and unripe fruits and take orally with water against painful urination, 161-Ayurveda-rejuvenating action on urinary system-useful in urinary problems, 161-Ayurveda-cystitis, 167-Ayurveda-root, 167-Ayurveda-root-Root powder is given with cow milk for micturition, 200-India, 217-Ayurveda, 285-Ayurveda-root-urinary disorders, 312-USA-Ayurveda-roots, 612-Ayurveda-root, 664-Ayurveda-root and bark-powder-with milk and sugar for frequent micturition,

Sida rhombifolia

Tr 51-India-whole plant?-urinary tract infections, 126-Colombia, 522-Guatemala-leaf and stem-decoction orally-urinary inflammation, 522-Peru-leaf-urinary bladder ailments, 522-Peru-leaf-Urethritis, 522-Ayurveda-roots and leaves-urinary complaints-urinary discharges-strangury.

Sida cordata

Tr 293-Ayurveda-root bark-hyperdiuresis, 496-Sida cordata-Pakistan-Siddha and Ayurveda-dysuria,

Sida indica

Tr 451-Thailand-seed, 678-Ayurveda-root-urethritis, 678-Ayurveda-root infusion-strangury, 678-Ayurveda-seeds, 678-Ayurveda-root-production of abnormally large volumes of dilute urine, 684-Ayurveda-urine output, 708-Ayurveda-root-in urethritis, 710-China-entire plant, 711-Ayurveda-seed, 712-India-roots-strangury, 712-India-roots-polyuria, 712-India-roots-urinary discharge, 712- India-roots-urethritis, 735-Ayurveda-review-roots-uretyhritis,

Sida rhomboidea **Tr** 280-Ayurveda, 288-Ayurveda, 320-Ayurveda, 520-India,

Sida spinosa **Tr** 55-India-root-decoction-irritability of bladder, 55-India-leaves-bruised in water and the filtrate is administered-scalding urine, 99-India-leaf-scalding urine,

Blood, Anti-diabetic

Diabetes in present scenario is the most common non-communicable disease worldwide. Due to its high prevalence, morbidity and mortality, diabetes is the third killer of mankind after cancer and cardiovascular disease. [171] Many oral agents for the treatment of DM are expensive and cause adverse effects. Furthermore, none of the oral synthetic hypoglycemic agents have been successful in maintaining euglycemia and controlling long-term microvascular and macrovascular complications. As a result, attempts have been made to discover new antidiabetic regimens derived from plants. Many traditional plant treatments for diabetes are used throughout the world, which are frequently considered to be less toxic and results in fewer side effects than synthetic compounds. [451] There are more than 1000 anti-diabetic plants have been described in the scientific literature. The plant kingdom is a wide field to search for a natural effective oral hypoglycemic or hypolipidemic agent that has slight or no side effects. Natural products with both hypoglycemic and hypolipidemic properties are useful anti-diabetic agents. [131]

Sida acuta Tr 609-India, 201-review from Ghana-whole plant,

Sida cordifolia 180-rats-aerial parts-acqueous extract-The three weeks treatment at 1000 mg/kg bw showed a significant reduction in cholesterol, triglycerides, LDL-C and VLDL-C in treated rats when compared with metformin at 500 mg/kg bw ($P<0.05$). HDL-C was significantly improved by treatment of extract. Body weight decreased 9%,

Tr 180-India-These results could explain the basis for the use of this plant extract to manage serum glucose level and cholesterolemia associated with diabetes mellitus, 502-Saudi Arabia-used in herbal medicines for the treatment of different diseases, including diabetes

Sida rhombifolia Tr 59-Brazil, 131-Ayurveda-leaves-diabetes mellitus, 134-India, 150-Ethiopia-leaves, 522-Central Africa-dried leaf-infusion, 622-India,

Sida cordata Tr 496-seeds-Pakistan-Siddha and Ayurveda-diabetes mellitus, 549-Ayurveda,

Sida spinosa Tr 434-India- ethno botanical survey conducted revealed that root is used in the treatment of diabetes (2011),

Sida rhomboidea

134-mice-whole plant?-methanol extract?-This study is a first scientific report on protective role of S. rhomboidea ROXB. extract against HFD induced insulin resistance in C57BL/6J mice and strengthens the folklore claim of use of SR leaves as alternative medicine against diabetes and obesity.

Tr 130-NE India, 134- Sida rhomboidea-India-this study... strengthens the folklore claim of use of SR leaves as alternative medicine against diabetes and obesity, 320-Ayurveda-leaves-decoction-eaten, 520-India-is being used by the populace of North-East India to alleviate symptoms of diabetes and obesity,

Sida retusa

131-leaves-acqueous extract- a dose of 200 mg/kg of aqueous extract has shown reduction in glucose level 0%)- When tested in STZ-induced diabetic rats the reduction in plasma glucose was 17%.

Tr 131-Sida retusa-Ayurveda- It is also reported that Sida retusa extract is traditionally used by diabetic patients to lower their blood glucose levels-(this) investigation provides biochemical evidence to validate the use of Sida retusa as anti-diabetic by Ayuvedic physicians.

Sida indica

451-rats-leaves/twigs/roots-boiling water extract-In conclusion, this study demonstrated that the aqueous extract derived from the whole plant Sida indica manifested 2 important antidiabetic properties in rodents: the inhibition of glucose absorption and the stimulation of insulin secretion. Its activity on the inhibition of glucose absorption, in particular, supports the use of the extract as an adjuvant to the treatment of diabetes and/or a health promoting agent for the prevention of diabetes,

Tr 445-USA-This plant has a long history of being used medicinally as an antidiabetic remedy-known to contain an active ingredient against diabetes and is believed to reduce some symptoms of diabetic complications, 448-Ayurveda, 451-Thailand-has a long medical history of being used as an antidiabetic remedy--contains an active ingredient against diabetes and was believed to reduce some symptoms of diabetic complications, 452-Bangladesh, 454-India-leaves-local practitioners have claimed that the leaves are highly useful in controlling diabetes mellitus, 454-India-Since all the extracts of the leaves are found to possess hypoglycemic activity, it is difficult to attribute this activity to any one of the constituents. But the present study justifies the claim of the local practitioner that the leaves are useful in controlling diabetes mellitus, 678-Ayurveda-root and bark, 684-Ayurveda, 711-Sida indica-Ayurveda-root and bark,

Blood Cleaner   No peer review

(Sida indica) Reported in the Siddha system as a remedy for jaundice, piles, ulcer, leprosy, rakttapitta dosha and blood purifier. [449]

Sida rhombifolia   **Tr** 150-Ethiopia-fruits, 279-Ethiopia-whole plant.

Sida indica **Tr** 443-Ayurveda, 449-Ayurveda-blood purifier,

Sida tiagii **Tr** 205-Sida tiagii-India, 551- Sida tiagii-India, 553-Sida tiagii-India and Pakistan,

143

Blood disorders

Sida acuta

103-rats-leaf-ethanolic and methanolic extracts-200 mg/kg bw- significantly (p<0.05) reversed the decrease in neutrophil count (white blood cells), **655**-invitro-leaves-absolute ethanol extract-The extract inhibits prostaglandin activity, phospholipase A2 activity and positive effect on platelet aggregation, membrane stabilization which showed a significant inhibition of in-vitro haemolysis {the rupture or destruction of red blood cells>blood clots} and could have a potential therapeutic effect on disease processes causing destabilization of biological membranes,

Tr 3-India-root, 18-India, 63-India, 90-Ayurveda- disorders of blood and bile, 111-India, 118-Ayurveda-bark-blood conditions, 217-Ayurveda, 270-India-root, 275-Colombia-leaves and stems-100% ethanolic extract, 361-Phillipines-vomiting of blood, 362-Phillipines-roots, 561-Ayurveda-root, 644-Ayurveda-root,

Sida cordifolia

Tr 32-Ayurveda-root infusion, 118-Ayurveda, 167-Ayurveda-root, 358-Kenya, 362-review-Malaysia-roots-infusion-for disorders of the blood and bile, 362-review-Malaysia-roots-disorders of the blood, 437-Ayurveda-roots-bily blood, 444-Ayurveda-Bala-Raktapittahara – relieves bleeding disorders, 561-Ayurveda-root, 664-Ayurveda-bark,

Sida rhombifolia **Tr** 167-Ayurveda-root, 190-India-hemothermia (helps regulate blood temp), 437-Ayurveda-roots-bily blood, 561-Ayurveda-root,

Sida cordata **Tr** 167-Ayurveda-root, 437-Ayurveda-roots-bily blood,

Sida indica **Tr** 437-Ayurveda-roots-bily blood, 444-Ayurveda-Pittasrahara-relieves bleeding disorders,

Sida veronicaefolia **Tr** 561-Ayurveda-roots?,

Blood, Diabetes mellitus

Diabetes mellitus (DM) is an impending public health challenge of the present century. It affects over 387 million people globally, and this number is projected to increase to 592 million by 2035. DM is currently the fourth leading cause of mortality in the world. It has also emerged as a major socioeconomic burden for developing countries. **[502]** Each class of drug carries the burden of drug-associated side effects. All oral anti-diabetic drugs therapies have limited efficacy, and mechanism based side effects. Presently, there is growing interest in herbal remedies due to the side effects associated with the oral synthetic hypoglycemic agents for the treatment of diabetes

144

mellitus. Herbal medicines have been long used for the treatment of diabetic patients and continue to be accepted as an alternative therapy. There are more than 1000 anti-diabetic plants have been described in the scientific literature. The plant kingdom is a wide field to search for a natural effective oral hypoglycemic or hypolipidemic agent that has slight or no side effects. [131]

Sida acuta   Tr   609-India,   201-review from Ghana-whole plant,

Sida cordifolia

148-rats-400mg/kg,   171-rats-water extract-aerial parts-400mg/kg wt, 180-rats-aerial parts-water extract-1gm/kg wt-this medicinal plant is considered to be effective and alternative treatment for diabetes,   641-seed-cold distilled methanol extract- Protein glycation in hyperglycemic conditions -82% Inhibition (at 2 mg/mL)-IC50 .63 (mg/mL),   171-invitro-aerial parts-water extract- bioactive component of plant mainly flavonoids and alkaloids produces antidiabetic activity- significantly (P<0.05) decreases total cholesterol (55.12±1.47mg/dl), triglycerides (45.95±1.56mg/dl), LDL (24.12±1.72mg/dl), plasma creatinine (0.54±0.07mg/dl), plasma urea nitrogen (58.59±3.25mmol/l), lipid peroxidation (5.90±0.34nmol MDA/ml) and significantly (P<0.05) increases HDL (34.76±1.66mg/dl), catalase (59.98±3.25Umol H2O2/min/mg of Hb) and superoxide dismutase (62.47±2.33U/mg of Hb) activity of group-D diabetic rats on day 29,

Tr   180-India-These results could explain the basis for the use of this plant extract to manage serum glucose level and cholesterolemia associated with diabetes mellitus,   502-Saudi Arabia-used in herbal medicines for the treatment of different diseases, including diabetes.

Sida rhombifolia

131-rats/mice-leaves-hot distilled water extract-has shown mild hypoglycemic and hypolipidemic activity. The results obtained from the experiment provided scientific evidence in favor of the traditional use of Sida rhombifolia ssp. retusa leaves for the treatment of diabetes mellitus,   134-mice-leaf-?extract-This study is a first scientific report on protective role of S. rhomboidea ROXB. extract against HFD induced insulin resistance in C57BL/6J mice and strengthens the folklore claim of use of SR leaves as alternative medicine against diabetes and obesity,   503-rats-methanol extract- has potential to alleviate the conditions of moderate diabetic, but not severe diabetes.

Tr   59-Brazil, 131-Ayurveda-leaves-The investigation provides biochemical evidence to validate the use of Sida retusa as anti-diabetic by Ayuvedic physicians, 134-India, 131-Ayurveda-leaves, 131-Ayurveda-diabetes mellitus, 150-Ethiopia-leaves, 522-Central Africa-dried leaf-infusion, 622-India,

....

Sida is one of the important medicinal plant species used to treat various diseases in Ayurveda and other traditional systems of medicine. [15]

Sida cordata

496-rats-whole plant-ethanol extract-We suggested that SCEE could be used as antidiabetic component in case of diabetes mellitus -which gives a possibility of regenerative action of SCEE on the islet of Langerhans.

Tr 496-Pakistan-Siddha and Ayurveda-diabetes mellitus-seeds, 549-Ayurveda,

Sida rhomboidea

Tr 130-NE India, 134-India-this study... strengthens the folklore claim of use of SR leaves as alternative medicine against diabetes and obesity, 320-Ayurveda-leaves-decoction-eaten, 520-India, 520-India-is being used by the populace of North-East India to alleviate symptoms of diabetes and obesity,

Sida indica

451-aqueous extract-whole plant-manifested 2 important antidiabetic properties in rodents: the inhibition of glucose absorption and the stimulation of insulin secretion. Its activity on the inhibition of glucose absorption, in particular, supports the use of the extract as an adjuvant to the treatment of diabetes and/or a health promoting agent for the prevention of diabetes, **454**-rats-invitro-leaves-400 mg/kg bw-extracts reduced blood glucose levels: ether 35%-benzene 46%-ethanolic 30%, acqueous 54%-comparable to tolbutamide 40 mg/kg bw 55%,

Tr 445-USA-This plant has a long history of being used medicinally as an antidiabetic remedy-known to contain an active ingredient against diabetes and is believed to reduce some symptoms of diabetic complications, 448-Ayurveda, 451-Thailand-has a long medical history of being used as an antidiabetic remedy--contains an active ingredient against diabetes and was believed to reduce some symptoms of diabetic complications, 452-Bangladesh, 454-India-leaves-local practitioners have claimed that the leaves are highly useful in controlling diabetes mellitus, 454-Since all the extracts of the leaves are found to possess hypoglycemic activity, it is difficult to attribute this activity to any one of the constituents. But the present study justifies the claim of the local practitioner that the leaves of Sida indica are useful in controlling diabetes mellitus, 678-Ayurveda-root and bark, 684-Ayurveda, 711-India-leaf?-antidiabetic,

Sida retusa
131-Ayurveda- It is also reported that Sida retusa extract is traditionally used by diabetic patients to lower their blood glucose levels-(this) investigation provides biochemical evidence to validate the use of Sida retusa as anti-diabetic by Ayuvedic physicians,

Tr 131-Ayurveda-validates the use as anti-diabetic by Ayuvedic physicians,

Sida spinosa
Tr 434- India-ethno botanical survey conducted revealed that Sida spinosa Linn. root is used in the c of diabetes (2011),

Blood, Haemolysis

Tr no reported use

The rupture or destruction of red blood cells

Sida acuta

655-invitro-leaves-absolute ethanol extract-showed a significant inhibition of in-vitro haemolysis and could have a potential therapeutic effect on disease processes causing destabilization of biological membranes.

Sida cordata 293-goat blood-leaves-acetone or methanol extract.

Sida indica

687-The phytocompounds present in leaf of S. indica such as flavonoids, phenolic compounds, terpenoids and also less amount of form forming compounds may be responsible for minimum lysis of erythrocyte-The acetone extract of S. indica leaf showed minimum haemolysis against human erythrocytes.

Blood, Hypoglycemic

Hypoglycemia (low blood sugar) is when blood sugar decreases to below normal levels. This may result in a variety of symptoms including clumsiness, trouble talking, confusion, loss of consciousness, seizures, or death. [1]

Sida acuta

103-rats-leaf-ethanolic and methanolic extracts-200 mg/kg bw-the hypoglycemic effects were comparable to that of glibenclamide,   **201**-aqueous and methanol extracts -review from Ghana,   **588**-rabbits-leaf-the aqueous extracts of S acuta (AESA) and the methanol extracts of S acuta (MESA) (400mg/kg) significantly increased the tolerance for glucose in glucose fed normal rabbits. Blood glucose was reduced significantly at 1 1 /2 hrs post-glucose load (p<0.05). This reduction was consistent and persisted to 2 1 /2 hrs. (400mg/kg p.o) produced significant decreases in blood sugar at 4hours with percentage glycemic change of 30% and 20% respectively. The anti-hyperglycemic action of AESA and MESA were sustained up to 8hours with significant percentage glycemic change of 46% and 45% respectively,

Tr   32-Ayurveda,   40-Brazil,   118-Ayurveda,   148-India,   161-Ayurveda, 580-India-whole plant-ethanol extract,   588-Nigeria,

Sida cordifolia

32-mice-root-40% ethanol extract-Mice pretreated with extract showed reduced blood glucose,   **45**-invitro-root-methanol extract-significant hypoglycemic activity,   **148**-aerial parts-alcoholic extract-400 mg/kg bw significantly decreased the blood glucose level in diabetic rats-200 mg/kg bw showed non-significant change in diabetic rats,   **171**-invitro-aerial parts-water extract- All parts of plant are utilized for hypoglycemic activity-400 mg/kg bw significantly decreases blood glucose level,   **285**-rats-root-methanol extract-600 mg/kg bw-showed a decrease in blood sugar levels in normal rats and also influenced the GTT curve, indicating good hypoglycemic activity, **408**-invitro-root-methanolic extract- was found to possess significant hypoglycemic activity, **533**-review-all parts?-any extract?-can increase blood pressure,

Tr   40-Brazil, 118-Ayurveda, 125-India,   148-India-aerial parts,   152-India-seed oil,   161-Ayurveda- Has a hypoglycemic (blood sugar lowering) effect,   162-Brazil,   171-India- All parts are utilized for hypoglycemic activity,   180-India-These results could explain the basis for the use of this plant extract to manage serum glucose level and cholesterolemia associated with diabetes mellitus,   312-USA-Ayurveda-hypoglycemic agent,   312-Brazil,   664-Ayurveda-whole plant?.

Sida rhombifolia

196-rats-200 mg/kg aqueous extract reduced glucose level (10%),   **522**-review- The pharmacological activities reported include hypoglycemic activity.   **Tr**   131-India,

Sida tiagii

553-rats-fruits-petroleum ether>ethanol extract>n-Hexane Extract/Ethyl Acetate Extract-Further, during chronic study in RES treated rats, at doses of 500 mg/kg, significant reduction in plasma glucose level was observed on 19 day of administration with 47.16 ± 3.41% reductions-Phytoconstituents responsible for the anti-hyperglycemic effects,   **553**-rats-fruit-95% ethanol extract-signifi-cantly reduced the blood glucose level at both 200 and 500 mg/kg doses.

Sida spinosa   Tr   217-Ayurveda,   434-India-Based on an ethno botanical approach, the plant Sida spinosa Linn. has been traditionally claimed to possess hypoglycemic property,

Sida indica

439-rats-leaves-Alcohol and water extracts of Sida indica leaves (400 mg/kg, p.o.) showed significant hypoglycemic effect in normal rats 4 h after administration (23.10% and 26.95%, respectively),   **448**-leaf-rats,   **454**-invitro-leaves-water extract-400 mg/kg bw-It was also observed that different extracts have shown significant hypoglycemic activity but aqueous extract was most potent in reducing the blood glucose levels,

Sida retusa

131-rats-leaves-aacqueous extract-The results of the present studies indicate that 300 mg/kg Sida retusa was found to reduce the glucose level in normal and the animals made diabetic with STZ-as effective as Glibenclamide,

Tr   131-Ayurveda-traditionally used by diabetic patients to lower their blood glucose levels,

Sida cordata

496--rats--whole plant--ethanol extract--liquid partition by using solvents in order of n-hexane, chloroform, ethyl acetate, and n-butanol-ethyl acetate fraction--Anti-hyperglycemic for both normal and hyperglycemic rats.

Sida tuberculata   Tr   490-Brazil-leaves and roots,

Cryptolepine   (S. acuta, cordifolia, rhombifolia, spinosa, and ?) **248**-invitro-first report that cryptolepine possesses ant hyperglycemic properties,

Blood, Stops Bleeding   No peer review

Sida acuta   Tr   88-Nigeria,   220-Nigeria,   221-India-leaf,

Sida cordifolia   Tr   161-Ayurveda-used in bleeding disorders,

Sida rhombifolia   Tr   51-India-cuts,   150-Ethiopia-leaf-cuts and skin bleeding,   524-Phillipines-whole plant?-poultice-cuts,   568-Nigeria,

Sida cardifolia   Tr   200-Ayurveda-whole plant-bleeding disorders,

Blood, Thrombolytic activity

Thrombolysis is the breakdown (lysis) of blood clots formed in blood vessels, using medication. **[1]**   Sida acuta flower extract possessed considerable thrombolytic activity. **[649]**

Sida acuta

115-invitro-leaf-methanol extract-human blood clots reduced 24.786 % by 100 ul of aqueous extract-extract has notable Thrombolytic activity-clot lysis increased with increase in concentration---reducing activity and absorption both increase with concentration but no mention of lysis at 500 ul tested, **649**-invtro- dried flowers-95% methanol extract-The thrombolytic potency of Sida acuta is found 48.87% and the standard have 80.22%. It seems good result or may be said significant as the extract was the mixture of many phytochemical, it shows nearby percent of clot lysis. The cytotoxic result obtained 67.5μg/ml (LC50) it so good, but proper isolation can make it more potent and useful,   **655**-invitro-leaves-absolute ethanol extract- as the extract concentration increases from 0.2 mg/ml to 0.5 mg/ml, it inhibited the capacity of the CaCl2 which induce aggregation of human platelets. Demonstration of inhibition of CaCl2-induced human platelet aggregation in vitro with ethanol extract of Sida acuta leaves suggest anti-platelet properties-The extract inhibits prostaglandin activity, phospholipase A2 activity and positive effect on platelet aggregation, membrane stabilization which showed a significant inhibition of in-vitro haemolysis and could have a potential therapeutic effect on disease processes causing destabilization of biological membranes,

Cryptolepine (S. acuta, cordifolia, rhombifolia, spinosa, and ?)

391-mouse-cryptolepine produced 25% maximal protection at 1 mg/kg while dipyridamole produced a 20% maximal effect at 2 mg/kg. Higher doses of cryptolepine showed a reduced effect-20% ethanol vehicle alone provided 45% protection.   **401**-invitro-exhibited antiplatelet effects in vitro in human, rabbit and rat-it exhibited an indirect fibrinolytic action in the rat.

Sida tiagii   Tr   552-India-antiplatlet.

Body, Adaptogenic   Tr   no reported use

An entire section of the Materia Medica of Ayurveda termed Rasayanas is devoted to the enhancement of the body resistance with immunomodulatory and adaptogenic activities. Rasayana generally means nourishing and rejuvenating drugs with multiple applications for longevity, memory enhancement, immunomodulation and adaptogenic.**[728]**

Sida cordifolia

32-mice-root-40% ethanol extract-possess antistress, and adaptogenic activity, hence can be categorized as plant adaptogen.-The stress induced increase in total white blood cell count is decreased indicating antistress, adaptogenic activity-Plant adaptogen are smooth prostressors which reduce the reactivity of host defense system. The mode of action of adaptogens is basically associated with stress system. Adaptogen increase the capacity of stress to respond to the external signals of activating and deactivating mediators of stress response subsequently. The stress induced increase in total WBC count is decreased by SCE, indicating antistress, adaptogenic activity,   **289**-invitro-root-Both sitoindoside IX and X (extracted from Sida cordifolia) exhibited significant adaptogenic effects in the battery of tests accepted for this purpose. The phagocytotic index determined for the two compounds in vitro and the dose-dependent blastogenic response produced in thymocytes and splenic lymphocytes suggest their strong potential as immunostimulatory agents. Sitoindoside X significantly inhibited the production of oxygen metabolites by activated PMN. These findings validate the use of the two plant drugs as health promotive agents in Ayurveda medicine.

Sida cordata

405-rats-whole plant-90% ethanol extract-100/200 mg/kg bw-the above study indicates positive adaptogenic activity of the extract by forced swim test and resultant biochemical studies-significant decrease in the immobility period with simultaneous increase in adrenaline and serotonin levels.

Body, Sedative

Sida rhombifolia
128-mice-root-crude acqueous extract-5mg/kg weight-abolished both conditioned and unconditioned avoidance response-the crude extract produced maximum behavioral changes.

Sida retusa
435-rats-roots-crude water extract-5/10 gm/kg bw-produced a sedative effect, characterized by a decrease in alertness, wakefulness and reactivity,   **529**-mice-root-crude extract-5/10 gm/kg bw-extract produced a sedative effect, characterized by a decrease in alertness, wakefulness and reactivity,

Body, Anti-convulsant

Sida retusa
435-rats-roots-crude water extract-5/10 gm/kg bw-did not possess any anticonvulsant activity,   **529**-mice-root-crude extract-no anticonvulsant activity,

Other Sida

128-Sida rhombifolia-mice-root-crude extract-possessed no anti-convulsant (induced) activity-,   **205-Sida tiagii**-mice-fruit-95% ethanolic extract, n-Hexane extract, ethyl acetate extract-50 and 100 mg/kg bw- In conclusion the EAS of S. tiagii possess sedative, depressant, anxiolytic and anti-seizure activity.,   **275-Sida acuta**-mice-ethanol extract-PTZ induced seizure 50 mg/kg = 100% protection-300 mg/kg = 75% protection,

Body, Antioxidant

An enzyme or other organic substance, as vitamin E or beta carotene, that is capable of counteracting the damaging effects of oxidation in animal tissues. **[dictionary.com]**   Medicinal plants are largely used either for the prevention, or for the curative treatment of several diseases. Among the properties behind these virtues, the antioxidant activity holds the first place. **[27]**   Antioxidants prevent the negative impacts of free radicals and reactive oxygen species and protect the body. However, the use of synthetic antioxidants has been debated due to their toxic and carcinogenic effects, which can result in liver damage, so the discovery of new, reliable and harmless antioxidants from natural resources has become a prominent research topic. **[638]**   All forms of life maintain a reducing environment through endogenously produced enzymes, body fluid, and diet. Disturbances in the normal redox state can cause toxic effects through the production of peroxides and free radicals that damage all components of the cell, including proteins, lipids, and DNA. The damage may cause cell injury and various degenerative disorders such as cardiovascular disease, aging, diabetes, Alzheimer's disease mutations, and cancer. **[716]**

Sida acuta

15-invitro-root-methanolic extract,   77-invitro-leaves-hot distilled water extract- The plant extract and its silver nanoparticles showed good potential as antioxidant agent,   89-invitro-whole plant-aqueous acetone extract (70%, v/v),   92-invitro-whole plant?-methanol extract- it seems that the extracts of S. acuta utilize their antioxidant properties by increasing SOD activity to nearly 1.8–2.2 its normal level in order to protect cells against negative effects of stress produced by the proliferation of HepG-2 cells, 103-invitro-ethanolic>methanolic extract,   114-invitro-whole plant?-80% acetone extract- The results of this study show that these Malvaceae species can be used as easily accessible source of natural antioxidants, natural lipoxygenase and xanthine oxidase inhibitories,   115-invitro-leaf-methanol extract-exhibited the potential free radical scavenging activity (antioxidant activity) having IC50 value of 86.34µg/ml. The reducing power of the extract was linearly proportional to the concentration of the sample,   141-whole plant?-methanol extract-The results of the antioxidant properties showed that theses extracts significantly increased SOD, CAT and GsT activity after 48 h,   237-invitro-leaf-water and methanol extracts- The photochemistry of the plant leaves revealed that S. acuta is laden with anti-oxidative compounds with remarkable concentrations of saponins (0.772 mg/100g), flavonoids (0.112 mg/100g), alkaloids (0.076 mg/100g) and tannins (0.0541mg/100g),   254-invitro-ethyl acetate and dichloromethane fractions most potent,   264-rats-leaf-100% ethanol extract-40-60mg/kg body weight-The result showed that ethanolic leaf extract of S. acuta possesses an antioxidant property which, in a dose dependent manner, reduces/ameliorates oxidative stress in rats-a significant increase (P < 0.05) in reduced glutathione in rats treated with 40 and 60 mg/kg of S. acuta leaf extract when compared to the control while catalase and superoxide dismutase activity showed significant increase (P < 0.05) in rats treated with 60mg/kg leaf extract of Sida acuta when compared to the control group., 270-The antioxidant effects demonstrated by these extracts may contribute to this protective effect, although ethanolic extract demonstrated better antioxidant activity than methanol extract,   292-invitro-The present study has shown that the whole plant of Sida acuta contains DEHP and the compound is a potent inhibitor of LOX. The enzyme inhibition may partially impart the anti-inflammatory property of the plant,   460-rats-ethanolic extract- NDEA and CCl4 induced hepatocellular cancers-200 mg/kg bw-28 days- antioxidant enzymes reduced oxidative stress induced damage exhibiting a potent antioxidant and anticancer activity, in a dose dependent manner,   460-rats-whole plant-70% ethanol extract-400mg/kg bw-significantly quenched the free radical damage- showed a significant increase in activities of antioxidant enzymes that reduces the oxidative stress induced damage exhibiting a potent antioxidant and anticancer activity,   565-invitro-whole plant-three compounds showed significant antioxidant effect (EC50 = 86.9, 68.2, and 70.9 µM, respectively) in the DPPH radicals scavenging activity assay,   644-invitro-whole plant- chloroform extract- in vitro free radical scavenging assays activity, the roots posses moderate antioxidants activities when compared with standard drug of Ascorbic acid. Therefore, based on the results it can be concluded that the chloroform extract of Sida acuta may hold enormous resource of pharmaceutical properties, **653**-invitro-leaves-chloroform and ethanolic extracts-In all tests inhibition percentages increased with increasing concentrations of the extracts. The chloroform extract was somewhat stronger than the alcoholic extract in all tests. Sida acuta shows good activity in all the tested methods at 100μg/ml concentration...Phenolic content shows good scavenging of all the tested methods at 100μg/ml concentration, when compared to that of whole extracts...The results of free radical scavenging activity showed that the leaves have significant antioxidant activity.

Tr 89-Burkina Faso, 221-India, 264-Nigeria, 609-India,

Sida cordifolia

14-invitro-highest total phenolic content of any sida, **15**-invitro-root-methanolic extract-most antioxidants of all sidas, **24**-roots-80% ethanol extract-as the concentration of the extract increased, activity was found to increase. The IC50 value for the extract was 50 μg/mL and for ascorbic acid standard was 1.16 μg/mL, **26**-rats-water extract-100 mg/kg bw-Rotenone induced oxidative damage was attenuated by the water extract- The maximum effect in all the above activities was observed in the water extract (100mg/kg) treated group, which was comparable to l-deprenyl treated group, **27**-invitro-whole plant?-80% acetone extract>chloroform extract for alkaloid compounds-The antioxidant activity of the samples was significant using three separate methods--DPPH 6.63±0.10 mmoL AAE/g fractions-Quercetin 13.76±0.26 mmoL AAE/g fraction—FRAP 3.47±0.001 mmoL AAE/g fraction-Trolox 7.46±3.38 mmoL AAE/g fraction—ABTS 3.90±0.03 mmoL AAE/g fraction- Quercetin 7.81±0.21 mmoL AAE/g fraction,, **28**-rats?-50 % ethanolic extract- The activity of antioxidant enzymes and glutathione content, which was lowered due to alcohol toxicity, was increased to a near-normal level, **31**-rats-root-ethanolic extract- In short, the study revealed that 50% ethanolic extract of Sida cordifolia has got potent antioxidant and antiinflammatory activity and the activity is comparable with the standard drug deprenyl, **33**-rats-leaves-hydroalcoholic extract-100 and 500 mg/kg- both doses significantly increased endogenous antioxidants in heart tissue homogenate. Moreover, biochemical findings were supported by histopathological observations, **42**-rats-the results from the ABTS assay showed that the ethanolic extract of Sida cordifolia was IC50 16.07 mcg/ml- The relative antioxidant capacity for the water infusion was IC50 342.82 μg/ml-The results on lipid peroxidation was IC50 126.78 μg/ml, **67**-rats-neurotoxicity-ethanolic extract of root-50 mg/100gm bw/day-comparable with the standard drug deprenyl, **115**-invitro-leaf-methanol extract-The methanol extract of the plant exhibited the potential free radical scavenging activity (antioxidant activity) having IC50 value of 86.34μg/ml. The reducing power of the extract was linearly proportional to the concentration of the sample, **117**-invitro-whole plant?-80% acetone extract- Antioxidant capacity noticed that the reduction capacity of DPPH radicals obtained the best result comparatively to the others methods of free radical scavenging (but scored on all three antioxidant tests, **120**-aerial parts-aqueous and hydroalcoholic extracts-test results indicate that S. cordifolia has a rich content of antioxidant compounds, mostly saponins-low correlation between antioxidant activity and saponins content, **121**-invitro-roots-All extracts of Sida cordifolia. (SC) have effective reducing power and free-radical scavenging activity. Only the root extract exhibited superoxide-scavenging activity and inhibited lipid peroxidation in rat liver homogenate. All these antioxidant properties were concentration dependent, **123**--rats--whole plant--ABTS assay--ethanolic extract of Sida cordifolia =IC50 16.07 mg/ml--water infusion=IC50 342.82 mg/ml, **146**-invitro-whole plant-ethanol and acqueous extract (10, 20, 30, 40 mg/ml)-possesses potent antioxidant activity-ethanolic extract almost quantitatively equivalent to the standard ascorbic acid, **148**-rats-leaves-alcoholic extract-400mg/kg weight-significant increase in antioxidant enzymes such as catalase and superoxide dismutase levels, **163**-rats-leaves-petroleum ether and methanol extract-it was evident from our study that 500 mg/kg, and 500 mg/ kg, causes significant inclination in endogenous antioxidant enzyme activities such as SOD and catalase when compared to ISO/IRI control group, **169**-rats-whole plant?-ethanol extract- Oxidative stress was increased in alcohol-treated rats as evidenced by the lowered activities of antioxidant enzymes, decreased level of reduced glutathione (GSH), increased lipid peroxidation products, and decreased expression of γ-glutamyl cysteine synthase in liver. The co-administration of Sida cordifolia with alcohol almost reversed these changes, **171**-rats-aerial parts-water extract-an increase in antioxidant enzymatic activity (SOD, CAT) and decrease in lipid peroxidation indicating Sida cordifolia prevent oxidative damage of diabetic rats-400mg/kg is sufficient to increase the antioxidant enzymatic (SOD, CAT) activities through free radicals scavenging, **175**-rats-water extract-200&400 mg/kg bw-the flavonoids and phenols present in Sida cordifolia contribute for antioxidant potentiality that exhibits nephroprotective activity, **182**-invitro-root-50% ethanol extract-has potent anti-oxidant and anti-inflammatory activity-has a protective effect on quinolinic acid-induced neurotoxicity, which was comparable with the standard drug deprenyl--exerts an antioxidant effect by decreasing lipid peroxidation, increasing GSH level and maintaining a normal level of antioxidant enzymes-The activity of antioxidant enzymes and glutathione content, which was lowered due to alcohol toxicity, was increased to a near-normal level, **200**-invitro-had maximum amount of polyphenols and flavonoids which is directly related to their greater antioxidant activity, **211**-invitro- aerial parts?- 80% acetone extract (400 ml acetone + 100 ml water) for 24 h under mechanic agitation at room temperature-DPPH 6.63± mmoL/g-Quercetin DPPH 13.76± mmoL/g--FRAP 3.47± mmoL/g-Trolox FRAP 7.46± mmoL/g--ABTS 3.90± mmoL/g-Quercetin ABTS 7.81± mmoL/g, **289**-invitro-roots-it significantly inhibited the production of oxygen metabolites by activated PMN, **470**-invitro-roots-ethanol extract- The antioxidant property of ethanolic extract of S. cordifolia was assessed by DPPH free radical scavenging activity-the IC50 value was found to be 50 µg/mL which was not comparable to the standard ascorbic acid, **502**-invitro- Sida cordifolia exhibited a potent anti-oxidant activity in both DPPH and superoxide anion radical scavenging assays IC50 = 0.005 ± 0.0004, and 0.078 ± 0.002 mg/mL, respectively, **641**-seed-cold distilled methanol extract- exhibited a potent anti-oxidant activity in both DPPH and superoxide anion radical scavenging assays (IC50 = 0.005 ± 0.0004, and 0.078 ± 0.002 mg/mL, respectively), **644**-invitro-whole plant- chloroform extract- in

154

vitro free radical scavenging assays activity, the roots posses moderate antioxidants activities when compared with standard drug of Ascorbic acid. Therefore, based on the results it can be concluded that the chloroform extract of Sida acuta may hold enormous resource of pharmaceutical properties.

Tr 148-India-all parts of the plant are used as (an) antioxidant,

Sida rhombifolia

15-invitro-root-methanolic extract, **46**-rats-stems and roots-extracts- In induced arthritis in experimental rats the altered levels of hematological parameters were reverted to near normal levels-The free radical scavenging activity of the plant was further evidenced by histological and transmission electron microscopy observations made on the hind limb tissue, **49**-rats-seed-free radical scavenging activity, **57**-rats-The comparative antioxidant potentials of ethanol extract of roots, stems, leaves, and whole plant were studied-All extracts of this plant showed effective free radical scavenging activity, reducing power, and superoxide scavenging activity. Only root extract inhibited lipid peroxidation in rat liver and brain homogenate. All these antioxidant properties were concentration dependent, **75**-invitro-All extracts of this plant showed effective free radical scavenging activity, reducing power, and superoxide scavenging activity. The highest antioxidant activity was observed in root extract-All these antioxidant properties were concentration dependent, **127**-invitro-rats-superoxide scavenging activity-free radical scavenging activity, **155**-rats-IP (85 mg/kg, s.c.) induced myocardial necrosis in rats-significant increase in cardiac endogenous enzymatic and non-enzymatic antioxidants, **170**-invitro-water and methanolic extracts-the methanolic extract of Sida rhombifolia Linn. exhibited better antioxidant activity (IC50: 10.77 and 42 µg/mL) than aqueous extract (IC50: 44.36 and 62.68 µg/mL) in DPPH scavenging assay, **195**-invitro-ethyl acetate extract-had the highest content of phenolic compounds (88.311 ± 2.660 mg GAE/g) and the best antioxidant activity for the DPPH and TEAC assay (IC50 = 70.503 ±1.629 and 20.580 ± 0.271, respectively), **407**-rats-seed-80% methanol extract-Seed extract possibly due to its free radical scavenging property was capable in augmenting the deficient functioning of impaired enzymes of antioxidant defense system, **486**-invitro-whole plant?- water, ethanol 70%, alkaloid and flavonoid extracts-From several extracts of sidaguri, the strongest and the weakest of LC50 value were ethanol extract of leaves (1780 ppm) and water extract of herbs (148 ppm), respectively. Most of the extracts examined could inhibit the activity of xanthine oxidase and the strongest inhibitor was alkaloid extract of herbs (400 ppm) followed by flavonoid extract of herbs (400 ppm), **536**-rats-whole plant?-ethanol extract- causes myocardial adaptation by augmenting endogenous antioxidants and protects rat hearts from decline in cardiac function and oxidative stress associated with ISP induced myocardial injury, **538**-rats-root-ethanol extract-The protective effect of Sida rhombifolia. L root might be attributed to the antioxidant elements present in it, **541**-rats-roots-alcoholic extract- The biological defense system constituting the superoxide dismutase, glutathione peroxidase, ascorbic acid showed a significant increase while the lipid peroxide content was found to decrease to large extent on SRE treatment thereby indicating the extracts free radical scavenging property, **619**-whole plant-ethyl acetate extract-scavenging DPPH radicals and ferrous ions with EC50 of 380.5 and 263.4μg/mL, respectively, **662**-invitro-leaves-cold distilled water extract-the biofunctionalized AgNPs displayed remarkable antioxidant activities-The AgNPs exhibited higher phosphomolybdate reducing power (2127 AEAA) when compared to the aqueous extract (1428AEAA)and standard (742AEAA).The ferric reducing power of AgNPs (1.83AU at a concentration of 1000 mg/ml) was estimated by the reduction of Fe3þ/ferricyanide complex and it was higher than the standard ferulic acid (1.61AU)as well as aqueous extract (1.27AU).The AgNPs exhibited higher superoxide radical scavenging activity (IC50 value46.25 mg/ml) when compared to aqueous extract (IC50 value 81.99 mg/ml) and standard (IC50value202.2 mg/ml). The DPPH radical scavenging activity of AgNPs was found to be dose-dependent and higher (IC50 value 50.12 mg/ml) when compared to aqueous extract (IC50 value 77.48 mg/ml) and standard (IC50value 153.4 mg/ml).

Tr   524-Phillipines-roots,

Sida spinosa

15-invitro-root-methanolic extract,   **114**-invitro-whole plant?-80% acetone extract- The results of this study show that these Malvaceae species can be used as easily accessible source of natural antioxidants, natural lipoxygenase and xanthine oxidase inhibitories,   **254**-invitro-ethyl acetate and dichloromethane fractions most potent,   **433**-invitro-whole plant-80% ethanol extract-50 ug/ml-Free radicals scavenging activity was comparable to ascorbic acid (standard). The crude ethanolic extract of whole plant of Sida spinosa exhibited significant inhibition of nitric oxide & superoxide scavenging activity. The study reveals in-vitro antioxidant activity of Sida spinosa-Hydroxyl radicals scavenging activity was dose dependent and less than half of standard,   **566**-invitro-whole plant-80% ethanolic extract- The study reveals in-vitro antioxidant activity of Sida spinosa.

Sida cordata

15-invitro-root-methanolic extract,   **282**-invitro-leaf-methanol extract-The plant extract show moderate free radical scavenging (IC50 190μg/ml) compared with standard ascorbic acid (IC50 10 μg/ml),   **293**-invitro-goat blood-methanol and acetone extracts have maximum activity,   **405**-rats-whole plant-+90%ethanol extract- The animals treated with total extract (100mg/kg) and (200mg/kg) showed significant increase in anti oxidant markers,   **494**-rats-whole plant-methanol extract- Although the extract and all its derived fractions exhibited good antioxidant activities however, the most distinguished scavenging potential was observed for the ethyl acetate fraction,   **496**-rats-whole plant-methanolic extract- ethyl acetate fraction-This may be related to its anti-oxidative properties.

Sida rhomboidea

288-rats-leaves-ethanol extract-a potent antioxidant and free radical scavenger-pre-treatment improves cardiac antioxidant status in IP induced Myocardial infarction by effective scavenging of free radicals generated during oxidation of catecholamines thus collectively contributing to its overall antioxidant and anti ischemic activity, **320**-invitro-leaves-methanol extract-possesses potent antioxidant and free radical properties that have been demonstrated using a variety of in vitro experimental models-higher reducing potential OD max=1.20±0.27), **323**-invitro-leaf-?extract, **288**-rats-leaves-ethanol extract-a potent antioxidant and free radical scavenger-Results clearly indicated that SR was capable of reducing LDL oxidation and formation of intermediary oxidation products. Also, SR successfully attenuated peroxyl radical formation, mitochondrial dysfunction, nuclear condensation, and apoptosis in Ox-LDL-exposed human monocyte-derived macrophages, **547**-invitro-leaf-Results clearly indicated that SR was capable of reducing LDL oxidation and formation of intermediary oxidation products.

Sida retusa

15-invitro-root-methanolic extract, **57**-rats-The comparative antioxidant potentials of ethanol extract of roots, stems, leaves, and whole plant were studied-All extracts of this plant showed effective free radical scavenging activity, reducing power, and superoxide scavenging activity. Only root extract inhibited lipid peroxidation in rat liver and brain homogenate. All these antioxidant properties were concentration dependent, **461**-rats-roots-methanol extract-The quantity of S. retusa root extract required for 50% inhibition of lipid peroxidation, scavenging hydroxyl radical and superoxide radical was 1130.24 ug/ml respectively, **464**-mice/rats-seed-80% methanol extract- We report for the first time that chemopreventive and anti-hepatotoxic potentials of S. rhombifolia ssp. retusa seed extract of is due to free radical scavenging activity and restoration and maintenance of cellular integrity... Seed extract possibly due to its free radical scavenging property was capable in augmenting the deficient functioning of impaired enzymes of antioxidant defense system.

Tr 131-Ayurveda, 461-invitro-Ayurveda-root-possesses significant antioxidant activity

Sida indica

15-invitro-root-methanolic extract, **674**-invitro-leaf-boiling distilled water extract- polyphenol stabilized gold nanoparticles displayed good in vitro free radical scavenging activities as indicated in various in vitro antioxidant assays, **677**-invitro-fruits-80% ethanol extract/Petroleum ether extract/ Chloroform extract/Ethyl acetate extract/Butanol extract/Aqueous extract-- Ethyl acetate fraction of Sida indica has produced highly significant antioxidant activity followed by chloroform extract. The both extracts are rich in total phenol and flavonoid content (and) can be considered as new source of natural antioxidant (the other extracts all have lesser amounts as well), **686**-invitro-leaf and seed-methanol extract-the current findings reconfirmed those of earlier studies that found S. indica to be a reliable natural antioxidant that can safely be used in the pharmaceutical and food industries to prevent the effects of reactive oxygen species and reduce the risks of cardiovascular disease-- the extracts obtained from S. indica seed treated with CAN, NPK or grown on control soils had little tendency to scavenge DPPH radicals compared to the other extracts. When leaves grown on CAN- and NPK-treated and control soils were compared, the control leaf extract showed the highest DPPH radical scavenging activity at all of the studied concentrations. Among the fertilizer applications, leaves treated with NPK showed higher DPPH scavenging activity than leaves treated with CAN. When roots treated with CAN and NPK and the control were compared, the CAN and NPK root extracts showed higher DPPH scavenging activities than the control root extract, **705**-leaf-aqueous extract-exhibits good free radical scavenging activities, **707**-leaf-aqueous extract-exhibits good free radical scavenging activities, **716**-invitro-whole plant-methanol extract> butanol > ethyl acetate > chloroform > n-hexane and butanol > chloroform > hexane > ethyl acetate fractions-the antioxidant/radical scavenging capacity of the extracts was found to be a dose-dependent activity-potential sources of natural antioxidants, **719**-invitro-leaf-methanolic extract-Maximum scav-enging of nitric oxide and superoxide radical found were 28.74 % and 49. 62 % respectively at 250 µg/ml concentration,

Sida cardifolia

177-rats-whole plant?-50% ethanol extract- potent anti-antioxidant and anti-inflammatory activity when compared with standard drug deprenyl, **200**-invitro-leaf-acetone extract-Thus acetone leaf extract of Sida cardifolia had maximum amount of polyphenols and flavonoids which is directly related to their greater antioxidant activity also. Thus active molecules present in the acetone leaf extract of Sida cardifolia has antioxidant property which may be useful in targeting the release of free radical intermediates along with the generation of ROS from various metabolic activities,

Other Sidas

15-Sida mysorensis-invitro-root-methanolic extract, **318-Sida pilosa**-whole plant?-water extract/ethyl acetate-highest antioxidant activity, **350-Sida veronicaefolia**-invitro-meristem and leaves-ethanolic extract-strength in decreasing order-Ascorbic acid>ESV (0.3mg/kg)>ESV (0.2 mg/kg)> ESV (0.1 mg/kg)-exhibits free radical scavenging activity, **490- Sida tuberculata**-leaves and roots-water and ethanol extracts-all extracts are a considerable source of ecdysteroids and possesses a significant antioxidant property with low toxic potential- hydroethanolic extracts of leaves were most effective compared to roots and presented a higher IC50 antioxidant than aqueous extracts.

Body, Arthritis and Osteoarthritis

The non-steroidal anti-inflammatory drugs (NSAIDs) are the main drugs of choice in modern medicine which has lots of side effects; therefore they are not safe for long-term therapy. Sandhigatavata (Osteoarthritis) is a chronic, progressive and degenerative disorder of the joints. In modern medical science, a lot of research works have been conducted but still no radical therapy is available for Sandhigata Vata (Osteoarthritis). Some drugs like NSAIDs, Corticosteroids and Opoid analgesics are used in routine practice to provide some relief in signs and symptoms. These medications usually provide quick relief in symptoms but causes a number of unpleasant and intolerable side effects. Osteoarthritis is the most common articular disorder begins asymptomatically in the 2nd & 3rd decades and is extremely common by age 70. Almost all persons by age 40 have some pathologic change in weight bearing joint, 25% females & 16% males have symptomatic osteoarthritis. Allopathic treatment has its own limitation in managing this disease. It can provide either conservative or surgical treatment and is highly symptomatic and with troublesome side effects. Whereas such type of conditions can be better treatable by the management and procedures mentioned in Ayurvedic classics. [161]   Radiological and histological studies revealed that near a normal structure of paw and knee joint respectively with the high dose of the extract in FA induced arthritis. Phytochemical constituents like flavonoids, saponins, glycosides and alkaloids were already reported for their anti-arthritic activity and these constituents were present in Ethanolic extract of Sida cardifolia. Hence these chemical constituents can be accounted for the observed anti-arthritic activities. [177]   250 mcg/ml. concentrations of Sida indica were used and results were better than acetyl salicylic acid. [715]

Sida acuta   Tr   32-Ayurveda-aches and pains- joints and bones, 161-Ayurveda-aches and pains,   161-Ayurveda-root extract-medicated enema, 568-Nigeria,

Sida cordifolia

23-osteoarthritis-rats,   **177**-rats-anti-arthritic,   **317**-osteoarthritis-rats?-whole plant?-dried powder (270 mg/kg b. wt.)- possesses potent anti-osteoarthritic activity-Results clearly indicate that S. cordifolia (is) responsible for preventing the structural loss of the knee joint and joint space, which is an important aspect in this disease,-The anterior posterior radiographs showed a protective effect against OA. Histopathology revealed protection in the structure of the articular cartilage and in chondrocyte pathology as well as reduced clefting. Treatment with herbs has shown chondroid matrix within normal limits.

Tr   28-India-aches and pains,   32-Ayurveda-aches and pains,   118-Ayurveda-allieviates local pain-as oil,   125-India-seed-oil applied to sore muscles and joints,   161-Ayurveda-osteoarthritis,   317-Ayurveda-Among many herbs that have been used for ages in Ayurveda to treat the inflammatory conditions like OA, Sida cordifolia L. (Bala),   664-India-oil-extract-aches and pains,

Sida rhombifolia

46-rats-stems and roots-extracts- induced arthritis in experimental rats. The altered levels of hematological parameters were reverted to near normal levels-Oral administration significantly increased the levels of thiobarbituric acid reactive substances and activities of catalase and glutathione peroxidase and decreased the levels of reduced glutathione and superoxide dismutase activity in arthritis induced rats,   **73**-rats?- ethanol and aqueous extracts-

159

useful in the treatment of arthritis, **127**-rats?-root and stem-The altered levels of hematological parameters were reverted to near normal levels, especially the elevated rate of erythrocyte sedimentation was significantly reduced by S. rhombifolia extracts in experimental rats. Oral administration of root and stem of S. rhombifolia extracts significantly increased the levels of thiobarbituric acid reactive substances and activities of catalase and glutathione peroxidase and decreased the levels of reduced glutathione and superoxide dismutase activity in arthritis induced rats,, **292**-review, **541**-rats-roots-90% alcoholic extract- The biological defense system constituting the superoxide dismutase, glutathione peroxidase, ascorbic acid showed a significant increase while the lipid peroxide content was found to decrease to large extent on SRE treatment thereby indicating the extracts free radical scavenging property. Histopathological studies too supported anti-rheumatic potential of the roots of Sida rhombifolia. The compete repair of synovial membrane by SRE in Histopathological parameter further proved the anti-arthritic potential of SRE.

Tr 46-India, 190-India, 522-India-decoction of entire plant reduces rheumatic pain, 522-India-decoction of entire plant mixed with equal proportion of cow's milk and taken every morning for about a week reduces rheumatic pain

Sida cardifolia
177-mice-whole plant-50% ethanolic extract-potent anti-antioxidant and anti-inflammatory activity when compared with standard drug deprenyl--500mg/kg bw exhibited a significant anti-arthritic activity by reducing serum biochemical parameters like ALP, SGOT, SGPT levels and reduced the hematological parameters like ESR and WBC and increases the RBC and Hb levels in FA induced arthritis models in rats-Radiological and histological studies revealed that near a normal structure of paw and knee joint respectively with the high dose of the extract in FA induced arthritis,

Sida indica
715-invitro-whole plant?-water extract-100m cg/ml and 250 mcg/ml. concentrations were used and results were better than acetyl salicylic acid (250 mcg/ml.). **Tr** 678-Ayurveda-root,

Sida cordata
Tr 497-India-whole plant- decoction of the whole plant is given daily for one week to relive from joint pain,

Body, Chemoprotective
In the treatment of cancer, chemoprotective agents are drugs which protect healthy tissue from the toxic effects of anticancer drugs. **[1]** We report for the first time that chemopreventive and anti-hepatotoxic potentials of S. rhombifolia ssp. retusa seed extract of is due to free radical scavenging activity and restoration and maintenance of cellular integrity. **[464]**

Sida acuta   cytoprotective (protects cell against harmful agents)

64-review-widely used in cancer treatment was recently screened for cytoxicity against Hep G2 hepatocarcinoma cells-showed moderate anti-proliferative effects,   **253**-invitro-whole plant-EtOAc extract-10 microg/mL-exhibits 75% inhibition of induced preneoplastic lesions,

Tr   82-India-cytoprotective (protects cell against harmful agents),   211-Burkana Faso-cancer treatment,

Sida cordifolia   (neurotoxicity)

31-rats-root-50% ethanolic extract-quinolinic acid (QUIN) induced neurotoxicity and to compare its effect with the standard drug deprenyl in rat brain-has got potent antioxidant and antiinflammatory activity and the activity is comparable with the standard drug deprenyl,   **64**-review-widely used in cancer treatment was recently screened for cytoxicity against Hep G2 hepatocarcinoma cells-showed moderate anti-proliferative effects,   **67**-rats-root-50% ethanolic extract-quinolinic acid induced neurotoxicity- 50 mg/100 g bw/day-potent antioxidant and antiinflammatory activity-the activity is comparable to deprenyl,   **182**-rats-roots-50 % ethanolic extract-quinolinic acid-induced neurotoxicity-has potent anti-oxidant and anti-inflammatory activity-protective effect comparable to deprenyl.

Sida rhombifolia

64-review-widely used in cancer treatment was recently screened for cytoxicity against Hep G2 hepatocarcinoma cells-showed moderate anti-proliferative effects.

Sida retusa

464-mice-seeds-methanol-80% methanol extract-We report for the first time that chemopreventive and anti-hepatotoxic potentials of S. rhombifolia ssp. retusa seed extract of is due to free radical scavenging activity and restoration and maintenance of cellular integrity.... Remarkable changes viz; enhanced cell to cell adhesion among adjacent cells, compact junctional complexes, restoration of morphological architecture and intimate cell contacts with well defined cell boundaries resembling to normal hepatocytes were noticed. This suggests that the seed extract helps in repair of cellular damage and prevents the formation of preneoplastic histopathological changes. In conclusion, the chemopreventive and antihepatotoxic effects of seed extract are attributed for its suppression of lipid peroxidation, free radical scavenging activity, ability to induce GST and other phase II enzymes involved in carcinogen detoxification and maintenance of structural integrity of the hepatocyte. Therefore, the present study validates the potential usefulness of seeds as a promising hepatoprotectant--the chemo-preventive and hepatoprotective potentials of seed extract are due to free radical scavenging activity and restoration of cellular structural integrity--the results of the present study indicates significant inhibitory effects of seed extract on the development of preneoplastic foci.

Sida is one of the important medicinal plant species used to treat various diseases in Ayurveda and other traditional systems of medicine. [15]

Body, Chills
No peer review

Sida acuta   Tr   32-Ayurveda,   161-Ayurveda,

Sida cordifolia   Tr   32-Ayurveda, 118-Ayurveda, 161-Ayurveda,

Body, Depression
Tr   no reported use

A state of low mood and aversion to activity that can affect a person's thoughts, behavior, feelings, and sense of well-being. People with a depressed mood may be notably sad, anxious, or empty; they may also feel notably hopeless, helpless, dejected, or worthless. [1]

Sida acuta

14--mice--leaf--ethanol extract—18-25g--contains analgesic and antidepressant-like properties which may be beneficial in the management of pain, **690**-invitro-the beneficial effects of Loliolide in depression treatment are also significant,

Sida tiagii

205--invitro--fruit--ethanolic/ethyl acetate extract--sedative, depressant, anxiolytic and anti-seizure activity--50-500 mg/kg,   **607**-mice-fruit-hot 95% ethanol extract-the monamine oxidase inhibiting effect and lipid peroxidation inhibiting effect may contribute favorably to an antidepressant like activity-may have potential therapeutic value for the management of depressive disorders,

Body, Detoxification

Sida cordifolia   **182**-rats-roots-50 % ethanolic extract-GSH is a tripeptide antioxidant critical for cellular protection such as detoxification of reactive oxygen species. Depletion of GSH in tissue leads to impairment of the cellular defense against reactive oxygen species and may lead to peroxidative injury... increased GSH level with S. cordifolia is in agreement with earlier studies- potent hepatoprotective action against alcohol-induced toxicity, which was mediated by lowering oxidative stress and by down-regulating the transcription factors.

Tr   161-Ayurveda-root extract-used for all kinds of detoxification-like medicated enema,   444-Ayurveda-Bala-Balya-tonic, improves strength

Sida rhombifolia   Tr   587-Bangladesh-stems and roots-depurative,

162

Sida cardifolia
177-mice/rats-whole plant-50% ethanolic extract-500mg/kg bw-potent anti-antioxidant and anti-inflammatory activity when compared with standard drug deprenyl.-5gm/kg wt,

Body, Edema
An abnormal accumulation of fluid in the interstitium, located beneath the skin and in the cavities of the body, which can cause severe pain. [1]

Sida acuta
186-rats-whole plant-methanolic extract-400mg/kg-the PI with indomethacin and Sida acuta in carrageenan induced paw edema at the dose level 400 mg/kg were 60% and 52.5% at the end of 5 hr, 581-invitro-whole plant-methanolic extract- The PI with indomethacin and Sida acuta in carrageenan induced paw edema at the dose level 400 mg/kg were 60% and 52.5% at the end of 5 hr... The methanolic extract possesses anti-inflammatory and analgesic activity, 651-invitro-leaves-ethanol extract-The edema reductions were more than that obtained for phenylbutazone; the standard anti-inflammatory agent,

Tr 32-Ayurveda, 161-Ayurveda, 270-India-boiled in gingelly oil-testicular swellings and elephantiasis, 361-India- leaves are boiled in oil and applied to testicular swellings and elephantiasis, 362-India- leaves are boiled in oil and applied to testicular swellings and elephantiasis, 358-review-leaves,

Sida cordifolia
36-rats/invitro-a new alkaloid-produced 16.93 and 24.43 % inhibition of paw edema at the doses of 25 and 50 mg/kg body weight respectively at the third hour of study, 43-rats-leaf-water extract-400 mg/kg bw- significant inhibition of carrageenin-induced rat paw edema but did not block the edema induced by arachidonic acid. 61-rats-leaf-water extract-400 mg/kg bw- a significant inhibition of carrageenin-induced rat paw but did not block the edema induced by arachidonic acid, 116- new flavonol glycoside-rats-80% ethanolic extract>n-hexane/dichloromethane/ethyl acetate/n-butanol-In carrageenan induced rat paw edema the compound produced 16.15 and 28.52% inhibition of paw edema at doses of 25 and 50 mg kg body weight at the 3rd h of study, 133-rats-whole plant-water extract-successively extracted with chloroform (3x72 h), methanol (3x72 h) and 80% ethanol (3x72 h)-showed significant inhibition of writhing reflexes...extracts exhibited sufficient inhibition of paw edema of 32.97 - 40.85%, at the end of the fourth hour. The activities of the extracts were comparable to the standard drug, phenylbutazone. In this experiment, the lower dose 100 mg/kg did not show any significant antiinflammatory activity (data not given). The exact mechanism(s) of the analgesic and antiinflammatory activities of the extracts is/are yet to be elucidated, 152-rats-seed oil- petroleum ether (40-600C) extract-displayed significant anti-inflammatory activity at a dose of 400 mg/Kg bw-possesses anti-inflammatory activity against carrageenan induced

paw edema, **154**-mice-acqueous extract-leaves-400 mg/kg- a significant inhibition of carrageenin-induced rat paw edema-but did not block the edema induced by arachidonic acid, **183**-mice-aerial parts-chloroform (3 × 72h)/methanol (3 × 72h)/80% ethanol (3 × 72h) extract>ethyl acetate-50 mg/ kg bw-compound also exhibited significant (p<0.01) inhibition of rat paw edema induced by carrageenan, **537**-rat-whole plant?-80% ethanolic extract- percentage reduction in the paw edema was 58.13% with Indomethacin, 48.83% and 53.48% with 100 mg/kg and 200 mg/kg Sida cordifolia Linn respectively.

Tr 32-Ayurveda, 118-Ayurveda-Oil preparation is also cure (for) swelling disorder, 161-Ayurveda, 358-Senegal, Côte d'Ivoire, Burkina Faso, Burundi, Kenya, Papua New Guinea and the Philippines-pounded leaves are applied as a poultice to sprains and swellings,

Sida rhombifolia

127-rats-stems and roots-successive extracts of petroleum ether, chloroform, ethyl acetate and ethanol, **136**-rats-roots-water and ethanol extracts-200/400/600 mg/kg bw-the time dependent inhibition of edema was observed starting from 2 hours. The ethanolic extract produced most effective inhibition of edema, **185**-leaves-butanolic extract-200mg/kg-comparable to that of phenylbutazone, 100 mg/kg inhibition, **194**-rats-whole plant?-80% acetone extract-100/200/400 mg/kg bw-dose-dependent inhibition of edema was observed at 1; 2 and 3 hours-extracts showed a dose-dependent inhibition of croton oil induced ear edema, at doses of 200; 300 and 500 μg/ear, **201**-rats-aerial parts-methanolic extract- The methanolic extract of the aerial parts showed significant edema suppressant activity in rats- The edema suppressant activity the drug may be due to the inhibitory effects on the release of histamine like substances, **281**-rats-leaves-ethanol: water 3:7-400 mg/kg orally- significant edema suppressant activity in rats, **324**-whole plant-methanolic extract-significant edema suppressant activity in rats-may be due to the inhibitory effects on the release of histamine like substances.

Tr 51-India-whole plant?-poulticing swellings, 150-Ethiopia-root and leaf, 150-Ethiopia-leaf, 522-Ayurveda-leaves-The Mundas apply the pounded leaves on swellings, 522-Guatemela-dried leaf-hot aqueous extract-externally-scrofula, 524-Phillipines-whole plant?-poultice, 543-Ayurveda, 634-Sri Lanka-upper root,

Sida rhomboidea

185-invitro-leaf-Percentage inhibition of edema by butanolic extract (33.05, P<0.001) is comparable to that of phenylbutazone, 100 mg/kg inhibition (38.83%).

Other Sida

448-**Sida Indica**-rats-whole plant-Pet. ether, Chloroform, Ethanol & Aqueous extracts-400 mg/kg bw-reduced Carragenan induced paw edema, **551**- **Sida tiagii**-rats?-fruits-95% ethanol extract>n-Hexane/Ethyl acetate extract>Residual ethanolic extract-There was decrease in edema volume in administered animals in carrageenan and egg-albumin induced edema models,   **Tr**   568- Sida ovata Forssk-Nigeria,

Cryptolepine   (S. acuta, cordifolia, rhombifolia, spinosa, and ?)

386-rats-10–40 mg/kg i.p.- produced significant dose-dependent inhibition of the carrageenan-induced rat paw edema,   **583**-invitro-Carrageenan induced edema in the rat hind paw was inhibited by Cryptolepine (1, 5, 10 and 20 mg/kg-1).

Body, Fever (Antipyretic)
Substances that reduce fever [1]

Sida acuta

3-rats-leaf-acetone extract-showed significant antipyretic activity,   **110**-rats-leaves-all extracts lowered the temperature with the passage of time (cited in 107),

Tr   3-India-root or whole plant,   6-Ayurveda,   7-Burkina Faso/Italy, 7-Central America,   21-Ayurveda-root,   52-India-whole plant-hot water extract,   76-W Africa,   82-India,   101-India,   88-Nigeria-Ayurveda, 93-Italy/Burkina Faso-leaves,   101-Nicaragua,the decoction of the entire plant is taken orally,   107-India,   107-Nicaragua,   110-India,   138-India-whole plant-hot water extract,   168-Nicaragua-decoction of the entire plant taken orally,   168-India-dried entire plant-hot water extract,   174-India, 186-India,   203-Burkina-Faso-children,   214-India-febrile illness,   217-Ayurveda,   219-Nigeria-leaf usually used,   220-Burkina Faso,   220-Nicaragua/Guatemala,   220-India,   220-Nigeria,   220-BurkinaFaso, 220-SriLanka,   221-India,   223-India,   238-Sri Lanka-roots and leaves, 270-India-root,   271-Nicaragua-decoction of the entire plant,   271-India-hot water extract of the dried entire plant-taken orally,   273-Nigeria,   358-review-roots,   361-review,   362-review-leaves-fever in small children-root-for high fever,   377-Ayurveda-root,   485-Nigeria-survey,   523-India-leaves,   526-Phillipines-Decoction of roots and leaves-taken internally,   526-Phillipines-roots,   549-Ayurveda,   571-India,   588-Nigeria-decoction of whole plant,   596-Nigeria-leaf/root,   609-India, 619-Malaysia,   644-Ayurveda-root,   646-Nigeria,   653-Ayurveda,

Sida cordifolia

34-rats-aerial parts-methanolic extract-500 mg/kg bw-significantly reduced pyrexia induced by TAB vaccine,   **70**-rats-aerial parts-methanolic extract-Oral dose of 500 mg/kg- significantly reduced pyrexia induced by TAB vaccine.

Tr   27-Burkina Faso-leaf decoction,   40-Brazil,   76-W Africa,   88-Ayurveda-juice of plants with water, 117-Burkina-Faso-leaf decoction,   118-Ayurveda-Decoction of the root of bala and ginger is given in intermittent fever attended with cold shivering fits,   120-Columbia-internal fever, 124-India-decoction of roots,   125-India,   148-India-aerial parts,   156-

Brasil, 162-Brazil, 167-Ayurveda-leaves, 180-India, 200-India, 203-Burkina-Faso-children, 285-Ayurveda, 312-USA-Ayurveda, 312-Brazil, 167-Ayurveda-Root decoction-mixed with ginger is effective in curing intermittent fever, 358-review-Benin-roots, 358-review-DR Congo-leaf infusion, 362-review-leaves-fever in small children-root-for high fever, 377-Ayurveda-root, 437-India-bark, 537-India-intermittent fever, 609-India, 619-Malaysia, 664-Ayurveda-root-decoction-with ginger is given for intermittent fever attended with cold shivering fits,

Sida rhombifolia 522-review-pharmacological activities reported include antipyretic activities,

Tr 47-India-roots and stems, 51-India-roots and stems, 57-Ayurveda, 75-Ayurveda, 88-Ayurveda, 126-Colombia-Analgesic to control fever, 127-India-as a febrifuge with pepper, 128-Ayurveda-roots, 150-Ethiopia-root and leaf, 194-Gabon, 131-Ayurveda, 197-Ayurveda, 217-Ayurveda, 362-review-leaves-fever in small children-root-for high fever, 377-Ayurveda-with pepper, 377-Ayurveda-root, 437-India-bark, 522-Nicargua-leaf-decoction-orally, 522-Ayurveda-roots and leaves, 522-India-entire plant-hot aqueous extract-orally-in treatment of fever, 522-Nicaragua-leaf-decoction-taken orally, 522-Guatemela-leaf-decoction-orally, 524-Phillipines-roots-decoction-bitter bark, 524-Phillipines-Juice of pounded leaves-or roots, 524-Phillipines-root-decoction, 524-India-Hindus, 524-Ayurveda- widely used, 545- Bangladesh-stems-with pepper, 609-India, 619-Malaysia, 634-Sri Lanka-upper root,

Sida retusa 128- Sida retusa-mice-root-the crude extract lowered yeast-induced pyrexia-10g/kg bw lowered temperature than aspirin (150mg/kg) after 3 hours.

Tr 75-India, 131-Ayurveda-widely used in Ayurveda in the treatment of fever, 196-Ayurveda, 529-Ayurveda-attended with shivering and fits, 435-Ayurveda-fevers attended with shivering and fits, 527-Sida retusa,

Sida cordata Tr 288-Ayurveda, 293-Ayurveda-roots, 437-India-bark, 496-Sida cordata-Pakistan-Siddha and Ayurveda, 549-Ayurveda, 603-Himalayas,

Sida rhomboidea Tr 320-Ayurveda, 520-India,

Sida spinosa

Tr 11-Burkina-Faso, 55-India-root-in mild cases, 88-Ayurveda-roots, 99-India-root-given in mild cases of debility and fever, 217-Ayurveda, 362-review-fever in small children, 433-India-Decoction of the root-bark and root is used in mild cases, 609-India, 619-Malaysia,

Sida indica

Tr 377-Ayurveda-root, 437-Ayurveda-bark-febrifuge, 437-Ayurveda-Sida indica-seeds and roots-decoction, 444-Ayurveda-Vishamajwarahara-

166

useful against recurrent fever,   445-India and China-high fever,   445-Thailand,   448-Ayurveda-high fever,   451-Thailand-seeds,   451-Thailand-leaf extract, 452-Bangladesh-high fever, 678-Ayurveda-bark,   678-Ayurveda-root infusion-in fevers as a cooling medicine,   684-Ayur-vedic, 708-Ayurveda-bark,   710-Ayurveda-leaf-decoction,   710-Ayurveda-bark, 710-China-entire plant,   711-Chinese-bark and root,   711-India-leaf extract-inflammation of the bladder,   711-India-seed-chronic dysentery, 712-India-roots or leaves,   712-India-roots or leaves,   735-Ayurveda-review-bark,   737-India-root-decoction--root-infusion-a good cooling remedy in fevers--seeds-infusion in water-a cooling drink,

Other Sidas   Tr   200-Sida cardifolia-Ayurveda-whole plant, 499- Sida urens-Burkina Faso,

Body, Gout

The earlier research reported that flavonoid crude extract from this plant could inhibit in vitro the activity of xanthine oxidase (xanthine:oxygen oxidoreductase, EC 1.2.3.2) up to 55% and could be an antigout. [187]

Sida cordifolia   Tr   444-Ayurveda-Bala-Vatasrahara-Relieves gout

Sida rhombifolia

187--invitro--crude extract--roots?--inhibitory effect 48 to 71%--100-800 mg l-1, 486-invitro-whole plant?- water, 70% ethanol extract- alkaloid and flavonoid extracts-From several extracts of sidaguri, the strongest and the weakest of LC50 value were ethanol extract of leaves (1780 ppm) and water extract of herbs (148 ppm), respectively. Most of the extracts examined could inhibit the activity of xanthine oxidase and the strongest inhibitor was alkaloid extract of herbs (400 ppm) followed by flavonoid extract of herbs (400 ppm)-strength of inhibition=ethanolic extract LC50 1780 ppm>alkaloid extract LC50 400 ppm>flavenoid extract LC50 400 ppm >acqueous extract LC50 148 ppm.

Tr   187-Indonesia, 243-Indonesia, 524-Indonesia, 622-India,

Sida indica   Tr   712- India-root,

Body, Immuno-stimulant

Sida cordifolia has strong potential as an immunostimulatory agent... These findings validate its use as health promotive agents in Ayurvedic medicine. [289]

Sida acuta

79-invitro-isolated from Sida acuta-Scopoletin induced cell proliferation on normal T lymphocytes (Proliferation stimulation index: 1 µg/ml scopoletin:

1.26 ± 0.1; 10 μg/ml scopoletin: 3 ± 0.25; 100 μg/ml scopoletin: 1.86 ± 0.08)-a stimulatory action. **Tr** 107-India-immunomodulator,

Sida cordifolia

27-invitro-whole plant?-80% acetone extract>chloroform extract for alkaloid compounds- Our results showed a low immunostimulatory effect and this result could be explained by the lack of biologically active antioxidants such as polyphenol compounds lowly contained in the alkaloid compounds, **289**-invitro-root-suggest their strong potential as immunostimulatory agents. Sitoindoside X significantly inhibited the production of oxygen metabolites by activated PMN. These findings validate the use of the two plant drugs as health promotive agents in Ayurvedic medicine,

Tr 444-Ayurveda-Bala-Ojovardhaka-improves immunity.

Sida indica

449-mice-leaves-400 mg/kg/day bw- was found to have a significant immunostimulatory activity on both the specific and non-specific immune mechanisms. The significant increase in the immunostimulatory activity of AI could be attributed to the presence of flavonoids (quercetin), alkaloids, tannins, saponin glycosides and phenolic compounds-neutrophil adhesion-both have a significant immunostimulatory activity on both the specific and non-specific immune mechanisms,

Tr 444-Ayurveda-Ojovardhaka-improves immunity,   678-Ayurveda-whole plant?-immune stimulant,   711-Ayurveda-immune stimulant,

Body, Immuno-supportive

Sida cordifolia has strong potential as an immunostimulatory agent. These findings validate the use of the two plant drugs as health promotive agents in Ayurvedic medicine. **[289]**   **Tr   no reported use**

Sida cordifolia

27-invitro-whole plant?-80% acetone extract>chloroform extract for alkaloid compounds- Our results showed a low immunostimulatory effect and this result could be explained by the lack of biologically active antioxidants such as polyphenol compounds lowly contained in the alkaloid compounds--Indeed, surely this low immune power could be also explained by the low bioavailability of the extracts administered orally. It is worth noting that the intestinal absorption of plant extracts through the intestinal absorption is often low and weak,

Sida rhombifolia

267- cited by **[239]** -has immune enhancing properties,

Sida humilis

469-mice- shows immunomodulatory activity by showing immune response to SRBCs by increasing paw volume in mice. Immunomodulatory activity of drug was compared to disease control group,

Body, Inflammation   Anti-inflammatory

Inflammation is a local response of living mammalian tissues to injury. It is a body defense reaction in order to eliminate or limit the spread of injurious agent. There are various components to an inflammatory reaction that can contribute to the associated symptoms and tissue injury... Aging is also considered to be inflammatory response... Currently available anti-inflammatory agents are associated with unwanted side effects and have their own limitations. About 34-46% of the users of NSAIDs usually sustain some gastrointestinal damage due to the inhibition of the protective cyclo-oxygenase enzyme in gastric mucosa. Therefore, new anti-inflammatory and analgesic drugs lacking these side effects are being researched as alternatives to NSAID and opiates. Attention is being focused on the investigation of the efficacy of plant based drugs used in the traditional medicine because they are cheap, have little side effects and according to WHO, about 80% of the world population still rely mainly on herbal remedies. **[186]**

Sida acuta

84-mice/rats-whole plant-crude extract- exhibited significant (p< 0.001) analgesic and anti-inflammatory activities,   **186**-invitro-whole plant-methanolic extract- The PI with indomethacin and Sida acuta in carrageenan induced paw edema at the dose level 400 mg/kg were 60% and 52.5% at the end of 5 hr... The methanolic extract possesses anti-inflammatory and analgesic activity,   **315**- vasicine (in S acuta and S cordifolia)-chloroform extract- significant anti-inflammatory activities,   **571**-mice-whole plant-methanolic extract-100, 200 and 400 mg/kg bw po-400 mg/kg caused significant (p<0.01) decrease in paw edema compared to vehicle while lower dose 100 mg/kg did not show any effect,   **593**-Cienfuegosia digitata Cav (along with Sida spinosa)-invitro-whole plant-?extract-exhibited the best and significant results in polyphenol contents, antioxidants properties and anti-inflammatory activity (over S acuta, S cordifolia, S rhombifolia, S urens), **651**-invitro-leaves-ethanol extract- showed a good anti-inflammatory activity against acute inflammation -reduced paw edema induced-inflammation to some extent,   **739**-berberine-review,

Tr   52-India-whole plant-hot water extract,   76-W Africa,   82-India, 84-Nigeria,   88-India,   93-Italy/Burkina Faso-leaves-renal inflammation, 107-India,   220-Nigeria,   221-India-leaf,   224-Nigeria,   361-Philippines-seeds-used to cure enlarged glands and inflammatory swellings, 361-inflammation,   362-review-Philippines-seed-cure enlarged glands and inflammatory swellings, 588-Nigeria,   609-India,   619-Malaysia,   646-Nigeria-leaves and stem,

Sida cordifolia

31-rats-root-50% ethanolic extract-has got potent antioxidant and antiinflammatory activity and the activity is comparable with the standard drug deprenyl, **36**-rats/invitro-a new alkaloid-produced 16.93 and 24.43 % inhibition of paw edema at the doses of 25 and 50 mg/kg body weight respectively at the third hour of study, **42**-rats-the results from the ABTS assay showed that the ethanolic extract of Sida cordifolia was IC50 16.07 microg/ml- The relative antioxidant capacity for the water infusion was IC50 342.82 microg/ml-results of water infusion on lipid peroxidation were IC50 126.78 microg/ml, **43**-rats-leaf-water extract-400 mg/kg bw- significant inhibition of carrageenin-induced rat paw edema but did not block the edema induced by arachidonic acid, **45**-rats?-root and aerial parts-ethyl acetate extract-600 mg/kg bw-showed comparable antiinflammatory activity with indomethacin and possessed significantly higher activity when compared with that of the methanol extract of the root part, **61**-rats-leaf-water extract-400 mg/kg bw- a significant inhibition of carrageenin-induced rat paw but did not block the edema induced by arachidonic acid, **67**-rats-neurotoxicity-50% ethanolic extract of root-50 mg/100 g bw, **61**-rats-leaf-water extract-400 mg/kg bw-potent antioxidant and antiinflammatory activity and the activity is comparable with the standard drug deprenyl, **116**- new flavonol glycoside-rats-80% ethanolic extract>n-hexane/dichloromethane /ethyl acetate/n-butanol-In carrageenan induced rat paw edema the compound produced 16.15 and 28.52% inhibition of paw edema at doses of 25 and 50 mg kg^{-1} body weight at the 3rd h of study, **133**-rats/mice-aerial parts-butanol extract and methanol extract (after acid base treatment)-200 mg/kg bw-exhibited sufficient inhibition of paw edema of 40.85 and 39.35 % respectively at the end of the fourth hour. The activities of different extracts were comparable to the standard drug, phenylbutazone, **152**-rats-seed oil-petroleum ether (40-600C) extract-displayed significant anti-inflammatory activity at a dose of 400 mg/Kg bw-possesses anti-inflammatory activity against carrageenan induced paw edema, **153**-rats-leaf-alcoholic extract-proved to be anti-inflammatory, **154**-mice-acqueous extract-leaves-400 mg/kg- a significant inhibition of carrageenin-induced rat paw edema-but did not block the edema induced by arachidonic acid, **182**-rats-roots-50% ethanolic extract-potent antiinflammatory, **183**-mice-aerial parts-chloroform (3 × 72h)/methanol (3 × 72h)/80% ethanol (3 × 72h) extract>ethyl acetate-50 mg/kg bw exhibited 25.65% (p <0.01) inhibition of paw volume-80 mg/kg phenylbutazone produced 31.94% inhibition, **235**-invitro- a new alkaloid, 1,2,3,9-tetrahydro-pyrrolo [2,1-b] quinazolin-3-ylamine—Carrageenan induced rat paw edema produced 16.93 and 24.43 % inhibition of paw edema at the doses of 25 and 50 mg/kg body weight respectively at the third hour of study, **285**-rats-root-ethyl acetate extract-150, 300, 600 mg/kg bw-demonstrated mild to moderate antiinflammatory activity. The activity of SCR-E at a dose of 600 mg/kg is equivalent to that of indomethacin and exhibited no ulcerogenicity indicating its safety on the gastrointestinal tract, **292**-invitro-The present study has shown that the whole plant of Sida corsifolia contains the most DEHP and the compound is a potent inhibitor of LOX. The enzyme inhibition may partially impart the anti-inflammatory property of the plant, **408**-

invitro-root-ethyl acetate extract-showed comparable anti-inflammatory activity with indomethacin and possessed significantly higher activity when compared with that of the methanol extract of the root part,   537-rats-whole plant?-80% ethanol extract- showed statistically significant acute & sub- acute anti-inflammatory effects-It was found that percentage reduction in the paw edema was 58.13% with Indomethacin, 48.83% and 53.48% with 100 mg/kg and 200 mg/kg bw-Percentage reduction in the granuloma formation was 60.2% with Indomethacin, 54.7% and 56% with 100 mg/kg and 200 mg/kg Sida cordifolia Linn respectively,

Tr   28-India-inflammation of oral mucosa,   40-Brazil,   43-Brazil-inflammation of oral mucosa,   45-India-aerial and root parts,   61-Brazil-inflammation of the oral mucosa,   118-Ayurveda,   120-Brazil,   125-India, 152-India,   153-Brasil,   156-Brasil,   158-India,   159-Ayurveda,   160-Brazil,   161-Ayurveda- has an anti-inflammatory effect,   162-Brazil,   161-Ayurveda,   180-India,   182-India-used in folk medicine for the treatment of the inflammation of oral mucosa,   200-India,   224-Nigeria,   312-Brazil,   317-India-(has) been widely used in traditional medicine for (its) anti-inflammatory activity,   619-Malaysia,   664-Ayurveda-whole plant?,

Sida rhombifolia

46-rats-stems and roots-extracts-induced arthritis in experimental rats. The altered levels of hematological parameters were reverted to near normal levels, Oral administration significantly increased the levels of thiobarbituric acid reactive substances and activities of catalase and glutathione peroxidase and decreased the levels of reduced glutathione and superoxide dismutase activity in arthritis induced rats,   **127**-rats?-root and stem-The free radical scavenging activity of the plant was further evidenced by histological and transmission electron microscopy observations made on the hind limb tissue, **136**-rats-roots-water   and   ethanol   extracts-200/400/600 mg/kg bw-produced significant (P< 0.05) and a dose dependent anti-inflammatory activity-ethanolic best-extracts were 80-100% of effect of Indomethacin (5 mg/ kg bw),   **144**-rats-leaf-95% ethanol extract- exhibited significant (p<0.05) anti-inflammatory activities in a dose-dependent manner,   **149**-rats?-leaf-95% ethanol extract-30/100/300 mg/kg bw- all doses of the extract, administered intraperitoneally IP, exhibited significant (p<0.05) antinociceptive and anti-inflammatory activities in a dose-dependent manner,   **183**-mice-aerial parts-chloroform (3 × 72h)/methanol (3 × 72h)/80% ethanol (3 × 72h) extract>ethyl acetate-50 mg/kg bw exhibited 25.65% (p <0.01) inhibition of paw volume-80 mg/kg phenylbutazone produced 31.94% inhibition,   **185**-animals-comparable to phenylbutazone, **194**-rats-whole plant?-80% acetone extract-100/200/400 mg/kg bw-produced significant and a dose-dependent anti-inflammatory activity, **201**-rats-aerial parts-methanolic extract- showed significant edema suppressant activity,   **281**-rats-leaves-ethanol: water 3:7-400 mg/kg orally,324-whole plant-methanolic extract- significant edema suppressant activity in rats,   **324**-rats-aerial parts-methanol extract-showed significant edema suppressant activity on carrageenan induced paw edema in rats, **522**-review-The pharmacological activities reported include anti-inflammatory activity,   **619**-whole plant--n-hexane, ethyl acetate and methanol extracts-strongest anti-inflammatory activity with IC50 of 52.16 and 146.03 µg/mL for NO and protein denaturation inhibition assays, respectively, **672**-invitro-root-ethanol extract- extract produced a dose-dependent inhibition of carrageenan (1%) which was comparable with indomethacin anti-inflammatory drugs. The extract produced significant anti-inflammatory activity. Significant reduction of paw edema was observed at 0.6 g/kg bw still 2.4 g/kg bw,

Tr 47-India-roots and stems-some inflammations, 51-India-roots and stems-all kinds of inflammation, 88-India, 136-India-root and leaves-various inflammation conditions, 144-Malaysia, 149-Malaysia, 150-Ethiopia-leaves, 190-Ayurveda, 192-Burkina-Faso-a remedy for inflammatory disorder, 194-Gabon, 197-Ayurveda, 522-Ayurveda-roots and leaves-all kind of inflammations, 522-Guatemela-dried leaf-hot aqueous extract-externally, 524-Phillipines-roots, 543-Ayurveda, 619-Malaysia,

Sida cordata
293-goat blood-methanol and acetone extracts have maximum activity,

Sida indica

448-rats-whole plant-Pet. ether, Chloroform, Ethanol & Aqueous extracts-400 mg/kg bw-The dose of various extracts was found to be more (or) less similar-with significant anti-inflammatory activity comparable with positive control Diclofenac (10 mg/kg bw)-On the basis of the results of this study, it is possible to conclude that all the effects observed are true anti - inflammatory effects, **682**-rats-roots/seeds-alcoholic extract-shows considerable effect on inflammation, however seed extract produces more activity compared to root extract....400 mg/kg seed extract produces significant activity as that of standard drug (Diclofenac sodium 10 mg/kg), **706**-invitro-aerial parts-methanol extract-significant anti-inflammatory activity of this medicinal plant,

Tr 445-Thailand, 454-India-leaf-alll kinds of inflammation, 678-Ayurveda-whole plant?, 706-India-widely used by Ayurveda and Unani practitioners as an anti-inflammatory drug in various inflammatory conditions, 710-Ayurveda-leaves-all kinds of inflammation, 711-Ayurveda, 712-India-leaves,

Sida rhomboidea

185-rats?-leaf- butanolic extract-200 mg/kg bw- Percentage inhibition of edema (33.05, P<0.001) is comparable to that of phenylbutazone, 100 mg/kg inhibition (38.83%),

Tr 288-Ayurveda-all kinds of inflammation, 288-Ayurveda, 520-India-works against all kinds of inflammation,

Sida spinosa

11-review-whole plant-acetone extract-previous studies performed in our laboratory showed that aqueous acetone extract of Sida alba L. possesses antioxidant properties, **593**-invitro-whole plant-?extract- exhibited the best

172

and significant results in polyphenol contents, antioxidants properties and anti-inflammatory activity (over S acuta, S cordifolia, S rhombifolia, S urens).

Tr   11-Burkina Faso-inflammatory related ailments,   619-Malaysia,

Sida tiagii

551-rats?-fruit-95% ethanolic extract>n-Hexane Extract and ethyl acetate extract-showed significant (P<0.01) antiphlogistic effect against xylene-induced ear edema-percentage inhibition of inflammation in EAS (34.15%) and RES (39.66%) was found comparable with that of the standard drug, diclophenac sodium (46.69%)-Thus the plant can be used as a potential anti-inflammatory candidate in animals.   Tr   552-India,

Sida cardifolia

177-rats-whole plant?-50% ethanol extract-potent anti-antioxidant and anti-inflammatory activity when compared with standard drug deprenyl.

Tr   177-India-used in folk medicine for the treatment of inflammation, 200- Ayurveda-whole plant.

Other Sida

Tr   490-Sida tuberculata-Brazil-leaves and roots,   496-Sida cordata-Pakistan-Siddha and Ayurveda-seeds- inflammation of eye conjunctitis.

Cryptolepine   (S. acuta, cordifolia, rhombifolia, spinosa, and ?)

386-rats-10–40 mg/kg i.p.- produced significant dose-dependent inhibition of the carrageenan-induced rat paw edema, and carrageenan-induced pleurisy in rats. These effects were compared with those of the non-steroidal anti-inflammatory drug indomethacin (10 mg/kg),.

Body, Jaundice   No peer review

A yellowish or greenish pigmentation of the skin and whites of the eyes due to high bilirubin levels. Causes of jaundice vary from non-serious to potentially fatal [1]   In spite of the availability of more than 300 preparations for the treatment of jaundice and chronic liver diseases in Indian systems of medicine using more than 87 Indian medicinal plants, only four terrestrial plants have been scientific-ally elucidated. [484]

Sida acuta   Tr   588-Nigeria,

Sida linfolia   Tr   358-Benin,

Sida indica   Tr   443-Ayurveda,   445-India and China,   674-Siddha,

Body, Leprosy   No peer review

A long-term infection by the bacteria Mycobacterium leprae or Mycobacterium lepromatosis. [1]

Sida cordifolia, Sida rhombifolia, Sida cordata

Tr 437-Ayurveda-roots-powder,

Sida indica

Tr 238-Sri Lanka-roots, 437-Ayurveda-root powder-leprosy, 443-Ayurveda, 444-Ayurveda-Atibala-leprosy, 449-Ayurveda, 450-India-root, 451-Thailand-root-also effective in the treatment of leprosy, 674-Siddha, 678-Ayurveda-root infusion, 711-India-root, 712-India-roots, 735-Ayurveda-review-root,

Sida spinosa   **Tr** 217-Ayurveda,

Body, Muscles

Sida acuta

275-mice-leaves and stems-100% ethanolic extract-500 and 1000 mg/kg-retained muscle coordination while under CNS-no decrease in motor coordination at all used doses, except 750 mg/kg, **500**-invitro-root-extract did not produce any impairment in muscle relaxant activity (rota-rod test), which indicate that SA does not act on skeletal muscles,

Sida cordifolia   **148**-rats-aerial parts-alcoholic extract-400 mg/kg bw- helps to check muscle wasting

Tr 118-Ayurveda-sore muscles, 125-India- seed oil -sore muscles and joints in rheumatism and arthritis, 664-Ayurveda-oil-extract-sore muscles,

Sida rhombifolia   **Tr** 358-Fiji and Papua New Guinea-leaves-strained muscles, 361-Fiji and Papua New Guinea-leaves-strained muscles, 362-review-Fiji and Papua New Guinea-leaves-strained muscles,

Body, Obesity

(Sida rhomboidea) Obesity, a fast spreading epidemic, is a major contributor to the global burden of chronic disease and disability. Currently, more than one billion adults worldwide are overweight and at least, 300 million of them are clinically obese. Such individuals are maximally prone to type-2 diabetes, cardiovascular disease and hypertension in the long run. Induction of obesity in humans is either 'genetic' of 'lifestyle' related. The latter is however a complex intermix of sedentary lifestyle and a high calorie diet amounting to nutritional overload. Synthetic anti-obesity drugs have often been reported to be very costly with some of them also beset with undesirable side effects, thereby necessitating a need to screen natural/ herbal products for treating obesity. In recent times, many traditional herbal preparations have been put through a detailed scrutiny to explore their anti-obesity potential and the underlying mechanism of action. **[520]**

Sida acuta   Tr   609-India

Sida cordifolia   Tr   161-Ayurveda-tea,

Sida rhombifolia   Tr   134-India,

Sida rhomboidea

128-rats-leaf-?extract-200 & 400 mg/kg bw- Results clearly substantiate the antihypertriglyceridemic potential of S. rhomboidea. Roxb leaf extract mediated via decreased intestinal absorption and increased catabolism of TG. The present study is of merit in providing pharmacological evidence for use of SR leaf extract as a folklore medicine for controlling obesity amongst north-eastern population of Indian subcontinent,   **130**-rats-leaf-boiling distilled water extract-Overall, the present study has revealed the highly potent ability of Sida rhomboidea leaf extract in controlling dyslipidemia and hence portends a strong potential for use as a therapeutic agent in lipid disorders and obesity,   **134**-mice-whole plant?-? extract-first scientific report on protective role against HFD induced insulin resistance in C57BL/6J mice and strengthens the folklore claim of use of SR leaves as alternative medicine against diabetes and obesity,   This study is the first report on role of SR in controlling hypertriglyceridemia thus confirming its folklore use by North Eastern population for obesity,   **287**-rats-leaves-boiling distilled water extract- This study is the first report on role of SR in controlling hypertriglyceridemia thus confirming its folklore use by North Eastern population for obesity,   **520**-rats?-leaves-boiling distilled water extract-SRLE induced prevention of pre-adipocytes differentiation, and leptin release further substantiated these findings and scientifically validates the potential application of SRLE as a therapeutic agent against obesity,

Tr   128-leaf-extract,   130-NE India,   134-India-leaves,   287-India, 320-Ayurveda-leaves-decoction-eaten,   520-India-leaf extract-is being used by the populace of North-East India to alleviate symptoms of diabetes and obesity,

Body, Rheumatism   No peer review

Sida root is extensively used in the treatment of rheumatism in Ayurveda. **[668]**

Sida acuta

Tr   3-India-leaves-rheumatic afflictions,   21-Ayurveda-leaves,   21-Ayurveda-root,   82-India,   107-India-leaf,   107-Ayurveda,   109-Siddah, 174-India,   186-India,   214-India,   220-SriLanka, Decoction also used as demulcent; for rheumatism,   238-Sri Lanka-roots and leaves,   361-rheumatism,   526-Phillipines,   568-Nigeria,   571-India-rheumatic conditions,   609-India,

Sida cordifolia

Tr 27-Burkina Faso-whole plant decoction?-rheumatic pain, 28-India, 40-Brazil, 53-root bark tea-Ayurveda, 71-Ayurveda-root, 116-Bangladesh, 117-BurkinaFaso-rheumatic pain, 118-Ayurveda-juice of whole plant-sore muscles and joints, 118-Ayurveda-Juice of the whole plant pounded with a little water is given in doses of ¼ seers, 125-India-seed-oil applied to sore muscles and joints, 133-invitro-whole plant-water extract, 148-India-all parts, 156-Brasil, 160-Brazil, 161-Ayurveda-one of the best medicines, 162-Brazil, 167-Ayurveda-whole plant-water extract, 180-India, 182-India, 217-Ayurveda, 218-Ayurveda-decoction of the root bark, 285-Ayurveda, 312-USA-Ayurveda, 312-Brazil, 358-DR Congo-leaf-water infusion-given to children in case of rheumatism, 408-India-whole plant-water extract, 537-India, 548-India, 561-Ayurveda-root, 596-Nigeria-leaf/root/seed, 612-Ayurveda-root, 664-Ayurveda-whole plant?-extract, 664-Ayurveda-whole plant-pounded with a little water-juice-doses of ¼ seers,

Sida rhombifolia

Tr 49-Ayurveda, 88-Europe, 88-Ayurveda-root, 127-India-roots of these herbs are held in great repute in treatment of rheumatism, 128-Ayurveda-root-held in high repute by practitioners, 136-India-stem and root, 149-Malaysia, 190-India, 197-India-roots, 202- ethyl acetate and aqueous fractions-exhibited significant antifungal activity against Aspergillus niger, Candida albicans and Microsporum gypseum, 217-Ayurveda-children-decoction, 292-India, 292-Indonesia-juice of whole plant, 407-Ayurveda -holds a remarkable reputation among the medical practitioners for its anti-rheumatism activity, 435-Ayurveda-roots- An infusion made from the roots of this plant is held in great repute by the local ayurveda physicians in the treatment of rheumatism, 464-India-This indigenous plant holds a remarkable reputation among the medical practitioners for its anti-rheumatism activity, 522-Ayurveda-roots-The root is held in great repute in the treatment of rheumatism, 522-Europe-whole plant?-In Europe, the plant has been regarded as a valuable remedy in pulmonary tuberculosis and rheumatism, 524-Phillipines, 524-Malaysia-whole plant?, 541-Siddha, 543-Ayurveda, 545- Bangladesh-roots, 561-Ayurveda-root, 568-Nigeria,

Sida cordata **Tr** 293-Ayurveda-roots, 496-Sida cordata-Pakistan-Siddha and Ayurveda, 549-Ayurveda,

Sida retusa

Tr 131-Ayurveda-rheumatoid arthritis , 435- Ayurveda-root, 461-invitro-(Bala) is a very important Ayurvedic medicinal plant, forms a chief ingredient of the famous medicine Kshirabala used in the treatment of rheumatism, 527-roots-Ayurveda-for rheumatism, 529-Ayurveda-an infusion made from the roots of this plant is held in great repute by the local ayurvedic physicians in the treatment of rheumatism,

176

Sida indica   **Tr**   445-India and China,   446-India,   712-India-leaves,

Sida spinosa   **Tr**   561-Ayurveda-root,

Body, Stimulant   Used like ephedrine

Bala roots, the parts traditionally used, reportedly accumulate high levels of ephedrine. [411]   Ephedrine a medication and stimulant. [1]

Sida acuta

315-invitro-vasicine-exhibited marked respiratory and uterine stimulant activity,   **362**-review-ephedrine-decrease of the sensation of fatigue and the need to sleep, and thus qualitatively it resembles an amphetamine.

Tr   88-China

Sida cordifolia

315-invitro-vasicine- exhibited marked respiratory and uterine stimulant activity,   **362**-review-ephedrine-decrease of the sensation of fatigue and the need to sleep, and thus qualitatively it resembles an amphetamine,   **533**-review- Country mallow can stimulate the body.

Tr   312-China, 362-India,   562-Ayurveda,

Sida rhombifolia

315-invitro-vasicine- exhibited marked respiratory and uterine stimulant activity,   **362**-review-ephedrine-decrease of the sensation of fatigue and the need to sleep, and thus qualitatively it resembles an amphetamine,

Tr   545- Bangladesh,

Sida retusa   **362**-review-ephedrine-decrease of the sensation of fatigue and the need to sleep, and thus qualitatively it resembles an amphetamine,

Sida cordata   **362**-review-ephedrine-decrease of the sensation of fatigue and the need to sleep, and thus qualitatively it resembles an amphetamine,

Sida indica

362-review-Sida retusa/ Sida indica/Sida rhomboidea-ephedrine-decrease of the sensation of fatigue and the need to sleep, and thus qualitatively it resembles an amphetamine,   **449**-mice-leaves-400 mg/kg/day bw- was found to have a significant immunostimulatory activity on both the specific and non-specific immune mechanisms. The significant increase in the immunostimulatory activity of AI could be attributed to the presence of flavonoids (quercetin), alkaloids, tannins, saponin glycosides and phenolic compounds-neutrophil adhesion-both have a significant immunostimulatory activity on both the specific and non-specific immune mechanisms.

Tr   449-Ayurveda,

Sida rhomboidea   362-review-ephedrine-decrease of the sensation of fatigue and the need to sleep, and thus qualitatively it resembles an amphetamine,

Sida spinosa   362-review-ephedrine-decrease of the sensation of fatigue and the need to sleep, and thus qualitatively it resembles an amphetamine,

Body, Strength   No peer review
(Traditional) Sida acuta 'Spiritual strength' – Bundugo is supplementary strength magically added to an individual, and this species is used for that. [326]

Sida acuta
Tr   220-India-The plant is used to prepare Bundugo", supplementary strength magically added to a person,   526-Phillipines-Decoction or infusion,   568-Nigeria,

Sida cordifolia   **Tr**   444-Ayurveda-Bala-Balya-tonic, improves strength,   521-Ayurveda-root-generalized weakness,

Sida spinosa   **Tr**   99-India-root-mild debility,   433-India-Decoction of the root-bark and root is used in mild cases

Sida cordata   **Tr**   496-Pakistan-Siddha and Ayurveda-whole plant?-general debility,   549-Ayurveda-general debility,

Sida indica   **Tr**   437-Ayurveda-tonic for strengthening the body, 444-Ayurveda-Atibala-body strengthening,

Sida tiagii   **Tr**   553- Sida tiagii-India and Pakistan-strengthens muscles.

Body, Thirst   No peer review
Traditionally, various plants of Abutilon species are used in relieving thirst (Sida indica) [721]

Sida cordifolia   **Tr**   437-Ayurveda-bark-allay thirst,

Sida rhombifolia   **Tr**   437- Ayurveda -bark-allay thirst,

Sida cordata   **Tr**   437- Ayurveda -bark-allay thirst,

Sida indica   **Tr**   437-Ayurveda-bark-to allay thirst,   451-Thailand-leaf extract-is used in relieving thirst,   684-Ayurveda-leaf juice,   711-India-leaf extract,

178

Body, Tonic   General nutritive tonic and prolonged life

(**See also:** Nerves, Nervous disorders; Reproduction, (several categories); Body, Strength)   Present preliminary studies confirm better cardiotonic activity of Sida cordifolia than digoxin. [534]

Sida acuta

22-historical research-Soma (food of the immortals)-proposed to be major constituent,   **210**-invitro- exceptionally high concentrations of minerals, **313**-vascine-uterotonic,

Tr   3-India-decoction of leaves and roots,   3-India-root,   52-India-whole plant-hot water extract,   82-India-bitter tonic,   107-India,   174-India-bitter tonic,   186-India-bitter tonic,   217-Ayurveda,   275-Brazli-leaves and stems-100% ethanolic extract,   326-review-'PhD thesis Germany-Spiritual strength'-supplementary strength magically added to an individual, and this species is used for that,   361-Indo-China and Philippines-roots-tonic,   377-Ayurveda-root,   526-Phillipines-Decoction of roots and leaves- taken internally,   561-Ayurveda-roots-fresh juice,   571-India-bitter tonic,   644-Ayurveda-root,

Sida cordifolia   **148**-rats-aerial parts-alcoholic extract-muscle wasting-400mg/kg,   **313**-vascine-uterotonic,   **534**-root-infusion with distilled water-cardiotonic,

Tr   53-Ayurveda,   88-Ayurveda-root bark,   118-Ayurveda-roots-alternative tonic,   132-Brazil-roots,   151-Ayurveda-increased energy,   161-Ayurveda-rejuvenative-root extract-medicated enema,   217-Ayurveda-rejuvenative,   218-Ayurveda,   285-Ayurveda-root,   312-USA-Ayurveda-root bark,   377-Ayurveda-root,   437-Ayurveda-tonic for strengthening the body,   437-India-roots-nervine tonic,   444-Ayurveda-Bala-Balya-tonic, improves strength-Kshayahara-Relieves emaciation,   561-Ayurveda-roots-fresh juice,   664-Ayurveda-whole plant?,

Sida rhombifolia   **313**-vascine-uterotonic.

Tr   136-India- root and leaves,   150-Ethiopia-fruit-fatigue,   150-Ethiopia-root and leaf-tonic,   361-Malaysia-It is considered a plant with magical properties,   362-review-Malaysia-whole plant?-considered a plant with magical properties,   377-Ayurveda-root,   407-Ayurveda-an important ingredient in polyherbal formulations. Being a Rasayana drug they are rejuvenating and age-sustaining tonics for promoting vitality and longevity, 437-Ayurveda-tonic for strengthening the body,   437-India-roots-nervine tonic,   464-India-is an important ingredient in polyherbal formulations. Being a Rasayana drug they are rejuvenating and age-sustaining tonics for promoting vitality and longevity,   522-Ayurveda-roots and leaves,   522-Ayurveda-dried leaf and root-hot aqueous extract,   524-Phillipines-roots, 545- Bangladesh,   545-India-stimulant tea,   561-Ayurveda-roots-fresh juice,

Sida Tiagii   Tr 551-India, 553-India and Pakistan,

Sida cordata

Tr 293-Ayurveda-roots,   405-Ayurveda-whole plant material rejuvenates,   405-Ayurveda-root-rejuvenates,   405-Ayurveda-antiaging,   437-Ayurveda-tonic for strengthening the body,   437-India-roots-nervine tonic,   496-Sida cordata-Pakistan-Siddha and Ayurveda-general debility,

Sida indica

Tr 377-Ayurveda-root,   437-Ayurveda-tonic for strengthening the body,   437-Ayurveda-roots-nervine tonic,   443-rats-leaves-methanol extract-gives excessive tonic strength,   443-rats-leaves-methanol extract-is a stronger heart tonic,   444-Ayurveda-Balya-tonic, improves strength,   443-Ayurveda-Atibala- excessive tonic strength,   445-Thailand-blood tonic,   710-Ayurveda-seeds,   712-India-seeds,   737-India-root-decoction-nerve tonic,

Sida spinosa   Tr 55-India-root,   99-India-root,   561-Ayurveda-roots-fresh juice,

Other Sidas   Tr 131-Sida retusa-Ayurveda,   561- S. veronicae-folia-Ayurveda-roots-fresh juice,

Body, Weight Change

Sida acuta   229-weaner rabbits-aerial parts?-sole source of food-gained weight.   Tr 151-Ayurveda-fat loss,   161-Ayurveda,   609-India,

Sida cordifolia

122-rats-appetite suppressant-reduces both food intake and body weight (dose dependent),   148-rats-Alcoholic extract of S. cordifolia at 400 mg/kg significantly improved the body-weight,   180-Streptozotocin (STZ)-induced rats-aerial parts-methanol and aqueous extracts-1000 mg/kg, b.w.-(a) check on the loss of body weight was also observed,

Tr 53-review-In western world ephedrine once upon a time was widely used for weight loss,   118-Ayurveda,   120-Colombia-slimming,   158-India-fat reducer,   161-Ayurveda-Use as a weight loss supplement-herbal extract or tea is used for obesity and obesity related disorders, especially in western countries-weight loss as the ephedrine alkaloids control metabolism in human body,   411-invitro-root- used in food supplements for loosing weight,   312-USA-Ayurveda,   548-Ayurveda-roots-used as a food supplement for fat loss,   664-Ayurveda-whole plant?-extract,

Sida rhombifolia   276-chickens-this study showed that feeding 5% of sidaguri had an effect (P>0,05) on feed consumption, average daily weight gain and feed conversion ratio of broiler chicken,

180

Sida rhomboidea
286-rats?-leaf-water extract-3000 mg/kg bw-decrement in food intake and body weight gain,

Sida cardifolia
157-mice-water crude extract-500/1000mg/kg wt-dose dependent loss of total body weight and reproductive organ weight,

Body, Wound healing

Sida acuta
237-The strong anticoagulase activity of S. acuta, and it's efficacy in inhibiting coagulase elaboration by Staph aureus especially Staph. aureus SS-3SW isolated from septic wound forms the basis of it's use in folk medicine for wound treatment.

Tr 3-India-fresh juice of roots, 21-Siddha (Tamil)-leaves, 21-India-root, 107-India-leaves, 214-India-the leaf extract combined with turmeric, 217-Ayurveda-juice of roots, 219-Nigeria-leaf usually used-wound infections, 220-Nigeria, 221-India-leaf, 234-Nigeria, 237-it's use in folk medicine for wound treatment, 273-Nigeria-wound infection, 428-survey-first aid-India-farmers- used for first aid in the treatment of some minor injuries like sunstroke, scorpion and snake bites, headache and indigestion, 508-India-leaf paste, 561-Ayurveda-fresh juice of root, 597-India-root, 599-India-root-wound healing, 601-Nigeria-leaf-crushed leaves are applied over wounds, fresh cuts and bruises, 601-Nigeria-leaf-Leaves are squeezed and placed at the nostril-nosebleed,

Sida cordifolia
Tr 53-Ayurveda-root juice-unhealthy sores, 88-Konkan, 88-Ayurveda-seeds, 118-Ayurveda-root juice-Root juice is also used to promote healing of wounds, 120-Colombia (flavenoids), 124-India-apply pounded leaves on cuts, 124-India-root juice, 124-India-wound dressing, 125-India-crushed leaves, 127-Ayurveda-root juice-unhealthy sores, 167-Ayurveda-Root decoction-mixed with ginger is effective in healing of wounds, 218-Ayurveda-root juice-unhealthy sores, 277-Ayurveda-fracture healing-leaf paste along with egg yolk, 444- Ayurveda-Kshatahara-useful in injuries, 537-India, 561-Ayurveda-fresh juice of root, 596-Sida pilosa-Nigeria-leaves-cuts, 597-India-root, 599-India-root-wound healing, 601-Nigeria-leaf-crushed leaves are applied over wounds, fresh cuts and bruises, 664-Ayurveda-root-juice-promote healing of wounds, 664-Ayurveda-crushed leaves-poultice-external wounds,

Sida rhombifolia
Tr 47-Camaroon and Madagascar-antiseptic, wound-healing activities, 51-India-whole plant?-cuts, 51-India-whole plant?- broken bones, 150-Ethiopia-leaf-skin bleeding, 150-Ethiopia-leaf and stem bark-treatment of wound, 150-Ethiopia-leaf-cuts and wounds, 358-Africa-leaves or leaf sap-antiseptic, 522-review-The infusion of this plant is applied locally for the treatment of skin diseases and infected wounds, 524-Phillipines-whole

plant?-poultice-broken bones,   561-Ayurveda-fresh juice of root,   596-Nigeria-leaves,

Sida cordata   Tr 498-India,   603-Himalayas-leaf-Poultice applied to cuts & bruises,

Sida spinosa   Tr 561-Ayurveda-fresh juice of root,   597-India-root, 599-India-root-wound healing,

Sida indica Tr 444- Ayurveda-Kshatahara-useful in injuries,   451-Thailand-leaf extract-wound cleaning, 684-Ayurveda-leaf juice-wound cleaning,   735-Ayurveda-review-leaves-as a poultice to painful parts of the body,

Other Sidas   Tr 595-Sida mysorensis-India-leaves-powder (external use)-healing wounds,   596-Sida pilosa-Nigeria-leaves,

Brain, Myocardial injury (MI)

Myocardial infarction (MI) and the resultant complication in cardiac function represent the leading cause of morbidity and mortality in developed countries. The use of complementary and alternative medicines is burgeoning globally for MI, especially in developed countries including US. Attempts are being made globally to get scientific evidences for these traditionally reported herbal drugs. **[163]**   The result confirm, at least in part, for the use of Sida cordifolia in folk medicine to treat MI. **[33]**

Sida cordifolia

33-rats-leaves-hydroalcoholic extract-100 and 500 mg/kg- both doses significantly increased endogenous antioxidants in heart tissue homogenate. Moreover, biochemical findings were supported by histopathological observations.- The result confirm, at least in part, for the use of Sida cordifolia in folk medicine to treat MI,   **163**-rats-petroleum ether +methanol extract-leaves-pretreatment offers dose-dependent protection from myocardial injury,

Tr   33-India- The result confirm, at least in part, for the use of Sida cordifolia in folk medicine to treat MI,   69-India,   163-India-the results confirm, at least in part, for the use of Sida cordifolia in folk medicine to treat MI,

Sida rhombifolia

536-rats-whole plant?-ethanol extract-100&200 mg/kg-causes myocardial adaptation by augmenting endogenous antioxidants and protects rat hearts from decline in cardiac function and oxidative stress associated with ISP induced myocardial injury.

Sida rhomboidea

155-rats-whole plant-extract-cardioprotective effect against isoproterenol induced myocardial necrosis, **288**-rats-leaves-ethanol extract-a potent antioxidant and free radical scavenger-pre-treatment improves cardiac antioxidant status in IP induced Myocardial infarction by effective scavenging of free radicals generated during oxidation of catecholamines thus collectively contributing to its overall antioxidant and anti ischemic activity.

Brain, Neurodamage   Tr   no reported use

A number of Indian medicinal plants have been used for thousands of years in the traditional system of medicine (Ayurveda). Amongst these are plants used for the management of neurodegenerative diseases ... ABTS assay showed that the ethanolic extract of Sida cordifolia was found to be most potent (IC50 16.07 microg/ml). **[42]**

Sida acuta

140-rats-Ethanolic Leaf Extract-cerebral astrocytes-hyperplasia at 200mg/kg-hypertrophy and hypoplasia of astrocytes at 400mg/kg-hypoplasia of astrocytes at 600mg/kg, **266**-rats-Cerebral Cortex of Adult Wistar Rats. Hypoplasia of cells in the cortical, Intermediate and sub-ventricular zones was intense in group that received 200mg/kg of leaf extract Animals that received 400mg/kg of the extract showed hypertrophy of cell in the intermediate and sub- ventricular layers. This result suggests that high doses of ethanolic leaf extract of Sida acuta may cause some neurological disorders. {200 mg/kg probably upper limit for regular consumption}.

Sida cordifolia   **42-invitro**-ABTS assay showed that the ethanolic extract of Sida cordifolia was found to be most potent (IC50 16.07 microg/ml),

Brain, Neurotoxicity   Tr   no reported use

Sida cordifolia is a plant belonging to the Malvaceae family used in many ayurvedic preparations. This study aimed at assessing the effects of ethanolic extract of Sida cordifolia root on quinolinic acid (QUIN) induced neurotoxicity and to compare its effect with the standard drug deprenyl in rat brain... the activity is comparable with the standard drug deprenyl. **[31]**

Sida acuta

275-mice-leaves and stems-100% ethanolic extract-500 and 1000 mg/kg-the extract protects against seizures induced by PTZ

Sida cordifolia

31-rats-root-50% ethanolic extract-quinolinic acid (QUIN) induced neurotoxicity and to compare its effect with the standard drug deprenyl in rat brain-has got potent antioxidant and antiinflammatory activity and the activity is comparable with the standard drug deprenyl, **67**-rats-root-50% ethanolic extract-quinolinic acid induced neurotoxicity- 50 mg/100 g bw/day-potent antioxidant and antiinflammatory activity-the activity is comparable to deprenyl, **182**-rats-roots-50% ethanolic extract-quinolinic acid-induced neurotoxicity-has potent anti-oxidant and anti-inflammatory activity-protective effect comparable to deprenyl.

Sida rhombifolia

619-whole plant--n-hexane extract-anti-cholinesterase- AChE enzyme inhibition was 58.55%,

Brain, Other conditions   No peer review

Sida acuta

Tr   123-Ayurveda-extensively used in the Indian traditional (Ayurveda) system of medicine for the management of neurodegenerative diseases, 124-India-roots orally with sugar-sun stroke,   428-India-sun stroke,

Sida cordifolia

Tr   42-Ayurveda-neurodegenerative diseases,   161-Ayurveda- It is used in neurological ailments, especially in Stroke rehabilitation,   362-ephedrine crosses the blood-brain barrier, it has a stimulating psychic effect: stimulation of the attention and concentration, decrease of the sensation of fatigue and the need to sleep,   521-Ayurveda-root-mental exhaustion,

Sida rhombifolia

Tr   435-Ayurveda-roots- An infusion made from the roots of this plant is held in great repute by the local ayurvedic physicians in the treatment of a variety of neurological complaints including epilepsy,   545-Mexico-leaves-smoked-mental exhaustion,

Sida retusa   **Tr**   131-Ayurveda-neurodegenerative diseases,   527-Ayurveda-variety of neurological problems,

Children, Child's remedy   No peer review
The leaves are used for cooling of fever in small children. [Tr-362]

Sida acuta

Tr   203-Burkina-Faso-children-fever, malaria, or smallpox.   362-review-leaves-fever in small children-root-for high fever,

Sida cordifolia

Tr   88-Portugese,   203-Burkina-Faso-children-fever,   203-Burkina-Faso-children-pain,   203-Burkina-Faso-children,   358-DR Congo-leaf-water infusion-given to children in case of rheumatism,   217-Ayurveda-

184

children-decoction-rheumatism, 217-Ayurveda-blockage of the bile ducts-children, 358-DR Congo-leaf-water infusion-given to children in case of rheumatism, 362-review-leaves-fever in small children-root-for high fever, 522-New Guinea-fresh leaf juice-children-diarrhea, 524-Cuba-roots-decoction-for infantile diarrhea,

Sida indica

Tr 712-India-seeds-rectum of children affected with thread worms, 737-India-whole plant-juice-applied as an emollient to relieve soreness of the nates in young children-emollient.

Other Sida

Tr 11-Sida spinosa-Burkina Faso-whole plant-hot water extract?-infectious diseases in children, 192-Sida rhombifolia-Burkina Faso-infectious diseases in children, 362-Sida veronicaefolia-review-fever in small children,

Choline   A water-soluble vitamin-like essential nutrient [1]

Choline and its metabolites are needed for three main physiological purposes: structural integrity and signaling roles for cell membranes, cholinergic neurotransmission (acetylcholine synthesis), and a major source for methyl groups via its metabolite, trimethylglycine (betaine), which participates in the S-adenosylmethionine (SAMe) synthesis pathways. **[1]**

Sida veronicaefolia

806-invitro-whole plant?-ethanolic extract>water-soluble fraction-detected,

Companion/Catch Plant

Research has shown that Sida plants do not negatively affect a commercial crop, once it is established. Thus it could be a second crop. More important, since it has such a high protein content it should make a good catch crop (if it isn't deemed the more important crop.

Sida rhombifolia

465-field study- Thirty days after coffee seedling transplantation into 12 L pots, weeds were transplanted into or sown in those pots- Effects of competition by S. rhombifolia against coffee plants were among the lowest, since only a slight decrease in all the characteristics evaluated in coffee plants was observed,

Sida spinosa   **517**-field study-prickly sida competition 4 to 6 weeks after cotton emergence until harvest did not reduce the seed cotton yields,

Ear and Nose Problems

Folk use: Leaves are used to treat bleeding nose and for treating eye pain. Preparation of Remedy: Leaves are squeezed and placed at the nostril and the stem is cut into small pieces and soaked into water for some hours and later used as eye drop. Dosage: The squeezed leaves with the juice are put at the nostril to stop nasal bleeding and it is dropped in the eye twice daily. [601]

Sida acuta 237-invitro-leaf-water extract-strong bactericidal effect on Otitis media (OM). **Tr** 601-Nigeria.

nasal congestion **Tr** 28-india, 32-Ayurveda, 40-Brazil, 41-Brazil, 43-Brazil, 61-Brazil, 88-Brazil, 118-Ayurveda, 154-Brazil, 161-Brazil, 161-Ayurveda, 182-India,

Sida cordifolia

Tr 28-India, 32-Ayurveda, 28-India, 40-Brazil, 41-Brazil, 43-Brazil, 61-Brazil, 118-Ayurveda, 120-Colombia, 125-India, 132-Brazil, 132-Brazil, 153-Brasil, 154-Brazil, 156-Brasil, 160-Brazil, 161-Brazil, 162-Brazil, 182-India, 312-USA-Ayurveda,

Sida indica

Tr 445-India and China-some ear problems, 448-Ayurveda-deafness and/or tintinitis,, 684-Ayurveda-deafness and/or tintinitis, 712-India-leaves-earache,

Eye Problems

Sida acuta

Tr 238-SriLanka-cataracts, 358-review-Leaf mucilage used for getting foreign objects out of the eye, 600-root-conjunctivitis, Pinkeye-India-root-two drops of juice are put in the eye, 601-Nigeria-stem-the stem is cut into small pieces and soaked into water for some hours and later used as eye drop-dropped in the eye twice daily,

Sida cordifolia

Tr 88-Konkan, 118-Ayurveda, 124-India-leaves-applied in ophthalmic diseases, 127-Ayurveda-leaf paste, 358- conjunctivitis, Pinkeye-Burkina Faso a root macerate is applied to the eyelids, 378-medical website-a paste made from bala leaves has been applied to the affected eye, 437-eye diseases-Ayurveda-roots, 568- eye infections, 664-Ayurveda-whole plant?-extract,

Sida rhombifolia

Tr 150-eye problems-Ethiopia-roots or leaf, 150- conjunctivitis, Pinkeye-Ethiopia-roots, 437-eye diseases-Ayurveda-roots, 522- conjunctivitis, Pinkeye-Guatemala-dried leaf-hot aqueous extract-externally,

186

Sida indica anti-cataract activity

685-invitro-leaf-ethanol, water and hydro-ethanol solvents-The amount of protein, SOD and AR inhibition were found to be increased in the lens incubated with the plant extract and enalapril and were found to suppress the formation of cataract which is evident from the above results- The results showed a reduction in the opacity of the lens incubated with the plant extract- the hydro-ethanolic leaf extract of possesses the anti-cataract activity,

Tr 437-Ayurveda-Sida indica-root-eye diseases, 437-a wash in eye diseases-Ayurveda-Sida indica-roots, 450-eye wash-India-Sida indica-leaf, 711-India-leaf-eye wash, 737-India-seeds-decoction-eye sores,

Sida cordata Tr 437-eye diseases-Ayurveda-roots, 496- conjunctivitis, Pinkeye-Pakistan-Siddha and Ayurveda-seeds, 549-Ayurveda,

Fat/lipids - Increases HDL

This inventory scrutinizes the effect of methanolic extract of Sida rhomboidea on high fat diet-induced hyper-lipidemia in male Charles foster rats... Plasma TC, TG, low density lipoproteins (LDL), very low density lipoproteins (VLDL) and free fatty acids (FFA) levels were decreased along with significantly increased plasma HDL levels. **[319]**   **Tr** no reported use

Sida acuta

753-berberine-0.5 g to 1.5 g per day-The results showed that berberine intake was associated with a significant decrease in blood TC (0.61 mmol/L), TG (0.50 mmol/L), and LDL-C (0.65 mmol/L) concentrations compared with the control group. A small but significant increase in blood HDL-C (0.05 mmol/L) concentration after berberine treatment was also found,

Sida cordifolia

148-rats-leaves-alcoholic extract-400mg/kg weight- significant decrease in total cholesterol, triglycerides, low density lipids, plasma-creatinine, plasma-urea nitrogen and lipid-peroxidation and a significant increase in high density lipid-level, **159**-rats-leaves-petroleum ether+methanol-400mg/kg bw-lowered their serum TC, TG and LDL-C significantly, while raised the serum HDL-C, **171**-rats-water extract-aerial parts- -significantly (P<0.05) decreases total cholesterol (55.12±1.47mg/dl), triglycerides (45.95±1.56mg/dl), LDL (24.12± 1.72mg/dl), plasma creatinine (0.54±0.07mg/dl), plasma urea nitrogen (58.59± 3.25mmol/l), lipid peroxidation (5.90±0.34nmol MDA/ml) and significantly (P<0.05) increases HDL (34.76±1.66mg/dl), catalase (59.98±3.25Umol H2O2/ min/mg of Hb) and superoxide dismutase (62.47±2.33U/mg of Hb) activity of group-D diabetic rats on day 29, **180**-rats-aerial parts-acqueous extract-The three weeks treatment at 1000 mg/kg bw showed a significant reduction in cholesterol, triglycerides, LDL-C and VLDL-C in treated rats when compared with metformin at 500 mg/kg bw (P<0.05). HDL-C was significantly improved by treatment of extract,

187

Sida rhombifolia

155-rats-root?-extract?-400 mg/kg per day-significant (p<0.05) decrease in plasma lipid profile and cardiac lipid peroxidation-significant increase in plasma HDL.

Sida rhomboidea

130--rats--leaves--freeze-dried--distilled water extract-400 mg/kg bw-a comparison of results obtained in this study with lipid lowering potential of lovasatin suggests that the freeze-dried water extract is more effective in elevating circulating HDL levels and maintain tissue TG metabolism. Overall, the present study has revealed the highly potent ability of SR leaf extract in controlling dyslipidemia and hence portends a strong potential for use as a therapeutic agent in lipid disorders and obesity-can significantly elevate plasma DHL level and reduce LDL, TC, TG and TL levels without significantly influencing the lipid profile of normolipidemic rats, **287**-rats-leaf-acqueous extract-200mg/kg-significant decrement in plasma TC (p<0.05), TG (p<0.05) while HDL (p<0.05) was increased, **319**-invitro-leaves-methanol extract-plasma TC, TG, low density lipoproteins (LDL), very low density lipoproteins (VLDL) and free fatty acids (FFA) levels were decreased along with significantly increased plasma HDL levels- an excellent lipid lowering potential and also possess curative properties in conditions of hyperlipidemia and related disorders

Fat/lipids – Inhibit lipid peroxidation

The oxidative degradation of lipids. The process in which free radicals "steal" electrons from the lipids in cell membranes, resulting in cell damage. [1]

Sida acuta

103-rats-leaf- ethanolic and methanolic extracts (200 and 400 mg kg-10)-Both extracts significantly reduced plasma total cholesterol (p<0.05) and triglyceride (p<0.001)-the hypolipidaemic effects were comparable to that of glibenclamide, **460**-rats-whole plant-70% ethanol extract-400 mg/kg completely reversed lipid peroxidation-showed a marked decrease or restoration of serum markers to near normal level in a dependent manner, **739**-berberine-review-anti-hyperlipidemia,

Sida cordifolia

28-Sida cordifolia-50 % ethanolic extract-Lipid peroxidation products were reduced, **31**- ethanolic extract-root-lipid peroxidation products decreased, **42**-Sida cordifolia-water infusion- lipid peroxidation was reduced-IC50 126.78 microg/ml, **67**-Sida cordifolia-root-ethanolic extract-the lipid peroxidation products decreased, **121**-rats-root-ethanolic extract- Only the root extract exhibited superoxide-scavenging activity and inhibited lipid peroxidation in rat liver homogenate, **123**-rats-whole plant- water infusion-IC50 value for inhibitory action on lipid Peroxidation was 126.78 mg/ml; R2_/0.9808), **148**-rats-leaves-alcoholic extract-400mg/kg weight-significant decrease in total cholesterol, triglycerides, low density lipids, plasma-creatinine, plasma-urea nitrogen and lipid-peroxidation and a significant increase in high density lipid-level, **171**-rats-water extract-aerial parts-400mg/kg wt-significantly (P<0.05) decreases total cholesterol (55.12±1.47mg/dl), triglycerides (45.95±1.56mg/dl), LDL (24.12± 1.72mg/dl), plasma creatinine (0.54±0.07mg/dl), plasma urea nitrogen (58.59± 3.25mmol/l), lipid peroxidation (5.90±0.34nmol MDA/ml) and significantly (P<0.05) increases HDL (34.76±1.66mg/dl), catalase (59.98±3.25Umol H2O2/ min/mg of Hb) and superoxide dismutase (62.47±2.33U/mg of Hb) activity of group-D diabetic rats on day 29, **180**-rats-aerial parts-water extract-1 gm/kg bw-significant improvement (P<0.05) in lipid profile, **182**-rats-roots-50% ethanolic extract-Administration of alcohol induces lipid peroxidation-S. cordifolia exerts an antioxidant effect by decreasing lipid peroxidation,

Tr 180-India-These results could explain the basis for the use of this plant extract to manage serum glucose level and cholesterolemia associated with diabetes mellitus.

Sida rhombifolia

49-Sida rhombifolia-seed-ethanol extract-significantly limited lipid peroxidase, **75**-root-only root extract inhibited lipid peroxidation in rat liver and brain homogenate, **503**-rats-70% methanol extract- A long-term trial in the moderately diabetic group showed a normal lipid profile, **541**-rats-roots-90% ethanolic extract-100 mg- the lipid peroxide content was found to decrease to large extent on SRE treatment- showed remarkably reduced lipid peroxide activity, which was comparable to that of standard drug treated group.

Sida retusa

57-rat-root extract-Only root extract inhibited lipid peroxidation in rat liver and brain homogenate, **196**-mice-leaves-acqueous extract 200 mg/kg bw-reduction in triglycerides (TG) (16%), cholesterol (4%)- mild hypolipidemic activity, **461**-roots-methanol extract-found to inhibit lipid peroxidation-The quantity required for 50% inhibition of lipid peroxidation, scavenging hydroxyl radical and peroxide radical was 1130.24 ug/ml, **464**-Sida retusa-invitro-seed extract-significantly inhibited lipid peroxidase.

Sida cordata
540-rats-leaf-ether wash-95% ethanolic extract-Carbon Tetracholoride induced toxicity-Treatment significantly reversed all the changes.

Sida rhomboidea

280-rats/invitro-leaves-water extract- Nephrotoxicity was induced in rats with gentamicin (100 mg/kg bw(i.p.) for 8 days), then treated with Sida rhomboidea extract (200 and 400 mg/kg bw (p.o.) for 8 days)- lowered lipid peroxidation levels is attributable to the free radical scavenging ability of Sida rhomboidea that prevents membrane lipid peroxidation, **288**-rats-?extract-Pre-treatment with SR extract (400 mg/kg per day, p.o.) for 30 consecutive days followed by isoproterenol injections on days 29th and 30th, showed significant (p00.05) decrease in... plasma lipid profile, **319**-rats-leaves-methanolic extract-400 mg/kg BW)-experimentally induced hyper-lipidemia-has an excellent lipid lowering potential and also possess curative properties in conditions of hyperlipidemia and related disorders, **320**-invitro-leaves-methanol extract-Lipid peroxidation assay showed a dose dependent (50-600 µg/ml) response of MESR (p<0.05) with 800 ug/ml being the optimal concentration,

Sida Cardifolia **200**-invitro-leaf-acetone extract- showed the highest reducing power activity, Free radical scavenging potential and inhibition of lipid peroxidation.-100 µg concentration=87% inhibition of lipid peroxide generation.

Fat/lipids – Lowers cholesterol

An essential structural component of all animal cell membranes; essential to maintain membrane structural integrity and fluidity. [1] **Tr** no reported use

Sida acuta

753-berberine-0.5 g to 1.5 g per day-The results showed that berberine intake was associated with a significant decrease in blood TC (0.61 mmol/L), TG (0.50 mmol/L), and LDL-C (0.65 mmol/L) concentrations compared with the control group. A small but significant increase in blood HDL-C (0.05 mmol/L) concentration after berberine treatment was also found.

Sida cordifolia

148-rats-leaves-alcoholic extract-400mg/kg weight- significant decrease in total cholesterol, triglycerides, low density lipids, plasma-creatinine, plasma-urea nitrogen and lipid-peroxidation and a significant increase in high density lipid-level, **159**-rats-leaves-petroleum ether+ methanol-lowered their serum TC, TG and LDL-C significantly, while raised the serum HDL-C, **171**-rats-water extract-aerial parts-400mg/kg wt-significantly (P<0.05) decreases total cholesterol (55.12±1.47mg/dl), triglycerides (45.95± 1.56mg/dl), LDL (24.12± 1.72mg/dl), plasma creatinine (0.54±0.07mg/dl), plasma urea nitrogen (58.59± 3.25mmol/l), lipid peroxidation (5.90±0.34nmol MDA/ml) and significantly (P<0.05) increases HDL (34.76±1.66mg/dl), catalase (59.98±3.25Umol H2O2/ min/mg of Hb) and superoxide dismutase (62.47±2.33U/mg of Hb) activity of group-D diabetic rats on day 29, **180**-rats-aerial parts-acqueous extract-The three weeks treatment at 1000 mg/kg bw showed a significant reduction in cholesterol, triglycerides, LDL-C and VLDL-C in treated rats when compared with metformin at 500 mg/kg bw (P<0.05). HDL-C was significantly improved by treatment of extract,

Sida rhomboidea

130-rats-leaves-freeze-dried water extract-A comparison of results obtained in this study with lipid lowering potential of lovasatin suggests that the freeze-dried water extract (400 and 800 mg/kg bw) is more effective in elevating circulating HDL levels and maintain tissue TG metabolism. Overall, the present study has revealed the highly potent ability of SR leaf extract in controlling dyslipidemia and hence portends a strong potential for use as a therapeutic agent in lipid disorders and obesity-can significantly elevate plasma DHL level and reduce LDL, TC, TG and TL levels without significantly influencing the lipid profile of normolipidemic rats,   **287**-rats-leaf-acqueous extract-400mg/kg-decreased cholesterol in Triton WR 1339 induced rats-comparable lovastatin.

Sida retusa

131-mice-leaves-acqueous extract- a dose of 200 mg/kg of aqueous extract has shown reduction in triglycerides (TG) (16%), cholesterol (4%),

Fat/lipids – Lowers LDL   Tr   no reported use

Low-density lipoprotein particles pose a risk for cardiovascular disease when they invade the endothelium and become oxidized. [1]

Sida acuta

753-berberine-0.5 g to 1.5 g per day-The results showed that berberine intake was associated with a significant decrease in blood TC (0.61 mmol/L), TG (0.50 mmol/L), and LDL-C (0.65 mmol/L) concentrations compared with the control group. A small but significant increase in blood HDL-C (0.05 mmol/L) concentration after berberine treatment was also found

Sida cordifolia

148-rats-leaves-alcoholic extract-400mg/kg weight- significant decrease in total cholesterol, triglycerides, low density lipids, plasma-creatinine, plasma-urea nitrogen and lipid-peroxidation and a significant increase in high density lipid-level,   **159**-rats-leaves-petroleum ether+ methanol-lowered their serum TC, TG and LDL-C significantly, while raised the serum HDL-C, **171**-rats-water extract-aerial parts-400mg/kg wt-significantly (P<0.05) decreases total cholesterol (55.12±1.47mg/dl), triglycerides (45.95±1.56mg /dl), LDL (24.12± 1.72mg/dl), plasma creatinine (0.54±0.07mg/dl), plasma urea nitrogen (58.59± 3.25mmol/l), lipid peroxidation (5.90±0.34nmol MDA/ml) and significantly (P<0.05) increases HDL (34.76±1.66mg/dl), catalase (59.98±3.25Umol H2O2/ min/mg of Hb) and superoxide dismutase (62.47±2.33U/mg of Hb) activity of group-D diabetic rats on day 29,   **180**-rats-aerial parts-acqueous extract-The three weeks treatment at 1000 mg/kg bw showed a significant reduction in cholesterol, triglycerides, LDL-C and VLDL-C in treated rats when compared with metformin at 500 mg/kg bw (P<0.05). HDL-C was significantly improved by treatment of extract,

Sida rhomboidea

130-rats-leaves-freeze-dried water extract-A comparison of results obtained in this study with lipid lowering potential of lovasatin suggests that the freeze-dried water extract (400 and 800 mg/kg bw) is more effective in elevating circulating HDL levels and maintain tissue TG metabolism. Overall, the present study has revealed the highly potent ability of SR leaf extract in controlling dyslipidemia and hence portends a strong potential for use as a therapeutic agent in lipid disorders and obesity-can significantly elevate plasma DHL level and reduce LDL, TC, TG and TL levels without significantly influencing the lipid profile of normolipidemic rats.

Fat/lipids – Lowers Triglycerides

The main constituents of body fat in humans and other animals, as well as vegetable fat. [2]   They are also present in the blood to enable the bidirectional transference of adipose fat and blood glucose from the liver, and are a major component of human skin oils. [1]   Tr   **no reported use**

Sida acuta

753-berberine-0.5 g to 1.5 g per day-The results showed that berberine intake was associated with a significant decrease in blood TC (0.61 mmol/L), TG (0.50 mmol/L), and LDL-C (0.65 mmol/L) concentrations compared with the control group. A small but significant increase in blood HDL-C (0.05 mmol/L) concentration after berberine treatment was also found.

Sida cordifolia

148-rats-leaves-alcoholic extract-400mg/kg weight- significant decrease in total cholesterol, triglycerides, low density lipids, plasma-creatinine, plasma-urea nitrogen and lipid-peroxidation and a significant increase in high density lipid-level,   **159**-rats-leaves-petroleum ether+ methanol-lowered their serum TC, TG and LDL-C significantly, while raised the serum HDL-C, **171**-rats-water extract-aerial parts-400mg/kg wt-significantly (P<0.05) decreases total cholesterol (55.12±1.47mg/dl), triglycerides (45.95± 1.56mg/dl), LDL (24.12±1.72mg/dl), plasma creatinine (0.54± 0.07mg/dl), plasma urea nitrogen (58.59± 3.25mmol/l), lipid peroxidation (5.90±0.34nmol MDA/ml) and significantly (P<0.05) increases HDL (34.76±1.66mg/dl), catalase (59.98±3.25Umol H2O2/ min/mg of Hb) and superoxide dismutase (62.47±2.33U/mg of Hb) activity of group-D diabetic rats on day 29,   **180**-rats-aerial parts-acqueous extract-The three weeks treatment at 1000 mg/kg bw showed a significant reduction in cholesterol, triglycerides, LDL-C and VLDL-C in treated rats when compared with metformin at 500 mg/kg bw (P<0.05). HDL-C was significantly improved by treatment of extract,

Sida retusa

131- mice-leaves-acqueous extract- a dose of 200 mg/kg of aqueous extract has shown reduction in triglycerides (TG) (16%), cholesterol (4%),

Sida rhomboidea

128-rats-leaf-extract-Results clearly substantiate the anti-hypertriglycer-idemic potential,   **130**-rats-leaves-freeze-dried water extract-A comparison of results obtained in this study with lipid lowering potential of lovasatin

192

suggests that the freeze-dried water extract (400 and 800 mg/kg bw) is more effective in elevating circulating HDL levels and maintain tissue TG metabolism. Overall, the present study has revealed the highly potent ability of SR leaf extract in controlling dyslipidemia and hence portends a strong potential for use as a therapeutic agent in lipid disorders and obesity-can significantly elevate plasma DHL level and reduce LDL, TC, TG and TL levels without significantly influencing the lipid profile of normolipidemic rats.

Fiber

Species	Parts Used	Mode of Use
Sida indica	Stem	Cordage and also mixed with jute
Sida acuta	Stem, leaf	Jute fiber
Sida cordata	Shoot, bark	Rope
Sida cordifolia	Stem	Fiber, Jute
Sida Mysorensis	Stem	Fiber used for rope
Sida rhombifolia	Stem	Fiber [557]

Sida acuta   97-invitro-pulp and paper making fiber.

Tr   90-Ayurveda-also yields a good fibre,   109-Siddah-fiber plant,   212-India-brooms,   255-India-brooms,   270-India-It is commonly known as broom weed,   283-Australia-Chinese prospectors used the tough, fibrous stems to make brooms,   358-fiber-tooth cleaners, chew sticks – stems: brushes/brooms, stems, baskets – bark: netting, cord/string/twine – stems: ropes, mats, cord, string, twine.   Tough fibres used for making twine -- In Yucatan the bark-fibre is used for the manufacture of twine and hammocks -- Branches of this, and other, species of Sida often used in Mexico for making rough brooms -- Used as brush fibre in East Africa,   361-stems-brushes/brooms,   361-bark-fishing lines,   361-stems-basketry,   361-bark-cord/string/twine/ropes,   361-wood-constructions,   362-Mexico-fiber crop,   557-India-stem/leaf-jute fiber, 656-India-reinforced epoxy composite,

Sida cordifolia

Tr   88-India,   358-review,   167-India,   358- Mozambique and Zimbabwe- bark yields fibres that are used for making cordage,   358-Congo-stems are used in basketry,   358-Africa, China- Use of the entire plant or branched stems as brooms is widespread,   557-India-stem-fiber, jute,

Sida rhombifolia

358-In DR Congo fibre yields of 1300 kg/ha have been recorded. In experiments in Rwanda in the 1950s fibre yields of 240 kg/ha were obtained, with the fresh, defoliated stems yielding 4.0% fibre after 6 days of retting. Extraction of the fibre is difficult, but these problems should be easily overcome through experimentation. In the Central African Republic the stems are left to dry for 10–12 days and retting in water takes another 20 days, **426**-invivo-The stem flexibility was expressed as the stem breaking angle and leaf tensile strength as the ratio of the leaf breaking load to the DW of a 5 cm length of leaf - The stems of Sida rhombifolia did not break or collapse at any degree of bending up to 180°, over the period of the experiment... S. rhombifolia leaves had the lowest tensile strengths, **489**-India-plant fiber raised from irradiated seeds are stronger, **506**-review-This plant yields a good fiber. Because of this reason the cultivation of Sida rhombifolia has been encouraged in India (Bailey,1958), **669**- Sida rhombifolia-stem-perennial shrub from which high stiffness natural fibers can be extracted. The physico-chemical properties of Sida rhombifolia fibers (SRFs), crystallinity index (56.6%), higher cellulose (75.09 wt.%) content, and lower density (1320.7 kg/m3) were revealed and compared to those properties of other natural fibers.

Tr 524-Fiber-Stem yields a good fiber-considered a good substitute for jute, 361-Yields fibre rated better in quality than jute, 362-India, Australia, Africa and America-fibre crop, 367-review-The bark of Sida rhombifolia yields fibres that are used in the same way as those of jute (Corchorus spp.). In Niger the fibres are used to make fishing-lines and nets and in the Central African Republic for making large hunting-nets. The stems are woven to produce wattle-work doors. The whole plants are used as brooms in DR Congo, the Central African Republic and Gabon, 524-Phillipines-stem, 557-India-stem-fiber,

Sida hermaphrodita

471-review-mainly used in industry as... a source of fibers, **477**- Poland -the pulp obtained may be used as an insulating material and in the production of agglomerated materials- do not differ much from boards made entirely from wood particles,

Sida spinosa

Tr 358-review-The bark fibre is used for cordage, the stems are used for cleaning teeth and stems tied together are used as brooms. In Malawi the stems are used for tying in roof construction,

Other Sidas

Tr 358- Sida linifolia-Gabon- the stems are used for brooms, 358-Sida urens-Africa, India, West Indies- bark yields a good quality fibre, 557-India-Sida indica-stem-cordage and also mixed with jute, 557-Sida cordata-India-shoot or bark-rope, 557-Sida Mysorensis Wight&Arn-India-stem-fibre used for rope.

Fiberglass   Tr   no reported use

Sida hermaphrodita

477-Poland-invitro-wood particles-the degree of substituting wood particles with Sida was 25% in case of UF and MUPF resins, 10% in case of PMDI resin and 100% for all the investigated resins. The obtained results lead to the conclusion that low-density particleboards produced with use of Sida hermaphrodita Rusby do not differ much from boards made entirely from wood particles.... For all the investigated values of density, the increase in the amount of Sida does not deteriorate these values, but it even improves them.

Food storage protection Tr no reported use
Sida acuta
416-invivo-leaf-made into a paste-damage to grains of wheat and maize by Sitophilus oryzae and Prostephanus truncates was reduced 10% when the grain was admixed with sida leaves. Slurries, produced by adding distilled water to the powder and stirring so that a smooth paste was obtained, were generally more effective than powders, especially against Sitophilus oryzae.

Food, for Humans
Traditional leafy vegetables are those plants whose leaves or aerial parts have been integrated in a community's culture for use as food over a long span of time. These vegetables are highly recommended due to their relatively high nutritional value compared to the introduced varieties, and are also important in food security. [213]   Investigation into proximate and micronutrients composition of Sida acuta leaves in this study has shown S. acuta to be composed of significant amounts of essential food nutrients. These food nutrients are in amounts comparable to those of leafy vegetables which are commonly consumed for good nutrition. The phytochemical constitution and composition of S. acuta are in amounts to be responsible for diverse medicinal and therapeutic purposes. Sida acuta leaves would provide nutritional benefits and medicinal value. [223]   Three varieties of Sida were ingredients in Soma, the legendary food of the gods. [22] {There is some toxicity, see **Toxicity, Toxic to living things** for details.}

Sida acuta
258-Kenya-leaves-a local food,   **415**-invitro-had the highest crude protein amongst pasture plants,

Tr   223-review-traditional food plant of western Kenya,   258-leaves-a local food-perennials of local abundance,   358-review-leaf-food or condiments/ relishes/chutneys,   671-Australia-A tea made from fresh leaves and then chilled is a perfect beverage for hot and humid days,

Sida cordifolia
Tr   71-Ayurveda-root- food supplement for fat loss,   88-China,   158-invitro-seed-protein=22%,   161-Ayurveda-nutritive, 217-Ayurveda,   358-Nigeria- the leaves are cooked as a vegetable,   411-invitro-root- used in food supplements for loosing weight,   548-Ayurveda-roots-used as a food supplement for fat loss,

Sida rhombifolia

Tr   47-Camaroon-human food,   362-South America-leaves and shoots-vegetable,   358-In South Africa the leaves are preserved by drying before storing to be consumed later as a vegetable,   358-the leaves and shoots are used as a vegetable in Middle and South America, as well as South Africa. In Indo-China, the roasted leaves are used for making a refreshing drink. The dried leaves are also used as tea.   367-review-The leaves and shoots are used as a vegetable in South Africa and South America,   595-India-leaves-appetiser,

Sida spinosa

Tr   358-review-Leaf used as food in West Nile and Madi districts in Uganda-Used by Gwembe Tonga of Zambia as a vegetable relish-Leaves are used as condiments/relishes/chutneys,   358-In Malawi the leaves are cooked and eaten as a vegetable -- In Senegal an infusion of leaves and roots is drunk to cure dysentery and to increase the energy of recovering patients.

All Sidas   **Tr**   22-review- We propose that Soma (food of the gods) was a combination... with an ephedrine and phenylethylamine-rich Sida spp. Extract.

Food, Other than human

Illinois-food source-migratory shorebirds-Plants composed 35% of the aggregate weight of food found in spring migrating blue-winged teal (Anas discors) collected in Missouri. Genera found included... Sida. **[604]**

{See also Insects, Food and Sustenance}

Sida acuta

60-observation-Nigeria-goats-However, the RS showed greater preference (P<0.05) for Danilia olivery, Sida acuta and dry Gmelina leaves than the other breeds,   **204**- S. acuta is widely employed as livestock and poultry feed [Egunjobi, J.K. Some common weeds of West Africa, Bulletin of Research Division Ministry of Agriculture, Natural Resources Western State. Ibadan, Nigeria. (1969) - cited in 204],   **210**-goats,   **229**-weaner rabbits-aerial parts-sole source of food-gained weight,   **358**-review-seeds and flower buds-primates/baboons,   **358**- sheep-leaves --camels, horses, goats and game mammals-forage-stems,   **361**-Game mammals: Minor food plant for rhino; eaten by nyala, bushback and warthog,   **362**-review-not good forage when overgrazed-the stems are unpalatable to cattle,   **415**-invivo-goats-Protein content, cell wall fractions and mineral concentrations of some minor plant species collected in pastures grazed by goats in the Philippines were examined. Legumes and herbs had higher CP, especially S. acuta. S. acuta had exceptionally high concentrations of minerals. The results showed that some minor plant species could extend the range of concentration of some nutrients (CP and minerals) beyond that normally found in conventional pasture species,   **420**-citing another-widely employed as livestock and poultry feed (Egunjobi, 1969),   **427**-invivo-aerial parts-Sida acuta and S. rhombifolia showed higher digestibility, CP and acid detergent lignin contents and lower acid detergent fibre, Si and neutral detergent fibre than other Ecuadorean forage - in the dry season cattle did not eat this, **604**-Illinois-invivo-food source-migratory shorebirds, **643**-invivo-aerial parts-wild forage-utilized for goat reproduction, **694**-field study-whole plant?-dried plant supplement- Total feed intake and feed conver-sion ratio of the rabbits fed Sida acuta were significant (P > 0 01) higher than for rabbits fed poultry growers mash alone,

Tr 61-leaves-grazing food-cattle/Equidae/game mammals/pigs/sheep/ goats-Minor food plant for rhino/nyala/bushback/warthog, 204-Nigeria, 220-Nigeria, 258-Kenya-leaves a local food-perennials of local abundance, leaves most luxuriant in the rainy season, 420-Nigeria-widely employed as livestock and poultry feed.

Sida cordifolia

122-rats-leaf?-water extract- was found to be more effective in reducing the food intake and body weight, **276**-invivo-livestock feed for broiler chicken-added 5% of Sida cordifolia to feed for chickens with no negative results, **358**-review-The foliage is eaten by livestock throughout West Africa and in northern Nigeria it is valued as a fattening feed for horses, **362**-review-not good forage when overgrazed-the stems are unpalatable to cattle, **410**-seeds-commercial carp fed 2% of body weight per day for 60 days - Specific growth rate, food conversion ration and gross conversion efficiency were all improved compared to control-the fingerlings receiving Bala mixed diet were visible more healthy and active. Statistical analysis of results showed that the fish growth was significantly influenced by this herb, **608**-rats-aerial parts?-whole plant as food supplement,

Sida rhombifolia

130-rats-acqueous extract-leaves-weight stayed the same but ate less, **276**-chickens-this study showed that feeding 5% of sidaguri had an effect (P>0,05) on feed consumption, average daily weight gain and feed conversion ratio of broiler chicken, **286**-rats?-leaf-water extract-3000 mg/kg body weight-significant decrement in food intake and body weight gain, **362**-review-not good forage when overgrazed-the stems are unpalatable to cattle, **367**-review-Like most Sida species, Sida rhombifolia is appreciated as a fodder, **427**-invivo-aerial parts-Sida acuta and S. rhombifolia showed higher digestibility, CP and acid detergent lignin contents and lower acid detergent fibre, Si and neutral detergent fibre than other Ecuadorean forage - in the dry season cattle did not eat this, **520**-mice-leaf-boiling distilled water extract-reduced food intake,

Tr 358-South Africa-leaves are preserved by drying before storing to be consumed later as a vegetable,

Sida rhomboidea

134-mice-whole plant?-? extract-high fat diet-reduced bodyweight (p<0.05), food intake (p<0.05) and feed efficiency ratio (p<0.05), **367**-review-Like most Sida species, Sida rhombifolia is appreciated as a fodder,

Sida spinosa

358-review-roots-pigs-browse, **358**-review-stems-forage-goats, **358**-review-The leaves are browsed by goats (Kenya), horses, donkeys (Sudan), camels, and game animals, **358**-review-primates/baboons-roots/fruits/seeds/flower buds.

Food, Tea   No peer review

Sida acuta

Tr   270-India-It is commonly known as tea weed,   361-Mexico-Leaves used in some parts of Mexico as a substitute for Chinese tea,   362-In general, the decoction, infusion or pressed juice of the mucilaginous leaves and bitter roots of Sida are used for cooling, emollient, diuretic and febrifuge purposes, to treat gonorrhoeae and rheumatism and externally as a poultice for boils, ulcers, swellings, cuts, coughs and chickenpox,   671-In India a tea is prepared from the fresh or dried leaves which is very refreshing and also stimulating,

Sida cordifolia

Tr   32-Ayurveda-root infusion- given in nervous and urinary diseases and also in disorders of the blood and bile,   118-review- The root infusion is given in nervous and urinary diseases and also in disorders of the blood and bile,   161-Ayurveda- Its herbal extract or tea is used for obesity and obesity related disorders, especially in western countries,   362-review-An infusion of the roots is given for diseases such as hemiplegia or facial paralysis, for asthma as well as in disorders of the blood and bile,   358-DR Congo-leaf-water infusion-given to children in case of rheumatism,

Sida rhombifolia

Tr   51-India-whole plant?- An infusion of the root is given in dysentery, 362-Indo-China-leaves-roasted-make a refreshing drink,   367-review-Indo-China-roasted leaves-used for making a refreshing drink,   522-review- The infusion of dried leaf of S. rhombifolia in Central Africa is used for diabetes, chest pain and diarrhea on oral administration. The infusion of this plant is applied locally for the treatment of skin diseases and infected wounds, 524-Phillipines-leaves-tea,   524-Mexico-tea substitute,   671-In India a tea is prepared from the fresh or dried leaves which is very refreshing and also stimulating,

Other Sidas

Tr   358-Sida spinosa-In Senegal an infusion of leaves and roots is drunk to cure dysentery and to increase the energy of recovering patients,   435-Sida retusa-Japan-An infusion made from the roots of this plant is held in great repute by the local Ayurvedic physicians in the treatment of rheumatism and a variety of neurological complaints including epilepsy, 613-Sida tuberculata-leaves and roots-hot water infusion-how it is usually taken,

198

Fuel, Heat production   Tr   no reported use

Although, this species comes from the United States of America, research on height of yield and quality of its raw material for energy purposes is being carried out in Poland exclusively... To obtain similar yield levels from sewage sludge in light soil seems possible. Considering the high combustion heat, this would let us achieve energy productivity higher than from any other plant cultivated in such conditions. A valuable merit is that Sida hermaphrodita plantations do not need any yearly cultivation treatment typical for annual plants. Difficult is only the year of establishing the plantation as the first year of cultivation with no biomass yield, which is very typical for perennial species. [473]

Sida hermaphrodita

472-invivo-whole living plant-Considering the energetic purposes, the height of the crop of Sida stems is also important. Other studies indicated good combustion heat efficiency of this material, expressed in kJ/kg. This efficiency reached 88.0% of pine wood efficiency and 80.1% of beech wood, **473**-field study-whole plant-twice or three times as much energy was obtained than, on average, during a year from several years old pine or spruce forest (annual average – 25-year-old pine forest – 69 GJ, 35-yearold spruce forest– 93 GJ·ha-1)... In the third and fourth years of production an average yield of dry matter of over 11 t·ha-1 was obtained; energy productivity level was 219.5 GJ·ha-1,   **474**-Poland- Based on averages from three years of tests, significantly higher yields (5 t/ha) of dry matter and more production of energy per hectare (30.5%), were obtained from Virginia fanpetals' trials, than that of the tested willow,   **475**-Germany-invivo-Since more drought spells will occur in the future climate and the availability of productive land will be reduced permanent bioenergy cultures will have to be based on marginal agricultural production systems. The perennial species addressed here are potentially suited candidates because they have high water use efficiency and do not need to be grown under highly intensive conditions.

GI tract, Abdominal pains   No peer review

{GI tract is stomach to anus. Mouth and throat are in different sections}

Sida acuta

Tr   3-India-root,   76-Burkina Faso- abdominal infections and associated diseases,   82-India,   88-India,   90-India?-chronic bowel complaints, 106-Cameroon,   174-India,   186-India-disorders of bile, chronic bowel complaints,   201-leaf-review from Ghana,   203-Burkina Faso- abdominal infections and associated diseases,   270-India-stomachic in chronic bowel complaints,   362-review-colic and chronic bowel complaints,   377-Ayurveda,   561-Ayurveda-root,   571-India-chronic bowel complaints,

Sida cordifolia

Tr 27-Burkina Faso-whole plant decoction?, 117-BurkinaFaso-decoction-abdominal pain, 203-Burkina Faso- abdominal infections and associated diseases, 285-Ayurveda-seeds-bowel complaints, 362-review-colic and chronic bowel complaints, 561-Ayurveda-root, 571-India-chronic bowel complaints,

Sida rhombifolia

Tr 51-India-root infusion-abdominal complaints, 362-review-colic and chronic bowel complaints, 522-Australia-dried root-used by traditional people for abdominal upset, 524-Phillipines-juice swallowed-abdominal cramps, 524-Phillipines-root-decoction-absominal troubles, 571-India-chronic bowel complaints,

Sida spinosa **Tr** 571-India-chronic bowel complaints, 561-Ayurvedic-root.

Other Sidas

Tr 318-Sida pilosa-whole plant?-lower abdominal pains and intestinal helminthiasis, 362-Sida indica-review-colic and chronic bowel complaints,

GI tract, Colic No peer review
{GI tract is stomach to anus. Mouth and throat are in different sections}

Sida acuta **Tr** 85-India-Tribal people of Chhattisgarh use for colic pain, 362-review-colic and chronic bowel complaints,

Sida cordifolia

Tr 88-Ayurveda-seeds, 118-Ayurveda, 124-India-root, 158-India, 167-Ayurveda-seeds-colic pain, 312-USA-Ayurveda-seeds, 358-Mauritius-plant sap is diluted and drunk to relieve colic, 362-review-Malaysia-seeds, 664-Ayurveda-whole plant?-extract,

Sida rhombifolia **Tr** 362-review-colic and chronic bowel complaints, 407-Ayurveda-seeds,

Sida cordata **Tr** 496-Sida cordata-Pakistan-Siddha and Ayurveda-seeds,

Sida indica **Tr** 362-review-colic and chronic bowel complaints,

GI tract, Constipation No peer review
{GI tract is stomach to anus. Mouth and throat are in different sections}

Sida acuta **Tr** 362-review,

200

Sida cordifolia

Tr 40-Brazil-laxative, 120-Columbia, 125-India-laxitive, 148-India-aerial parts-laxative, 152-India, 161-Ayurveda-root extract-laxative, 162-Brazil-laxative, 180-India-laxitive, 285-India-root-laxitive, 285-Ayurvdic-seeds-laxative, 312-Brazil-laxitive, 312-USA-Ayurveda-laxative, 362-review, 437-India-seeds-laxative, 437-India-leaves-decoction-enema,

Sida rhombifolia

Tr 362-review, 437-India-seeds-laxative, 437-India-leaves-decoction-enema, 524-Phillipines-root-decoction of old root, 568-Nigeria,

Sida cordata

Tr 437-Ayurveda-seeds-laxative, 437-India-leaves-decoction-enema, 496-Sida cordata-Pakistan-Siddha and Ayurveda-seeds or roots-laxative.

Sida indica

Tr 362-review, 437--Ayurveda--seeds-laxative--leaves-decoction-enema, 708-Ayurveda-seed, 711-India-seed-a laxative for those having hemor-rhoids, 712-India-stem bark or seeds-laxative, 437-Ayurveda, 445-Thailand-laxative, 451-Thailand-leaf extract-can also be used as an enema, 451-Thailand-seeds-can be used as an enema or laxative for those having hemorrhoids, 678-Ayurveda-seeds, 684-Ayurveda-leaf juice, 711-India-leaf?, 735-Ayurveda-review-seeds,

GI tract, Diarrhea

{GI tract is stomach to anus. Mouth and throat are in different sections} It has been reported that diarrhea is the most infant mortality disease in the world, mostly in developing countries. Each year, this disease kills more than 6 million of children in the world with 7.7% and 8.5% respectively in Africa and South East of Asia. In Cameroon, diarrheic infection is involved in high mortality and morbidity of the children and accounts for thirty thousand deaths among children each year. [47]

Sida acuta

Tr 7-W Africa, 52-India-whole plant-hot water extract, 106-Cameroon, 107-India, 220-India, 220-BurkinaFaso, 221-India, 270-India-chew fresh root, 361-diarrhea, 361-Costa Rica-Roots-diarrhea-a decoction of the roots-infantile diarrhea, 523-India-leaves, 601-Nigeria-during pregnancy, 609-India, 619-Malaysia, 646-Nigeria,

Sida cordifolia

Tr 27-Burkina Faso-whole plant decoction?, 117-BurkinaFaso, 124-India-during pregnancy, 161-Ayurveda, 444-Ayurveda-Bala-Pitta Atisaranashan-relieves diarrhea of Pitta origin, 541-Siddha, 568-Nigeria, x619-Malaysia,

Sida rhombifolia

47-invitro-methanolic extract-A single oral dose of Sida rhombifolia extract of 400 mg/kg body weight produced a significant decrease in the severity of diarrhea, **199**-rats--methanolic extract-400mg/kg-single dose comparable to Diphenoxylate (50 mg/kg),

Tr 47-Camaroon and Madagascar, 126-Colombia, 150-Ethiopia-roots decocted, 190-India, 199-India, 522-Central Africa-dried leaf-infusion, 522-Cameron-leaf and root infusions-orally, 522-Mozambique-leaf and root infusions-as emollient, 522-New Guinea-fresh leaf juice-children, 522-Australia-dried root, 522-Nicaragua-leaf-decoction-taken orally, 524-Cuba-roots-decoction-for infantile diarrhea, 524-Australian aborigines, 541-Siddha, 543-Ayurveda, 545-Australian aborigines, 596-Nigeria-leaves, 619-Malaysia,

Sida indica

437-review-invitro-roots-powder-cited another study--leaves-methanolic extract and aqueous extract showed significant anti-diarrheal activity in vitro,

Tr 450-India-leaf-bilious diarrhea, 451-Thailand-leaf extract, 452-Bangladesh, 684-Ayurveda-leaf juice, 711-India-leaf extract, 712-India-leaves-Catarrhal bilious diarrhea,

Other Sida

Tr 293-Sida cordata-India-leaf, 596-Sida pilosa-Nigeria-leaves, 619-Sida spinosa-Malaysia,

GI tract, Digestive Problems   No peer review

{GI tract is stomach to anus. Mouth and throat are in different sections}

Sida acuta   **Tr** 150-Ethiopia-roots, 192-BurkinaFaso-gastrointestinal disturbances.

Sida rhombifolia

Tr 150-Ethiopia-root-stomach disorders, 150-Ethiopia-roots and leaves-irritable bowel syndrome, 358-DR Congo-general stomach complaints.

GI tract, Dysentery   Inflammation of the intestine

{GI tract is stomach to anus. Mouth and throat are in different sections}

Sida acuta   **14**-mice-leaf-ethanol extract-The results revealed a reduction in the frequency of abdominal constrictions induced by acetic acid,

Tr 52-India-whole plant-hot water extract, 101-Papua New Guinea-fresh root is chewed, 107-India-demulcent, 151-Ayurveda-chronic dysentery, 168-Papua New Guinea-fresh root-chewed, 201-roots-review from Ghana, 203-Burkina Faso-abdominal infections and associated diseases, 220-

India, 221-India, 270-India-chew fresh root, 362-review, 523-India-leaves, 609-India, x619-Malaysia, 646-Nigeria,

Sida cordifolia

Tr 116-Bangladesh, 167-Ayurveda-root-chronic dysentery, 167-Ayurveda-leaves, 180-India-chronic dysentery, 182-India, 312-USA-Ayurveda-roots/leaves/stems-chronic dysentery, 358- Senegal, Côte d'Ivoire, Burkina Faso, Burundi, Kenya, Papua New Guinea and the Philippines-leaves are taken, 362-review-Papua New Guinea and Philippines-leaf-juice-mixed with honey, 408-India-roots/leaves/stems /seeds, 568-Nigeria, 609-India, 612-Ayurveda-root-chronic dysentery,

Sida rhombifolia

Tr 47-India, 51-India-root infusion, 88-Madagascar, 107-India-demulcent, 150-Ethiopia-roots and leaves-inflammation of the intestine, 150-Ethiopia-root, 151-Ayurveda-chronic dysentery, 220-India, 270-India-chew fresh root, 358-DR Congo-a watery maceration of the leaves, 361-Fiji and Papua New Guinea-Roots-chewed against dysentery, 362-review-Fiji and Papua New Guinea-Roots-chewed, 522-Madagascar-whole plant?- the infusion of the root is given in dysentery, 522-Cameron-leaf and root infusions-orally, 522-Mozambique-leaf and root infusions-as emollient, 522-India-leaf paste-taken orally with milk, 522-Madeira-flower-infusion-used as an emollient, 609-India, 619-Malaysia,

Sida cordata   **Tr** 498-India,

Sida indica   **Tr** 362- review, 451-Thailand-seeds-chronic dysentery, 711-India-seed-chronic dysentery, 737-India-seeds-decoction-chronic dysentery,

Sida schimperiana   **Tr** 631-Sida schimperiana-Ethiopia-Powder is mixed with melted butter and drunk.,

Sida spinosa   **Tr** 358-Senegal-root/leaf infusion-drink,

GI tract, Flatulence (farts)   No peer review
{GI tract is stomach to anus. Mouth and throat are in different sections}

Sida cordifolia   **Tr** 88-Ayurveda-root bark,

Sida rhombifolia   **Tr** 150-Ethiopia-roots decocted, 150-Ethiopia-roots and leaves, 190-India,

Sida indica   **Tr** 445-Thailand-carminative, 452-Bangladesh,

GI tract, Gastric disorders   No peer review

{GI tract is stomach to anus. Mouth and throat are in different sections}

Sida acuta

Tr 52-India-leaf juice, 88-India, 101-Nicaragua, 101-India-leaf juice, 107-India-leaf juice, 168-India-leaf juice-vomiting and gastric disorders, 361-seeds-Digestive System Disorders, 377-Ayurveda-stomach ache, 526-Phillipines-Decoction or infusion-indigestion, 609-India, 646-Nigeria-leaves and stem,

Sida cordifolia   **Tr** 29-Ayurveda-indigestion,

Sida rhombifolia

Tr 126-Colombia-gastritis, 150-Ethiopia-root-stomach disorders-stomach pain, 150-Ethiopia-roots and leaves-gastritis-enteritis, 568-Nigeria-stomach cramps, 524-Phillipines-pulped leaves-applied externally-stomach ache, 524-Phillipines-leaves and juice-taken by mouth-for stomach cramps.

Sida indica   **Tr** 443-Ayurveda,

GI tract, Hemorrhoids   No peer review
{GI tract is stomach to anus. Mouth and throat are in different sections}

Sida acuta

Tr 3-India-decoction of leaves and roots, 201-leaf-review from Ghana, 220-SriLanka, 238-Sri Lanka-roots and leaves, 270-India-leav/root tea as emollient, 361-Indo-China and Philippines-leaves and roots-hemorrhoids, 362-review-Indo-China and Philippines-leaf/root-decoction, 526-Phillipines-Decoction of roots and leaves,

Sida cordifolia   **Tr** 664-Ayurveda-bark-piles, 664-Ayurveda-leaves-cooked and eaten-bleeding piles,

Sida rhombifolia

Tr 47-India-roots and stems-piles, 51-India-roots and stems, 150-Ethiopia-piles-roots and leaves, 292-India-piles, 437-Ayurveda-leaves-cooked and eaten-bleeding piles, 437-Ayurveda-roots-piles, 522-Ayurveda-roots and leaves-piles, 522-Ayurveda-dried leaf and root-hot aqueous extract, burning sensation of the body, 545- Bangladesh-leaves and roots-piles,

Sida cordata

Tr 293-India-flower and ripe fruits-relieves burning sensation, 437-Ayurveda-leaves- cooked and eaten-bleeding piles, 437-Ayurveda-roots-piles, 496-Pakistan-Siddha and Ayurveda-seeds, 497-India-whole plant- The root paste along with cow s butter is applied locally to cure piles, 520-India-burning sensations-(had no specific ref to hemorrhoids but here is where burning occurs), 522-India-burning sensations-(had no specific ref to hemorrhoids but here is where burning occurs),

Sida indica

Tr 377-Ayurveda, 437-Ayurveda-leaves cooked and eaten-bleeding piles, 437-Ayurveda-roots-piles, 443- Ayurveda, 448- Ayurveda, 451-Thailand-leaf extract, 452-Bangladesh, 454-seeds-India, 454-India-leaf, 674-Siddha, 678-Ayurveda-seeds or whole plant?-piles, 684-Ayurveda-hemorrhoids, 708-Ayurveda-seed or fruit-in treatment of piles, 710-Ayurveda-leaves-bleeding piles, 711-Ayurveda, 711-India-seed-as a laxative, 711-India-leaf?, 711- India-seed-a laxative for those having hemorrhoids, 712-India-leaves/fruit and/or seed, 735-Ayurveda-review-seeds-piles, 737-India-leaves-cooked and eaten for bleeding piles--seeds-infusion in water,

Sida rhomboidea
Tr 288-Ayurveda-piles, 320-Ayurveda, 520-India-piles-and burning sensation,

GI tract, Stomachic
No peer review

{GI tract is stomach to anus. Mouth and throat are in different sections} Promotes appetite or assists digestion [1]

Sida acuta

Tr 3-India-root, 21-Ayurveda-root, 52-India-whole plant-hot water extract, 88-India, 107-India, 217-Ayurveda, 270-India-roots-in chronic bowel complaints, 358-roots, 361-Indo-China and Philippines-roots, 362-Phillipines-roots, 460-India, 526-Phillipines-roots, 644-Ayurveda-root,

Sida cordifolia
Tr 88-Ayurveda-root bark-stomachic, 118-Ayurveda-roots-stomachic, 312-USA-Ayurveda-root bark.

Sida rhombifolia

Tr 136-India- root and leaves, 150-Ethiopia-root-digestion problem, 524-Phillipines-roots-decoction-internally, as a stomachic, 545-Bangladesh, 561-Ayurveda-roots-fresh juice, 595- India-leaves-powder (external use)-appetizer,

Sida cordata
Tr 496-Pakistan-Siddha and Ayurveda-roots-stomachic,

Sida veronicaefolia
Tr 561-Ayurveda-roots-fresh juice-stomachic,

GI tract, Stomach, Ulcer

{GI tract is stomach to anus. Mouth and throat are in different sections} A number of drugs including proton pump inhibitors, prostaglandins analogs, histamine receptor antagonists and cytoprotective agents are available for the treatment of peptic ulcer. But most of these drugs produce several adverse reactions including toxicities and even may alter biochemical mechanisms of the body upon chronic usage. [4]   Hence, herbal medicines are generally used in such cases when drugs are to be used for chronic periods. Several natural drugs have been reported to possess anti-ulcerogenic activity by virtue of their predominant effect on mucosal defensive factors. Pretreatment of methanol extract of S. indica leaves showed significant ($P<0.05$) decrease in the gastric volume, total acidity and free acidity. [443]   Pylorus ligation induced ulcers are due to auto digestion of the gastric mucosa and breakdown of the gastric mucosal barrier. These factors are associated with the development of upper gastrointestinal damage.... The antiulcer property of S. indica in pylorus ligation model is evident from its significant reduction in free acidity, total acidity, number of ulcers and ulcer index. S. indica treated animals significantly inhibited the formation of ulcers in the pylorus ligated rats and also decreased both the concentration and increased the pH, it is suggested that S. indica can suppress gastric damage induced by aggressive factors. [445]

Sida acuta

84-mice-whole plant-crude extract- a marked protection against acetylsalicylic acid-induced gastric mucosal ulceration in rats ($p< 0.001$)-showed a reduction in gastric volume, free acidity, and ulcer index (53.69%)-markedly decreased the incidence of ulcers-not reduced the total acidity nor significant change in pH-protection index (24.4%), **109**-rats-leaves-ethanolic extract- significant antiulcer activity by reducing the ulcer index in the above model-200mg/kg equivalent to Famotidine 20mg/kg-the results obtained were found to be significant at ($p<0.001$),   **174**-rats-whole plant-ethanol extract-300 mg/kg wt-aspirin and pylorous ligation induced gastric ulcer-markedly decreased the incidence of ulcers-reduced ulcer index 53.69%-significant reduction in ulcer lesion,

Tr   3-India-whole plant or fresh juice of roots,   6-Ayurveda,   7-Central America,   84-Nigeria,   93-Italy/Burkina Faso-leaves,   101-Nigeria,   101-Nicaragua,the decoction of the entire plant is taken orally,   107-Nicaragua, 109-Siddah-leaves-smeared with gingelly oil and applied to suppurate ulcers, 168-Nicaragua-decoction of the entire plant taken orally,   174-rats-whole plant-ethanol extract-300 mg/kg wt,   217-Ayurveda,   219-Nigeria-leaf usually used,   220-Nicaragua/Guatemala,   220-India,   220-Nigeria, 221-India,   223-India,   264-Nigeria,   271-Nicaragua-decoction of the entire plant,   273-Nigeria, 361-review-leaves, 362- mucilaginous leaves and bitter roots-decoction, infusion or pressed juice-ulcers,   485-Nigeria-survey, 523-India-leaves,   526-Poultices made from boiled leaves are applied to ulcers,   561-Ayurveda-fresh juice of root,   588-Nigeria-decoction of whole plant,   596-Nigeria-leaf/root,   646-Nigeria-leaves and stem,   653-Ayurveda,

Sida cordifolia

34-rats-aerial parts-methanolic extract-500 mg/kg bw-significant anti-ulcerogenic effect,   **70**-rats-methanolic extract of aerial parts comparable to reference drugs,   **167**-rats–leaves-ethanolic extract-200mg/kg wt-showed a considerable degree of antiulcer activity in comparison to positive controlled treated group-Famotidine (20mg/kg)-significant to (p<0.001),   **285**-rats-root-methanol extract-600 mg/kg bw-exhibited no ulcerogenicity indicating its safety on the gastrointestinal tract-equivalent to that of indomethacin, **285**-rats-root/aerial parts-ethyl acetate extract-600 mg/kg bw- exhibited no ulcerogenicity indicating its safety on the gastrointestinal tract,

Tr   70-India,   93-Italy/Burkina Faso-leaves,   167-India-leaves-smeared with gingelly oil and applied to suppurate ulcers,   362-review,   437-Ayurveda-leaves,   561-Ayurveda-roots-fresh juice,

Sida rhombifolia

Tr   47-Camaroon and Madagascar,   51-India-poulticing ulcers,   358-DR Congo,   358-Africa-leaves or leaf sap,   362-review,   437-Ayurveda-leaves, 543-Ayurveda,   561-Ayurveda-fresh juice of root,   568-Nigeria-review,

Sida indica

443-rats-leaves-ether/95% methanol extract-500 mg/kg bw-56-75% ulcer inhibition-showed significant (P<0.05) decrease in number of ulcers and ulcer score index in pylorus ligation and ethanol induced ulceration models-evident from its significant reduction in gastric volume, free acidity, total acidity, number of ulcers and ulcer index-the methanol extract possesses significant antiulcer properties in a dose dependent manner,   **445**–leaves-rats-ether/95%methanol extract-500 mg/kg bw-56-75% ulcer inhibition-possesses significant antiulcer properties in a dose dependent manner, **712**- India-leaves,

Tr   238-Sri Lanka-leaf,   362-review,   437-Ayurveda-leaves or flowers, 443-Ayurveda-The present investigation...justify the traditional claims endowed upon this herbal drug as a rasayana,   444-Ayurveda,   451-Thailand-The juice from its leaves has been used to formulate into an ointment for quick ulcer healing,   674- Siddha,   678-Ayurveda-leaves, 684-Ayurveda-leaf juice-quick ulcer healing,   708-Ayurveda-leaves-internally for treatment of ulcer,   711-India-leaf?,   735-Ayurveda-review-leaves,   737-India-leaves-flowers-eaten raw.

Other Sidas

Tr   358-Sida linfolia-Nigeria-stem and root paste,   561-S. veronicaefolia-Ayurveda-fresh juice of root,   561-Sida spinosa-Ayurveda-fresh juice of root,   437-Ayurveda-Sida cordata-India-leaves,   527-Sida retusa-Leaves used for dressing ulcers,

GI tract, Tenesmus   No peer review

{GI tract in this book is stomach to anus. Mouth and throat are a different section.}   Continual or recurrent inclination to evacuate the bowels, caused by disorder of the rectum or other illness.

Sida cordifolia
Tr 88-Ayurveda-juice of plants with water, 88-Ayurveda-seeds, 312-USA-Ayurveda-seeds, 167-Ayurveda-seeds,

Dandruff No peer review

The cause is unclear but believed to involve a number of genetic and environmental factors... It is not due to poor hygiene. The underlying mechanism involves the over growth of skin cells. Diagnosis is based on symptoms. There is no known cure. Dandruff affects about half of adults [1]

Sida acuta
Tr 107-India-leaf juice poultice, 145-leaves-India- Paste of leaves is mixed with coconut oil and applied on head regularly for killing dandruffs, 214-India, 220-India-paste of leaves is mixed with coconut oil, 225-Nicaragua-leaf juice, 270-India-paste of leaves is mixed with coconut oil, 523-India-leaves-paste mixed with coconut oil-applied regularly,

Sida rhombifolia
Tr 524-Phillipines-plant parts-with coconut oil-applied externally for scurf (dandruff)

Hair loss No peer review

Sida cordifolia
Tr 120-Colombia-used for treating hair loss,

Sida rhombifolia
Tr 362-review, 522-Mexico-flower, fruit and leaf-infusion-externally-hair loss, 522-Peru-leaf-alopecia,

Strengthening Hair No peer review

Sida acuta
Tr 145-Paste of leaves is mixed with coconut oil and applied on head regularly for killing dandruffs and also for strengthening hair, 220-India-paste of leaves is mixed with coconut oil and applied on head regularly for strengthening hair, 270-India-paste of leaves is mixed with coconut oil and applied on head regularly, 523-India-leaves-paste mixed with coconut oil-applied regularly strengthens hair,

Head, Headache No peer review

Sida acuta
Tr 3-India-leaves and roots paste applied to forehead, 5-Togo, 6-Ayurveda-headache and migraine, 7-Central America, 52-India-whole plant-hot water extract, 82-India, 85-India- Chellipale community of Tamil Nadu use it for headache, 93-Italy/Burkina Faso-leaves, 107-

India, 174-India, 186-India, 220-Nicaragua/Guatemala, 220-Togo, 221-India-leaf, 223-India-migraine, 264-Nigeria, 362-Sida spp.-review, 428-India, 508-India-leaf paste, 571-India, 646-Nigeria, 653-Ayurveda-also migraine,

Sida cordifolia Tr 32-Ayurveda, 161-Ayurveda, 362-review.

Sida cordata Tr 496-Sida cordata-Pakistan-Siddha and Ayurveda-roots, 549-Ayurveda,

Sida indica Tr 238-Sri Lanka-leaf, 362-Sida spp.-review, 444-Ayurveda- headache,

Heart, Arrhythmia   Irregular heart beat

Sida acuta

732-berberine-dogs and cats-antagonizes arrhythmias-beneficial effect of berberine on ischemia-induced arrhythmias- Frequency and complexity of ventricular premature beats were decreased and the left ventricular ejection fraction were increased by berberine at a daily oral dose of 1.2 g for 2 weeks-these changes have been correlated with plasma concentrations of berberine, **739**-berberine-review-anti-arrhythmia,

Heart, Bradycardia   slow heart action

Sida acuta

160-rats-vasicine produces hypotension and bradycardia, which appears to be due to a direct and indirect stimulation of cardiac muscarinic receptors, and by a decrease of the total peripheral resistances- In isolated rat mesenteric artery rings, vasicine (0.03, 0.1, 0.3, 1, 3, 10, 30, 100 and 300 µg/mL, cumulatively) induced concentration-dependent relaxation of phenylephrine-induced tone (IC50= 3.8±0.9 µg/mL; n = 6)

Sida cordifolia

40-rats-hydroalcoholic extract-produce hypotension and bradycardia, **156**-rats-leaves-95% ethanolic extract-results demonstrate that TAF (total alkaloid fraction) induces hypotension and bradycardia- our results demonstrate that the TAF of S. cordifolia induces hypotension and bradycardia, **160**-rats/invitro-a complex extraction of vasicine, an alkaloid isolated from the leaves of Sida cordifolia L-intense bradycardia, **311**-invitro+rats-leaves-95% EtOH/chloroform extract-vasicine as active agent-Vasicine induced intense bradycardia, **533**-review-all parts?-any extract?-can increase heart rate, **534**-invivo-roots-acqueous extract- Present preliminary studies confirm better cardiotonic activity of Sida cordifolia Linn than digoxin. A significant increase in height of force of contraction (positive ionotropic effect) and decrease in heart rate (negative chronotropic effect) was observed.

Tr 88-Ayurveda-juice of plants with water- cardio tonic in asthma, 161-Ayurveda-may decrease both blood pressure and heart rate, 534-India-cardiotonic activity, 562-Ayurveda-seeds-cardiac stimulant,

Sida rhombifolia

160-vasicine produces hypotension and bradycardia, which appears to be due to a direct and indirect stimulation of cardiac muscarinic receptors, and by a decrease of the total peripheral resistances.

Heart, Blood pressure depressant

(Sida acuta) The vasodilatory or hyptotensive effect of berberine can be attributed to multiple cellular mechanisms. **[732]**

Sida acuta

16-mice-anti-hyptotension, **160**-vasicine produces hypotension and bradycardia, which appears to be due to a direct and indirect stimulation of cardiac muscarinic receptors, and by a decrease of the total peripheral resistances, **315**-invitro-vasicine-a moderate degree of hyptotensive activity, **732**-berberine-invitro-vasodilatory and hyptotensive,

Tr 16-Nigeria-anti-hyptotensive, 107-India-roots, 118-Ayurveda-tones the blood pressure, 161-Ayurveda, 217-Ayurveda-lowers, 220-SriLanka, 609-India-cardiac problems,

Sida cordifolia

40-rats-hydroalcoholic extract-produce hypotension and bradycardia, **156**-rats-leaves-95% ethanolic extract-results demonstrate that TAF (total alkaloid fraction) induces hypotension and bradycardia- our results demonstrate that the TAF of S. cordifolia induces hypotension and bradycardia, **160**-rats/invitro-a complex extraction of vasicine, an alkaloid isolated from the leaves of Sida cordifolia L, **311**-invitro+rats-leaves-95% EtOH/chloroform extract-vasicine as active agent-Vasicine induced marked hypotension, **315**-invitro-vasicine-a moderate degree of hyptotensive activity,

Tr 118-Ayurveda, 158-India-hypotensive, 161-Ayurveda-may decrease both blood pressure and heart rate, 312-USA-elevates blood pressure, 358-DR Congo-whole plant?-extract-ethanolic extract-decrease of blood pressure in cats and dogs, 362-increasese blood pressure, 533-blood pressure increase-review, 664-Ayurveda-whole plant?-extract-tones the blood pressure.

Sida rhombifolia

160-vasicine produces hypotension and bradycardia, which appears to be due to a direct and indirect stimulation of cardiac muscarinic receptors, and by a decrease of the total peripheral resistances, **315**-invitro-vasicine-a moderate degree of hyptotensive activity, **522**-review-hypotensive, **622**-hypotensive-review-The pharmacological activities reported include hypotensive activity,

Tr 437-Ayurveda-roots-heart problems, 522-Ayurveda-dried leaf and root-hot aqueous extract-heart disease, 524-Phillipines, 609-India-cardiac problems, 622-India, 634-Sri Lanka-upper root-hypotension,

Sida spinosa   **Tr** 217-Ayurveda,

Cryptolepine   (S. acuta, cordifolia, rhombifolia, spinosa, and ?)
389-rats-antihyptotensive-antagonist of noradrenalin on the rat isolated vas deferens. It is of about the same potency as phentolamine (pA2 of phentolamine = 7.5 ± 0.40, pA2 of cryptolepine = 6.6 ± 0.35). We here report a potentiatory effect of small doses of cryptolepine (3.0 × 10-7-10-6M) on the effect of noradrenalin, an effect which has not been obtained with phentolamine, and methoxamine - induced contractions of the vas deferens.,

Heart, Cardioprotective

Encompasses several regimens that have shown to preserve function and viability of cardiac muscle cell tissue subjected to ischemic insult or reoxygenation. [1]   Recent research has shown that medicinal plants with antioxidant properties are also able to impart cardioprotection. **[288]**

Sida acuta   **Tr** 609-India-cardiovascular and cardioprotective,

Sida cordifolia

159-rats-leaves-petroleum ether extract(60 °C)>methanol extract-chronic administration in high dose up to 500 mg/kg has definite cardioprotective potential-is a powerful agent for combating elevated levels of lipids during CHD and other cardiac manifestation, **534**-invivo-roots-acqueous extract-frog heart-Present preliminary studies confirm better cardiotonic activity of Sida cordifolia Linn than digoxin. A significant increase in height of force of contraction (positive ionotropic effect) and decrease in heart rate (negative chronotropic effect) was observed.

Tr 88-Ayurveda-juice of plants with water-cardio tonic, 118-Ayurveda-improves cardiac irregularity, 159-Ayurveda- used as home remedy as cardioprotective agent without any scientific background, 161-Ayurveda-cardio tonic, 217-Ayurveda-cardiac tonic -improves cardiac irregularity, 534-India- cardiotonic activity, 562-Ayurveda-seeds-cardiac stimulant, 534-invivo-roots-acqueous extract- Present preliminary studies confirm better cardiotonic activity of Sida cordifolia Linn than digoxin. A significant increase in height of force of contraction (positive ionotropic effect) and decrease in heart rate (negative chronotropic effect) was observed-cardio tonic, 664-Ayurveda-whole plant?-extract-improves cardiac irregularity,

Sida rhombifolia

536-rats-whole plant?-ethanol extract- causes myocardial adaptation by augmenting endogenous antioxidants and protects rat hearts from decline in cardiac function and oxidative stress associated with isoproterenol (ISP) induced myocardial injury,

Sida rhomboidea

155-rats-whole plant-extract-cardioprotective effect against isoproterenol induced myocardial necrosis-IP (85 mg/kg, s.c.) induced myocardial necrosis in rats, **288**-rats--leaves-ethanol extract-400 mg/kg-pretreatment prevented isoproterenol induced myocardial necrosis via multiple mech-anisms-It can be concluded that SR pretreatment provides cardioprotection against IP induced MN

Sida indica   Tr   449-Ayurveda-stronger heart tonic,

Heart, myocardial infraction

Myocardial infarction (MI) and the resultant complication in cardiac function represent the leading cause of morbidity and mortality in developed countries. The use of complementary and alternative medicines is burgeoning globally for MI, especially in developed countries including US. Attempts are being made globally to get scientific evidences for these traditionally reported herbal drugs. [163]   A potent antioxidant and free radical scavenger-pre-treatment improves cardiac antioxidant status in IP induced Myocardial infarction by effective scavenging of free radicals generated during oxidation of catecholamines thus collectively contributing to its overall antioxidant and anti ischemic activity. [288]

Sida cordifolia

33-rats-leaves-hydroalcoholic extract-100 and 500 mg/kg- both doses significantly increased endogenous antioxidants in heart tissue homogenate. Moreover, biochemical findings were supported by histopathological observations-The aim of the present study was to evaluate the antioxidant and biochemical profile of hydroalcoholic extract of Sida cordifolia L. (HESC) leaves against myocardial infarction (MI) in rats... The result confirm, at least in part, for the use of Sida cordifolia in folk medicine to treat MI,

Tr   33-India-a widely allocated herb by folk tribes of Gujarat state of India for the treatment of coronary manifestations- The result confirm, at least in part, for the use of Sida cordifolia in folk medicine to treat MI,

Sida rhombifolia

536-rats-whole plant?-ethanol extract-100& 200 mg/kg/p.o-causes myocardial adaptation by augmenting endogenous antioxidants and protects rat hearts from decline in cardiac function and oxidative stress associated with ISP induced myocardial injury,

212

Sida rhomboidea

155-rats-leaves-ethanol extract-pre-treatment with SR extract (400 mg/kg per day, p.o.) for 30 consecutive days-this study is the first scientific report on cardioprotective effect of Sida rhomboidea against isoproterenol induced myocardial necrosis in rats,

Tr   288-India-This study validates traditional use of SR extract for treating heart ailments thus confirming its folklore claim,

Heart disease

Sida acuta   **Tr**   107-India-roots,   220-SriLanka,   609-India-cardiac problems,

Sida cordifolia

Tr   33-India- treatment of coronary manifestations,   71-Ayurveda-root, 118-Ayurveda-Oil preparation-Gritha cures Heart diseases,   148-India-aerial parts,   158-India,   163-India- widely allocated herb by folk tribes of Gujarat state of India for the treatment of coronary manifestations,   173-India-root- cardiac diseases,   217-Ayurveda,   548-India,   437-Ayurveda-roots-heart problems,   609-India-cardiac problems,

Sida rhombifolia

Tr   47-India-roots and stems-heart disease,   51-India-roots and stems-heart disease,   217-Ayurveda-children,   437-Ayurveda-roots-heart problems,   522-Ayurveda-dried leaf and root-hot aqueous extract-heart disease,   524-Phillipines,   609-India-cardiac problems.

Sida rhomboidea

288-rats-leaves-ethanol extract-This study validates traditional use of SR extract for treating heart ailments thus confirming its folklore claim.

Tr   288-Ayurveda-heart disease,   320-Ayurveda,   520-India-heart diseases,

Sida cordata   **Tr**   437-Ayurveda-roots-heart problems,

Sida indica

Tr   437-Ayurveda-root-heart problems,   609-India-cardiac problems, 710- China-root-pulmonary sedative,   711-Chinese-bark and root-pulmonary sedative,

HIV/AIDS   **Tr   no reported use**

Sida cordifolia   **68**-invitro-HIV-unprecedented NES non-antagonistic inhibitor for nuclear export of Rev, {2010 study, no follow up found}

Insect, Anti-sida

All Sidas

362-review- A common insect found on Sida is whitefly (Bemisia tabaci), which transmits a range of viruses, including Sida golden mosaic virus, cassava mosaic virus, okra leaf curl, tobacco leaf curl and tomato yellow leaf curl. Sida acuta is a host for Aphis gossypii, which transmits cotton leaf roll disease. Mycoplasm-type organisms cause yellow symptoms on Sida cordifolia and Sida rhombifolia in Burkina Faso. Sida cordifolia is a common host for several nematodes, including Meloidogyne incognita,

Sida acuta

283-field study-aerial parts-Calligrapha pantherina-A reduction in grazing pressure by the beetle can then allow a rapid return to high weed densities. By 1999 however the sida densities had been reduced by between 84% and 99% of the original densities and introduced pastures and native herbs and grasses dominated the sites,   423-field study-aerial parts- Most of the 20 insect species on S. acuta and the 23 on S. cordifolia were rarely or only occasionally encountered and tended to be native or naturalized, polyphagous, ectophagous chewing or sucking species. S. cordifolia was more fully exploited by insects than S. acuta,

Sida cordifolia

423-field study-aerial parts- Most of the 20 insect species on S. acuta and the 23 on S. cordifolia were rarely or only occasionally encountered and tended to be native or naturalized, polyphagous, ectophagous chewing or sucking species. S. cordifolia was more fully exploited by insects than S. acuta

Insects, Beneficial

The bees use these plants as principal pollen source while wasps and butterflies use them as nectar source. The Sida species with their luxuriant growth play a key role in maintaining the populations of bees and butterflies by providing them both with pollen and nectar. [654]

All Sidas

487-field observation-aerial parts-several types use the Sida family as hosts, S rhombifolia in particular with Pyrgus oileus,   635-invivo-bee plant-apifauna,   654-field observation-aerial parts-With these characteristics, the Sida species attract bees, wasps and butterflies to their flowers as soon as they are open in the morning and the foragers collect the forage with great ease for a brief period due to closure of the petals by noon. The bees use these plants as principal pollen source while wasps and butterflies use them as nectar source during which they contact the anthers and stigmas and pollinate the flowers-S. acuta, S. cordata and S. cordifolia are simultaneously pollen and nectar sources for honey bees... The Sida species with their luxuriant growth

214

play a key role in maintaining the populations of bees and butterflies by providing them both with pollen and nectar.

Sida acuta

635-field study-Brazil-bee plant, **654**- field study/invitro-Honey bees collect Sida pollen voraciously and deposit it in their hives. Ceratina bees, small carpenter bees, also gather pollen for use in brood development.... DeGroot (1953) reported that honey bees require ten essential amino acids, six out of which are present in the pollen of these plants, plus some non-essential amino acids... The pollen grains are sources of six (of the ten needed) essential amino acids, and eight non-essential amino acids... The bees use these plants as principal pollen source while wasps and butterflies use them as nectar source. The Sida species with their luxuriant growth play a key role in maintaining the populations of bees and butterflies by providing them both with pollen and nectar, **658**-invivo-The Simpson diversity index values for both woody and herbaceous plant species are indications of high diversity of forage species for honeybees...Sida acuta ranks high among all bee plants in Nigeria...utilized very frequently (by bees), **660**-invivo-bees-Floral Sucrose Content.-Volume/mm 17.7 (range 3.2-36)--% Mass sucrose concentration=11.7 (range 10.2-33.8), **692**-field study-aerial parts-bee plant-apifauna, **693**-field study-aerial parts-both nectariferous and polleniferous for bees in Nigeria, **697**-field study-India, West Bengal-butterfly nectar and host- Lemon Pansy, Grey Pansy, Lime Blue, Common Pierrot, Indian Skipper,

Sida cordifolia

654- field study/invitro-Honey bees collect Sida pollen voraciously and deposit it in their hives. Ceratina bees, small carpenter bees, also gather pollen for use in brood development.... DeGroot (1953) reported that honey bees require ten essential amino acids, six out of which are present in the pollen of these plants, plus some non-essential amino acids... The pollen grains are sources of six [of the ten needed] essential amino acids, and eight non-essential amino acids... The bees use these plants as principal pollen source while wasps and butterflies use them as nectar source. The Sida species with their luxuriant growth play a key role in maintaining the populations of bees and butterflies by providing them both with pollen and nectar,

Sida rhombifolia

487-field observation-aerial parts-butterflies and moths-several types use the Sida family as hosts, S rhombifolia in particular with Pyrgus oileus, **635**-field study-Brazil-bee plant, **697**-field study-India, West Bengal-butterfly nectar and host- Lemon Pansy, Grey Pansy, Lime Blue, Common Pierrot, Indian Skipper,

Sida cordata

654- field study/invitro-Honey bees collect Sida pollen voraciously and deposit it in their hives. Ceratina bees, small carpenter bees, also gather pollen for use in brood development.... DeGroot (1953) reported that honey

215

bees require ten essential amino acids... The pollen grains are sources of six [of the ten needed] essential amino acids, and eight non-essential amino acids... The bees use these plants as principal pollen source while wasps and butterflies use them as nectar source. The Sida species with their luxuriant growth play a key role in maintaining the populations of bees and butterflies by providing them both with pollen and nectar,

Sida spinosa

692-field study-aerial parts- The flowers attract various bees, including bumblebees, little carpenter bees, and Halictid bees, as well as small to medium-sized butterflies and skippers. Charles Robertson observed the following Lepidopteran species on the flowers of Prickly Sida: Colias philodice (Clouded Sulfur), Eurema lisa (Little Yellow), Pieris rapae (Cabbage White), Pontia protodice (Checkered White), and Pyrgus communis (Common Checkered Skipper). The foliage is not known to be toxic and it may be eaten occasionally by mammalian herbivores.

Insects, Healing from   No peer review

Sida acuta   Tr   88-Ayurveda-scorpion bites,   220-BurkinaFaso-insect bites,

Sida rhombifolia

Tr   150-Ethiopia-flowers-stings and bites of scorpion, snake and wasp, 192-BurkinaFaso-insecticide,   278-Ethiopia-used for treating stings and bites of scorpion, snake and wasp (its flowers),   361-Philippines and Indonesia-flowers-applied to wasp stings,   362-review-Philippines and Indonesia-flowers-wasp stings,   524-Phillipines-flowers-wasp stings, 524-Phillipines-fresh leaves-emollient-scorpion stings,   545- Bangladesh-stems-mucilage for scorpion stings.

Other Sida   Tr   527-Sida retusa-Poultice of leaves used for insect bites,   595-Sida spinosa-root-India-scorpion bite,

Insects, Pest Control

The protection of stored grains from insect damage is currently dependent on synthetic pesticides. The repeated use of synthetic insecticides for insect pests and vectors control has disrupted natural biological control systems. It has also resulted in the development of resistance, undesirable effects on nontarget organisms and fostered environmental and human health concern, which initiated a search for alternative control measures... Plants are considered as rich sources of bioactive chemicals and they may be an alternative source of insect control agents... Pest control strategies, especially those that are effective, cheap and environmentally non-hazardous are needed. Hence, crude plant extracts have played an important role in this aspect. **[98]**

Most Sidas

422-invitro and invivo-leaf- ether and ethyl alcohol extracts- exhibited strong feeding deterrence and toxicity against the larvae of Earias vittella.

Sida acuta

Deterrent/Insecticidal   **265**-leaf-80% ethanol extract- Acanthscelides obtectus (bean weevil)-4% solution-1.5 hours-mortality 48%+--this study suggested that S. acuta possesses insecticidal properties and can be used to control variety of insect pests and vectors-the bioassay has indicated that the toxic effect of the extracts was proportional to the concentration and higher concentration has stronger effect. The observed overall mean mortality also increased with increase in time intervals after treatment,   **422**-invivo-leaf-solvent ether and ethyl alcohol-extracts exhibited strong feeding deterrence and toxicity against the larva,   **463**-leaf and root-methanol extract-this integrated application could be useful as alternative synthetic insecticides,- Phytochemical screening revealed the presence of some vital insecticidal and antiplasmodial constituents such as terpenoids, flavonoids and alkaloids,

Tr   265-possesses insecticidal properties and can be used to control variety of insect pests and vectors-bean weevil,

Larvicidal   **354**-invivo-leaf-?extract-synthesized silver nanoparticles-larvicidal-the use of S. acuta synthesized silver nanoparticles can be a rapid, environmentally safer biopesticide which can form a novel approach to develop effective biocides for controlling the target vector mosquitoes. This is the first report on the mosquito larvicidal activity of the plant aqueous extract and synthesized nanoparticles,   **362**-review-leaf-? extract-exhibits strong feeding deterrence and toxicity against the larvae of the insect pest Earias vittella-a serious pest of cotton and okra among other commercial crops, **463**-leaf and root-methanol extract-showed significant antiplasmodial activity-showed markedly significant antimalarial activity and antivectorial activity effects even at low concentrations-Phytochemical screening revealed the presence of some vital insecticidal and antiplasmodial constituents such as terpenoids, flavonoids and alkaloids,   **516**-Finland-invivo-leaf-Eleven indigenous Ghanaian plant species were tested for their toxicity to 3 storage pest species compared to Neem-least effective was S. acuta,

Tr   362-Phillipines-roots- expelling intestinal worms,   422-India-invitro and invivo-leaf- ether and ethyl alcohol extracts- exhibited strong feeding deterrence and toxicity against the larvae of Earias vittella,

Sida rhombifolia

51-invitro-fruit-Petroleum ether (C2H5-O- C2H5), chloroform (CHCl3) and methanol (CH3OH) fruit extracts-possesses insecticidal properties,   **545**-Culex quinquefasciatus mosquito-stem-isolated pure compound phenyl ethyl β-D glucopyranoside from the stem-larvicidal.

Tr   192-BurkinaFaso-insecticide,

Sida indica

441-invitro- Anopheles stephensi Liston- crude hexane, ethyl acetate, petroleum ether, acetone and methanol extracts- All extracts showed moderate larvicidal effects; however, the highest larval mortality was found in petroleum ether extract,

Sida corymbosa   Tr   568-kills flies-Nigeria,

Insects, Food and Sustenance for

However, in all three Sida species (Sida acuta, S. cordata and S. cordifolia), the flowers without perceptible smell are yellow, shed pollen during the forenoon period, provide landing platform and offer traces of nectar that is covered by thin hairs at the base of sepals. With these characteristics, the Sida species attract bees, wasps and butterflies to their flowers as soon as they are open in the morning and the foragers collect the forage with great ease for a brief period due to closure of the petals by noon. The bees use these plants as principal pollen source while wasps and butterflies use them as nectar source during which they contact the anthers and stigmas and pollinate the flowers. Since nectar is produced in traces at flower and even plant level, these insects in a quest for nectar move quickly from flower to flower within and between populations and in effect, promote crosspollination... Nevertheless, Sida species with their huge population size and profuse flowering during the wet season are potential pollen and nectar sources for all these honey bees. Honey bees also collect Sida pollen voraciously and deposit it in their hives. Ceratina bees, small carpenter bees, also gather pollen for use in brood development. The pollen contains the same amino acids in all three Sida species. The pollen grains are sources of six essential amino acids: threonine, valine, methionine, iso-leucine, lysine, and phenylalanine, and eight non-essential amino acids: alanine, aspartic acid, cysteine, cysteine, glutamic acid, hydroxyproline, proline, and serine. DeGroot (1953) reported that honey bees require ten essential amino acids, six out of which are present in the pollen of these plants, plus some non-essential amino acids. The pollen also has a small amount of protein content. It is thus nutritionally important. These bees use Sida species as important pollen sources and their pollen collecting activity **[654]**   S. acuta, S. cordata and S. cordifolia are simultaneously pollen and nectar sources for honey bees. **[654]**   Most Sidas-invivo-bee plant **[635]**

Sida acuta

635-invivo-bee plant,   **654**-invivo-simultaneously pollen and nectar sources for honey bees,   **658**-invivo-The Simpson diversity index values for both woody and herbaceous plant species are indications of high diversity of forage species for honeybees...Sida acuta ranks high among all bee plants in Nigeria...utilized very frequently (by bees),   **660**-invivo-bees-Floral Sucrose Content.-Volume/mm 17.7 (range 3.2-36)--% Mass sucrose concentration=11.7 (range 10.2-33.8).   **695**-bee plant-field study-Pollen analysis of 34 samples of honey from three apiaries in the northwest Benin, combined with direct observations around each apiary within 1000 m radius were realized per month. In total 129 species were censised including 109 species inventorized on the field and 73 taxa identified through pollen analysis.

Sida cordifolia

635-invivo-bee plant-apifauna, **654**-invitro-simultaneously pollen and nectar sources for honey bees... The Sida species with their luxuriant growth play a key role in maintaining the populations of bees and butterflies by providing them both with pollen and nectar.

Sida rhombifolia

487-reference-Several types of butterflies use the Sida family as hosts, S rhombifolia in particular with Pyrgus oileus, **635**-invivo-bee plant,

Sida cordata

635-invivo-bee plant-apifauna, **654**-invitro-simultaneously pollen and nectar sources for honey bees... The Sida species with their luxuriant growth play a key role in maintaining the populations of bees and butterflies by providing them both with pollen and nectar.

Sida rhomboidea **635**-invivo-bee plant-apifauna,

Sida spinosa

635-invivo-bee plant, **654**-invitro-simultaneously pollen and nectar sources for honey bees... The Sida species with their luxuriant growth play a key role in maintaining the populations of bees and butterflies by providing them both with pollen and nectar.

Sida hermaphrodita **564**-Hungary-used as a fodder crop, honey crop, ornamental plant, or in public gardens.

Kidney, Nephroprotective

Protective of the kidneys. Produced significant nephroprotective activity in Gentamicin induced nephrotoxicity models. **[139]**

Sida acuta

530-rats-leaf-ethanol extract->100 mg/kg bw- notwithstanding that Sida acuta extract may not impair liver and kidney functions, possible effects on fluid and electrolyte balance should be seriously monitored, **531**-rats-leaf-ethanol extract-200mg/kg bw-could have adverse effects on the kidney electrolytes- sodium, chloride and creatinine showed higher levels that are significant--100 mg/kg bw-creatinine was actually slightly lower than control-any adverse effects on creatine come between 100-200 mg,

Tr 7-Central America, 93-Italy/Burkina Faso-leaves, 137-leaf-Guatemala, 220-Nicaragua/Guatemala, 568-Nigeria-kidney problems, 580-India-whole plant-ethanol extract-kidney diseases, 609-India,

Sida cordifolia

139-rats-leaves-water and ethanol extracts-both the extracts produced significant nephroprotective activity in Gentamicin induced nephrotoxicity models-Gentamicin induced glomerular congestion, blood vessel congestion, and epithelial desquamation, accumulation of inflammatory cells and necrosis of the kidney cells were found to be reduced in the groups receiving extracts of Sida cordifolia, 174-animals-water extract-400 mg/kg wt-antioxidant potentiality that exhibits nephroprotective activity,

Sida rhombifolia Tr   126-Colombia-treatment of kidneys,

Sida rhomboidea

280-rats-leaves-water extract-200 and 400 mg/kg bodyweight (400 best)-Nephrotoxicity was induced in rats with gentamicin (100 mg/kg bw(i.p.) for 8 days), then treated with Sida rhomboidea extract (200 and 400 mg/kg bw (p.o.) for 8 days)- lowered lipid peroxidation levels is attributable to the free radical scavenging ability of Sida rhomboidea that prevents membrane lipid peroxidation.

Sida indica

679-rats-root-ethanolic extract-These findings confirm the nephroprotective effect of Sida indica root in animal model of ARF. The nephroprotection was better with 300 mg/kg of Sida indica root than 150 mg/kg.

Kidney, Stones

(Sida indica) Urolithiasis constitutes as a global health problem with an incidence of up to 5% in the general population, but its prevalence is even greater in specific geographic regions such as 20% in Gulf countries, 15 % in U.S. and Turkey, 11% in India and 4-8% in U.K. The condition is approximately twice as common in males as in females and its incidence increases with age in adults. It is a disorder of the urinary tract in which insoluble mineral and salt concretions develop and aggregate around a nidus of proteinaceous material mainly within the bladder or urethra but it can occur anywhere in the urinary tract...One of the most significant clinical problems of urolithiasis is the high recurrence rate incidence without preventive measures after first stone. After 3 years this is about 40%, by 10 years up to 75% and by 25 years virtually every patient has formed at least one more stone, due to imbalance between promoters and inhibitors in the kidneys [688]

Sida acuta

90-invitro-root- successively extracted with petroleum ether (40°- 60°C), benzene, chloroform, methanol and water-the crystal growth after the addition of the methanolic and aqueous extracts in 20 mg/5 ml and 10 mg/5 ml doses was studied. In both the extracts there were reductions in sizes of calcium oxalate crystal columns and also the size of the individual calcium oxalate crystals when compared to that of the controls.... Aqueous extract showed a marked reduction in the tendency to form crystal aggregates and also resulted in corrosion, crevices in the crystals which could indicate a dissolution effect for drug.   650-rats-aerial parts-acqueous extract-200 mg/kg, 400 mg/kg -prevents kidney stones,

Decreased uric acid   103-rats,100-rats-acetone extract-whole plant-administration. Urea is a production of protein metabolism that is excreted in urine and its retention in the body may indicate renal damage.

Tr   5-Togo,   100-rats-acetone extract-whole plant-decreases uric acid, 220-Togo,   221-India-leaf,

Sida rhombifolia   Tr   127-India-useful in calculus troubles,   545-Bangladesh-stems-calculus problems,

Sida retusa   Tr   435-Ayurveda, 527-used as a diuretic,   529-Ayurveda-used in calculus troubles as a diuretic ,

Sida indica

640-leaves-cold distilled water extract-Percent Inhibition (PI) of CaOx crystals using Dot blot assay technique--20(mg/ml)=13.5%--40(mg/ml) =21.16%—60(mg/ml)=27.16%—80(mg/ml)=34.66%--100(mg/ ml)=42.33%, 688-rats-whole plant?-cold 70% ethanolic extract-ethylene glycol and vitamin D3 induced urolithiasis-notable anti-urolithiasis action -diminution of stone formation.

Liver, Bile disorders

Sida acuta

650-rats-aerial parts-ethanolic extract- Sida acuta produced a dose-dependent increase in urine output, with no effect on sodium excretion,

Tr   3-India-root-urinary problems,   6-Ayurveda-urinary diseases,   90-India?-chronic bowel complaints,   111-India- management of liver disorders, 174-India-urinary disease,   270-India-root-disorders of the bile,   275-Brazil-leaves and stems-100% ethanolic extract-bile disorders,   644-Ayurveda-root- diuretic,

Sida cordifolia

Tr   32-Ayurveda-root infusion,   118-Ayurveda,   167-Ayurveda-root, 358- Central African Republic and Kenya,   362-review-Malaysia-roots-infusion,

Sida rhombifolia   Tr   217-Ayurveda-blockage of the bile ducts-children,

Sida indica   Tr   437-Ayurveda-root- bily blood,   712-Ayurveda-alleviates bilious (excess secretion of bile),

Liver Disorders

No peer review

Conventional or synthetic drugs used in the treatment of liver diseases are sometimes inadequate and can have serious adverse effects. On the other hand, Ayurveda, an indigenous system of medicine in India, has a long tradition of treating liver disorders with plant drugs. [549]

Sida acuta

Tr 6-Ayurveda, 18-India, 63-India, 111-India, 114-Burkina Faso-hepatitis, 217-Ayurveda, 223-Ayurveda, 264-Nigeria, 275-Brazil-leaves and stems-liver disorders, 358-review-leaves-hepatitis (viral), 644-Ayurveda-root, 653-Ayurveda,

Sida rhombifolia
Tr 192-liver diseases-Burkina Faso,

Sida spinosa
Tr 11-Burkina-Faso-hepatitis,

Sida cordata

Tr 405-Ayurveda-whole plant-chronic liver disorders, 494-Pakistan-liver diseases, 497-India- chronic liver disorders, 506-Ayurveda-roots-liver disease, 497-India-whole plant-chronic liver disorders, 498-India,

Sida indica
Tr 444-Ayurveda-Atibala-liver disorders,

Liver, Hepatoprotective

protective of the liver

The liver is an organ of paramount importance, which plays an essential role in the metabolism of foreign compounds entering the body. Human beings are exposed to these compounds through environmental exposure, consumption of contaminated food or during exposure to chemical substances in the occupational environment. In addition, human beings consume a lot of synthetic drugs during diseased conditions which are alien to body organs. All these compounds produce a variety of toxic manifestations. Conventional drugs used in the treatment of liver diseases are often inadequate. Therefore it is necessary to search an alternative drug for the treatment of liver diseases to replace the currently used drugs of doubtful efficacy and safety. [347]

Sida acuta

18-rats-root-methanolic extract- significantly hepatoprotective, 169-rats-ethanolic extract-protects against alcohol-induced oxidative stress in liver, 303-rats-leaf-ethanloic extract-the administration of ethanolic leaf extracts of Sida acuta on the liver showed no structural or functional derangement on it, as it presented a normal cytoarchitecture of the liver, 460-rats-whole plant-70% ethanol extract-400mg/kg bw-in a dose dependent manner-significantly quenched the free radical damage-showed a significant increase in activities of antioxidant enzymes that reduces the oxidative stress induced damage exhibiting a potent antioxidant and anticancer activity.

222

Tr   15?-Ayurveda,   18-Ayurveda,   52-India-whole plant-hot water extract,   76-W Africa,   82-India,   107-India,   203-Burkina-Faso, 580-India-whole plant-ethanol extract,

Sida cordifolia

28-rats?-50 % ethanolic extract-has a potent hepatoprotective action against alcohol-induced toxicity, which was mediated by lowering oxidative stress and by down-regulating the transcription factors,   **37**-rats-leaves-acqueous extract-100mg/kg aqueous solution stimulates 90%+ liver regeneration after 67% partial hepatectomy in rats,   **153**-rats-leaves-100mg/kg-liver regenerating process,   **182**-rats-roots-50% ethanolic extract-alcohol induced liver damage ameliorated by extract,   **135**-rats-whole plant-aqueous extract-significant antihepatotoxic activity-comparable to that of silymarin,   **181**-rats-powdered aerial and root parts>methanolic and aqueous extract-significant hepatoprotective activity,   **182**-rats-ethanolic extract-50 % ethanolic extract-roots-has a potent hepatoprotective action against alcohol-induced toxicity-Fumaric acid isolated from S. cordifolia showed hepatoprotectiveactivity comparable with silymarin,   **218**-review-recently it has been banned due to reported hepatotoxicity (injurious to the liver)-animal experiments however report hepatoprotective effect of Sida cordifolia,   **406**-invitro- methanolic/aqueous/total aqueous extracts- comparable to silymarin,

Tr   15-Ayurveda,   76-W Africa,   118-Ayurveda,   152-India,   158-India,   203-Burkina-Faso,   312-USA-Ayurveda,   664-Ayurveda-whole plant?,

Sida rhombifolia

324-rats-whole plant-acqueous extract-the powdered roots aerial parts and their aqueous extract showed significant hepatoprotective activity. The hepatoprotective activity of the powdered drug and its extract may be due the stimulatory effects on hepatic regeneration or free radical scavenging effects, etc.,   **407**-rats-seed-80% methanol extract-The chemopreventive and hepatoprotective potentials of seed extract are due to free radical scavenging activity and restoration of cellular structural integrity-the results of the present study indicates significant inhibitory effects of seed extract of S. rhombifolia ssp. retusa on the development of preneoplastic foci.

Tr   15-Ayurveda,   88-Ayurveda-root,   197-roots-hepatonic-as part of Ayurveda mixtures-India,   524-Phillipines-roots.

Sida spinosa   **Tr**   11-BurkinaFaso,   15-Ayurveda-hepatoprotective.

Sida cordata

494-rats-methanolic extract-These results revealed the presence of some bioactive compound in the ethyl acetate fraction, confirming the utility of S. cordata against liver diseases in folk medicine,   **549**-rats-leaf-95% ethanol extract-100-400 mg/kg bw-The results of this study strongly indicate the protective effect of SCLE against CCl4 induced acute liver toxicity in rats-significantly (up to $P<0.001$) reduced the lipid peroxidation in the liver tissue and restored activities of defense antioxidant enzymes GSH, SOD and CAT towards normal levels, which was confirmed by the histopathological studies.

Tr   15-Ayurveda,   494-Pakistan,   549-Ayurveda,

Sida indica

440-rats-acqueous extract- exhibited significant hepatoprotective activity by reducing carbon tetrachloride- and paracetamol-induced change in bio-chemical parameters,   **714**-rats-leaves-acqueous extract-showed significant hepatopro-tective activity at 100 and 200 mg/kg dose levels in CCl4-treated rats,   Tr   15-Ayurveda,

Sida retusa

57-rats-root-?extract-only root extract inhibited lipid peroxidation in rat liver,   **75**-invitro-root-only root extract inhibited lipid peroxidation in rat liver,   **197**-rats-roots-aqueous extract-400mg/kg-hepato-protective activity-thioacetamide and allyl alcohol induced hepatic damage,   **464**-mice/rats,invitro- Sida rhombifolia ssp. Retusa-80% methanol extract-We report for the first time that chemopreventive and anti-hepatotoxic potentials of S. rhombifolia ssp. retusa seed extract of is due to free radical scavenging activity and restoration and maintenance of cellular integrity.... Remarkable changes viz; enhanced cell to cell adhesion among adjacent cells, compact junctional complexes, restoration of morphological architecture and intimate cell contacts with well defined cell boundaries resembling to normal hepatocytes were noticed. This suggests that the seed extract helps in repair of cellular damage and prevents the formation of preneoplastic histopathological changes. In conclusion, the chemopreventive and antihepatotoxic effects of seed extract are attributed for its suppression of lipid peroxidation, free radical scavenging activity, ability to induce GST and other phase II enzymes involved in carcinogen detoxification and maintenance of structural integrity of the hepatocyte. Therefore, the present study validates the potential usefulness of seeds as a promising hepatoprotectant,   **542**-rats-roots-acqueous extract-pretreatment with 400-800 mg/kg bw-significantly ameliorated the liver damage in rats exposed to the hepatotoxic compound thioacetamide and allyl alcohol-In another study with allyl alcohol (toxic), indicated that changes in body weight and in necrosis index were restored to normal by treatment with aqueous extract, the results, indicated that physical and biochemical changes along with change in necrosis index were restored to normal by treatment with aqueous extract,   Tr   15-Ayurveda, 131- Ayurveda,

Other Sida

806-S. **veronicaefolia**-invitro-whole plant?-acqueous and ethanolic extracts-both extracts produce significant hepatoprotective effect not only by decreasing serum transaminase (SGPT & SGOT), alkaline phosphate and total bilirubin, but also significantly increased the levels of total protein. The effects of *EESV* and *AESV* were comparable with standard drug silymarin.

Tr   15-Ayurveda-Sida mysorensis,   631-Sida schimperiana-Ethiopia-Root juice is mixed with milk and drunk for 5 days.,

Lungs, Asthma

Asthma is a common long term inflammatory disease of the airways of the lungs. Symptoms include episodes of wheezing, coughing, chest tightness, and shortness of breath... Bronchial asthma is a complex disease with several clinically well-defined pathogenic components, including recurrent reversible airway obstruction, chronic airway inflammation and development of airway hyperresponsiveness. [1] Currently available inhaled bronchodilators and anti-inflammatory drugs are effective in most asthmatics, but this palliative therapy requires long term daily administration and is associated with serious toxicities. As a result, there is high prevalence of usage of alternative and complementary medicines in the treatment of bronchial asthma. Several medicinal plants having spasmolytic or anti-inflammatory activity are being found to be effective in the treatment of bronchial asthma. [706]

Sida acuta

Tr 6-Ayurveda, 7-Central America, 93-Italy/Burkina Faso-leaves, 101-Nicaragua,the decoction of the entire plant is taken orally, 107-Nicaragua, 168-Nicaragua-decoction of the entire plant taken orally, 220-Nicaragua/Guatemala, 221-India-asthmatic bronchitis, 223-India, 270-India-extract, 271-Nicaragua-decoction of the entire plant, 523-India-leaves, 588-Nigeria-decoction of whole plant, 609-India, 619-Malaysia, 653-Ayurveda-asthma,

Sida cordifolia

Tr 40-Brazil, 41-Brazil, 93-Italy/Burkina Faso-leaves, 116-Bangladesh, 118-Ayurveda, 120-Columbia, 125-India, 148-India-aerial parts, 151-Ayurveda, 156-Brasil, 158-India, 160-Brazil, 161-Brazil, 162-Brazil, 182-India, 312-USA-Ayurveda-antiasthmatic-roots/leaves/stems, 312-Brazil, 358- Central African Republic and Kenya-root infusion, 362-review-Malaysia-roots-infusion, 408-India-roots/leaves/stems/seeds, 596-Nigeria-leaf/root/seed, 609-India, 612-Ayurveda-root, x619-Malaysia,

asthmatic bronchitis Tr 28-India, 32-Ayurveda-bronchial asthma, 43-Brazil, 61-Brazil, 32-Ayurveda, 88-Brazil, 118-Ayurveda, 132-Brazil-asthmatic bronchitis, 153-Brasil, 154-Brazil, 161-Ayurveda, 161-Brazil, 182-India, 312-USA-Ayurveda, 312-Brazil,

Sida rhombifolia

Tr 136-India-stem and root, 358-Senegal, the Central African Republic and Madagascar-leaves and roots, 407-Ayurveda, 464-India, 522-review-The pharmacological activities reported include respiratory disorders-antiasthmatic, 524-Phillipines-root-decoction, 609-India, 619-Malaysia,

Sida retusa   **Tr** 49-Ayurveda, 407-Ayurveda,

Sida indica

706-invitro-aerial parts-methanol extract-significant anti-inflammatory activity and mast cell stabilizing suggests the possible mechanism responsible for anti-asthmatic activity of this medicinal plant,

Tr 451-Thailand-leaf extract-asthmatic bronchitis, 735-Ayurveda-review -root infusion-bronchitis,

Sida rhomboidea   **Tr** 609-India

Sida spinosa   **Tr** 217-Ayurveda, 609-India, x619-Malaysia,

Other Sidas   **Tr** 609-Sida cordata, 609-Sida asiatica-India, 609- Sida veronicaefolia-India.

Lungs, Bronchitis   No peer review
Inflammation of bronchi (large and medium-sized airways) in the lungs. [1]

Sida acuta   **Tr** 220-India, 609-India, 221-India-asthmatic bronchitis,

Sida cordifolia   **Tr** 32-Ayurveda-bronchial asthma 61-Brazil, 118-Ayurveda-bronchial asthma, 120-Colombia,-bronchial disorders,

Sida rhombifolia   **Tr** 358-Senegal, the Central African Republic and Madagascar-leaves and roots, 524-Phillipines-root-decoction,

Sida indica

Tr 445-India and China, 451-Thailand, 452-Bangladesh, 454-seeds-India, 708-Ayurveda-root-in chest infection, 710-Ayurveda-seeds-or leaves-decoction, 711-India-leaf extract, 712-India-roots-chest infection-also bronchitis-or leaves, 735-Ayurveda-review-roots-chest infection,

Lungs, Cough and wheezing   No peer review

Sida acuta   **Tr** 6-Ayurveda, 223-India, 264-Nigeria, 361-aerial parts-coughs, 653-Ayurveda-cough,

Sida cordifolia

Tr 27-Burkina Faso-whole plant decoction?, 32-Ayurveda, 117-BurkinaFaso, 118-Ayurveda, 437-Ayurveda-seeds---flowers-as powder in ghee-blood vomiting---roots-powder-cough, 521-Ayurveda-root,

Sida rhombifolia

Tr   47-Camaroon and Madagascar,   437-Ayurveda-seeds,   437-Ayurveda-flowers-as powder in ghee-blood vomiting,   437-Ayurveda-roots-powder-cough,   522-Mozambique-entire plant-hot aqueous extract- for cough when given orally,   522-Nicaragua-leaf-decoction-taken orally

Sida cordata   Tr   437-Ayurveda-seeds--flowers-as powder in ghee-blood vomiting-- roots-powder-cough,

Sida indica

Tr   427-Ayurveda-flowers-powder in ghee-cough,   427-Ayurveda-root powder-cough,   437-Ayurveda-seeds-cough,   445-Thailand-carminative, 448-Ayurveda-cough,   450-India-fruit-coughs,   451-Thailand-seeds, 684-Ayurveda,   708-Ayurveda-fruit-cough treatment,   711-India-seed, 711-India-seed,   712-India-roots-dry cough,   712 India-root/fruit and/or seeds-coughs,   735-Ayurveda-review-root infusion-dry cough,   737-India-flowers-powdered and eaten with ghee-cough.

Other Sidas

Tr   568- Sida ovata Forssk-Nigeria-dry cough,   631-Sida schimperiana-Ethiopia-Fresh leaves are crushed and drunk with honey,

Lungs, Expectorant   No peer review

A medication that helps bring up mucus and other material from the lungs, bronchi, and trachea **[medicinenet.com]**

Sida cordifolia   Tr   437-Ayurveda-seeds,

Sida rhombifolia   Tr   437-Ayurveda-seeds,

Sida cordata   Tr   437-Ayurveda-seeds,

Sida indica   Tr   437-Ayurveda-seeds-expectorant,   678-Ayurveda-seeds,   708-Ayurveda-seed,   712-India-seeds,   735-Ayurveda-review-seeds,

Lungs, Pneumonia   No peer review!

{Pathogens causing pneumonia are in the **Pathogens** section: Klebsiella pneumonia, Streptococcus pneumoniae, and Scpulariopsis candida}

The term pneumonia is sometimes more broadly applied to any condition resulting in inflammation of the lungs... Pneumonia is due to infections caused primarily by bacteria or viruses and less commonly by fungi and parasites. Although there are more than 100 strains of infectious agents identified, only a few are responsible for the majority of the cases... Bacteria are the most common cause of community-acquired pneumonia (CAP), with

Streptococcus pneumoniae isolated in nearly 50% of cases (top four bacteria sources never been tested against any Sida)... In adults, viruses account for approximately a third and in children for about 15% of pneumonia cases. [1]

Sida acuta

Tr 51-India-whole plant?-tuberculosis, 107-Ayurveda-pulmonary tuberculosis, 217-Ayurveda-chest ailments, 220-BurkinaFaso, 361-review-aerial parts- Respiratory System Disorders, 609-India-respiratory problems,

Sida cordifolia

Tr 118-Ayurveda, 161-Brazil, 161-Africa-in many parts of Africa for various ailments, particularly for respiratory problems, 521-Ayurveda-root-bronchospasm (a sudden constriction of the muscles in the walls of the bronchioles. It causes difficulty in breathing which can be very mild to severe.)

Sida rhombifolia

Tr 358-Senegal, the Central African Republic and Madagascar-leaves and roots-respiratory diseases, 464-India-chest ailments, 522-Central Africa-infusion of dried leaf-chest pain, 522-Europe-whole plant?-In Europe, the plant has been regarded as a valuable remedy in pulmonary tuberculosis, 522-Nicargua-leaf-decoction-orally-respiratory disorder, 568-Nigeria-tuberculosis,

Sida retusa
Tr 407-Ayurveda-chest ailments, 684-Ayurveda-lung disease,

Sida indica
Tr 445-India and China, 448-Ayurveda, 708-Ayurveda-root-in chest infection,

Lungs, Tuberculosis (Phthisis)

Tuberculosis has been present in humans since antiquity, at the latest. The earliest unambiguous detection of *M. tuberculosis* involves evidence of the disease in the remains of bison dated to approximately 17,000 years ago. Skeletal remains show prehistoric humans (4000 BC) had TB and researchers have found tubercular decay in the spines of Egyptian mummies dating from 3000–2400 BC... Tuberculosis remains the largest cause of death in the world from a single infectious disease.... Ominously, multidrug-resistant tuberculosis (MDR-TB) strains have emerged in several countries, with case fatalities ranging from 40 to 60% in immunocompetent individuals and >80% in immunocompromised individuals... The anti mycobacterial screening showed that the ethyl acetate extract of *Sida rhombifolia* L. leaves has the potential to cure tuberculosis (and *M. tuberculosis* resistant to S, H, R & E) and is a promise for future therapeutic interventions. To our knowledge it is for the first time that it has been possible to demonstrate experimentally in the laboratory the promising antitubercular activity of *Sida rhombifolia* L. leaves. [544]

228

Sida acuta

Tr 107-review-Ayurveda-whole plant or roots-water extract?, 361-England-tuberculosis, 561-Ayurveda-root, 609-India,

Sida cordifolia

Tr 71-Ayurveda-root-pulmonary tuberculosis, 118-Ayurveda-bark, 217-Ayurveda-pulmonary tuberculosis, 167-Ayurveda-root-pulmonary tuberculosis or a similar progressive systemic disease, 548-India, 561-Ayurveda-root,

Sida rhombifolia

544-invitro-leaves and roots-the ethyl acetate extract of Sida rhombifolia L. leaves has the dose dependent potential to cure tuberculosis-This is even more significant as this activity was noted against a clinical strain which was resistant to S, H, R and E.

Tr 47-India, 51-India-whole plant?, 136-India- root and leaves, 358-Mayaysia, 361-Malaysia-whole plant?, 362-review-Malaysia-whole plant?, 522-India- decoction of root-orally, 561-Ayurveda-root, 568-Nigeria,

Sida retusa
436- invitro-seed-methanol extract- potent antitubercular activities,

Sida cordata
Tr 496-Pakistan-Siddha and Ayurveda, 549-Ayurveda,

Sida indica

Tr 448-Ayurveda-pulmonary tuberculosis, 452-Bangladesh, 684-Ayurveda-pulmonary tuberculosis, 708-Ayurveda-root-in chest infection,

Sida spinosa
Tr 561-Ayurveda-root,

Cryptolepine
(S. acuta, cordifolia, rhombifolia, spinosa, and ?)

384-invitro- cryptolepine hydrochloride-antitubercular drugs- MICs ranged over 2–32 µg/mL- Mycobacterium fortuitum/M. phlei/M. aurum/M. smegmatis/M. bovis BCG/M. abcessus-dose (16 µg/mL)

Metal, Anti-corrosion
Tr no reported use

Among the several methods of corrosion control and prevention, the use of corrosion inhibitors, is very popular...Unfortunately, the use of some chemical inhibitors have been limited because of some reasons namely their synthesis is very often expensive and they can be toxic and hazardous for human beings environment as well. This has prompted the search for eco-friendly corrosion inhibitors as an alternative to replace inorganic and organic inhibitors to foster sustainable greenness to the environment. **[642]**

Sida acuta

77-invitro (imbrued with silver nanoparticles, with Artemisia annua),   227-invitro-it is noted that the inhibition efficiency of the leaves extract at all experimental temperatures was higher than that of the stem extract both in the presence of the extracts alone and on the addition of iodide ions. This seems to suggest that the leaves extract is a better corrosion inhibitor than the stem extract and may be attributed to higher concentration of the phytochemical constituents of the leaves extract compared to that of the stem extract-inhibition efficiency increases with increase in the iodide ion concentration,   307-invitro-leaves and stems-cold distilled water extract-The results presented in this work show that Sida acuta extract inhibits corrosion of Al-Cu-Mg alloy in HCl medium at room temperature... Therefore, in textile and food industries where processing plants make use of Al-Cu-Mg in the machine parts, the process of cleaning, pickling and descaling can be done using HCl with Sida acuta as the inhibitor. This will be more economical and efficient, and play a vital role in reducing corrosion rate,   642-invitro-leaves and stems- absolute ethanol extract-inhibited the acid induced corrosion of mild steel. The inhibition efficiency increases with increase in concentration of the extracts but decrease with rise in temperature,   696-invitro-leaves-HCl acid- The maximum inhibition efficiency of 71.16% was attained when the crushed leaves of Sida Acuta were added at 15g per liter of 0.7M HCl whilst the corrosion rate reduced from 1.0485 to 0.3006mgcm-2h-1--protective film formed on the mild steel surface,

Mineral accumulator, Chelator

Plant species should be able to produce high yields of mass in conditions of a deposit substrate, and take out substantial amount of harmful components from that deposit... The results confirmed, great diversification of the element contents which depends not only on the species but also on the part of individual plants. Analysis of the data revealed also another dependence: increased concentration of heavy metals in the soil corresponded to a higher content of heavy metals in the plants. **[554]   Tr no reported use**

Sida acuta

415-invitro- S. acuta had exceptionally high concentrations of minerals, calcium, magnesium and sodium, phosphorous, copper, molybdenum, 421-invitro-leaf-Nigeria roads,   532-invitro-leaves-acqueous extract-We have found that Sida Acuta Burm f. are useful to reduced fluoride content from water... The fluoride content in water sample of some villages of Bhiloda taluka was (about 1.55mg/l).with the help of extract (Fig. 2) fluoride content came down to (1.42mg/l),   657-invivo-whole plant- tolerated the 1150 mg Zn kg-1 soil level,

Phytoextraction   78-invitro,   94-invitro-India,   112-invitro -phytoremediation- removes heavy metals-suitable for phytostabilization of Cr, Cd and Zn in cement-polluted soil while Cr and Cd can be phytoextracted by these two weed species from cement-polluted soil without much

230

restriction,   **231**-invitro-zinc polluted soil-can survive up to 1150 mg of zinc contamination per kg of soil,   **356**-invitro-whole plant-found suitable for the decontamination of most of the metals from tannery waste contaminated sites,   **654**-invivo-The ability of these plants to grow on a wide range of soil types, both in polluted and non-polluted areas, is another advantage in considering them as initial stabilizers of degraded habitats and indicators of pollution levels... Therefore, further studies into the herbaceous weeds, including Sida species, are suggested, in order to use them as indicators of pollution levels in industrial or urban areas and subsequently for considering their roles in combating environmental pollution. True that Sida species are weeds and thus are risky, but they still have unappreciated roles in the restoration of degraded, damaged and polluted areas.

Sida cordifolia   **654**-see listing under Sida acuta above.

Sida rhombifolia

538-rats-roots-95% ethanol extract-500, 750 and 1000 mg/ kg bw-30 days-negative effect of cadmium chloride on body weight was significantly (P 0.05) ameliorated by Sida rhombifolia. L root extract in a dose dependent manner, **670**-invitro-The objective of this work was to identify and describe several plants that survived in a soil polluted with hydrocarbons in a former refinery-tolerated Benzene, toluene, xylen, polysyclic aromatic hydrocarbons, tetraethyl lead, methyl tert-butyl ether.

Sida cordata   **654**-see listing under Sida acuta above.

Sida hermaphrodita

472-Poland-invivo-whole living plant-Previous research proved the great ability of Sida hermaphrodita to take up many elements and to cumulate them in stems. During the 3 years of the experiment, similar amounts of Co, Cd, Pb, and Ni were taken up from the sludge, regardless of the propagation method, while significantly higher amounts of Fe were taken up by the Sida of the vegetative propagation-The greatest density of plants (III) caused a significant increase in the amount of cobalt and iron taken up from the sludge. The smallest amount of nickel was taken up by the stems of plants growing in medium density,   **476**-Significantly more phosphorus, magnesium and sulphur was contained by Virginia fanpetals biomass from the municipal sewage sludge compost than without,   **475**-Germany-invivo-Since more drought spells will occur in the future climate and the availability of productive land will be reduced permanent bioenergy cultures will have to be based on marginal agricultural production systems. The perennial species addressed here are potentially suited candidates because they have high water use efficiency and do not need to be grown under highly intensive conditions, **482**-invitro-whole living plant- highest tolerated level of soil contamination-top accumulator of Cadmium, lead, nickel, copper, and zinc,   **484**-invivo-cultivated in Soil Contaminated with Heavy Metals--the results from growing in heavy metal soil: Mg .30-1.42% -- Na .008-.047% -- K .87-4.76% -- Ca .86-5.06% -- Mn 6.82-108.3 mg,   **554**-invitro-the highest yield of dry mass was obtained from Sida hermaphrodita grown on sewage sludge. It took the highest amounts of Pb, Zn, Fe, Cr, Cu, an Ni from sewage sludge. The obtained results prove that Sida hermaphrodita is a valuable species to grow on sewage sludges in order to derive substantial amounts of heavy metals, **623**-invitro-absorbed high levels of zinc, lower levels of lead, copper, and nickel, and absorbed cadmium at least, **629**-field experi-ment/invitro-can be used for phytoremediation (phytoextraction) of heavy metals contained in sewage sludge, **630**-Sida hermaphrodita-field trial/ nvitro-can successfully be grown on moderately contaminated soil with heavy metals,

Sida rhomboidea   320-whole plant?-methanol extract-effective metal chelation (IC50=65.69±1.22µg/ml)

Minerals, Nanoparticles   Tr no reported use

Nanoparticles can be synthesized by chemical processes like pyrolysis, hydrothermal method, chemical precipitation etc. But these chemical processes cause pollution and are costly practices...However using "green" methods in the synthesis of Zinc nanoparticles has increasingly become a topic of interest. Nanoparticles in recent days have revolutionized the modern medicinal practices because of their potential activities in treatment of various diseases. **[683]**   The advantage of using plants for the synthesis of nanoparticles is that they are easily available, safe to handle and possess a broad variability of metabolites that may aid in reduction... [silver nanoparticles offer] copious benefits of eco-friendliness and compatibility for pharmaceutical and biomedical applications as they do not use toxic chemicals in the synthesis protocols... [they are] cost effective, environment friendly, easily scaled up for large scale synthesis and in this method there is no need to use high pressure, energy, temperature and toxic chemicals.**[77]** These results suggest that the use of S. acuta synthesized silver nanoparticles can be a rapid, environmentally safer biopesticide which can form a novel approach to develop effective biocides for controlling the target vector mosquitoes. This is the first report on the mosquito larvicidal activity of the plant aqueous extract and synthesized nanoparticles. **[253]**

Sida acuta

77-invitro-leaves-hot distilled water extract-imbrued with silver nanoparticles-20g of ground leaves added to 200mL of distilled water-boiled for 15 minutes-used immediately after- Candida albicans Zones of inhibition-just leaves (no activity)-with silver nanoparticles 21mm-silver nitrate alone 10mm,   **253**-Considerable mortality was evident after the treatment of S. acuta for all three important vector mosquitoes. The LC50 and LC90 values of S. acuta aqueous leaf extract appeared to be most effective against A. stephensi (LC50, 109.94 µg/mL and LC90, 202.42 µg/mL) followed by A. aegypti LC50 (119.32 µg/mL and LC90, 213.84 µg/mL) and C. quinque-fasciatus (LC50, 130.30 µg/mL and LC90, 228.20 µg/mL). Synthesized AgNPs against the vector mosquitoes of A. stephensi, A. aegypti, and C. quinquefasciatus had the following LC50 and LC90 values: A. stephensi had LC50 and LC90 values of 21.92, and 41.07 µg/mL; A. aegypti had LC50 and LC90 values of 23.96, and 44.05 µg/mL; C. quinquefasciatus had LC50 and LC90 values of 26.13 and 47.52 µg/m,   **354**-invivo-leaf-?extract-

232

synthesized silver nanoparticles-larvicidal-the use of S. acuta synthesized silver nanoparticles can be a rapid, environmentally safer biopesticide which can form a novel approach to develop effective biocides for controlling the target vector mosquitoes. This is the first report on the mosquito larvicidal activity of the plant aqueous extract and synthesized nanoparticles,

Sida cordifolia

662-invitro-leaves-cold distilled water extract-recorded impressive anticancer effect against two different types of cancer cells-In vitro cytotoxicactivity of AgNPs was evaluated at different concentrations and it showed a dose dependent activity against EAC and HT-29 cell lines with IC50 value of 204.7and129.3 mg/ml, respectively,

Sida indica

674-invitro-leaf-boiling distilled water extract- polyphenol stabilized gold nanoparticles displayed good in vitro free radical scavenging activities as indicated in various in vitro antioxidant assays, **683**-invitro-leaves-cold distilled water extract- The Zn nanoparticles synthesized using S. indica, showed positive results for cytotoxic activity with an IC50 value of 45.82 μg/ml. These positive results confirmed the cytotoxic potential of the Zn nanoparticles against cervical cancer. Thus Zn nanoparticles can be used as a potent drug in alternative therapy for treating the cervical cancer patients in the near future, **705**- leaf-aqueous extract- report the biological synthesis of Sida indica silver nanoparticles (AIAgNPs)-the biological properties of AIAgNPs were free radical scavenging activity, antibacterial effect and anti-proliferative activity, **707**-leaf-aqueous extract-the biological properties of AIAgNPs were free radical scavenging activity, antibacterial effect and anti-proliferative activity,

Mollusks, Molluscicide   Tr   no reported use

Pesticides against mollusks, which are usually used in agriculture or gardening, in order to control gastropod pests specifically slugs and snails which damage crops or other valued plants by feeding on them. [1]

Cryptolepine   (S. acuta, cordifolia, rhombifolia, spinosa, and ?)
309-review-Neocryptolepine,

Mouth, Demulcent   No peer review

An agent that forms a soothing film over a mucous membrane, relieving minor pain and inflammation of the membrane. [1]

Sida acuta

Tr 21-Siddha (Tamil)-leaves, 29-Ayurveda, 88-Portuguese-demulcent in gonorrhea, 88-Ayurveda-root, 107-India-leaves, 107-India-in gonorrhea, 109-Siddah-leaves, 217-Ayurveda, 220-SriLanka-

Decoction also used as demulcent for rheumatism,   270-India-leaves, 358-review-leaves-demulcent,   377-Ayurveda-root,   561-Ayurveda-root,

Sida cordifolia

Tr   28-India-inflammation of the oral mucosa,   43-Brazil,   61-Brazil-inflammation of the oral mucosa,   88-Ayurveda-root bark-inflammation of the oral mucosa,   120-Columbia,   154-Brazil,   161-Brazil,   167-Ayurveda-leaves,   182-India-inflammation of the oral mucosa,   285-India-seeds, 312-USA-Ayurveda-root bark,   377-Ayurveda-root,   437-Ayurveda-leaves, 561-Ayurveda-root,

Sida rhombifolia

Tr   47-India-stem,   51-India-stem,   88-Ayurveda-root,   107-India-demulcent,   127-India,   136-India- root and leaves,   217-Ayurveda,   220-SriLanka-Decoction also used as demulcent for gonorrhea,   377-Ayurveda-root,   437-Ayurveda-leaves,   522-Ayurveda-stems-The stems are abound in mucilage and are employed as demulcent and emollients both for external and internal use,   524-Phillipines,   524-India-roots,   545- Bangladesh-stems-abound in mucilage,   561-Ayurveda-root,

Sida retusa   Tr   527-Stems-demulcent-for external and internal use,

Sida cordata   Tr   437-Ayurveda-leaves,   496-Sida cordata-Pakistan-Siddha and Ayurveda-roots or seeds,

Sida indica

Tr   377-Ayurveda-root,   437-Ayurveda-leaves-demulcent,   561-Ayurveda-root,   678-Ayurveda-root,   708-Ayurveda-root,   710-China-seeds,   711-Chinese-seed,   712-India-seeds,   735- Ayurveda-review-roots,

Sida spinosa

Tr   3-India-leaves,   55-India-leaves-bruised in water and the filtrate is administered,   99-India-leaf-generally demulcent-plus a decoction of it is said to be given as a demulcent in irritability of bladder and in gonorrhea, 217-Ayurveda,   433-India,   561-Ayurveda-root,

Mouth, Dental hygiene

Antibiotic resistance in microorganisms recovered from the acute dental abscess has been reported to be increasing in some populations studied over the last few decades. The resistance problem demands that a renewed effort be made to seek antibacterial agents effective against pathogenic bacteria resistant to current antibiotics. [556-2007]

Sida acuta

234-invitro-dental plaque-The leaves of Sida acuta displayed good antibacterial activity against Streptococcus mutans and Streptococcus sanguis

234

which are both Gram positive microorganisms. Sida acuta showed promising antibacterial activities and thus can be employed as an effective anti-plaque agent and can be used in the prevention of dental caries, 237-leaf-water extract-strong bactericidal effect on buccal cavity-Staph. aureus SS-5BC, 598-review-chewing sticks-despite the recent civilization... in Nigeria, teeth are first cleaned with chewing sticks prior to the use of modern tooth paste and brush-the importance of chewing sticks, particularly to the relative low cases of dental caries and maintenance of strong teeth, are often unrecognized and/or pronounced.

Tr 234-Ghana-dental plaque, 361-review-stems-chew sticks, 532-India-very useful to remove fluoride content, 580-India-whole plant-ethanol extract-strengthen gums, 598-Nigeria-stem-chewing sticks, 602-Nigeria.twig/stem-teeth cleaning,

Sida cordifolia

208-invivo-stem?-axqueous extract- reduce the virulence of these periodontophathic bacteria and to reduce the rate of dental plaque formation,

Tr 88-Kenya-dental hygiene, 208-Kenya-chewing sticks (mswaki), 312-Kenya

Sida rhombifolia

672-invitro-root-ethanol extract-these results suggest that ethanol extract of S. rhombifolia roots have potential to be developed as dentistry formula.

Tr 150-Ethiopia-stem-toothbrush, 367-review-they are used for cleaning the teeth in Gabon and Kenya, 522-India-twig of the plant used as a toothbrush to strengthen gums. 522-Rotuma (Fiji)-stem chewed for dental hygiene.

Sida urens

499-invitro-mice-this plant possesses compounds with high antibacterial and analgesic properties that can be used as antibacterial and analgesic agents in developing new drugs for the therapy of dental caries bacteria,

Tr 499-Burkina Faso-dental caries bacteria,

Sida corymbosa

598-review-chewing sticks-despite the recent civilization... in Nigeria, teeth are first cleaned with chewing sticks prior to the use of modern tooth paste and brush-the importance of chewing sticks, particularly to the relative low cases of dental caries and maintenance of strong teeth, are often unrecognized and/or pronounced. Tr 598-review-chewing sticks,

Sida spinosa   Tr 568-Nigeria-cleaning the teeth,

....

(Sida acuta) This plant is used as a complementary treatment for malaria or other febrile illnesses and the leaf extract combined with turmeric applied for chronic wound and poisonous bite. [214]

Mouth, Inflamed stomatitis

Sida acuta

Tr　80-India-whole plant-toothache-strengthen gums,　568-Nigeria-catarrh (excessive discharge of mucus),　602-Nigeria.twig/stem-chewed for sore gum,

Sida cordifolia

208-invivo-stem?-axqueous extract-reduce the virulence of these periodontophathic bacteria and to reduce the rate of dental plaque formation.,

Tr　153-Brasil,　161-Brazil,　180-India-stomatitis,　312-Brazil,　437-Ayurveda-leaves-decoction-tender gums,

treat oral mucosa　**Tr**　28-India-inflammation of the oral mucosa,　43-Brazil-inflammation of the oral mucosa,　61-Brazil-inflammation of the oral mucosa,　88-Ayurveda-root bark-inflammation of the oral mucosa,　120-Columbia-treat oral mucosa,　154-Brazil,　161-Brazil,　182-India-inflammation of the oral mucosa,　312-USA-Ayurveda-inflammation of oral mucosa,　312-Brazil-inflammation of oral mucosa,

Inflamed throat　**Tr**　118-Ayurveda-bark-throat conditions,　167-Ayurveda-root-throat diseases,　664-Ayurveda-bark-throat troubles,

Sida rhombifolia　**Tr**　150-Ethiopia-root and leaf-gum infection, 437--Ayurveda-leaves-decoction-tender gums,

Sida cordata　**Tr**　437-Ayurveda-leaves-decoction-tender gums,

Sida indica

Tr　437-Ayurveda-leaves-decoction-tender gums,　450-India-leaf-mouthwash,　450-India-leaf-catarrh (excessive discharge of mucus),　454-India-leaves-mouthwash,　678-Ayurveda-leaves-decoction-tender gums,　708-Ayurveda-leaves-decoction is used in toothache and tender gums,　712-India-leaves-toothache and tender gums,　712-India-leaves-mouth wash, 735-Ayurveda-review-decoction of the leaves-tender gums,

Mouth, Toothache No peer review

Sida acuta

Tr　362-India-crushed leaves on gums,　580-India-whole plant-ethanol extract,　602-Nigeria-twig/stem-chewed for toothache,

Sida cordifolia　**Tr**　362-India-crushed leaves on gums,　437-Ayurveda-leaves-decoction,

236

Sida rhombifolia

Tr 126-Colombia, 150-Ethiopia-root, 358-Camaroonand Indonesia-roots-chewed, 362-India-crushed leaves on gums, 437-Ayurveda-leaves-decoction, 524-Phillipines-roots-decoction-used as a gargle for toothaches, 524-Phillipines-pulped leaves-to the gums for toothaches, 524-Phillipines-roots-crushed with or without ginger-held in the mouth, 524-Indonesia-crushed roots-chewed with ginger, 568-Nigeria,

Sida indica

Tr 362-India-crushed leaves on gums, 437-Ayurveda-leaves-decoction-toothache, 454-India-leaf-mouthwash for toothache, 678-Ayurveda-leaves-decoction, 708-Ayurveda-leaves-decoction is used in toothache and tender gums, 710-Ayurveda-leaves, 735-Ayurveda-review-decoction of the leaves,

Other Sidas   **Tr** 362-Sida spinosa-India-crushed leaves on gums, 437-Ayurveda-Sida cordata-India-leaves-decoction,

Nausea, Antiemetic   No peer review

A drug that is effective against vomiting and nausea. Typically used to treat motion sickness and the side effects of opioid analgesics, general anesthetics, and chemotherapy directed against cancer. [1]

Sida acuta

Tr 21-Ayurveda-leaves, 52-India-leaf juice, 101-India-leaf juice-for vomiting and gastric disorders, 107-India-leaf juice, 168-India-leaf juice-vomiting and gastric disorders, 361-Phillipines-vomiting of blood, 362-review-Philippines-leaf/root-decoction-for vomiting of blood, 370-Benin-anti-vomitive,

Sida cordifolia, Sida rhombifolia, Sida cordata, Sida indica

Tr 437-Ayurveda-bark or flowers-as powder in ghee-blood vomiting.

Nerves, CNS depressant (central nervous system)

Physiological depression of the central nervous system that can result in decreased rate of breathing, decreased heart rate, and loss of consciousness possibly leading to coma or death. [1]

Sida acuta

275-mice-leaves and stems-100% ethanolic extract-500 and 1000 mg/kg-sedative effect-causes effects on the central nervous system in experimental animals, **500**-mice-hydroalcoholic extract-shows general central nervous system inhibitory action-does not act on skeletal muscles.

Sida cordifolia

41-mice-leaves- hydroalcoholic extract- dose of 1000 mg/kg (i.p.)-Depressive activity on CNS was demonstrated by several alterations in mice's behavior in the pharmacological screening, **132**-mice-leaf-70% ethanol extract-Depressive activity on CNS was demonstrated by several alterations in mice's behavior in the pharmacological screening,-1000 mg/kg bw-at a dose of 1000 mg/kg (i.p. and p.o.) produced sedation, decrease of the ambulation, reduction of answer to the touch, analgesia and decrease of urination. The effects were more pronounced in animals treated intraperitoneally-caused significant reduction (p < 0.001) of the spontaneous locomotor activity in comparison with the control group-did not produce a significant alteration of the latency and the time of sleep of the treated animals in comparison with those from the control group-did not cause a significant difference in the motor coordination of the treated animals in comparison with the control group,

Tr 118-Ayurveda, 120-Colombia-CNS stimulant, 148-India-aerial parts, 158-India, 161-Ayurveda-exerts a positive influence on the central nervous systems, 378-medical website-may cause CNS (central nervous system) depressant effects, 664-Ayurveda-whole plant?,

Sida indica

454-invitro-leaves-400 mg/kg bw-water, ether and benzene extracts- all the extracts have shown CNS depressant activity,

Sida tiagii
205-invitro-anxiolytic-fruit-ethanolic/ethyl acetate extract,

Nerves, Nervous disorders

Sida acuta

275-Colombia/Spain-rats-leaves and stems-100% ethanolic extract-500 mg/kg-nervous diseases-sedative, depressive, anxiolytic and anticonvulsant effects; in addition, a potentiation of hypnosis induced by pentobarbital.,

Tr 3-India-root, 18-India-nervous diseases, 63-India, 82-India, 90-India?-root, 111-India, 118-Ayurveda-nerve tonic, 174-India-nervous disease, 186-India-nervous diseases, 217-Ayurveda, 270-India-tonic-root, 275-Colombia/Spain-Ayurveda-leaves?-nervous diseases-sedative agent, 358-review-roots, 561-Ayurveda-roots-nervous disorders, 571-India-nervous disease, 609-India-neuroprotective, 644-Ayurveda-root,

Sida cordifolia

533-medical site review-all parts?-any extract?- might cause side effects such as jitteriness, nervousness and anxiety,

Tr 32-Ayurveda-root infusion-nervous diseases, 87-India, 118-Ayurveda-Oil prepared from the decoction of root bark mixed with milk and sesame oil, 118-Ayurveda-root infusion-nervous diseases-nerve tonic, 120-Colombia- central nervous system stimulant (alkaloids), 124-India-root bark,   161-Ayurveda-rejuvenating-in medicated enema where its root extract is used for all kinds of nervous disorders like paralysis, arthritis etc-nerve tonic,   173-India,   285-India-root, 312-USA-Ayurveda-roots-nervous disorders,   358- Central African Republic and Kenya-root infusion-hemiplegia and facial paralysis, 378-medical website-can induce nervousness, 521-Ayurveda-root-nervousness,   561-Ayurveda-roots-nerv-ous disorders, 664-Ayurveda-whole plant?-extract-also fits,   664-Ayurveda-root bark-decoction-oil-mixed with milk and sesame oil-nervous system diseases,

Sida rhombifolia

Tr   522-India-hot aqueous extracts of dried leaf and root of the plant are used to treat nervous diseases,   524-India-Hindus-nervous disease,   561-Ayurveda-roots-nervous disorders,

Sida indica

Tr   445-India and China-some nervous problems,   678-Ayurveda-root and bark-nervine tonic,   711-Ayurveda-root and bark,

Other Sida

Tr   561-S. spinosa-Ayurveda-roots-nervous disorders,   496-S. cordata-Pakistan-Siddha and Ayurveda-seeds- the dry, nervous qualities of the Vata type,   561- S. veronicaefolia-Ayurveda-roots-nervous disorders,

Nerves, Neurodegenerative diseases

The progressive loss of structure or function of neurons, including death of neurons. Many neurodegenerative diseases including amyotrophic lateral sclerosis, Parkinson's, Alzheimer's, and Huntington's occur as a result of neurodegenerative processes. Such diseases are incurable, resulting in progressive degeneration and/or death of neuron cells [1]

Sida acuta

266-Nigeria-rats- administered with 200mg/kg, and 600mg/kg, showed hyperplasia of cells in the cortical, intermediate and sub-ventricular layers, respectively. Animals that received 400mg/kg of the extract showed hypertrophy of cell in the intermediate and sub- ventricular layers. This result suggests that high doses of ethanolic leaf extract of Sida acuta may cause some neurological disorders.   **Tr** 609-India-neural problems,

Sida cordifolia

26-rats-water extract-100 mg/kg bw-Rotenone induced oxidative damage was attenuated by the water extract- The maximum effect in all the above activities was observed in the water extract (100mg/kg) treated group, which was comparable to l-deprenyl treated group,

Tr   32-India-degeneration of nerve,   42-Ayurveda-degeneration of nerve-loss of memory and other neuronal disorders -Alzheimer's,   44-Ayurveda (with 3 other herbs),   71-Ayurveda-roots,   88-India-degeneration of nerve,

123-Ayurveda, 161-Ayurveda-root extract-neurological ailments, especially in Stroke rehabilitation, 167-Ayurveda-root, 180-Ayurveda, 312-USA-Ayurveda-roots/leaves/stems-degeneration of nerve-reduce severity of Parkinsonism, 548-India, 612-Ayurveda and Siddha-root-neurological problems,

Sida rhombifolia

Tr 127-India-degeneration of nerve, 522-Ayurveda-dried leaf and root-hot aqueous extract-nervous diseases,

Sida retusa

Tr 131-Ayurveda, 197-India?-roots-neurological complaints including epilepsy, 435-Ayurveda-An infusion made from the roots of this plant is held in great repute by the local ayurvedic physicians in the treatment of rheumatism and a variety of neurological complaints including epilepsy, 529-Ayurveda-root infusion-is held in great repute by the local ayurvedic physicians for a variety of neurological complaints including epilepsy

Sida cordata
Tr 496-Pakistan-Siddha and Ayurveda-seeds, 549-Ayurveda,

Sida tiagii
Tr 552-India-anti-seizure-neurological disorders.

Nerves, Paralysis

A loss of muscle function for one or more muscles. Paralysis can be accompanied by a loss of feeling (sensory loss) in the affected area if there is sensory damage as well as motor. About 1 in 50 people in the U.S. have been diagnosed with some form of paralysis. [1]

Sida acuta
Tr 88-Gold Coast, 107-Ayurveda-facial paralysis,

Sida cordifolia

146-Indian earthworm-whole plant-ethanol and acqueous extract (10, 20, 30, 40 mg/ml)- time of paralysis of the worms. Albendazole was included as reference standard. The most activity was observed with aqueous extract as compared to standard drug,

Tr (Facial paralysis) 88-Ayurveda-juice of plants with water- facial paralysis-hemophlegia (paralysis of one side of the body), 118-Ayurveda-Oil prepared from the decoction of root bark mixed with milk and sesame oil, 132-Brazil-roots-hemiplegia and facial paralysis, 161-Ayurveda-in medicated enema where its root extract is used for all kinds of nervous disorders like paralysis, arthritis etc, 167-Ayurveda-root bark-mixed with sesame oil and cow milk in curing facial paralysis, 285-India-root-hemiplegia and facial paralysis, 161-Ayurveda-rejuvenating-in medicated enema where its root extract is used for all kinds of nervous disorders like paralysis, arthritis etc, 312-USA-Ayurveda-roots-hemiplegia (paralysis of one side of the body), 358- Central African Republic and Kenya-root infusion-hemiplegia and facial paralysis,   362-Malaysia-infusion of the roots-hemiplegia or facial paralysis,   664-Ayurveda-root bark-decoction-oil-mixed with milk and sesame oil.

Sida cordata   (Facial paralysis)
Tr   496-whole plant?-Pakistan-Siddha and Ayurveda-hemiplegia and facial paralysis,   549-Ayurveda,   549-Ayurveda-hemiplegia, facial paralysis,

Nerves, Sciatica   No peer review
Characterized by pain going down the leg from the lower back. This pain may go down the back, outside, or front of the leg. Typically, symptoms are only on one side of the body. About 90% of the time sciatica is due to a spinal disc herniation pressing on one of the lumbar or sacral nerve roots. [1]

Sida acuta   **Tr**   53--Ayurveda-decoction of the root bark,   88-Ayurveda-juice of plants with water,   107-Ayurveda,   218-Ayurveda-decoction of the root bark,

Sida cordifolia
Tr   118-Ayurveda-Oil prepared from the decoction of root bark mixed with milk and sesame oil,   312-USA-Ayurveda-root?-pain reliever,   167-Ayurveda-root bark-mixed with sesame oil and cow milk in curing sciatica pain,   664-Ayurveda-root bark-decoction-oil-mixed with milk and sesame oil,

Sida cordata   **Tr** 496-Pakistan-Siddha and Ayurveda,   549-Ayurveda,

Nerves, Sedative
Various extracts of Sida retusa root that were tested on gross behavior of mice, only the crude extract produced a sedative effect, characterized by a decrease in alertness, wakefulness and reactivity. The maximum effect was noted 2 to 3 hours after drug treatment (5 and 10 g/kg). The crude extract of Sida retusa root (5 and 10 g/kg) produced a significant potentiation of the pentobarbitone (pentobarbitol) sleeping time in mice, and abolished both the conditioned and unconditioned avoidance response. It did not have any protective effect against amphetamine or leptazol-induced toxicity, nor did it possess any analgesic effect or anticonvulsant activity. [529]

Sida acuta   **Tr** 6-Ayurveda,   223-India,   275-Colombia,   601-Nigeria-leaf-treatment of hysteria,   653-Ayurveda,

Sida rhombifolia
Tr   358-Camaroon-leaves-a watery maceration of the leaves is drunk as an antihypertensive agent, as a sedative,   407-Ayurveda-seeds-tenseness,   522-Peru-leaf,

Sida retusa

128-mice-root-only the crude extract produced a sedative effect, **435**-rats-roots-crude water extract-5/10 gm/kg bw- produced a sedative effect, characterized by a decrease in alertness, wakefulness and reactivity, **529**-mice-root-crude extract-5 gm/kg bw-the crude extract produced a sedative effect, characterized by a decrease in alertness, wakefulness and reactivity. The crude extract of Sida retusa root produced a significant potentiation of the pentobarbitone sleeping time in mice, and abolished both the conditioned and unconditioned avoidance response.

Sida tiagii **205**-invitro-anxiolytic-fruit-ethanolic/ethyl acetate extract.
Tr 552- India,

Sida cordata **Tr** 496-Pakistan-Siddha and Ayurveda-seeds-tenseness--seeds-sedative,

Noise Reduction

Sida hermaphrodita

479-Results of research concerning use of Sida hermaphrodita as biological acoustic screen along communication routes, show that most effective noise suppression, by means of above mentioned plant screen, was observed at measurement height of 0.5 m, from May to October. Greatest noise reduction, reaching 13.4 dB, was noted for measurement profile C, 35 m from source of noise.

Pain, Analgesic

An analgesic or painkiller is any member of the group of drugs used to achieve analgesia, relief from pain. [1] Writing test (analgesic) = Analgesic activity of the ethanolic extract of S. cordifolia was tested using the model of acetic acid induced writhing in mice. The test consists of injecting 0.7% acetic acid solution and observing the animal for specific contraction of body referred as 'writhing'. [24]

Sida acuta

14-mice-leaf-ethanol extract-contains psychoactive substances with analgesic and antidepressant-like properties which may be beneficial in the management of pain, **76**-rats/mice-whole plant?-aqueous acetone extract-The extract has produced significant analgesic effects by the acetic acid writhing test and by the hot plate method (p <0.05) and a dose-dependent inhibition was observed, **84**-mice-whole plant-crude extract- exhibited significant (p< 0.001) analgesic and anti-inflammatory activities, **186**-rats-whole plant-methanolic extract-400mg/kg- possesses anti-inflammatory and analgesic activity-The effects were comparable with that of reference standard, indomethacin that showed 78.97% inhibition of writhing-In the

242

acetic acid induced writing test, the extract at the dose level 400 mg/kg showed 83.78% inhibition of writing. In radiant heat tail- flick method the extract at the dose 400 mg/kg showed reaction time 4.902 ± 0.545 (p<0.001)-a dose-dependent inhibition was observed, **203**-mice/rats-aqueous acetone extract-significant analgesic effects by the acetic acid writing test and by the hot plate method (p <0.05) and a dose-dependent inhibition was observed, **571**-mice-whole plant-methanolic extract-100, 200 and 400 mg/kg bw po--maximum inhibition was noted for MESA 400mg/kg (83.78%). The effects were comparable with that of reference standard, indomethacin that showed 78.97% inhibition of writing-400 mg/kg showed significant (P<0.01-0.001) increase in reaction time but the dose of 100 mg/kg did not produce any effect compared to control (P>0.05). The effects very much comparable with pentazocin 10 mg/kg, **580**-India-whole plant-ethanol extract-100mg/kg bw?-Analgesic activity,

Tr 3-India-whole plant, 76-W Africa, 84-Nigeria, 101-Nicaragua,the decoction of the entire plant is taken orally, 107-Nicaragua, 109-Siddah-leaf juice-chest pain, 168-Nicaragua-decoction of the entire plant taken orally, 194-Gabon, 203-Burkina-Faso, 257-Phillipines-Crushed leaves are rubbed on painful muscles, 271-Nicaragua-decoction of the entire plant, 523-India-leaves, 580-India-whole plant-ethanol extract, 588-Nigeria-decoction of whole plant, 596-Nigeria-leaf/root, 609-India, 646-Nigeria-leaves and stem,

Sida cordifolia

24-roots-80% ethanol extract-500 mg/kg bw-The crude extract produced 44.30% inhibition of writing which is statistically significant (P>0.001)- The results of the test showed that S. cordifolia ethanol extract at a dose of 500 mg/kg exhibited highly significant (P<0.001) inhibition of writing reflex by 44.30% while the standard drug diclofenac inhibition was found to be 45.22% at a dose of 25 mg/kg body weight, **36**-rats/invitro-a new alkaloid- In the acetic acid induced writing model, the compound 1 showed 25.4 (P<0.05) and 52.43% (P<0.01) inhibition of writing response at doses of 25 and 50 mg/kg body weight respectively, **43**-rats-leaf-water extract-400 mg/kg bw-increased the latency period for mice in the hot plate test, and inhibited the number of writhes produced by acetic acid **45**-rats?-root and aerial parts-ethyl acetate extract-600 mg/kg bw-showed very good central and peripheral analgesic activities **61**-rats-leaf-water extract-400 mg/kg bw- increased the latency period for mice in the hot plate test, and inhibited the number of writhes produced by acetic acid, **116**- new flavonol glycoside-rats-In the acetic acid induced writing model, the drug at a dose of 25 and 50 mg kg^{-1} body weight showed statistically significant (p<0.0001) inhibition of writing response of 25.12 and 52.30%, respectively, **133**-rats,mice-aerial parts-chloroform/methanol/ 80% ethanol extract-50mg/kg reduced writing 52.3% in dose dependent manner-aminopyrine 50 mg/kg reduced writing 67.9%-radiant heat tail-flick latency showed significant increase in a dose dependent manner, **154**-mice-acqueous extract-leaves-400 mg/kg- increased the latency period for mice in the hot plate test, and inhibited the number of writhes produced by acetic acid at the oral dose, **183**-mice-aerial parts-chloroform (3 × 72h)/methanol (3 × 72h)/80% ethanol

(3 × 72h) extract>ethyl acetate-50 mg/ kg bw caused 47.03% (p< 0.01) reduction in writhing-50 mg/kg bw aminopyrine produced 67.57% reduction—also caused significant increase in the tail flick latency, **235**-invitro- a new alkaloid, 1,2,3,9-tetrahydro-pyrrolo [2,1-b] quinazolin-3-ylamine-- showed 25.4 (P<0.05) and 52.43% (P<0.01) inhibition of writhing response at doses of 25 and 50 mg/kg body weight respectively, **285**-rats-root/aerial parts-ethyl acetate extract-600 mg/kg bw-showed very good central and peripheral analgesic activities, **358**-invivo?-aerial parts and roots-show analgesic activity, **362**-aerial parts and roots-? extract-shows analgesic activity, **408**-invitro-root and aerial parts-ethyl acetate/merhanol extracts-showed good analgesic activity, **470**-invitro-roots-ethanol extract-The crude extract produced 44.30% inhibition of writhing at the dose of 500 mg/kg body weight which is statistically significant (P>0.001),

Tr 24-Bangladesh-leaf-water extract, 32-Ayurveda, 40-Brazil, 45-India-aerial and root parts, 76-W Africa, 118-Ayurveda, 125-India-crushed leaves, 148-India-aerial parts, 152-India, 156-Brazil, 158-India, 160-Brazil, 161-Ayurveda-increases pain tolerance, 162-Brazil, 173-India, 180-India, 203-Burkina-Faso-children, 217-Ayurveda, 230-Burkina-Faso, 312-USA-Ayurveda, 312-Brazil, 408-India, 437-Ayurveda-leaves-fermented-painful parts of the body, 664-Ayurveda - whole plant?-crushed leaves-poultice-local pains,

Sida rhombifolia

128-mice-crude extract of root-did not reduce pain, **194**-rats-whole plant?-80% acetone extract-100/200/400 mg/kg bw- extracts produced significant analgesic effects in acetic acid writhing and hot plate method (p≤0.05) and in a dose-dependent inhibition was observed, **545**-mice-aerial parts-80% ethanol extract-500 mg bw-70% writhing inhibition in acetic acid-induced writhing in mice--comparable to the standard drug diclofenac sodium at the dose of 25 mg/kg of body weight, **672**-invitro-root-ethanol extract-Analgesic Test the result of the hot plate test revealed that latency time was significant (p<0.05). The extract showed dose-dependent inhibition and the effect of extract at the dose of 3.36 mg/kg bw was better than that of extract at the below-dose and negative control when given orally on mice. The extract possesses anti-inflammation and analgesic activities.

Tr 126-Colombia, 194-Gabon, 407-Ayurveda-chest ailments, 437-Ayurveda-leaves-fermented-painful parts of the body, 464-India-chest ailments, 522-Argentina-leaf-menstrual pain, 522-Nicaragua-leaf-decoction-taken orally, 522-Guatemela-leaf-decoction-orally-aches and pains, 522-Central Africa-infusion of dried leaf -chest pain, 522-Peru-leaf, 524-Phillipines, 543-Ayurveda-antinociceptive,

Sida spinosa **Tr** 11-BurkinaFaso-whole plant-hot water?-analgesic activities.

....

Now-a-days, the search for new active compounds from the plants depends on ethnic and folk informations obtained from traditional healers and is still considered as an important source for new drug discovery. **[522]**

Sida retusa

435-rats-roots-crude water extract-5/10 gm/kg bw-did not possess any analgesic effect {apparently using distilled water}, **529**-mice-root-crude extract-nor did it possess any analgesic effect.

Sida cordata   **Tr**   437-Ayurveda-leaves-fermented-painful parts of the body, 161-Ayurveda-Increases pain tolerance,

Sida indica

442-invitro-eugenol-At doses of 10, 30, and 50 mg/kg body weight, eugenol exhibited 21.30 (p < 0.05), 42.25 (p < 0.01) and 92.96% (p < 0.001) inhibition of acetic acid induced writhing in mice. At a dose of 50 mg/kg body weight, eugenol showed 33.40% (p < 0.05) prolongation of tail flicking time determined by the radiant heat method, **448**-rats-whole plant-analgesic activity after 4 hours-water extract-400 mg/kg-12.08±0.24--ethanol extracts-400 mg/kg-11.68±0.16--Pentazocine 4 mg/kg-14.32±0.21-- The dose of various extracts was found to be more (or) less similar-with significant anti-inflammatory activity comparable with positive control Diclofenac-On the basis of the results of this study, it is possible to conclude that all the effects observed are true analgesic or anti-inflammatory effects. It seems safe to conclude that these parts do possess biological activities following oral administration, **452**-invitro-leaf-methanol extract-Bioactivity guided isolation of Sida indica yielded eugenol (4-allyl-2-methoxyphenol), which was found to possess significant analgesic activity, **454**-invitro-leaves-400 mg/kg bw-ether and benzene extracts-very good analgesic activity without causing narcosis,

Tr   437-Ayurveda–fermented leaves-painful parts of the body, 678-Ayurveda-leaves-as poultice for painful parts of the body, 678-Ayurveda-root-chest infection, 710-Ayurveda-leaves-lumbago, 712-India-leaves-leg pain, 712-India-leaves-Fomentation to painful parts of the body, 712-India-leaves-lumbago,

Sida urens

499--mice—whole plant?—hot water extract?--rich fractions produced significant analgesic effects in acetic acid-induced writhing method--polyphenol-rich fractions more effective against all bacterial strains than Gentamicin,

Tr   499-Burkina Faso-pain,

Sida tiagii   **552**-albino mice-fruit-90% ethanolic extract-reduced pain and was found to have good analgesic activity, **Tr**   552-India,

Sida linfolia   **Tr**   358-Togo-leaf decoction-drunk to relieve lumbar pain,

Cryptolepine   (S. acuta, cordifolia, rhombifolia, spinosa, and ?)

386-rats-10 to 40 mg/kg bw i.p.-Analgesic activity was also exhibited by cryptolepine through a dose-related (10–40 mg/kg i.p.) inhibition of writhing induced by i.p. administration of acetic acid in mice-compared to indomethacin (10 mg/kg).

Pain, Antinociceptive   inhibits the sense of pain

Stimulation of sensory nerve cells called nociceptors produces a signal that travels along a chain of nerve fibers via the spinal cord to the brain. Nociception triggers a variety of physiological and behavioral responses and usually results in a subjective experience of pain in sentient beings. [1]

Sida acuta

203-mice/rats-whole plant?-aqueous acetone extract-we obtained 13.42% yield for S. acuta-the oral administration of the aqueous acetone extracts from S. acuta produced significant inhibition of the acetic acid-induced abdominal writhing in dose-dependent manner. This inhibition was lesser than that produced by paracetamol.,

Sida cordifolia

30-mice-leaves- ethanol extract>chloroform CF>methanol fractions MF--a pronounced antinociceptive activity on orofacial nociception- significantly reduced the orofacial nociceptive behavior with inhibition percentage values of 48.1% (100 mg/kg, CF), 56.1% (200 mg/kg, CF), 66.4% (400 mg/kg, CF), 48.2 (200 mg/kg, MF) and 60.1 (400 mg/kg, MF),   **116**-rats-aerial parts-80% ethanolic extract-significant antinociceptive activity   **203**-mice/rats-whole plant?-aqueous acetone extract-we obtained 13.42% yield for S. acuta-the oral administration of the aqueous acetone extract from S. cordifolia produced significant inhibition of the acetic acid-induced abdominal writhing in dose-dependent manner. This inhibition was lesser than that produced by paracetamol.,

Sida rhombifolia

144-rats-leaf-95% ethanol extract-30/100/300 mg kg-1 body weight all doses of the extract, administered intraperitoneally, exhibited significant (p<0.05) antinociceptive and anti-inflammatory activities in a dose-dependent manner,   **149**-rats-ethanolic extract-leaves-IP-30mg/kg wt+-works in dose dependent manner,   **185**-leaves-ethyl acetate extract-200mg/kg,   **194**-rats-whole plant?-80% acetone extract-100/200/400 mg/kg bw- extracts produced significant analgesic effects in acetic acid writhing and hot plate method (p≤0.05) and in a dose-dependent inhibition was observed,   **545**-mice-aerial parts-80% ethanol extract-acetic acid-induced writhing model 43.84% and 69.95% writhing inhibition at the dose of 250 and 500 mg/kg bw-comparable to diclofenac sodium where inhibition was 82.27% at the dose of 25 mg/kg bw,

Sida rhomboidea
185-invitro-leaf-ethyl acetate extract-200 mg/kg bw-has shown significant (P<0.01) antinociceptive activity.

Other Sida
499-Sida urens-mice-aerial parts-80% acetone extract-Acetic acid-induced writhing test- significant analgesic effects in acetic acid-induced writhing method and in a dose-dependent inhibition was observed -200 mg/kg bw dose had stronger effect than 100 mg/kg bw dose of Paracetamol, **552-Sida tiagii**-rats-fruit-ethanolic extract>n-hexane extract/ethyl acetate extract-ethanol extreact-200 mg/kg and 500 mg/kg-produced dose dependent antinociceptive activity in two thermal models for nociception,

Parasites, Anthelmintic
A group of antiparasitic drugs that expel parasitic worms (helminths) and other internal parasites from the body by either stunning or killing them and without causing significant damage to the host. [1]

Sida acuta
Tr 3-India-leaf juice, 6-Ayurveda, 7-Burkina Faso/Italy-worms, 7-Central America, 7-South America, 8-Guatemala, 9-Nicaragua, 21-Siddha (Tamil)-leaves, 82-India, 85-India-ringworm, 88-Bengal, 93-Italy/Burkina Faso-leaves, 101-Nicaragua-decoction of the entire plant-anti-worm medication, 101-Nicaragua-the decoction of the entire plant is taken orally, 107-India-leaves, 107-Nicaragua, 168-Nicaragua-decoction of the entire plant taken orally, 174-India-intestinal worms, 186-India, 201-leaves-review from Ghana-ringworm, 220-Nicaragua/Guatemala, 223-India, 270-India-root, 271-Nicaragua-entire plant-taken orally-antiworm medication, 361-Phillipines/Indo-China- decoction of the leaves and roots-expelling intestinal worms, 362-Phillipines/Indo-China- decoction of the leaves and roots-expelling intestinal worms, 523-India-leaves, 568-Nigeria-commonly used for GI parasitic infections-leaves used as an antihelminthic, 571-India-intestinal worms, 580-India-whole plant-ethanol extract, 596-Nigeria-leaf/root, 646-Nigeria-leaves and stem, 653-Ayurveda, 523-India-leaves, 571-India-intestinal worms, 646-Nigeria-leaves and stem, 653-Ayurveda,

Sida cordifolia
146-invivo-Pheretima posthuma (worm)-whole plant-R>E>A extracts—ethanol extract-10 mg/ml bw-kill time 34 min—acqueous extract-10 mg/ml bw-kill time 30 min—Albendazole-26 mg/ml bw-kill time 30 min-possesses potent antioxidant and anthelmintic activity,

Tr 93-Italy/Burkina Faso-leaves, 358- Senegal, Côte d'Ivoire, Burkina Faso, Burundi, Kenya, Papua New Guinea and the Philippines- a leaf decoction is drunk for control of intestinal worms, 437-Ayurveda-bark,

Sida rhombifolia
Tr 377-Ayurveda-roots, 437-Ayurveda-bark, 587-Bangladesh-stems and roots-ringworm,

Sida cordata
497-worms- Pheretima posthuma-stem/leaf-all extracts 5 mg/ml bw--aqueous extract-kill time=148min—ethanol extract-kill time=160min—Albendazole-kill time=135min--the aqueous extract of stem exhibited a significant anthelmintic activity effect over other extracts at the given experimental concentrations. Dose dependent activity was observed in both leaf and stem extracts but leaves extract showed more significant activity than stem extracts. **Tr** 437-Ayurveda-bark

Sida indica
Tr 437-Ayurveda-bark-anthelmintic, 452-Bangladesh-for various types of worm infections, 454-India-bark, 678-Ayurveda-bark, 708-Ayurveda-bark, 710-Ayurveda-bark, 711-Chinese-bark and root, 712-India-stem bark, 712-India-seeds-rectum of children affected with thread worms, 735-Ayurveda-review-bark,

Sida schimperiana
Tr 631-Ethiopia-Dried root and leaf powder are mixed with water and drunk before breakfast for 3 days,

Cryptolepine
(S. acuta, cordifolia, rhombifolia, spinosa, and ?)

172-invitro-presents antiparasitic properties, **245**-cryptolepine-mice-50 mg/kg bw/day-parasitaemia was suppressed by 80.5% of that of the untreated control animals. However, with chloroquine diphosphate at 5 mg/kg/day parasitaemia was suppressed by 93.5%.

Parasitic protozoa, Malaria

A number of protozoan pathogens are human parasites, causing diseases such as malaria (by Plasmodium), amoebiasis, giardiasis, toxoplasmosis, cryptosporidiosis, trichomoniasis, Chagas disease, leishmaniasis, African trypanosomiasis (sleeping sickness), amoebic dysentery, acanthamoeba keratitis, and primary amoebic meningoencephalitis (naegleriasis). **[1]** Malaria, by far the most important tropical parasite, causes an estimated annual 2.7 million deaths among the 300–500 million people suffering from the disease per year. Africa accounts for over 90% of reported cases, with an annual 20% increase of malaria-related illness and death. Malaria is responsible for as many deaths per annum as AIDS for all of the last 15 years. Drug resistance to malaria has become one of the most significant threats to human health and the search for new effective drugs is urgent. **[244-2001]**

Sida acuta
Antimalarial 4-invitro-Culex quinquefasciatus, Aedes aegypti and Anopheles stephensi, **12**-invitro-whole plant?-extract?-$IC_{50}<5$ µg/ml- was related to its alkaloid contents-Plasmodium falciparum, **19**-invivo-whole

248

plant?-water decoction/ethanol extract-two chloroquine-resistant strains-Plasmodium falciparum FcM29-Cameroon and a Nigerian chloroquine-sensitive strain-IC50 values obtained for these extracts ranged from 3.9 to -5.4 microg/ml, **20**-invitro- its alkaloid contents-Plasmodium falciparum-IC50< 5 microg/ml, **108**-invitro-multidrug resistant (K1) strain of Plasmodium falciparum- highly active with an IC50 value of 0.031±0.0085 (SE) µg/mL, equivalent to 0.134±0.037 µM (n = 3), **214**-invitro-complementary treatment for malaria, **220**-review, **252**-invivo-acqueous extract+ethanolic extract- FcM29-Cameroon (chloroquine-resistant strain) and a Nigerian chloroquine-sensitive strain-antiplasmodial-IC50 values 3.9 to −5.4 µg/ml, **354**-invivo-leaf-?extract-synthesized silver nanoparticles-larvicidal-bet use of S. acuta synthesized silver nanoparticles can be a rapid, environmentally safer biopesticide which can form a novel approach to develop effective biocides for controlling the target vector mosquitoes. This is the first report on the mosquito larvicidal activity of the plant aqueous extract and synthesized nanoparticles, **463**-leaf and root-methanol extract-showed significant antiplasmodial activity-showed markedly significant antimalarial activity and antivectorial activity effects even at low concentrations-Phytochemical screening revealed the presence of some vital insecticidal and antiplasmodial constituents such as terpenoids, flavonoids and alkaloids-showed higher mortality against mosquito larvae-lethal dose Lc50,

Larvicidal 77-invitro (imbrued with silver nanoparticles, with Artemisia annua)-The LC50 and LC90 values of S. acuta aqueous leaf extract appeared to be most effective against A. stephensi (LC50, 109.94 µg/mL and LC90, 202.42 µg/mL) followed by A. aegypti LC50 (119.32 µg/mL and LC90, 213.84 µg/mL) and C. quinquefasciatus (LC50, 130.30 µg/mL and LC90, 228.20 µg/mL), **253**-invitro-leaf-aqueous extract-silver nanoparticles extracted from S. acuta leaf-Synthesized AgNPs against the vector mosquitoes of A. stephensi, A. aegypti, and C. quinquefasciatus had the following LC50 and LC90 values: A. stephensi had LC50 and LC90 values of 21.92, and 41.07 µg/mL; A. aegypti had LC50 and LC90 values of 23.96, and 44.05 µg/mL; C. quinquefasciatus had LC50 and LC90 values of 26.13 and 47.52 µg/mL. These results suggest that the use of S. acuta synthesized silver nanoparticles can be a rapid, environmentally safer biopesticide,

Tr 7-W Africa, 12-BurkinaFaso, 19-W Africa, 20-Burkina Faso, 76-W Africa, 88-BurkinaFaso-Ivory Coast-Mexico, 93-Italy/Burkina Faso-leaves, 107-Nigeria-leaf decoction, 203-Burkina-Faso-children, 219-Nigeria-leaf usually used, 220-Nigeria, 221-India-leaf, 224-Nigeria, 252-Ivory Coast, 264-Nigeria, 273-Nigeria, 485-Nigeria-survey, 568-Nigeria, 588-Nigeria, 594-Nigeria-stem, 596-Nigeria-leaf/root, 609-India, 619-Malaysia,

Sida cordifolia
Tr 76-W Africa, 93-Italy/Burkina Faso-leaves, 203-Burkina-Faso-children, 224-Nigeria, x619-Malaysia,

Sida rhombifolia

74-stem-?extract-larvicidal, 522-review-The pharmacological activities reported include antimalarial activity, 540-invivo-leaves-80% cold methanolic extract-hydro alcoholic extracts of Sida rhombifolia showed a very good activity against the P berghei malaria parasite-400 mg/kg bw-parasitemia = 26.1%-percentage of inhibition = 52.3%--Chloroquine at 10 mg/kg bw-parasitemia = 0- percentage of inhibition = 100%, 605-[cited by 522] The methanol-water extract (1:1) of dried fruit of the plant was reported to have antimalarial activity against Plasmodium berghei at 100 µg/ml, while the ethanol/water extract (50%) showed weak antimalarial activity against the same strain at 1 gm/kg for 4 days treatment. 606-[cited by 522] Valsaraj found that the ethanol-water extract (1:1) exhibited antimalarial activity against Plasmodium berghei at the dose of 10µg/ml and poor antimalarial activity at the dose of 1 gm/kg.

Tr 150-Ethiopia-root decocted, 522-India-root-aqueous extract-orally, 619-Malaysia,

Sida spinosa Tr 11-BurkinaFaso-whole plant-anti-malarial-frequently and widely used, 619-Malaysia,

Cryptolepine (S. acuta, cordifolia, rhombifolia, spinosa, and ?)

73-invitro-antiparasitic, 73-neocryptolepine-invitro-antiparasitic, 108-invitro-multidrug resistant (K1) strain of Plasmodium falciparum- highly active with an IC50 value of 0.031±0.0085 (SE) µg/mL, equivalent to 0.134±0.037 µM (n = 3), 172-invitro-presents antiparasitic properties, 244--invitro—cryptolepine--the crystal structure of this antimalarial drug–DNA complex provides evidence for the first nonalternating intercalation and, as such, provides a basis for the design of new anticancer or antimalarial drugs, 245-cryptolepine-mice/invitro-(strain K1)-orally-50 mg/kg/day-parasitemia was suppressed by 80%-similar activity to that of chloroquine, 247-invitro-the data suggest that all cryptolepine compounds and in particular 2,7-dibromocryptolepine cause DNA damage and therefore may not be suitable for pre clinical development as antimalarial agents, 251-invitro- this compound appears to intercalate with DNA and this may explain the high degree of antimalarial activity demonstrated in vitro, 252-invivo-acqueous extract+ethanolic extract- antiplasmodial-IC50 values 3.9 to −5.4 µg/ml, 308-invitro-bind tightly to DNA and behave as typical intercalating agent- The poisoning effect is more pronounced with cryptolepine-Cryptolepine-treated cells probably die via necrosis rather than via apoptosis, cryptolepine-mice/invitro-(strain K1)-orally-50 mg/kg/day-parasitemia was suppressed by 80%-similar activity to that of chloroquine, 309-review-Neocryptolepine, 396-invitro-DNA damage-treatment of mammalian cells with cryptolepine can lead to DNA damage-cryptolepine did not appear to be mutagenic in the dosage range used (up to 2.5 µM, equivalent to 1.1 µg/ml)-after 24 h treatment of V79 cells cryptolepine induced a dose-dependent increase in micronuclei, 247-invitro- this compound appears to intercalate with DNA and this may explain the high degree of antimalarial activity demonstrated in vitro.

250

Parasitic protozoa, Other   Tr   no reported use

Cryptolepine   (S. acuta, cordifolia, rhombifolia, spinosa, and ?)
309-review-Neocryptolepine-antitrypanosomal-against unicellular parasitic flagellate protozoa causing sleeping sickness and Chagas disease,   **309**-review-Neocryptolepine-antileishmanial-disease   caused   by   protozoan parasites, **309**-review-Neocryptolepine-antischistosomal - parasitic flat-worms responsible for a highly significant group of infections in humans.

Poison, Alexeritic   No peer review
A substance to counteract infection or poison.   [http://www.ebbd.info/pharmacological-dictionary.html]

Sida acuta   Tr   221-India-leaf-poisoning,   224-Nigeria,

Sida cordifolia   Tr   437-Ayurveda-roots-remove poison,

Sida rhombifolia   Tr   437-Ayurveda-roots-remove poison,

Sida cordata   Tr   437-Ayurveda-roots-remove poison,

Sida indica

Tr   437-Ayurveda-root,   437-Ayurveda-root bark-alexteric,   437-Ayurveda-roots-remove poison,   454-India-bark,   678-Ayurveda-bark, 708-Ayurveda-bark,   710-Ayurveda-bark,   712-India-stem bark,   735-Ayurveda-review-bark,

Poison, Neutralizes poison

Sida acuta

10-mice-whole plant-ethanolic extract-partial protection from Bothrops atrox venom-anti-lethal effect-devoid of antiphospholipase A2 activity-when tested against one minimum indirect hemolytic dose of B. atrox venom (2 microg) in agarose-erythrocyte-egg yolk gels,   **206**-mice-Partial protection from Bothrops atrox venom -whole plant,

snake bite   Tr   3-India-whole plant,   6-Ayurveda,   7-Columbia,   10-Colombia,   88-Ayurveda-scorpion bites,   186-India- traditional healing for snakebites,   206-Colo9mbia,   214-India-chronic wound and poisonous bite, 220-W Columbia,   220-BurkinaFaso-insect bites,   220-Nigeria-whole plant or leaves-poisoning,   221-W Colombia,   223-India,   358-review,   361-snake bites,   428-India- scorpion and snake bites,   568-Nigeria-snake bite, 601-Nigeria-root and leaves-with black pepper are ground and applied locally in snake bite,   653-Ayurveda,

Sida cordifolia   Tr   568-Nigeria-snake bite,

Sida rhombifolia

Tr   150-Ethiopia-flowers-stings and bites of scorpion, snake and wasp, 278-Ethiopia-flowers-used for treating stings and bites of scorpion, snake and wasp,   361-Philippines and Indonesia-flowers-applied to wasp stings, 362-review-Philippines and Indonesia-flowers-wasp stings,   522-Madagascar-aerial parts-The hot aqueous extract of dried aerial parts are used for snake bite in East Africa,   522-East Africa-hot aqueous extract-dried aerial parts-snake bite,   522-India-leaf juice mixed with sesame oil for the treatment of snake bite,   522-Peru-snake bite,   524-Phillipines-flowers-wasp stings,   524-Phillipines-fresh leaves-emollient-scorpion stings,   545-Bangladesh-stems-mucilage for scorpion stings,

Sida spinosa

Tr   358-Kenya- leaves are chewed and the sap is swallowed after a snakebite,   568-Nigeria-antidote for snake bite,   595- India-leaves-powder (external use)- scorpion bite,

Sida indica   Tr 712- India-leaves-Antidote for the treatment of snakebite

Other Sidas   Tr   527-Sida retusa-Poultice of leaves used for insect bites,   568- Sida ovata Forssk-Nigeria-snake bite,

Reproduction, Abortifacient

A substance that induces abortion [1]

Sida acuta

Tr   6-India,   21-Ayurveda,   23-Ayurveda,   52-India-hot water extract of the dried entire plant,   88-Gold Coast,   96-gold Coast,   101-India, 107-India,   109-Africa-leaves,   138-Ayurveda-whole plant-hot water extract,   168-India-dried entire plant-hot water extract,   219-Nigeria-leaf usually used,   220-Nigeria,   224-Nigeria,   270-Africa-leaves,   271-India-hot water extract of the dried entire plant-taken orally,   273-Nigeria, 358-S acuta- Gold Coast-leaves,   362-Borneo, Vietnam and Central Africa, the leaves or roots are used as an abortifacieant,   609-India,   653-Ayurveda,

Sida cordifolia

Tr   358-Central African Republic and in Kenya the root extract is drunk to induce abortion,   362-Borneo, Vietnam and Central Africa, the leaves or roots are used as an abortifacieant,

Sida rhombifolia

Tr   358-roots and leaves (DR Congo) or the leaves alone (Gabon) are used as an abortifacieant,   362-Borneo, Vietnam and Central Africa, the leaves or roots are used as an abortifacieant,   522-Borneo/Central Africa-entire plant-hot aqueous extract-used as an abortifacieant when it is taken orally by pregnant women--eaten by pregnant women during third or fourth month of pregnancy in Borneo for abortion,   522-Central Africa-root-aqueous extract, 524-Borneo,

Sida spinosa   Tr   362-Borneo, Vietnam and Central Africa, the leaves or roots are used as an abortifacieant,

Other Sidas

157- **Sida cardifolia**-mice-sterile distilled water extract-500mg/kg wt-% fertility on female mice for control, 500 mg/kg and 1000 mg/kg were 100%, 20 % and 33.33% respectively.-no abnormalities in either case-produced mainly abortifacieant activity and antiimplantation activity,   **345, 550-Sida veronicaefolia** -rats- Oral doses producing the abortifacieant effects were 32 ml/kg bw when administered from the 15th–17th day of pregnancy

Tr   138- Sida carpinifolia-India-whole plant-hot water extract,   362-Sida indica-Borneo, Vietnam and Central Africa, the leaves or roots are used as an abortifacieant,   754-Sida linifolia-Côte d'Ivoire-contraceptive,   631-Sida schimperiana-Ethiopia-Fruit are tied around forehead.

Reproduction, Anti-fertility

Infertility is the inability of a person, animal or plant to reproduce by natural means. It is usually not the natural state of a healthy adult organism. **[1]**

Sida acuta

96-invitro-leaf-95% ethanolic extract-50 and 100 mg/kg bw-was found to be most effective in causing significant antiimplantation activity-the adverse effects on fertility are reversible upon withdrawal of the extract treatment is observed.

Tr   6-Ayurveda,   82-India,   223-India,   653-Ayurveda.

Sida cordifolia   157-rats-water extract-500mg/kg wt.

Sida carpinifolia

138-rats-Antifertility activity of indigenous plants Sida carpinifolia Linn- **186**-The plant is reported to have antifertility activity,   **178**-rats-anti fertility activity-no abstract but cited frequently.

Other Sida

157- Sida cardifolia-mice-sterile distilled water extract—Percentage of fertility-control=100%,   500   mg/kg=23%,   1000   mg/kg=33%-no abnor-malities in either case-produced mainly abortifacieant activity and antiimplantation activity.

Tr   568-Sida linifolia Juss. ex Cav-Côte d'Ivoire-contraceptive.

Reproduction, Aphrodisiac No peer review

Sida acuta   **Tr** 21-Ayurveda-root,   88-Mohammadans,   107-India-roots,   217-Ayurveda,   270-India-root,   561-Ayurveda-root,

Sida cordifolia

Tr 40-Brazil,   53-Ayurveda,   88-Ayurveda-seeds,   118-Ayurveda-seeds, 120-Colombia,   124-India-roots,   125-India,   127-Ayurveda,   167-Ayurveda-seeds,   312-USA-Ayurveda-roots/leaves/stems/seeds-induce/promote aphrodesia,   312-Brazil,   362-review-Malaysia-seeds, 437-Ayurveda-seeds,   444-Ayurveda-Bala-Vrushya-natural aphrodisiac, 561-Ayurveda-root,   664-Ayurveda,

sexual strength   **Tr** 118-Ayurveda,   124-India-seeds as general tonic, 217-Ayurveda-expressed juice of whole plant,   664-Ayurveda-whole plant?-extract,

Sida rhombifolia

Tr 47-India-leaf-infusion,   407-Ayurveda-seeds,   437-Ayurveda-seeds, 522-Ayurveda-roots and leaves,   522-India-entire plant-hot aqueous extract-orally-aphrodisiac,   522-Ayurveda-dried leaf and root-hot aqueous extract,   545- Bangladesh-leaves and roots,   561-Ayurveda-root,

Sida cordata   **Tr** 437-Ayurveda-seeds,   496- Pakistan-Siddha and Ayurveda-roots,

Sida indica   **Tr** 678-Ayurveda-seeds or root and bark,   711-Ayurveda-root and bark, or seed,   712-India-stem bark or seeds,

Sida spinosa   **Tr** 561-Ayurveda-root,

Reproduction, During labor

Sida acuta

652- -rats-leaf-ethanol extract-the extract at .4 ug/ml had a 92% rise in amplitude, adrenaline at .4 ug/ml had a 92% rise in amplitude, Oxytocin at 20ug/ml had a 114% rise in amplitude, and Acetylcholine at .40 ug/ml had a 150% rise in amplitude,

Tr 88-Assam,   107-Nigeria-leaf infusion,   201-roots-review from Ghana-dystocia (obstructed labor),   305-Nigeria,   588-Nigeria-hasten delivery,   609-India,   646-Nigeria-leaves and stem- also used by traditional birth attendants (TBAS) to quicken delivery,

Sida rhombifolia

Tr 257-Phillipines-Leaf decoction is given to mothers during delivery to relieve muscle pain. Crushed leaves are massaged on painful muscles,   361-

Philippines and Indonesia-flowers-eaten with wild ginger to ease labor pains, 361-Fiji and Papua New Guinea-leaves-labor pains,   362-review-Philippines and Indonesia-flowers-eaten with wild ginger to ease labor pains,   362-review-Fiji and Papua New Guinea-leaves-labor pains,   522-Ayurveda-roots-In Assam the roots are taken internally to help child birth-The herb is also tied round the abdomen for the same purpose,   522-Ayurveda-leaf and root-decoction-orally to facilitate child birth,   522-Nicaragua-leaf-decoction-taken orally,

Sida indica   Tr   451-Thailand-seed-puerperal disease,   711-India-seed-puerperal disease,

Sida veronicaefolia   Tr   550-a fraction from an alcoholic extract of Sida veronicaefolia, previously reported to be a potent oxytocic,

Reproduction, estrogenic activity

A chemical having estrogenic activity mimics human estrogen, by binding to the cell's normal estrogen receptor location. **[808]**   Tr   **no reported use**

Sida acuta

96-rats-leaf-ethanol extract- possesses estrogenic activity, the imbalance caused in progesterone and estrogen levels might be the reason for interruption of pregnancy. Withdrawal of these treatments to adult rats has resulted in normal reproductive activities,   313-vascine-different species of animals-It was observed that the uterotonic effect of vasicine was influenced by the degree of priming of the uterus by estrogens (known to enhance the synthesis of prostaglandins in the uterus) and it was markedly reduced after pretreatment of the uterus with aspirin and indomethacin. This indicated that the uterotonic effect of vasicine was at least partly mediated through the release of prostaglandins,

Sida cordifolia

313-vascine-different species of animals-It was observed that the uterotonic effect of vasicine was influenced by the degree of priming of the uterus by estrogens (known to enhance the synthesis of prostaglandins in the uterus) and it was markedly reduced after pretreatment of the uterus with aspirin and indomethacin. This indicated that the uterotonic effect of vasicine was at least partly mediated through the release of prostaglandins,   608-rats-aerial parts?-whole plant as food-appeared to contain estrogen-like activity which could have induced an increase in uterine weight as well as induced vaginal opening in the plant-fed rats- appear insufficient to cause peripheral eosinophilia as well as eosinophilic uterine infiltration.

Sida rhombifolia

313-vascine-different species of animals-uterotonic activity was similar to that of oxytocin and methyl ergometrine, It was observed that the uterotonic effect of vasicine was influenced by the degree of priming of the uterus by estrogens (known to enhance the synthesis of prostaglandins in the uterus) and it was markedly reduced after pretreatment of the uterus with aspirin and indomethacin. This indicated that the uterotonic effect of vasicine was at least partly mediated through the release of prostaglandins,

Sida indica

681-rats-whole plant-80% ethanol extract with distilled water- possesses significant and potent anti-estrogenic activity as it presented significant and positive results in both of the test methods used in the evaluation...only the 400mg/kg body weight dose had significantly reduced all the investigated serum hormones significantly ($p < 0.05$) compared to the control group. The administration of the extract at a dose of 100 mg/kg body did not produce any significant change ($p > 0.05$) in the concentration of the three hormones (follicle stimulating hormone, estrogen and progesterone). However, with administration of the extract at a dose of 200mg/kg of body weight, the concentrations of estradiol and progesterone were reduced significantly, while for administration at a dose of 400 mg/kg, there was a significant reduction in the levels of the three hormones under investigation

Reproduction, Female sexual problems

Sida acuta   **237**-invitro-leaf-water extract-strong bactericidal effect on vaginal candidiosis-Staphylococcus aureus SS-1VC, Staph. aureus SS-2VM,

Tr 6-Ayurveda-female disorders, 106-Cameroon-female infertility,   223-India-female disorders,   358-S acuta- Gold Coast-whole plant possesses antifertility activity,   653-Ayurveda- female disorders,

Sida cordifolia

Tr 43-Brazil,   61-Brazil-blenorrhea,   88-Brazil,   120-Columbia, 153-Brasil,   154-Brazil,   161-Brazil,   312-Brazil,   358- Central African Republic and Kenya-bark-chewed to encourage menstruation,   437-Ayurveda-leaves-decoction-vaginal infections.

Sida rhombifolia

Tr   47-India-urogenital diseases,   136-India-stem and root-sexual disorders,   524-Phillipines-pulped roots applied to sore breasts,   596-Nigeria-leaf/root/seed-urogenital disorders,

Vaginal infections Tr 437-Ayurveda-leaves-decoction,   522-Guinea-leaf juice-in vagina as an antiseptic,

Irregular menstruation   Tr   522-Malaysia-whole plant?-hot aqueous extract is used for irregular menstruation when taken orally by adult females, 522-Peru-leaf-emmenagogue-stimulates vaginal bleeding,   524-Phillipines-roots-decoction-any plant part-irregular menses

Sida cordata   **Tr** 437-Ayurveda-leaves-decoction-vaginal infections

Sida indica

Tr 437-Ayurveda-seeds- gleets, 678-Ayurveda-seeds-gleets, 708-Ayurveda-seed-in treatment of gleets,

Tr vaginal infections 437-Ayurveda-leaves-decoction, 451-Thailand-leaf extract, 448-Ayurveda-Menorrhoea, 684-Ayurveda-leaf juice-Menorrhoea, 711-India-leaf?, 735-Ayurveda-review-seeds, 737-India-seeds-infusion in water,

Sida spinosa
Tr 55-India-leaves-bruised in water and the filtrate is administered-gleets, 99-India-leaf, 433-India-gleets,

Sida linifolia

Tr 358- Côte d'Ivoire-aerial parts-women-cure for uterine fibroma-noncancerous growths of the uterus that often appear during childbearing years.

Reproduction, Leucorrhoea

A thick, whitish or yellowish vaginal discharge. [1]   **No peer review**

Sida acuta
Tr 29-Ayurveda, 107-Ayurveda, 107-India-roots,

Sida cordifolia
Tr 53-Ayurveda, 124-India-root bark, 127-Ayurveda, 218-Ayurveda, 362-review-Malaysia-root bark powder-with milk and sugar, 167-Ayurveda-root-Root powder is given with cow milk,

Sida cordata
Tr 293-Ayurveda-root bark, 496-Pakistan-Siddha and Ayurveda, 549-Ayurveda, 603-Himalayas-root bark,

Reproduction, Low or no sperm

Sida acuta

Tr 201-leaf-review from Ghana- azoospermia (man with no measurable level of sperm in his semen)-oligospermia (low sperm concentration in the semen), 217-Ayurveda- augments the seminal fluids.

Sida cordifolia
Tr 217-Ayurveda-augments the seminal fluids, 541-Siddha-seminal weakness, 543-Ayurveda-seminal weakness.

Sida linifolia
Tr 358-Côte d'Ivoire-whole plant-is considered as a cure for male sterility, 568-Côte d'Ivoire-male sterility-Nigeria.

Other Sida

Tr 407-Sida retusa-Ayurveda-seeds-spermatic tonics, 444-Ayurveda-Sida indica-Shukra Vruddhikari-Increases quality and quantity of semen.

Cryptolepine   (S. acuta, cordifolia, rhombifolia, spinosa, and ?)

247- invitro-the above results suggest that cryptolepine and the analogues cause some DNA damage in lymphocytes but appear to have no effect on human sperm,   **389**-rats-small doses of cryptolepine (3.0×10-7-10-6M) - Contractions of the vas deferens (among others) push fluids into the prostatic urethra. The semen is stored here until ejaculation occurs. During ejaculation, the smooth muscle in the walls of the vas deferens contracts reflexively, thus propelling the sperm forward. This is also known as peristalsis. The sperm is transferred from the vas deferens into the urethra, collecting secretions from the male accessory sex glands such as the seminal vesicles, prostate gland and the bulbourethral glands, which form the bulk of semen,

Reproduction, Male sexual problems
No peer review

Sida acuta   **Tr**   107-Ayurveda-spermatorrhea,

sexual impotence   **Tr**   3-India-decoction of leaves and roots,   106-Cameroon,   201-root or shoot-Ghana-male impotence,   220-SriLanka, 238-Sri Lanka-roots and leaves,   270-India-leaf/root tea,   361-Indo-China and Philippines-leaves and roots-impotency,   362-review-Indo-China and Philippines-leaf/root-decoction,   526-Phillipines-Decoction of roots and leaves-taken internally

testicular swellings   **Tr**   107-juice of the leaves is boiled in oil,   109-Siddah -juice of the leaves is boiled in oil,   361-India-leaves-are boiled in oil and applied to testicular swellings,   362-review-India-leaves-boiled in oil and applied to testicular swellings,

Sida cordifolia

Tr 53-Ayurveda-juice of whole plant-premature ejaculation, 218-Ayur-vedic-juice of whole plant-premature ejaculation,

Spermatorrhea   **Tr**   88-Ayurveda-juice of roots,   118-Ayurveda-Juice of the whole plant pounded with a little water is given in doses of ¼ seers, 127-Ayurveda-diuretic spermatorrhoea,   358-Malaysia- The juice of the whole plant pounded with a little water,   362-review-Malaysia-whole plant-juice pounded with a little water,   537-India,   596-Nigeria-leaf/root/seed, 167-Ayurveda-whole plant-water extract,   664-Ayurveda-whole plant-pounded with a little water-juice-doses of ¼ seers,

Sida rhombifolia

Tr   47-India-urogenital diseases,   136-India-stem and root-sexual disorders,   522-India-leaf-juice-orally-spermatorrhea,   596-Nigeria-leaf/root/seed-uro-genital disorders,

Sida linifolia   **Tr**   568-sexual impotence-Nigeria,

258

Reproduction, Miscarriage

Herbal plants used as a remedy against threatened miscarriage... The alkaloid, saponins, resins, flavonoids content of these plants mainly control the miscarriage without any side effects as they are of natural products. So the proper conservation of such precious medicinal plants is required for future use as these are in a verge of extinction due to various environmental constraints. **[230]** Sida L. has been used for centuries in traditional medicines in different countries for the prevention and treatment of... childbirth and miscarriage problems. **[609]**

Sida acuta

230-leaf-boiled leaves-Cook the leaves to a boiling point. Allow to cool very well-One tumbler 3 times daily-the alkaloid, saponins, resins, flavonoids content of these plants mainly control the miscarriage without any side effects as they are of natural products, **Tr** 609-India-miscarriage,

Sida cordifolia **Tr** 27-Burkina-Faso-leaf decoction-used to prevent miscarriage,

Sida rhombifolia **Tr** 522-the stem of the plant in Rotuma is chewed for dental hygiene and the infusion is used for prevention of miscarriage,

Sida indica **Tr** 451-Thailand-seeds-any bacterial infection of the female reproductive tract following miscarriage.

Reproduction, Pregnancy No peer review

Sida acuta

Tr 305-Nigeria-Bleeding after delivery-Oral consumption of juice extracted from squeezed leaves, 358-S acuta- Gold Coast-leaves when bruised are shiny and are put on the hands of midwives when they are about to remove dead children from the womb.

Sida cordifolia **Tr** 217-Ayurveda-boosts fetal growth, 521-Ayurveda-root-postpartum weakness,

Sida indica

Tr 201-review-Ghana-prenatal care, 451-Thailand-seeds-any bacterial infection of the female reproductive tract following childbirth or miscarriage, 601-Nigeria-leaf-decoction of the leaves is given for diarrhea during pregnancy,

Other Sidas

Tr 131-Sida retusa-Ayurveda-promotes reproduction, 603-Sida cordata-Himalayas-leaf-given to pregnant women to treat diarrhea, 358-Sida linifolia-Kenya-women chew the root bark daily during pregnancy to ease the expulsion of the placenta, 568- Sida ovata Forssk-Nigeria-placenta expellant-chew the root bark daily during pregnancy,

Reproduction, Uterine disorders

Sida acuta

313-vascine-different species of animals-Its uterotonic activity was found to be similar to that of oxytocin and methyl ergometrine, **315**-invitro-vasicine-exhibited marked uterine stimulant activity, **652**-rats-leaf-ethanol extract-uterine stimulant--in-vitro Contractile Effects on Isolated Uterine Rats--The extract at .4 ug/ml had a 92% rise in amplitude-adrenaline at .4 ug/ml had a 92% rise in amplitude--Oxytocin at 20ug/ml had a 114% rise in amplitude--Acetylcholine at .40 ug/ml had a 150% rise in amplitude.

Sida cordifolia

313-vascine-different species of animals-Its uterotonic activity was found to be similar to that of oxytocin and methyl ergometrine, **315**-invitro-vasicine-exhibited marked uterine stimulant activity, **608**-rats-aerial parts?-whole plant as food- caused a significant increase in the uterine weight (p<0.05)

Tr   437-Ayurveda-roots-uterine disorders,

Sida rhombifolia

313-vascine-different species of animals-Its uterotonic activity was found to be similar to that of oxytocin and methyl ergometrine, **315**-invitro-vasicine-exhibited marked uterine stimulant activity,

Tr   437-Ayurveda-roots-uterine disorders,

Sida cordata   **Tr**   437-Ayurveda-roots-uterine disorders,   496-Pakistan-Siddha and Ayurveda,   549-Ayurveda-uterine disorders,

Sida indica

Tr   437-Ayurveda-root-uterine disorders,   454-India-roots-uterine hemorrhagic discharges,   710-Unani-roots-used in uterine hemorrhagic discharges,   712-India-roots-uterine hemorrhagic discharge,   712-India-leaves-uterus displacement,

Sida linifolia   **Tr**   358-review-a cure for uterine fibroma,

Sanity, Delirium   No peer review

An organically caused decline from a previously baseline level of mental function. It often has a fluctuating course, attentional deficits, and disorganization of behavior. Delirium itself is not a disease, but rather a set of symptoms. [1]

Sida cordifolia   Tr   118-Ayurveda-bark-insanity,   118-Ayurveda-fits,   167-Ayurveda-root-insanity,   200-India-delirium,

Sida cardifolia   Tr   200-Ayurveda-whole plant-delirium,

Skin, Abscess   No peer review
A collection of pus that has built up within the tissue of the body. Signs and symptoms of abscesses include redness, pain, warmth, and swelling. [1]

Sida acuta   Tr   361-review-Flowers-abscesses-Flower tops or crushed leaves used as lotion for abscesses.

Sida rhombifolia
Tr   47-Camaroon and Madagascar-abscess and furuncle,   358-Africa-leaves or leaf sap,   522-Madagascar-leaf-juice externally applied,   522-Guatemela-dried leaf-hot aqueous extract-externally,   524-Phillipines-fresh leaves-poultice-to promote maturation of abscesses,

Sida linfolia   Tr   358- Togo- leaf pulp is applied to abscesses,
Plants have a limitless ability to synthesize aromatic substances, most of which are phenols or their oxygen substituted derivatives such as tannins. Many of the herbs and spices used by humans to season food yield have useful medicinal compounds including those having antibacterial activity. [556]

Skin, Astringent   No peer review
A chemical compound that tends to shrink or constrict body tissues. [1]

Sida acuta

Tr   3-India-root,   52-India-whole plant-hot water extract,   107-India,   217-Ayurveda,   270-India-root,   275-Colombial-astringent,   361-review-roots,   377-Ayurveda-root,   596-Nigeria-leaf/root,   644-Ayurveda-root,

Sida cordifolia
Tr   29-Ayurveda,   53-Ayurveda,   88-Ayurveda-root bark,   118-Ayurveda-roots,   161-Ayurveda,   217-Ayurveda,   285-Ayurveda-root,   312-USA-Ayurveda-root bark,   361-Mauritius,   377-Ayurveda-root,   437-Ayurveda-bark,   664-Ayurveda,

Sida rhombifolia   Tr   524-Phillipines-roots,   377-Ayurveda-root,   437-Ayurveda-bark,

Sida cordata   Tr   293-Ayurveda-roots,   437-Ayurveda-bark,   496-Pakistan-Siddha and Ayurveda-roots,

Sida indica
Tr   377-Ayurveda-root,   437-Ayurveda-bark-astringent , 452-Bangladesh, 678-Ayurveda-bark,   708-Ayurveda-bark,   712-India-stem bark,   735-Ayurveda-review-bark,

Skin, Boils   No peer review
A deep infection of the hair follicle. It is most commonly caused by infection by the bacterium Staphylococcus aureus, resulting in a painful swollen area on the skin caused by an accumulation of pus and dead tissue. [1]

Sida acuta   Tr   85-India-with lemon juice,   88-Konkan,   596-Nigeria-leaf/root,

Sida cordifolia   Tr   437-Ayurveda-leaves,

Sida rhombifolia
Tr   47-Camaroon-furuncle,   51-India-whole plant?,   437-Ayurveda-leaves, 522-Madagascar-leaf- The leaves are applied to boils,   522-Honduras-roots and leaves-poultice-applied externally on boils,   522-Nepal-whole plant?-juice-externally applied,   522-India-leaf paste-topically-applied externally, 522-Guatemela-dried leaf-hot aqueous extract-externally-furuncle,   524-Phillipines-whole plant?-poultice,

Sida cordata   Tr   437-Ayurveda-leaves,   497-India-whole plant-root paste is applied on boils khateera to take out pus (Panthi.M.P et al., 2009),

Sida indica   Tr   437-Ayurveda-leaves-flowers-boils,   452-Bangladesh-carbuncle,   737-India-leaves-flowers-eaten raw,

Skin, Cooling   No peer review
{Not sure what these entries refer to, but they all come from India. Cooling can be physical or an Ayurvedic process. Also have put other terms here: refrigerant, burning sensations. If you can clarify this, I would appreciate it.}

Sida acuta   Tr   52-India-whole plant-hot water extract,   644-Ayurveda-root,

Sida cordifolia   Tr   118-Ayurveda-roots,   444-Ayurveda-Bala-Sheetala-Coolant,   664-Ayurveda-bark,

lack of perspiration   Tr   32-Ayurveda,   118-Ayurveda,   161-Ayurveda,

Sida cordata   Tr   293-Ayurveda-flower and ripe fruits-refrigerant,

Sida rhomboidea

Tr 520-India-burning sensations-(had no specific ref to where burning), 522-Ayurveda-roots and leaves-burning sensations-(had no specific ref to where burning),

Sida spinosa **Tr** 55-India-leaves-bruised in water and the filtrate is administered, 433-India-refrigerant,

Skin, Diaphoretic/Sudorfic   No peer review

(chiefly of a drug) inducing perspiration [738]

Sida acuta

Tr 3-India-root, 21-Ayurveda-root, 137-leaf-Guatemala, 217-Ayurveda, 270-India, 361-Indo-China and Philippines-roots-diaphoretic, 362-Phillipines-roots, 644-Ayurveda-root-diaphoretic,

Sida cordifolia   **Tr** 32-Ayurveda-lack of perspiration,

Sida rhombifolia   **Tr** 136-India- root and leaves, 524-Phillipines, 545-Bangladesh-both diaphoretic and sudorific.

Skin, Emollient   No peer review

Moisturizer. Chemical agents specially designed to make the external layers of the skin (epidermis) softer and more pliable. [1]

Sida acuta

Tr 3-India-decoction of leaves and roots, 88-Ayurveda-leaves, 137-leaf-Guatemala, 361-emollient, 526-Phillipines-Decoction of roots and leaves, 601-Nigeria-leaf,

Sida cordifolia   **Tr** 53-Ayurveda, 118-Ayurveda, 127-Ayurveda, 664-Ayurveda,

Sida rhombifolia

Tr 47-India-stems, 51-India-stem, 358-Africa-roots and leaves, 377-Ayurveda, 522-Ayurveda-stems-The stems are abound in mucilage and are employed as demulcent and emollients both for external and internal use, 522-Madagascar-whole plant?- Madagascar the plant is mostly used as an emollient, 524-Phillipines-fresh leaves, 524-India-roots, 545-Bangladesh-stems-abound in mucilage, 596-Nigeria-leaves, 710-China-seeds,

Sida indica

Tr 711-Chinese-seed, 712-India-seeds, 737-India-whole plant-juice-applied as an emollient to relieve soreness of the nates in young children,

Sida retusa   **Tr**   527-Stems-for external and internal use,

Skin, Rashes and Inflammation

A change of the human skin which affects its color, appearance, or texture. The causes, and treatments for rashes, vary widely. **[1]**   **No peer review**

Sida acuta

Tr   358-Subcutaneous Cellular Tissue Disorders,   358-Soap, leaves, leafy stems/branches: Leaves and young shoots rubbed in water give a lather which may be used for shaving, especially in the case of a tender and irritable skin, 609-India-skin ailments,

Sida cordifolia   Tr   437-Ayurveda-roots-leucoderma,   664-Ayurveda-
crushed leaves-poultice-imperfections of the skin,

Sida rhombifolia

Tr   51-India-leaf,   150-Ethiopia-leaf,   361-Philippines and Indonesia-a paste of the leaves mixed with coconut oil applied to scurf and itch,   358-Africa-leaves or leaf sap-antiseptic,   362-review-Philippines and Indonesia-leaf-paste-mixed with coconut oil is applied to scurf and itch,   437-Ayurvedic-roots-leucoderma,   522-Guatemela-dried leaf-hot aqueous extract-externally-dermatitis,   524-Phillipines-plant parts-with coconut oil-applied externally for itches.

Sida cordata   Tr   437-Ayurveda-roots-leucoderma,

Other Sidas

Tr   358-Sida linfolia-Togo-leaf sap-skin rash caused by chickenpox, Leucoderma, also known as vitiligo, is a rare skin disease characterized by white spots and patches,   437-Ayurveda –S. indica-India-roots-leucoderma.

Skin, Skin beauty   No peer review

Bala is associated with Parvathi, the ancient Hindu goddess of beauty and grace. The herb is part of a trio of "beautifying" herbs, together with ashoka and shatavari, associated with women in Indian herbal folk medicine. **[2]**

Sida acuta   Tr   88-Ayurveda-juice of roots,

Sida cordifolia

Tr   2-Ayurveda-"beautifying" herb,   118-Ayurveda-imperfections of the skin,   379-Ayurveda-recommended for beautifying women,   444-Ayurveda-Bala-Kantivardhaka-improves skin texture and glow,

Sida indica   **Tr**   444-Ayurveda-Kantivardhaka-improves skin texture and glow,

Skin, Skin disease   No peer review

Sida acuta

Tr   52-India-whole plant-hot water extract,   107-India,   214-India, 220-India,   221-India,   264-Nigeria-skin infections,   270-India-root, 609-India-skin ailments,   646-Nigeria,   **Eczema:**   **Tr**   5-Togo, 88-Trininad & Tobago-leaf,   220-Togo,   221-India-leaves,

Sida cordifolia   **Tr**   125-India-crushed leaves,

Sida rhombifolia

Tr   47-India,   126-Colombia,   150-Ethiopia-stem-skin diseases and sores, 150-Ethiopia-leaf,   358-Africa-leaves or leaf sap-antiseptic,   522-Central Africa-dried leaf-infusion

Sida urens   **Tr**   535-Nigeria-leaves-decoction-skin infections,

Sida linifolia   **Tr**   568-treat skin diseases-Nigeria.

Skin, Sores   No peer review

Sida acuta

Tr   3-India-whole plant,   107-Philllipines-leaves as poultices,   109-Siddah-leaves as poultices,   221-India-leaf,   526-Phillipines-Poultices made from boiled leaves are applied to sores.

Sida cordifolia   **Tr**   167-Phillipines,

Sida rhombifolia

Tr   150-Ethiopia-stem,   358-Africa-leaves or leaf sap-antiseptic,   522-Madeira-flower-decoction-cleansing open sores,   522-Guatemela-dried leaf-hot aqueous extract-externally-skin eruption,   568-Nigeria-lumps,

Sida ovata   **Tr**   568- Sida ovata Forssk-Nigeria,

Skin, Lessens Perspiration   No peer review

Sida cordifolia   **Tr**   437-Ayurveda-bark-to lesson perspiration,

Sida rhombifolia   **Tr**   437-Ayurveda-bark-to lesson perspiration,

Sida cordata Tr 437-Ayurveda-bark-to lesson perspiration,

Skin, Wound healing

Sida acuta has been known to be medicinally important in many respects. However, this study has revealed that the leaves of Sida acuta have several active agents that are inhibitory to microorganisms. The significant activity of the ethanolic extract against microorganisms from infected skin, confirms their traditional usefulness in the cure of wound infections. **[102]**

Sida acuta

102-invitro-leaf-absolute ethanol and aqueous extracts-1000 mg/ml-has better ZI than gentamicin against B. subtilis and S aureus,   **104**-rats-whole plant?-methanol extract-The results showed that methanolic extract ointment possesses a definite prohealing action-comparable to nitrofurazone,   **237**-leaf-water extract-strong bactericidal effect on-septic wounds,

Tr 3-India-fresh juice of roots,   21-Siddha (Tamil)-leaves,   21-Ayurveda-root,   107-India-leaves,   214-India-the leaf extract combined with turmeric,   217-Ayurveda-juice of roots,   219-Nigeria-leaf usually used-wound infections,   220-Nigeria,   221-India-leaf,   234-Nigeria,   273-Nigeria-wound infection,   508-India-leaf paste,   561-Ayurveda-fresh juice of root,   597-India-root,   599-India-root-wound healing,   601-Nigeria-leaf-crushed leaves are applied over wounds, fresh cuts and bruises.

Sida cordifolia

25-rats-whole plant-ethanol-ointment-effectively stimulates wound contraction; increases tensile strength of excision, incision and burn wounds,

Tr 53-Ayurveda-root juice-unhealthy sores,   88-Konkan,   88-Ayurveda-seeds,   118-Ayurveda-root juice-Root juice is also used to promote healing of wounds,   120-Colombia (flavenoids),   124-India-apply pounded leaves on cuts,   124-India-root juice-wound dressing,   125-India-crushed leaves,   127-Ayurveda-root juice-unhealthy sores,   161-Ayurveda-used in bleeding disorders,   167-Ayurveda-Root decoction-mixed with ginger is effective in healing of wounds,   200-India-used in bleeding disorders,   218-Ayurveda-root juice-unhealthy sores,   277-Ayurveda-fracture healing-leaf paste along with egg yolk,   358-review-The powdered whole plant is applied to open wounds of horses in Niger,   537-India,   561-Ayurveda-fresh juice of root,   596-Sida pilosa-Nigeria-leaves-cuts,   597-India-root,   599-India-root-wound healing,   601-Nigeria-leaf-crushed leaves are applied over wounds, fresh cuts and bruises,   664-Ayurveda-crushed leaves-poultice-external wounds,   664-Ayurveda-root-juice-promote healing of wounds,

Sida rhombifolia

Tr 47-Camaroon and Madagascar-antiseptic, wound-healing activities,   51-India-whole plant?-cuts,   150-Ethiopia-root and leaf-skin bleeding,   150-Ethiopia-leaf and stem bark-treatment of wound,   150-Ethiopia-leaf-cuts and wounds, 358-Africa-leaves or leaf sap-antiseptic, 522-review- The infusion of dried leaf of S. rhombifolia in Central Africa is used for diabetes, chest pain and diarrhea on oral administration. The infusion of this plant is applied locally for the treatment of skin diseases and infected wounds, 561-Ayurveda-fresh juice of root, 596-Nigeria-leaves,

Sida cordata Tr 498-India, 603-Himalayas-leaf-Poultice applied to cuts & bruises,

Sida indica Tr 451-Thailand-leaf extract-wound cleaning, 684-Ayurveda-leaf juice-wound cleaning, 737-India-seeds-decoction-fistula,

Sida spinosa Tr 561-Ayurveda-fresh juice of root, 597-India-root, 599-India-root-wound healing,

Other Sidas Tr 595-Sida mysorensis-India-leaves-powder (external use)-healing wounds, 596-Sida pilosa-Nigeria-leaves,

Sleep, Sleeping time Tr no reported use

Sida acuta
275-mice-leaves and stems-100% ethanolic extract-500 and 1000 mg/kg-reduced the latency time (T1) and increased the sleeping time (T2) induced by pentobarbital, indicating a sedative and hypnotic effect of the plant's extract, **362**-review-ephedrine-decrease of the sensation of fatigue and the need to sleep, and thus qualitatively it resembles an amphetamine, **500**-invitro-root- significantly potentiation of phenobarbitone sodium-induced sleeping which indicate general depression of central nervous system,

Sida rhombifolia
128-mice-root-crude aqueous extract-5gm/kg weight-increased sleeping time 50%, **362**-review-ephedrine-decrease of the sensation of fatigue and the need to sleep, and thus qualitatively it resembles an amphetamine,

Sida retusa
362-Sida retusa/Sida indica/Sida rhomboidea-review-ephedrine-decrease of the sensation of fatigue and the need to sleep, and thus qualitatively it resembles an amphetamine, **529**-Sida retusa-mice-root-crude extract-5 gm/kg bw-the crude extract produced a sedative effect, characterized by a decrease in alertness, wakefulness and reactivity. The crude extract of Sida retusa root produced a significant potentiation of the pentobarbitone sleeping time in mice,

Sida cordifolia, Sida cordata, Sida rhomboidea, Sida spinosa
362-review-ephedrine-decrease of the sensation of fatigue and the need to sleep, and thus qualitatively it resembles an amphetamine,

Soap

Saponins possess the unique property of precipitating and coagulating red blood cells. **[687]**

Sida acuta

120-aerial parts-aqueous and hydroalcoholic extracts-good source of saponins with diverse chemical structures, mainly of steroidal nature, some of which may be hecogenin, diosgenin or a homologue, **559**-invitro-seed-the saponifiable fraction was found to have oleic, linoleic, palmitic, stearic, myristic and plamitoleic acids, whereas the unsaponifiable fraction contained β-amyrin, β-sitosterol and an unknown waxy nonsteroidal substance,

Tr 358-Soap, leaves, leafy stems/branches: Leaves and young shoots rubbed in water give a lather which may be used for shaving, especially in the case of a tender and irritable skin, 361-soap,

Sida rhombifolia **Tr** 358- Gabon and Kenya-leaves-soap, 367-review-Gabon and Kenya-leaves-used as a soap-substitute,

Soil, Rejuvenates degraded soil **Tr** no reported use

One of the cheapest, environmentally friendly methods for cleaning an environment polluted by heavy metals is phytoextraction. It builds on the uptake of pollutants from the soil by the plants, which are able to grow under conditions of high concentrations of toxic metals. **[623]** Apart from cleaning the substrate of the excess elements, the cultivation of Sida hermaphrodita had a positive effect on the granulometric composition of the sludge. Before the experiment, the sludge was an amorphous muddy mass, in which no structures typical of soil were stated. After 3 years of cultivation of Sida, aggregates of various size started to appear in the sludge. The fraction of 1-0.1 mm prevailed in the substrate (75-83% in the vegetative propagation and 81-87% in the generative one)... The up-to-date research indicate that the cultivation of *Sida hermaphrodita* on sewage sludge makes it possible not only to improve the physicochemical properties of this waste material, but can also be a source of renewable energy. **[472]**

Sida acuta

112-invitro- suitable for phytostabilization of Cr, Cd and Zn in cement-polluted soil while Cr and Cd can be phytoextracted from cement-polluted soil, **231**- Sida acuta can survive up to 1150 mg of zinc contamination per kg of soil respectively. This ability reveals the great potential of using it in stabilizing and recolonizing soils heavily polluted with zinc, **419**-invivo-plantations on degraded land-soil improvement, **657**-invivo-whole plant-tolerated the 1150 mg Zn kg-1 soil level, **670**-invitro-aerial parts or roots-survived in a soil polluted with hydrocarbons in a former refinery-tolerated Benzene, toluene, xylen, polysyclic aromatic hydrocarbons, tetraethyl lead, methyl tert-butyl ether.

Sida hermaphrodita

472-Sida hermaphrodita-invivo-whole living plant-The up-to-date research indicate that the cultivation of Sida hermaphrodita on sewage sludge makes it possible to improve the physicochemical properties of this waste material, **473**-invivo-whole living plant-those poor areas most often were excluded from cultivation for a long time, usually transformed into waste, margin land. Virginia fanpetals is one of the perennial species adjusted to over ten years of cultivation tolerant to quality of soil, **482**-invitro-whole living plant-highest tolerated level of soil contamination-top accumulator of Cadmium, lead, nickel, copper, and zinc, **484**-Conclusions: No regular influence of soil contamination with heavy metals on the contents of studied elements was found out. Under the influence of soil pollution with heavy metals the uptake of Mg, Na, K, Ca and Mn decreases, **623**-invitro-absorbed high levels of zinc, lower levels of lead, copper, and nickel, and absorbed cadmium at least-can successfully be grown on moderately contaminated soil with heavy metals, **629**-field experiment/invitro -can be used for phytoremediation (phytoextraction) of heavy metals contained in sewage sludge,

Toxicity, Low/no toxicity   Tr   no reported use

{See below for the other side of the story, Toxic to living things} Pharmacological substances whole LD50 is less than 5 mg/kg body weight are classified in the range of highly toxic substances, those with a LD50 between 5 mg/kg body weight and 5000 mg/kg body weight are classified in the range of moderately toxic substances and those with the lethal dose is more than 5000 mg/kg body weight not toxic 8. **[194,499]**

Sida acuta

60-the very weak toxicity values are interesting features which can securize the use of Sida acuta and Sida cordifolia in the traditional medicine of Burkina Faso. The low toxicity, evidenced by LD50 values, suggests a wide margin of safety for therapeutic doses. The extracts have no significant negative effect on biological parameters. Moreover we obtained good analgesic results by testing the two species aqueous acetone extracts against animal model. Both findings justify the therapeutic use of these plants in folk medicine of Burkina Faso, **76**-rats/mice-whole plant?-aqueous acetone extract-The low toxicity, evidenced by LD50 values (3.2 g/kg), suggests a wide margin of safety for therapeutic doses. The extracts have no significant negative effect on biological parameters, **96**-rats-No toxic effect was observed, **100**-rats-whole plant?- 80% aqueous acetone- The low toxicity evidenced by LD50 value (3200 mg/kg bw by ip injection) suggests a wide margin of safety for therapeutic doses. In sub-acute study, some effects were observed but there were no relevance of serious signs or significant changes in animal weights, effect of extract on animal organs and biochemical parameters. Briefly, these toxicity studies suggest that the extract of Sida alba is safe, **128**-mice-root-crude acqueous extract-no toxicity-15 g/kg.-72 hours -no excitement, convulsions, tremors or mortality, **186**-rats-whole plant-ethanol-Acute oral toxicity studies revealed that the extract was safe up to a

269

dose level of 2000 mg/kg of body weight (limit test) and LD50 is more than 2000mg/kg. No lethality or any toxic reactions or moribund state were observed up to the end of the study period,   **203**-mice/rats-aqueous acetone extract-LD50 value of 3.2 g/kg -The low toxicity, evidenced by LD50 values, suggests a wide margin of safety for therapeutic doses,   **427**-field-fresh plant-Ecuador- Grazing sida produced no signs of nutrient imbalance or toxicity in the cattle,   **460**-rats-whole plant-70% ethanol extract- The acute toxicity studies showed that there was no mortality in the animals administered up to a dose level 2000mg/kg bw,   **464**-mice/rats, invitro-80% methanol extract, 530-rats-leaves-ethanol extract-500 mg kg-1 bw-extract may not impair liver and kidney functions,   **571**-invitro-whole plant-ethanolic extract-LD50 is more than 2000mg/kg. No lethality or any toxic reactions or moribund state were observed up to the end of the study period, **651**-invitro-leaves-ethanol extract-The subjection of ethanol extract of Sida acuta to the acute toxicity studies showed the extract to be safe (non-toxic) up to 5000 mg/kg,   **679**-rats-root-ethanolic extract-No mortality or toxicity was observed up to 5000 mg/kg. Hence, extract was found to be safe,

Sida cordifolia

27-invitro-whole plant?-80% acetone extract>chloroform extract for alkaloid compounds- the value of LD50 was: 3.4 g/kg. The results of this study indicated that the extract of Sida cordifolia are low poisonous. During the 14 day period of acute toxicity evaluation, some signs of toxicity were observed, but they were all quickly reversible,   **32**-mice-root-40% ethanol extract-acute toxicity LD50 is more than a dose of 3 g/ kg,   **41**-mice-leaves-hydroalcoholic extract-low toxicity was observed in mice,   **42**-rats-water infusion?- infusions (up to 1 mg/ml) showed no toxic effects on the viability of PC12 cell line as judged by MTT-test,   **43**-mice-leaf-water extract-400 mg/kg bw-showed low acute toxicity,   **48**-rats-leaves-alcoholic extract-LD50>3000mg/kg weight,   **61**-rats-water extract-leaf-low acute toxicity, **60-**the very weak toxicity values are interesting features which can securize the use of Sida acuta and Sida cordifolia in the traditional medicine of Burkina Faso. The low toxicity, evidenced by LD50 values, suggests a wide margin of safety for therapeutic doses. The extracts have no significant negative effect on biological parameters. Moreover we obtained good analgesic results by testing the two species aqueous acetone extracts against animal model. Both findings justify the therapeutic use of these plants in folk medicine of Burkina Faso,   **76**-rats/mice-whole plant?-aqueous acetone extract-The low toxicity, evidenced by LD50 values (3.4 g/kg), suggests a wide margin of safety for therapeutic doses. The extracts have no significant negative effect on biological parameters,   **122**-rats-safe up to 2000 mg / kg body weight,   **123**-rats-ethanolic extract-At concentrations ranging from 25 mg/ml to 1 mg/ml of plant infusions, no toxic effect on the cell growth was observed,   **132**-mice-leaf-70% ethanol extract- a low toxicity was observed in mice-toxic at high doses administered (i.p.). The LD50 values were 2639 mg/kg with 95% confidence limits of 2068–3367 mg/kg for i.p. administration. Deaths were not observed among orally treated animals. **133**-mice-No adverse effect or mortality at 4 g/kg, p.o., for any extract during the 24 h observation period,   **152**-invitro-seed oil-petroleum ether (40-

270

600C) extract-no toxicity at 2000 mg/kg bw, **154**-mice-acqueous extract-leaves-the aqueous extract of S. cordifolia showed low acute toxicity in mice, **159**-rats-leaves-petroleum ether+methanol-5 g/kg bw safe, **161**-Ayurveda-root extract-used for all kinds of detoxification like medicated enema, **163**-rats-petroleum ether+methanol extract-leaves-nontoxic at 5gm/kg wt, **171**-rats-water extract-aerial parts-400mg/kg wt-can be used safely in medicinal practices without causing toxicity, **177**-rats-no effect at 5000 mg/kg, **180**-rats-aerial parts-methanolic extract-5gm/kg wt, **203**-mice/ rats-aqueous acetone extracts-The low toxicity, LD50 @ 3.4g/kg, suggests a wide margin of safety for therapeutic doses, **211**-mice-low toxicity-quickly reversible, **218**-review-recently it has been banned due to reported hepatotoxicity (injurious to the liver)-animal experiments however report hepatoprotective effect of Sida cordifolia, **591**-rats-whole plant-70% ethanol extract-The mortality rate was found nil and the herbal extract was found safe up to a dose level of 5000 mg/kg body weight,

Sida rhombifolia

47-invitro- methanolic extracts and water and methanol (1v:4v), (1v:1v), (3v:2v) extracts- Some toxic effects were found when rats received more than 8 g/kg bw of extract. For the acute toxicity study, no deaths of rats were recorded. However, significant increase of some biochemical parameters such as aspartate amino-transferase (AST), alanine aminotransferase (ALT), alkaline phosphatase (ALP) and creatinine (CRT) were found. The pathological examinations of the tissues on a gross basis indicated no detectable abnormalities at the end of the experiment. According to the OCED protocol S. rhombifolia extract can be classified as non toxic since the limited dose of an acute toxicity is generally considered to be 5.0 g/kg bw-This last result confirms that kidneys are slightly affected at the dose of 16 g/kg body weight of the extract, **126**-invitro-leaf-aqueous extracts were practically non-toxic (CL50 >1,000 ppm), suggesting that they can be safely used in infusions, **128**-mice-crude extract of root-nontoxic to 15mg/kg, **132**-mice-leaf-70% ethanol extract- a low toxicity was observed in mice-toxic at high doses administered (i.p.). The LD50 values were 2639 mg/kg with 95% confidence limits of 2068–3367 mg/kg for i.p. administration. Deaths were not observed among orally treated animals, **136**-rats-root-acqueous and ethanolic extracts-no toxicity to 2gm/kg, **147**-rats-root-water extract-oral administration at 5000 mg/kg bw for 90 days-did not cause acute or subchronic toxicities, **170**-invitro-water and methanolic extracts-low toxicity (LD50 >3 g/kg), **186**-rats-whole plant-ethanol-Acute oral toxicity studies revealed that the extract was safe up to a dose level of 2000 mg/kg of body weight (limit test) and LD50 is more than 2000mg/kg. No lethality or any toxic reactions or moribund state were observed up to the end of the study period, **192**-rats- aqueous acetone extract-No mortality was observed even at the highest dose of 6 g/kg (the value of LD50 is greater than 5000 mg/kg)-but was not without toxicity implication, **194**-mice-LD50 > 5000 mg/kg-aqueous acetone extract (SRE) no mortality at 400 mg/kg,-any toxicity is quickly reversed, **197**-rats-roots-aqyeiys extract-LD50 > 500 mg/kg, **199**-rats-root-methanolic extract @2000mg/kg wt not toxic, **427**-field study-fresh plant- no signs of nutrient imbalance or toxicity in the cattle,

540-mice-aerial parts-methanolic extract-exhibited safety profile at tested doses of 500 to 2000 mg/kg bw,   **541**-rats-roots-90% ethanolic extract-there was no mortality up to the dose of 3.2 g/kg body weight even after 7 days.

Sida retusa

435-rats-roots-crude water extract-5/10 gm/kg bw- did not have any protective effect against amphetamine or leptazol-induced toxicity,   **529**-mice-root-crude extract-nontoxic at 15 g/kg did not have any protective effect against amphetamine or leptazol-induced toxicity,

Sida cordata

177-rats-whole plant-ethanolic extract-5gm/kg wt,   **405**-rats-whole plant-+90%ethanol extract-LD50 of the test drug was found to be greater than 2000mg/kg,   **549**-leaves-95% (v/v) ethanol extract-produces no mortality at 2 000 mg/kg,

Sida indica

440-rats-whole plant?-acqueous extract- Acute toxicity studies revealed that the LD50 value is more than the dose of 4 g/kg body wt.,   **440**-rats-whole plant?-water extract-exhibited significant hepatoprotective activity-against carbon tetrachloride- and paracetamol-induced hepatotoxicities,   **443**-rats-leaves-methanol extract-Acute oral toxicity-safe at limit dose 2500 mg/kg and 5000 mg/kg with no mortality in studied subjects. 1/10th of these doses i.e. 250 mg/kg and 500 mg/kg were used in the subsequent study respectively,   **449**-mice/sheeps's blood-leaves (flowering stage)-distilled water extract (4000 mg/kg bw/day) and ethanolic extract (2000 mg/kg bw) were safe that dose with no mortality in studied subjects respectively,   **451**-rats-leaves,twigs, and roots-acqueous extract-5 g/kg not toxic,

Sida rhomboidea

280-rats-leaves-water extract-5 gm/kg bw,   **286**-mice-leaf-water extract-Oral administration of SR extract for 28 days did not induce any mortality with doses of 750, 1500 and 3000 mg\kg body weight-1500/3000 mg/kg bw-decrement in food intake and body weight gain,

Sida spinosa

100-rats-whole plant?- 80% aqueous acetone-the low toxicity evidenced by LD50 value (3200 mg/kg bw by ip injection) suggests a wide margin of safety for therapeutic doses. In sub-acute study, some effects were observed but there were no relevance of serious signs or significant changes in animal weights, effect of extract on animal organs and biochemical parameters. Briefly, these toxicity studies suggest that the extract of Sida spinosa is safe, **434**-rats-roots-ethanolic and acqueous extracts—non-lethal--Acute toxicity study revealed that animals showed good tolerance (up to 4000 mg/kg b.w) to single doses of ethanolic and aqueous extracts. Both extracts produced no noticeable effect on general behavior or appearance of the animals and all rats survived during and after the test period.,

Sida tiagii

551-rats?-fruit-95% ethanolic extract>n-Hexane Extract and ethyl acetate extract-5000 mg/kg-no deaths, **552**-mice-fruit-ethanolic extract>n-hexane extract/ethyl acetate extract-The filtrate was partitioned with n-hexane (n-hexane extract, HS) and ethyl acetate (ethyl acetate extract, the oral and *i.p.* LD50 in mice was found to be greater than 500 mg/kg.

Other Sidas

177- **Sida cardifolia**-rats-whole plant-ethanolic extract-5gm/kg wt, **490**-**Sida tuberculata**-leaves and roots-water and ethanol crude extracts-low toxic potential on A. salina-LD50 >1000 µg/mL, **499**-**Sida urens**-mice-aerial parts-acetone/water extract-LD50>5000 mg/kg-The results of the present study indicated that the extract of Sida urens is not poisonous. During the 14 day period of acute toxicity evaluation, some signs of toxicity were observed, but they were all quickly reversible

Toxicity, Protection from toxic metals

Sida rhombifolia

538-rats-root-ethanol extract- The current study was carried out with the aim to investigate the... possible protective role of Sida rhombifolia root on cadmium chloride (CdCl2) induced changes in body weight in Wistar rats... negative effect of cadmium chloride on body weight was significantly (P• 0.05) ameliorated by Sida rhombifolia. L root extract in a dose dependent manner. The protective effect of Sida rhombifolia. L root might be attributed to the antioxidant elements present in it.

Toxicity, Toxic to living things

{For a detailed study of the Sida acuta/Sida carpinfolia toxicity conundrum, see the section in **Sida as Weed/ Toxicity-Sida carpinfolia**} **Tr no reported use**

Sida acuta

213-brine shrimp-leaf+shoot- methanol+chloroform/methanol/chloroform extract (LC50 99.4 µg/ml) exhibited marked levels of toxicity-can cause acute or chronic toxicities when consumed in large quantities or over a long period of time, **274**-invitro-leaf-the high concentration of anti-nutrients in Sida acuta Burn.f. obtained from this locality might cause health hazard if consumed in large quantity over a long period of time, **362**-review-The water soluble portion of the alcoholic extract of Sida acuta exerts spasmodic action on the smooth muscle preparations of ileum, trachea, uterus and heart of experimental animals. Thus, the activity of the extract is similar to that of acetylcholine, **530**--rats--leaf--ethanol extract-->100 mg/kg bw--not-with-standing that Sida acuta extract may not impair liver and kidney functions, possible effects on fluid and electrolyte balance should be seriously monitored,   **531**-rats-leaf-ethanolic extract-The effect of the extract in the kidney electrolytes after the administration revealed that the extract of Sida acuta has adverse effect on the electrolytes of the kidney at the dose administered to the rats. In view of the above reports, it can be concluded that ethanolic extract of Sida acuta may be toxic when administered at a dose of 200mg/kg bw to Wistar rats,   **572**-rats-distilled water/ethanolic extract-200 mg/kg bw-In this study, the observed reduction and elevation in the activity of ALT, AST and ALP in the administered animals is indicative of the fact that the extract has an adverse effect on the liver enzymes as it is reported that below normal values of liver enzymes may suggest liver dysfunction or insufficient protein intake...100mg/kgbw-showed slight difference in their hepatic architecture. Nuclei were not prominent, but the overall integrity of the cells where maintained as compared to the control-200mg/kgbw-a distorted morphological features showing shrunken sinusoid, dilatation of the central vein and non prominent nuclei-it can be concluded that ethanolic extract of Sida acuta is toxic when administered at a dose of 200mg/kgbw to Wistar rats,

Sida acuta var. carpinfolia

{please refer to the section, **Toxicity-The Sida carpinfolia conundrum**, in the chapter, **Sida as Weed**, for the full story on this.}

242-in vivo-goats-aerial parts-poisonous to goats,   **418** -leaves- cattle - force-fed to five cattle at doses of 10 and 20 g/kg for 120 days, 40 g/kg for 30 days, and 30 and 40 g/kg body weight for 150 days. One animal died and the others were euthanatized at the end of the experiment. Clinical signs and lesions varied from mild to severe in the experimentally poisoned cattle and depended on dose and length of the period of consumption. It is concluded that ingestion of even small amounts S. carpinifolia for prolonged periods of time cause lisosomal storage disease in cattle,   **621**-invivo-goats-swain-sonine toxicosis and inherited mannosidosis-A neurologic disease characterized by ataxia, hypermetria, hyperesthesia, and muscle tremors of the head and neck,   **624**-invivo/invitro-sambar deer- The poisoning was characterized by emaciation and neurologic signs followed by unexpected death in some of the animals. Animals presented abnormal consciousness, posterior paresis, and musculoskeletal weakness; less evident were vestibulo-cerebellar signs. Histologically, there was vacuolation of neurons and epithelial cells of the pancreatic acines, thyroid follicules, and renal tubules. Furthermore, in the central nervous system were axonal degeneration, necrosis, and loss of neurons,   **625**-invivo/invitro- fallow deer (Dama dama)- a neurological syndrome characterized by muscular weakness, intention tremors, visual and standing-up deficits, falls, and abnormal behavior and posture,   **626**-invivo/invitro-pony horses-fatal-included multiple cytoplasmatic vacuoles in swollen neurons in the brain, cerebellum, spinal cord, autonomic ganglia (trigeminal and celiac ganglia), and submucosal and myenteric plexus of the intestines. In the kidneys, there was marked vacuolation of the proximal convoluted tubular cells,   **627**-invitro-The indolizidine alkaloid swainsonine has been identified as the toxic constituent-the swainsonine concentration was 0.006% on a dry weight basis, **628**-Saanen goats-typical of poisoning caused by plants of this group and were seen from the 37th day until seven days after withdrawal of the plant, when signs gradually became scarce and less evident, **629**-invivo/invitro-cattle-poisoning-no complete recovery,

Sida cordifolia

{Sida cordifolia by far has the most ephedrine of any Sida} **118**-review-when used excessively can cause ephedrine related side effects like insomnia, anxiety, nervousness, and increase in blood pressure, memory loss or even stroke. Ephedrine coupled with caffeine can prove fatal. Patients using MAO inhibitor medication (Antidepressants), having high blood pressure, heart disease, thyroid or prostrate condition along with pregnant or lactating women should not take this herb except under expert guidance, **378**-review-use cautiously in patients with heart disease, including arrhythmia, coronary artery disease, cerebrovascular disease, and a history of stroke or transient ischemic attack, due to potential side effects from the ephedrine constituent in bala. Use cautiously in patients using other energizing and diet supplements that may contain ephedrine, due to the potential for additive negative effects. Avoid use in patients taking ergot alkaloids and cardiac glycosides, due to the risk of irregular heart beat. Avoid in pregnant or breastfeeding women, due to a lack of available scientific evidence,

Tr   118-Ayurveda-Oil preparation-Gritha cures Heart diseases,

Sida rhombifolia

47-rats- methanolic extracts and water and methanol (1v:4v), (1v:1v), (3v:2v) extracts- Some toxic effects were found when rats received more than 8 g/kg bw of extract. For the acute toxicity study, no deaths of rats were recorded. However, significant increase of some biochemical parameters such as aspartate amino-transferase (AST), alanine aminotransferase (ALT), alkaline phosphatase (ALP) and creatinine (CRT) were found. The pathological examinations of the tissues on a gross basis indicated no detectable abnormalities at the end of the experiment. According to the OCED protocol S. rhombifolia extract can be classified as non toxic since the limited dose of an acute toxicity is generally considered to be 5.0 g/kg bw, **358**-Leaves-Toxic to stock---Reported that in Australia fowls are sometimes killed by eating the ripe carpels. The sharp points irritating the digestive canal and causing inflammation (Maiden, undated cited in Standley, 1920-1926) **427**-invivo-Ecuador- Grazing sida produced no signs of nutrient imbalance or toxicity in the cattle.

Other Sidas

205-Sida tiagii-India-fruit-95% ethanolic extract>n-Hexane extract>ethyl-acetate extract-LD50 2100mg/kg bw when ip-no toxicity at 5g/kb when op-behavioral toxic limit may be 200-500 mg/kg bw, **348-S. veronicaefolia**-mice-leaves-This study was carried out on the basis of OECD 423 guidelines, both extracts were non toxic up to 5000mg/kg hence the LD50 was 5000mg/kg and 1/10 LD50 was selected as dose for the study. **620-Sida rodrigoi Monteiro**-goats-toxic levels of swansonine were identified in the plant-poisoning as a plant induced α-mannosidosis animals showed weight loss, indifference to the environment, unsteady gait and ataxia,

Cryptolepine   (S. acuta, cordifolia, rhombifolia, spinosa, and ?)

{**Note:** Cryptolepine is toxic when isolated, but is not toxic in concentrations found in the plant.}

247-invitro-the data suggest that all cryptolepine compounds and in particular 2,7-dibromocryptolepine cause DNA damage and therefore may not be suitable for pre clinical development as antimalarial agents-on account of its toxicity, cryptolepine is not suitable for use as an antimalarial drug, **380**-invitro-Cryptolepine easily crosses the cell membranes and accumulates selectively into the nuclei rather than in the cytoplasm of B16 melanoma cells, **396**-invitro-DNA damage-treatment of mammalian cells with cryptolepine can lead to DNA damage- cryptolepine did not appear to be mutagenic in the dosage range used (up to 2.5 μM, equivalent to 1.1 μg/ml)-after 24 h treatment of V79 cells cryptolepine induced a dose-dependent increase in micronuclei,

Venereal Disease, Gonorrhea   No peer review

{See peer-review Neisseria gonorrhoeae in **Pathogens**}

At least three people worldwide are infected with totally untreatable "superbug" strains of gonorrhea which they are likely to be spreading to others through sex, the World Health Organization (WHO) said on Friday. Giving details of studies showing a "very serious situation" with regard to highly drug-resistant forms of the sexually-transmitted disease (STD), WHO experts said it was "only a matter of time" before last-resort gonorrhea antibiotics would be of no use.   **[July, 2017 742]**

Sida acuta

Tr   88-Portuguese-demulcent in gonorrhea,   107-Ayurveda,   107-India-in gonorrhea,   201-shoot-review from Ghana,   217-Ayurveda,   219-Nigeria-leaf usually used,   220-Nigeria,   220-SriLanka-Decoction also used as demulcent for gonorrhea,   221-India-leaf,   224-Nigeria,   238-Sri Lanka-roots and leaves,   273-Nigeria,   601-Nigeria-root bark-mixed with sugar and milk is taken orally,

Sida cordifolia

Tr   53-Ayurveda,   88-Cambodia-diuretic in gonorrhea,   88-Ayurveda-seeds,   116-Bangladesh,   118-Ayurveda-Juice of the whole plant pounded with a little water is given in doses of ¼ seers,   124-India-seeds,   151-Ayurveda, 158-India,   167-Ayurveda-root,   167-Ayurveda-seeds,   167-Ayurveda-whole plant-water extract,   180-India,   182-India,   217-Ayurveda, 218-Ayurveda, 312-USA-Ayurveda-roots/leaves/stems,   312-USA-Ayurveda-seeds,   362-review-Malaysia-seeds,   378-review-Natural Medicines Professional Database-whole plant juice has been pounded with water and taken by mouth as tea in doses of 1/4 seer (approximately one cup), 437-Ayurveda-seeds-also gleet,   408-India-roots/leaves/stems/ seeds, 537-India,   596-Nigeria-leaf/root/seed,   664-Ayurveda-whole plant-pounded with a little water-juice-doses of ¼ seers,

Sida rhombifolia

Tr 407-Ayurveda-seeds, 437-Ayurveda-seeds-also gleet, 522-Guatemela-infusion-taken orally, 522-Peru-leaf, 545- Bangladesh-leaves and roots, 587-Bangladesh-stems and roots,

Sida cordata

Tr 293-Ayurveda-root bark, 437-Ayurveda-seeds-also gleet, 496-Pakistan-Siddha and Ayurveda-seeds, 603-Sida cordata-Himalayas-root bark-leucorrhoea.

Sida indica

Tr 238-Sri Lanka-leaf, 437-Ayurveda-seeds-gonorrhoea and gleet, 445-India and China-gonorrhea, 450-India-fruit, 450-India-root, 451-Thailand-leaf extract, 454-seeds-India, 678-Ayurveda-seeds or whole plant?, 684-Ayurveda-leaf juice, 708-Ayurveda-seed or fruit-in treatment of gonorrhea, 710-Ayurveda-seeds, 710-Ayurveda-leaves-decoc-tion, 711-India-leaf extract, 712- India-root/fruit/leaves and/or seeds, 735-Ayurveda-review-seeds-gleet or gonorrhea, 737-India-seeds-infusion in water,

Sida spinosa

Tr 55-India-leaves-bruised in water and the filtrate is administered, 55-India-root-decoction-irritability, 99-India-leaf, 99-India-root-decoction as a demulcent in gonorrhea, 433-India,

Sida javensis

Tr 362-review-entire plant-decoction-used specifically against gonorrhea, 520-Phillipines-Entire plant or leaf decoction, 528-Phillipines-Entire plant or leaf decoction used as specific for gonorrhea.

Venereal disease   No peer review

{See peer-review studies of Neisseria gonorrhoeae in **Pathogens**}

Sida acuta

Tr 88-Gold Coast, 96-Gold Coast, 101-Nicaragua-a decoction of the dried entire plant is taken orally, 107-Nicaragua, 168-Nicaragua-decoction of the dried entire plant taken orally, 271-Nicaragua-decoction of dried entire plant, 523-India-leaves-decoction of dried plant-oral, 588-Nigeria-decoction of whole plant,

Sida cordifolia   **Tr** 120-Colombia-syphilis treatment (saponins),

Sida rhombifolia   **Tr** 522-Nicargua-leaf-decoction-orally

Sida indica

Tr 712-India-leaves-Syphilis of penis, 735-Ayurveda-review- leaves and seeds are crushed with water to form pastes which is applied to penis to cure syphilis,

Worms, Earthworm friendly

The aim of the study was to investigate the impact of the cultivation of newly introduced perennial bioenergy crops on earthworm species composition, number and biomass at an experimental site in Western Germany. **[480]**
Tr no reported use

Sida hermaphrodita 480-invivo-earthworms-on comparison within the (other bioenergy) perennial crops-highest earthworm number was found in soil cultivated with Sida hermaphrodita.

Other Uses

Sida acuta

514- mushroom cultivation-In this paper we report that weeds can be used as the substrate for cultivation of oyster mushroom (Pleurotus ostreatus). The main problem of oyster mushroom cultivation on weed substrates was found to be low yield in the second flush. Of 15 combinations of weeds with or without straw, Rice straw + Sida acuta (1:1) had a rank of B first flush, A for second flush. Sida acuta alone had a rank of C for first flush, and B for second flush, **532-reduces fluoride**-invitro-leaves-acqueous extract-We have found that Sida Acuta Burm f. are useful to reduced fluoride content from water... The fluoride content in water sample of some villages of Bhiloda taluka was (about 1.55mg/l).with the help of extract (Fig. 2) fluoride content came down to (1.42mg/l),

Tr 220- is used for spiritual practices, 358-leaf mucilage used for getting foreign objects out of the eye, 361-wood-charcoal gives a black dye, 361-Malasya-wood-charcoal gives a black dye to blacken teeth, 671-the leaves of Sida rhombifolia and Sida acuta are smoked in many countries for their stimulating and euphoric effect (especially in Mexico, where S. rhombifolia is regarded as the stronger species).

Sida cordifolia

Tr 358-glue-Pounding the leaves yields a glue that is used in Tanzania to seal leaking pots, while in Nigeria this glue is used as an ingredient of arrow-poison. 666-dye plant- gives various shades in green-yellow region on woolen fabric with the help of various chemical and natural mordants-good fastness.

Sida rhombifolia

Tr   362-India-wood charcoal-may be used for blackening teeth,   367-review-India-used for blackening teeth,   367-review-East Africa-the wood-tar is used as a dye,   545-Mexico-leaves-smoked-mental exhaustion,   671-the leaves of Sida rhombifolia and Sida acuta are smoked in many countries for their stimulating and euphoric effect (especially in Mexico, where S. rhombifolia is regarded as the stronger species),

Sida indica

479-noise reduction-results of research concerning use of Sida hermaphrodita as biological acoustic screen along communication routes, show that most effective noise suppression, by means of above mentioned plant screen, was observed at measurement height of 0.5 m, from May to October. Greatest noise reduction, reaching 13.4 dB, was noted for measurement profile C, 35 m from source of noise,   **636-wheat growth enhancer**-leaves-3% aqueous extract-wheat- This study indicates promotive potential of S. indica on seed germination and seedling growth of wheat-The root length increased to 153% of control-shoot length was 131%-dry weight also increased to 147% of control-significantly increased seedling growth-Seed germination was not affected,   **637-Pollutant absorbent**-invitro-acid activated leaves turned activated carbon-aqueous solution- an effective adsorbent for the abatement of many pollutants, including dyes,   **638-Oil plant** -- Seed crude oil yield was calculated on a 91% dry matter basis, extracted with *n*-hexane in a Soxhlet apparatus over 8 h at a constant temperature of 80 °C ....The crude oil content ranged from 13.6 to 14.7%, with the highest value observed with the NPK application. Different fertilizer applications had a statistically significant effect on seed crude oil acids, except for the palmitic and linolenic acids. Among the fertilizer applications that statistically affected the crude oil acid contents, NPK yielded the highest values,   **675-fabric finish**-cotton-leaves-80% methanol extract-to finish using Sida indica on the hundred percent cotton denim fabrics using dip method enhanced the wearing capacity of the denim fabric for an extended period without any skin/dermal irritations/infections, without any bad odor.

Conversion Factors

hectare = 10,000 square meters = 2.471 acres

hectare = 107,369 square feet   square meter = 10.7639 square feet

....

The use of plants for healing is as ancient and universal as medicine itself. Plants act generally to stimulate and supplement the body's healing forces, they are the natural food for human beings. Many infectious diseases are known to be treated with herbal remedies throughout the history of man kind. **[83]**

Sida Benefits Narrative

Research has shown that the Sida genus, with a few rare exceptions, is basically non-toxic and universally beneficial. Sidas do not have much in the way of warnings, contra-indications, or dose limitations. Of course, nothing is completely non-toxic, so do read the sections on **Toxicity** in **Benefits** and **Sida as Weed**. This book is a compilation of known peer-review research and is not to be considered medical advice.

Throughout the topics and sub-tropics (American tropics, African tropics, India, South-east Asia, Pacific ocean, Caribbean, SE US, etc.) Sidas are consumed by millions of people daily as a tea. People have been taking Sidas since time-out-of-mind for an amazing number of conditions, as you have seen in the previous **Benefits** section.

There has been relatively little scientific research on Sida, which is surprising since it has been used as a medicinal for thousands of years all over the tropical world. In these research studies a possible benefit is usually tested on just one variety of sida, often using only one part of the plant, perhaps employing only one means of extraction – I strongly recommend going back to the original research once you have found a topic that interests you.

The reported medicinal properties of Sida vary somewhat from variety to variety, but this research strongly indicates that the major medicinal varieties of Sida (S. acuta, S. cordifolia, S. rhombifolia, S. alba, and Sida indica, at least) all have enough of the same profound medicinal properties to be largely used interchangeably. My chapter on **Composition of Sida** displays the similarities in composition of the major Sidas. See the section on **Ayurvedic** medicine in the chapter on **Traditional Use** for the reasoning behind this.

There have been few negative results in Sida research, and many of them are due to procedural flaws. For example, many tests use distilled water as part of the extraction, but some of the most profound health compounds in Sida are the alkaloids, which are brought out by acidic water.

Most studies note that sida protection is dose dependent; usually more gives more benefits (in certain cases this is not so). Different extraction methods produce different results. Traditional methods of preparation are hot water infusion, and for the sophisticated, ethanol tincture. These listings indicate successful endpoints, but you will have to research the best method of preparing sida for any given circumstance.

Sida L. (Malvaceae) has been used for centuries in traditional medicines in countries around the world for the prevention and treatment of different diseases such as diarrhea, dysentery, gastrointestinal and urinary infections, malarial and other fevers, childbirth and miscarriage problems, skin ailments, cardiac and neural problems, asthma, bronchitis and other respiratory problems, weight loss aid, rheumatic and other inflammations, tuberculosis, etc.

Phytochemical investigation of this genus has resulted in identification of about 245 chemical constituents. The crude extracts and isolates have exhibited a wide spectrum of in vitro and in vivo pharmacological effects involving antimicrobial, analgesic, anti-inflammatory, abortifacient, neuroprotective, cardiovascular and cardioprotective, antimalarial, antitubercular, antidiabetic and antiobesity, antioxidant and nephroprotective activities among others.

Ethnopharmacological preparations containing Sida species as an ingredient in India, African and American countries possess good efficacy in health disorders. **[168]**

Synergy effects of the mixture of bioactive constituents and their byproducts contained in plant extracts are claimed to be responsible for the improved effectiveness of many extracts and conventional antimicrobial drugs. Such properties can be partly attributed to the diverse array of secondary metabolite such as alkaloids which are known to be essential for plants' defense against microbial attack or insect and animal predation. [27]

Medicinal plants are largely used either for the prevention, or for the curative treatment of several diseases. **Among the properties behind these virtues, the antioxidant activity holds the first place.** [27]

Many other compounds which are demonstrated to have interesting pharmacological properties alone have been isolated from the plant, in addition the plant may have many other properties since it has not been tested for all desired pharmacological activities. However it should be noted that all laboratory screenings have been carried out with laboratory classical extractions as it is often observed with other medicinal plants. No study has been conducted with traditional preparation; this must be the priority for two reasons. First people still use the plant even if laboratory screenings do not confirm the assumed activity, so the laboratory results in the conditions of the traditional usage is more pertinent and can directly improve this usage. Secondly most of these extracts act sometimes by synergistic effects so the fractionation may result in the lost of the activity, in addition the establishment of the drug from pure single compound may be too expensive so the drug may not be affordable for our populations. [220]

It may be concluded from this study that sida spinosa leaf extract has antimicrobial activity against certain bacteria and fungi. It is expected that using natural products as therapeutic agents will probably not elicit resistance in microorganisms. This can explain the rationale for the use of the plant in treating infections in traditional medicine. The plant could be a veritable and cheaper substitute for conventional drugs since the plant is easily obtainable and the extract can easily be made via a simple process of maceration or infusion. [55]

Q. What is the difference between a pure Herbal powder and a herbal extract? Our pure powders are the Whole Plant preparation. This means that the part of the plant that is used (e.g.: the bean, the root, the leaf, the bark etc.) is used completely. It is not an extract of this plant. This means that the chemical constituents that are present in the plant occur in their natural proportions rather than in a standardized percentage. The benefits of taking whole part plant preparations are numerous. Many people believe that taking the whole plant brings with it the naturally occurring "holistic" balance of medicine that nature provides. An extract is when a powder is processed, to extract the active phyto-chemical constituents from the plant matter, this means that the bulk matter is greatly reduced and it is more condensed. This means that a smaller quantity can be taken. [379]

Water was less able to extract the metabolite of interest, while methanol or its mixture with water showed greater extracting ability... It should be noted that although there may be several compounds with antioxidant properties in a plant sample, each one exhibits its own activity and kinetic characteristics, depending on the presence of one, two or more kinds of components. [172]

Sida cordifolia. Results revealed that maximum accumulation of alkaloids and phenols occurred in summer season... Peak concentrations of alkaloids and phenols were observed in flowering stage.... Interestingly, no alkaloids or phenols accumulated in the seedling stage. **[409]**

Methods of extraction

IC50 = The IC50 is a measure of how effective a drug is. It indicates how much of a particular drug or other substance is needed to inhibit a given biological process (or component of a process, i.e. an enzyme, cell, cell receptor or microorganism) by half. In other words, it is the half minimal (50%) inhibitory concentration (IC) of a substance (50% IC, or IC50). It is commonly used as a measure of antagonist drug potency in pharmacological research. [1]   The antiproliferative activity of each extract was expressed as CC50 (50 cytotoxic concentration values) with a lower CC50 value indicating a higher antiproliferative activity. **[92]**

In order to elucidate whether the observed antimicrobial effects were microbicide or microbiostatic, MBC/MIC ratios were calculated. Extracts with ratios greater than 1 were considered as microbiostatic, while the other extracts are microbicide. From these data, it can concluded that some extracts have either microbicide or microbiostatic activities on specific strains. **[89]**

In some cases it is preferable to evaporate the alcohol before taking the tincture or fluid extract. This is advised with babies, children, the elderly and if someone is sensitive to alcohol or recovering from an alcohol addiction. This can be done by putting the measure of tincture or fluid extract into a pan of boiling water, allow this to boil for 30 seconds, then turn off the heat and leave for 10 minutes to let all the ethanol in the tincture evaporate. This can be added to fruit juice or taken directly. **[379]**

The evaluation of herbal products face several major problems. The first is the use of mixed extracts (concoctions) and variations in methods of harvesting, preparing and extracting the herb, which can result in dramatically different levels of certain alkaloids. **[495]**

Traditional methods

Sida alba leaves are bruised in water and the filtrate is administered. **[55]** Leaves are bruised in water, strained through cloth and administered in the form of a draught. Root is used in decoction. **[433]**   Extracts of Sida acuta were obtained by preparing decoction in water of the powdered plant, the technique used by most of the traditional healers. **[19, 459]**   The powdered *Sida cordifolia* leaves were extracted several times by boiling with water for three hours. **[122]**

Preparation of Aqueous Extract: Aqueous extract was prepared by decoction process. One part of powdered root of *Sida rhombifolia* L. and four parts of sterilized water were taken in a boiling apparatus and boiled for 15 minutes. **[136]**

For preparation of extract, Sida rhombifolia leaves were shade dried, manually crushed and grinded in an electric grinder to obtain fine powder. Hundred gm of powdered leaves were boiled in 1000 mL of distilled water at 100 °C for 3 h and filtered using a sterilized muslin cloth. Resulting filtrate was collected in petri plates and concentrated by heating at 100 °C to form a semisolid paste. **[520]**

How to make a perfect herbal decoction

A herbal decoction is made from the roots, bark, seeds or other tough woody parts of a plant. These herbs won't yield their active ingredients as easily as leaves, flowers or aerial parts and need prolonged heating in order to extract them.

To make a perfect cup of herbal tea decoction for one person you will need a saucepan or coffee pot that can be heated in a stove, 500 ml of spring or filtered water and the required amount of quality cut, dried herbal roots, bark etc.

1. Add all the water and the herbs to the pan or pot. The exact quantity of herb will vary but a good amount for the average herbal tea is roughly 2 teaspoons

2. Place on a stove and bring the mixture to the boil. Once boiling turn down the heat and allow to simmer for 10 to 30 minutes.

3. Allow the mixture to cool a little then pour through a tea strainer into a cup

4. Drink and enjoy

Herbal tea decoctions can also be made in larger quantities and will keep for 3 days or so if covered and refrigerated.

{Indigo Herbs of Glastonbury has a marvelous website. they are in England but cover an excellent range of herbs including tropicals of merit like Sida. Check them out.} **[379]**

How to make a perfect herbal tea infusion

The word 'tea' here is a bit of a misnomer. Tea in this context refers, not to camellia sinensis (who's various leaves are used to make black tea, green tea and white tea) but to what a herbalist would call an infusion, tisane or ptisan. Making a herbal tea is effectively a method of extracting the active ingredients of a herb into an easy to digest form.

To make a perfect cup of herbal tea for one person, you will need a teapot or cafetiere, 750 ml of spring water (or filtered water will do) and enough top quality cut, dried herb depending on your herb of choice and how strong you want your tea to be.

284

1. Bring all the water to the boil

2. Add roughly a third of the water to your empty, clean teapot or cafetiere, replace the lid and allow the vessel to warm for a few moments.

3. Empty the teapot of its warming water and add the herbs. The amount you add will depend on which herbal tea you are making and how strong you want it but a good amount is usually about 2 heaped teaspoons.

4. Immediately pour over the remaining boiling water (make sure it is still boiling) and quickly and calmly put the lid on the teapot and cover with a tea cosy or other insulating cover.

5. Leave the tea for between 5 and 15 minutes allowing the herbs to infuse into the water.

6. Pour your delicious herbal tea into a clean cup, through a tea strainer and drink.

Larger volumes of herbal tea infusions can be stored for up to 3 days if kept covered and refrigerated. **[379]**

Scientific extraction

The leaves were crushed in an iron mortar. Crushed material was subjected to extraction by hot maceration at 60–70°C for 6h continuously in distilled water three times. The extract was filtered, combined, and evaporated to dryness. Dried extract was obtained by concentrating filtrate under reduced pressure in rotary evaporator. **[196]**   {note use of distilled water}

For aqueous extraction, 10 g of air-dried powder was added to distilled water and boiled on slow heat for 2 h. It was then filtered through 8 layers of muslin cloth and centrifuged at 5000g for 10 min. The supernatant was collected. This procedure was repeated twice. After 6 h, the supernatant collected at an interval of every 2 h, was pooled together and concentrated to make the final volume one-fourth of the original volume (Parekh et al., 2005). It was then autoclaved at 121 °C temperature and at 15 lbs pressure and stored at 4° C. For solvent extraction, 10 g of air-dried powder was taken in 100 ml of organic solvent (methanol or ethanol) in a conical flask, plugged with cotton wool and then kept on a rotary shaker at 190-220 rpm for 24 h. After 24 hours the supernatant was collected and the solvent was evaporated to make the final volume one-fourth of the original volume (Parekh et al., 2005) and stored at 4oC in airtight bottles. **[446-Sida indica, among others]**

The leaves, twigs, and roots of the Sida indica plant were collected from Mahidol University, Salaya Campus, Nakorn Pathom Province, Thailand, and were identified by Associate Professor ungravi Temsiririrkkul, Department of Pharmaceutical Botany, Mahidol University, Bangkok, Thailand. All fresh parts were dried at 50° C in a hot air oven and then pulverized by an electric blender. A crude extract was produced by boiling 1 kg of plant powder in 10 L of distilled water for 10 minutes. The boiling process was repeated twice, and the combined extract was filtered through cotton wool and gauze. The filtrate was lyophilized in freeze drying system, yielding a dark brown powder of 11.44% wt/wt. [451]

After separating the leaves from the plant, it was cut into small pieces and air dried for several days. The plant materials were then ground into coarse powder. The dried and ground plant powder (600g) was extracted with methanol (2.5 liters) in an air tight, clean flat bottomed container for 3 days at room temperature with occasional stirring and shaking. The extract was then filtered first through a fresh cotton plug and finally with a Whatman filters paper. The filtrate was concentrated using a rotary evaporator at low temperature (40-450C) and pressure. The weight of the crude extract was 23.65 gm. Solvent–solvent partitioning was done using the protocol designed by Kupchan [11] and modified version of Wagenen et al. [12]. The crude extract (5 gm) was dissolved in 10% aqueous methanol which was subsequently extracted first with n-hexane, then carbon tetrachloride and finally with chloroform. All the four fractions were evaporated to dryness by using rotary evaporator and kept in air tight containers for further analysis.... In terms of alcoholic concentration, the most efficient solvents were hydroethanolic solutions at 40% for leaves and at 70% for roots, when the dry residue parameter was considered alone. [452]

Phytochemical screening was performed with the ethanolic extract of the plant using Molish (carbohydrates), foam, Rosenthaler, hemolysis (saponins), Folin-Ciocalteu (polyphenols), chloride ferric salt gelatin (tannins), ammonia vapors, Shinoda (flavonoids), Arnow (phenylpropanoids), Bornträger (anthraquinone), Lieberman-Burchard, Salkowski (terpenes/steroids), vanillin/HCl (iridoids), Dragendroff, Mayer, Wagner, Tanred, Erhlic, Reineckato, Valser (alkaloids), Baljet, Kedde, m-dinitrobenzene (cardiotonic agents), NaOH/heat/UV light (coumarins), m-dinitrobenzene, Raymond, Mathoud and CCD (terpene lactones) tests. The crosses system was used to specify qualification of secondary metabolites. [120]

Preliminary Phytochemical Analysis: Qualitative phytochemical analysis of the crude powder of the twelve plants collected was determined as follows: Tannins (200 mg plant material in 10 ml distilled water, filtered). A 2 ml filtrate + 2 ml FeCl3, blue-black precipitate indicated the presence of Tannins. Alkaloids (200 mg plant material in 10 ml methanol, filtered). A 2 ml filtrate + 1% HCl + steam, 1 ml filtrate + 6 drops of Mayor's reagents/ Wagner's reagent/ Dragondroff's reagent, Creamish precipitate/ Browinsh-red precipitate/ orange precipitate indicated the presence of respective alkaloids. Saponins (frothing test: 0.5 ml filtrate + 5 ml distilled water. Frothing persistence meant saponins were present). Cardiac Glycosides (Keller-kiliani test: 2 ml filtrate + 1 ml glacial acetic acid + FeCl3 + conc. H2SO4). Greenblue color indicated the presence of cardiac glycosides. Steroids (Liebermann-Burchard reaction: (200 mg plant material in 10 ml chloroform, filtered). A 2 ml filtrate + 2 ml acetic anhydride +conc. H2SO4. Blue-green ring indicated the presence of terpenoids. Flavonoids (200 mg plant material in 10 ml ethanol, filtered). A 2 ml filtrate + conc. HCl +

286

magnesium ribbon. Pink-tomato red color indicated the presence of flavonoids. **[446-Sida indica, among others]**

For flavonoids, 0.5 g of the extract and few pieces of magnesium strips was mixed with concentrated HCl. An orange faint color of effervescence solution indicated the presence of flavonoids. For tannins, 0.5 g of the plant extract was stirred with 1 ml of distilled water, filtered and ferric chloride solution or reagent was added to the filtrate. A blue black or blue green precipitate was taken as evidence for the presence of tannins. For Anthraquinones, 0.5 g of the plant extract was boiled with 1 ml of 10% sulphuric acid and filtered. 2.5 ml of benzene was added to the filtrate and shaken. The benzene layer was separated and half its own volume, 10% ammonia solution was added. The presence of a pink or red-violet color in the lower ammonia phase indicated the presence of Anthraquinones. **[102]**

(Sida indica) The leaves were separated from the fresh stems and dried on filter paper sheets under shade at room temperature until with changing of color of filter papers. The shade-dried, coarsely powdered leaves (500 g) were successively extracted with petroleum ether (60-800C) for 8 hr. to remove fatty matter. The defatted marc was then subjected to soxhlet extraction with 95% methanol to obtain methanolic extract... The aqueous suspension of methanolic extract of leaves of Sida indica (MEAI) as prepared in 0.5 % carboxymethyl-cellulose (CMC) solution in distilled water prior to oral administration to animals. **[443]**

Ethyl acetate and dichloromethane fractions of sida acuta and sida alba aqueous acetone extracts elicit the highest polyphenol content, antioxidant and enzymatic activities. **[254]**

Extraction Longevity

Organic Bala Tincture is the active constituents of the Sida Cordifolia plant extracted into ethanol (medical alcohol)... This traditional method maintains and preserves the naturally-occurring constituents found in the plant. It extends the shelf life for up to 4 years. **[379]**

The results of susceptibility tests showed that freshly prepared extracts displayed different antimicrobial activities compared to stored extracts. From the time zero of polyphenols extraction, tests were made twice a week. (Sida acuta) Freshly prepared extracts ZI=0. Stored extracts for 21 days ZI=15mm **[89]**

Q. How long will my product last?

All of our products will have a best before date on the back of the pack when it is sent out. How long is on the product varies on the batch of the product. We do however guarantee the products will have the following time before they expire at a minimum when we send them to you:

Tinctures – 12 months minimum

Powders- 6 months minimum

Whole foods – 3 months minimum

Raw Chocolates – 3 weeks minimum

Tea Blends and loose teas – 6 months minimum

Oils blends and rollers – 6 months minimum

Essential Oils – 12 months minimum

In our experience however lots of our products have a much longer before they expire than these minimums.

{Indigo Herbs of Glastonbury has a marvelous website. they are in England but cover an excellent range of herbs including tropicals of merit like Sida. Check them out.} **[379]**

Toxicity

{I have been taking Sida acuta extract pretty continuously for over five years with no detrimental effect on my body chemistry}

Pharmacological substances whole LD50 is less than 5 mg/kg body weight are classified in the range of highly toxic substances, those with a LD50 between 5 mg/kg body weight and 5000 mg/kg body weight are classified in the range of moderately toxic substances and those with the lethal dose is more than 5000 mg/kg body weight not toxic 8. **[194,499]**

A. Sida is non-toxic

The very weak toxicity values are interesting features which can securize the use of **Sida acuta** and **Sida cordifolia** in the traditional medicine of Burkina Faso. The low toxicity, evidenced by LD50 values, suggests a wide margin of safety for therapeutic doses. The extracts have no significant negative effect on biological parameters. Moreover we obtained good analgesic results by testing the two species aqueous acetone extracts against animal model. **[203]**

The very weak toxicity values are interesting features which can securize the use of Sida acuta and Sida cordifolia in the traditional medicine of Burkina Faso. The low toxicity, evidenced by LD50 values, suggests a wide margin of safety for therapeutic doses. The extracts have no significant negative effect on biological parameters. Moreover we obtained good analgesic results by testing the two species aqueous acetone extracts against animal model. Both findings justify the therapeutic use of these plants in folk medicine of Burkina Faso. **[60]**

In this study, the results indicated that the extract of Sida alba is low poisonous. During the 14 day period of acute toxicity evaluation, some signs of toxicity were observed, but they were all quickly reversible. Recent studies showed that pharmacological substances whole LD50 is less than 5 mg/kg body weight are classified in the range of highly toxic substances, those with a LD50 between 5 mg/kg body weight and 5000 mg/kg body weight are classified in the range of moderately toxic substances and those with the lethal dose is more than 5000 mg/kg body weight not toxic. [17]

Consequently, if we refer to this classification we could say that the extract of Sida alba is moderately toxic and would be regarded as being safe or of low toxicity... (sub acute toxicity) However, the decrease in body weight observed in the rats treated with the doses of the extract at 4th week may be due to low feed intake and utilization... Certainly the tannins would be responsible in this fact; because, according to recent studies, tannins have been known to occur in high concentrations in the leaf extract of Sida The toxicological and pharmacology effects obtained in this study seem be interesting for the therapeutic use of Sida alba. The low toxicity evidenced by LD50 value suggests a wide margin of safety for therapeutic doses. In sub-acute study, some effects were observed but there were no relevance of serious signs or significant changes in animal weights, effect of extract on animal organs and biochemical parameters. Briefly, these toxicity studies suggest that the extract of Sida alba is safe. [100]

B. Sida may be toxic under certain conditions

{A high concentration of anti-nutrients in raw leaves limits their eating fresh} The result obtained revealed that the leaves of S. acuta contain appreciable amount of proteins, fat, fiber, carbohydrate and high calorific, mineral elements, vitamins and moderately high concentration of toxicant. Consumption of these leaves over a long period of time will lead to bioaccumulation of toxicants. However, S. acuta can be detoxified by soaking and boiling. The chemical constituents of S. acuta predicate that it may not only be useful due to its dietetic value but also medicinally and pharmacologically. [274]

(Sida Acuta) In view of the above reports, it can be concluded that ethanolic extract of Sida acuta is toxic when administered at a dose of 200mg/kgbw to Wistar rats... In this study, the observed reduction and elevation in the activity of ALT, AST and ALP in the administered animals is indicative of the fact that the extract has an adverse effect on the liver enzymes as it is reported that below normal values of liver enzymes may suggest liver dysfunction or insufficient protein intake... Group B and C received 100 and 200mg/kg body weight for three weeks... Group B (100mg/kgbw): The liver tissues from this administered animals showed slight difference in their hepatic architecture. Nuclei were not prominent, but the overall integrity of the cells where maintained as compared to the control. The liver section from group C (200mg/kgbw) administered rats revealed a distorted morphological features showing shrunken sinusoid, dilatation of the central vein and non prominent nuclei. **[256]**

(Sida acuta) Doses of the extract 100, 200, 300, 400 and 500 mg kg-1 bw, were administered daily for two weeks- Decreases ($p > 0.05$) in mean concentrations (mg dL-1) of both urea and creatinine were recorded for all the test groups, comparative to the control. Serum bilirubin concentrations (mg dL-1) were relatively nonsignificantly affected by the extract. Studies on electrolytes showed significant decreases in serum Na+ concentration (mmol L-1) for doses 300 mg kg-1 bw. and above. Similarly, K+ and HCO_3^- concentrations (mmol L-1) were reduced significantly whereas Cl concentrations (mmol L-1) were significantly increased for all the experimental groups, comparative to the control. However, notwithstanding that Sida acuta extract may not impair liver and kidney functions, possible effects on fluid and electrolyte balance should be seriously monitored. **[530]**

Many Sida species contain ephedrine, a pseudo-alkaloid, biosynthetically derived from the amino acid phenylalanine. Ephedrine acts as a sympathomimetic on the body, which means that its effects are similar to those of the sympathetic (adrenergic) neurotransmitters like noradrenalin and adrenalin (also known as norepinephrine and epinefrine). The mechanism of action of ephedrine is of the indirect type: the substance does not activate adrenergic receptors directly, but it facilitates the release of neurotransmitters from sympathetic nerves. Pharmacological effects of ephedrine include e.g. stimulation of the heart rate and cardiac output, together with a variable increase of the peripheral resistance; as a result it usually increases blood pressure. In the lungs, it promotes bronchodilatation, acceleration and intensification of respiration. It may increase the resistance to the outflow of urine in the bladder. Furthermore, ephedrine crosses the blood-brain barrier, it has a stimulating psychic effect: stimulation of the attention and concentration, decrease of the sensation of fatigue and the need to sleep, and thus qualitatively it resembles an amphetamine. Because of the numerous contraindications, drug interactions and required precautions, the compound is no longer used very often. **[362]**

Sida cordifolia when used excessively can cause ephedrine related side effects like insomnia, anxiety, nervousness, and increase in blood pressure, memory loss or even stroke. Ephedrine coupled with caffeine can prove fatal. Patients subjected to IOC drug testing, using MAO inhibitor medication (Antidepressants), having high blood pressure, heart disease, thyroid or prostrate condition along with pregnant or lactating women should not take this herb except under expert guidance. **[118]**

C. Sida has toxicity

(Toxic)This study was carried out to assess the effect of ethanolic leaf extract of Sida acuta on the kidney electrolytes of adult Wistar rats. Forty five rats weighing between 140-180g were assigned to three groups (A, B and C) with fifteen animals each. Group A served as the control while groups B and C served as the experimental groups and received 100mg/kgbw and 200mg/kgbw of the extract respectively for fourteen days. All the animals were sacrificed after fourteen days. Blood was collected by cardiac puncture for biochemical analysis of serum electrolytes. Serum chemistry revealed significantly raised sodium and decreased potassium levels in animals treated with 100mg/kgbw, but chloride, creatinine and potassium not significantly affected (P>0.05). Animals treated with 200mg/kgbw of the extract had significantly raised sodium levels, but reduced potassium, chloride and creatinine relative to control (P<0.05). From the result of this experiment, it is concluded that the administration of ethanolic extract of Sida acuta leaves could have adverse effects on the kidney electrolytes of Adult Wistar rats at the doses and duration used in the course of this experimentation.... The effect of the extract on the kidney electrolyte after administration revealed no marked differences in the potassium levels while sodium, chloride and creatinine showed higher levels that are significant when compared to their respective control groups.(p<0.05) From this observation, it can be suggested that the extract has adverse effect on some kidney electrolytes. It is on record that too much or too little sodium can cause cells to malfunction, and extremes in the blood sodium levels can be fatal. High levels of sodium in the blood causes the cells to be dehydrated leading to hypernatrema which can cause coma or death. Chloride balances sodium cations and helps to maintain proper water distribution outside the cell s and a high level of it causes certain kidney disease and over activity of parathyroid glands. Similarly, high levels of serum creatinine is of clinical importance since creatinine is used as a measure of renal functions. The only important pathological condition that causes high levels of serum creatinine is damage to large number of nephrons. Creatinine levels about 2.0mg/dL is suggestive of severe kidney impairment; hence any condition that impairs the function of the kidney is likely to raise the creatinine level in the blood. Therefore, this report is an indication that the ethanolic extract of Sida acuta has adverse effect on the kidney electrolytes. [531]

D. The Sida acuta/carpinfolia conundrum

The toxicological studies on Sida acuta are listed near the end of the **Benefits** chapter. At the end of the **Sida as Weed** chapter there is a detailed look at the Sida carpinfolia conundrum.

Dosage

{Many studies report a dose dependent action, that is, the larger the dose the stronger the effect. As usual with Sida, sometimes the larger dose in less effective.}

Typical Use

Ayurvedic Pharmacopoeia mentioned 3-6 gm of powder of S. cordifolia is effective & safe as well. The Quality Standards of Indian medicinal Plants have also mentioned 3-6 gm as safe dose. The toxicity study of

Standardization of Botanicals shows 3g/Kg dose of S, cordifolia is toxic in mice. In Indian Herbal Pharmacopoeia, the dose mentioned is 1-3 gm. Dr. Amritpal Singh reported 1-3 gm dose as a safe dose of S. cordifolia... The dose of S. rhombifolia is 3-6gm & the reported LD 50 is 8.5gm/kg in rats... Traditionally 2-4 gm is considered as safe dose of S. acuta. [88]

Bala fair trade Powder - Take 1/2 to 2 grams per day, use mixed with milk or fruit juice - can be split up over day. Bala / Sida cordifolia Fair trade Tincture - 5-10ml daily (can be split up into 2-3 doses per day) or as directed by an herbal practitioner. [379]

Sida indica Dosage

Plant Part or Derivative	Dosage
Roots Powder	3 to 6 grams
Seed Powder	1 to 3 grams
Root extract	250 mg to 750 mg
Seed extract	125 mg to 500 mg

The maximum dosage of Indian mallow (Sida indica) root or seed powder should not exceed 12 grams per day. [727]

Based on the data of present study, it is concluded that alcoholic extract of S. cordifolia at a dose of 400 mg/kg have potency to act as anti diabetic, hypoglycemic and anti oxidant properties and also helps to check muscle wasting. Further it also protects from LPO that damages the cell membrane. [148]

Dosing Sida cordifolia (Bala)

Adults (18 years and older)   Doses from clinical trials are lacking. One capsule containing 300 milligrams of bala has been taken by mouth. Five to 10 milliliters of a bala tincture diluted 1:3 in 25% alcohol has been taken by mouth daily in divided doses. Ten grams of bala per cup of water has been steeped for at least one hour and taken by mouth as tea.

For elephantiasis, the juice of the whole plant has been pounded with a little water, made into paste with the juice of the palmyra tree, and applied to the affected area.

For eye disease, a paste made from bala leaves has been applied to the affected eye.

For general musculoskeletal soreness, bala oil has been used to massage the affected area.

For gonorrhea, whole plant juice has been pounded with water and taken by mouth as tea in doses of 1/4 seer (approximately one cup).

For wound dressing, a paste made from bala leaves has been applied to the affected area.

Children (under 18 years old) There is no proven safe or effective dose for bala in children. [378]

Alcoholic extract of S. cordifolia at a dose of 400 mg/kg have potency to act as anti diabetic, hypoglycemic and antioxidant properties and also helps to check muscle wasting. Further it also protects from LPO that damages the cell membrane.... no such findings have been found in alcoholic extracts of S. cordifolia at dosage level of 200 mg/kg. [148]

Based on the data obtained, all doses (30-300mg) of the Sida rhombifolia extract (rats-ethanolic extract-leaves-administered intraperitoneally) exhibited significant (p<0.05) antinociceptive and anti-inflammatory activities in a dose-dependent manner. [149]

However at 400 mg/kg, the alcoholic extract of S. cordifolia showed beneficial effect indicating significant decrease in total cholesterol, triglycerides, low density lipids, plasma-creatinine, plasma-urea nitrogen and lipid-peroxidation and a significant increase in high density lipid-level in diabetic rats. Interestingly at 400 mg/kg, a significant increase in antioxidant enzymes such as catalase and superoxide-dismutase-activity was seen in the diabetic rats. The dose 200 mg/kg of alcoholic extract of S. cordifolia showed non-significant change in diabetic rats. [148]

Ayurvedic Pharmacopoeia mentioned 3-6 gm of powder of S. cordifolia is effective & safe as well. The Quality Standards of Indian medicinal Plants have also mentioned 3-6 gm as safe dose. The dose of S. rhombifolia is 3-6gm & the reported LD 50 is 8.5gm/kg in rats. Traditionally 2-4 gm is considered as safe dose of S. acuta. [88]

Size of the dose makes a difference

The successful application of sida is often dose dependent. Different extraction methods produce different results (water infusion, ethanol tincture, etc). This applies to traditional uses as well. The methods of preparation vary, and that has an effect on outcomes. These listings indicate successful endpoints, but you will have to research the best method of preparing sida for any given circumstance.

More is not always better. Sida cordifolia stimulated over 90% liver regeneration after a 67% partial hepatectomy in rats. This was done with an aqueous extract of 100mg/kg. Higher concentrations resulted in less regeneration, i.e., 200 mg/kg resulted in only 50% regeneration, and 400mg/kg resulted in only 40% regeneration. [37]

Sida tiagii-mice-fruit-95% ethanolic extract-Pentylenetetrazole-induced seizure. Diazepam (1 mg/kg bw) did not show convulsion. Sida tiagii-95% ethanolic extract-50 and 100 mg/kg bw induced 100% protection but significantly increase onset of seizures, 200 mg/kg bw induce 85.3% protection but also significantly increased onset of seizures, 500 mg/kg bw induced 69.3% protection with no onset of seizures compared to control. [205]

invitro-Staphylococcus aureas-MIC-leaves 50 and 500 ug=8mm - stem 50 and 500 ug=8mm - root 50 ug=11mm - root 500 ug = 12mm -- invitro-Pseudomonas aeruginosa-MIC-leaves 50 and 500 ug=7mm - stem 50 and 500 ug=6mm - root 50 g=9mm - root 500 ug =7mm the best dose is 50ug and anything more is less effective against Pseudomonas aeruginosa. [126]

Dose dependent, needs more

Antibacterial activity of *Sida acuta* against bacterial species tested by disc diffusion assay

Botanical Name	Concentration	MIC	Antibacterial Activity*
Escherichia coli	5 +g/ml	0.634±0.01	8.6±0.21
Escherichia coli	10 +g/ml	0.510±0.03	10.1±0.48
Escherichia coli	15 +g/ml	0.383±0.04	11.6±0.72
Escherichia coli	20 +g/ml	0.248±0.02	13.4±0.26
Vibrio cholerae	5 +g/ml	0.487±0.02	7.8±0.43
Vibrio cholerae	10 +g/ml	0.383±0.03	9.4±0.71
Vibrio cholerae	15 +g/ml	0.274±0.01	10.7±0.28
Vibrio cholerae	20 +g/ml	0.210±0.1	12.6±0.13
Staph. aureus	5 +g/ml	0.550±0.02	6.4±0.31
Staph. aureus	10 +g/ml	0.448±0.02	7.9±0.5
Staph. aureus	15 +g/ml	0.330±0.02	9.5±0.14
Staph. aureus	20 +g/ml	0.220±0.01	11±0.21
Proteus mirabilis	5 +g/ml	0.541±0.01	6.1±0.14
Proteus mirabilis	10 +g/ml	0.424±0.01	7.5±0.63
Proteus mirabilis	15 +g/ml	0.301±0.01	9.0±0.7
Proteus mirabilis	20 +g/ml	0.178±0.01	11±0.21
P. aeruginosa	5 +g/ml	0.571±0.03	5.5±0.26
P. aeruginosa	10 +g/ml	0.453±0.01	6.4±0.15
P. aeruginosa	15 +g/ml	0.301±0.01	7.4±0.41
P. aeruginosa	20 +g/ml	0.178±0.01	8.9±0.16

*The antimicrobial activity was determined by measuring the diameter of zone of inhibition, that is, the mean of triplicates ± SD of triplicates. P aeruginosa = Pseudomonas aeruginosa [214-Sida acuta]   MIC = the lowest concentration of a chemical which prevents visible growth of a bacterium. [1]

Alcoholic extract of S. cordifolia at a dose of 400 mg/kg have potency to act as anti diabetic, hypoglycemic and antioxidant properties and also helps to check muscle wasting. Further it also protects from LPO that damages the cell membrane.... no such findings have been found in alcoholic extracts of S. cordifolia at dosage level of 200 mg/kg. [148]

Sida cordifolia-aerial parts-alcoholic extract- Interestingly at 400 mg/kg, a significant increase in antioxidant enzymes such as catalase and superoxide-dismutase-activity was seen in the diabetic rats. The dose 200 mg/kg of alcoholic extract of S. cordifolia showed non-significant change in diabetic rats. [148]

Aqueous extracts of Sida cordifolia leaves show high antimicrobial activity and contains phytochemicals that are responsible for such an activity-Increasing concentrations of the extracts (aqueous and methanolic) exhibited increased zone of inhibition against the bacteria and fungi (7-20mm). Better antifungal activity was observed with aqueous extract even at low concentrations (zone diameter of 11 to 15 mm at 175 ug/disc) and at high concentrations-the activity was equivalent of fluconazole (20mm at 2mg/disc). Increasing concentrations of the extracts (aqueous and methanolic) exhibited increased zone of inhibition against the bacteria and fungi (7-20mm)-2 mg acqueous as powerful as Fluconazole 25 mcg. [125]

The influence of the concentration of ethanol (50, 60, and 70%, of the degree of grinding of the plant raw material, and of the time of maceration, on the yield of rutin from the epigeal part of Virginia sida, family Malvaceae has been studied. It has been established that the highest yield of rutin can be obtained from raw material ground to 2.5–3.0 mm with the use of 70% ethanol and a time of maceration of 12 h. In an investigation of the influence of the concentration of ethanol and the time of steeping on the yield of rutin from raw material ground to 2.5–2.0 mm, regression equations for 50, 60, and 70% ethanolic extractions have been derived. [483]

Different Parts Have Different Strengths

Methanolic root extracts (10% w/v) of Sida species, viz., S. acuta, S. cordata, S. cordifolia, S. indica, S. mysorensis, S. retusa, S. rhombifolia, and S. spinosa were analyzed. Sida cordifolia possessed highest total phenolic content and also possessed highest antioxidant activities. [15]   Alkaloids were extracted from each part of S. acuta. Alkaloid content estimated in each gram of dried plant material was recorded (Table1). Buds of the plant showed maximum amount of alkaloid content (7 mg/gm dw), followed by leaves (3.35 mg/gm dw), stem (1.1mg/gm dw) and roots (0.15 mg/gm dw). [221]   It is worth mentioning that most of the extracts exhibit very low MIC values (a desirable features). Two active extracts (Alkaloid extracts of buds and roots) were found to be bactericidal whereas remaining were found bacteriostatic in nature. [221]

The quantitative and qualitative variations of the three types of alkaloids, occurring in the roots and aerial portions of the *Sida* species and at different stages of vegetation are also noteworthy. ß –phenethylamines were found to constitute the major bases in the aerial parts, but occurred as minor components, or were absent in roots. It was further observed that the abundance of quinazoline alkaloids was greater in younger (about 6 months old) species. It was also observed that the roots of 6 months old plants afford quinazoline alkaloids as the major entities, while the carboxylated tryptamines were present only in traces. Older roots (about 2 years old) contained these two types of alkaloids in almost equal proportions. [217]

(S. rhombifolia) Absence of light favored germination and germination speed index. [198]

Phytochemicals analysis of acetone extracts of S. indica.

	Leaf	Stem	Flower	Pod
Alkaloids	+	+	+	++
Carbohydrates	++	+	+++	+
Glycosides	++	++	+++	++
Tannins	++	+	+	+
Phenols	++	++	++	++
Flavonoids	+	++	++	+
Coumarines	++	++	+++	+++
Saponins	+	++	+++	++
Quinones	++	++	++	++
Terpenoid	+++	+++	++	+
Phlobatanin	_	_	_	_
Anthraquinone	_	_	_	_
Steroids	+++	++	++	++

+++= (Highly present); ++= (Moderate); += (Mild); - = absent   [687]

Plant species, parts, weights of plant material, quantity of methanol used, the extract weights obtained and the percentage yields of the extracts of the plants

Species	Amt methanol (ml)	Extract wt (gm)	Yield of extracts %
Sida acuta whole plant	650	12.55	25.1
Sida acuta leaves	600	8.53	17.06
S. rhombifolia stems	700	2.94	5.88

weight of plant 50 gm   **[560]**

From several extracts of sidaguri (water, ethanol 70%, alkaloid and flavonoid), the strongest and the weakest of LC50 value were ethanol extract of leaves (1780 ppm) and water extract of herbs (148 ppm), respectively. **[486-S. rhombifolia]**

Dominance of Medicinal properties by parts of plant

Leaves   Demulcent   Laxative   Diuretic   Aphrodisiac   Sedative
Seeds   Laxative   Expectorant   Demulcent
Roots   Diuretic
Stem bark   Diuretic   Astringent   Mucilage*   Diuretic   Demulcent
* extracted from leaves   **[727- Sida indica]**

Phytochemical studies - Sida rhombifolia

Extracts	Leaves	Roots
Petroleum ether	Steroids, Terpenoids	(same)
Chloroform	Alkaloids, Phenol	(same)
Ethyl acetate	Saponins, Glycosides,	(same)
	Tannins, Flavanoids	(same)
Ethanol	Alkaloids, Glycosides,	(same)
	Tannins, Saponins,	(same)
	Terpenoids, Flavanoids	(same)

[544]

Phytoconstituents of different parts of *"Sida cordifolia"* plant

Plant parts	Phytoconstituents	Alkaloid %
Whole parts	Large amount of ephedrine	Extend of 0.085 %
Seeds	Sterculic, malvalic and coronaric acid along with other fatty acids.	0.32 %
Leaves	Ephedrine , pseudoephedrine	0.28 %
Stems	Ephedrine	0.22 %
Roots	Ephedrine, saponine, choline, vasicine, hypaphorine, pseudo-ephedrine, betaphenethyl-amine, ecdysterone and related indole alkaloides.	0.06 %
Aerial parts	Ephedrine, pseudoephedrine, Palmitic ,stearic and β – sitosterol, hexacosanoic acids, 6-phenyl ethyl amine, carboxylated tryptomines, qunazoline, hypaphorine, vasicinol	0.31%

[118,312]

Antitubercular activity of leaf and root extracts of *Sida rhombifolia* L. against clinical isolate of *M. tuberculosis* resistant to S, H, R & E.

Extract	Reduction in RLU	
	100 µg/ml	500 µg/ml
Leaf - Ethyl Acetate	67.18	83.61
Leaf - Ethanol	0	3.61
Root - Ethyl Acetate	29.02	62.37
Root - Ethanol	0	29.94 **[544]**

Quantitative estimation of flavonoids of *S. acuta*

	Free	Bound	Total
Root	4.25	0.5	4.75
Stem	5.0	0.45	5.45
Leaf	8.15	0.35	8.5
Bud	4.10	1.75	5.85

Flavonoids (mg/gm dw)   **[271]**

Minimum inhibitory concentration of parts of S. acuta against two micro-organisms

S. aureus Leaf .63 > Stem .31-.63 > Root .016-.019 > Bud no activity

All figures are in mg/ml **[271]**

Ethanol extracts were found to be a good scavenger of DPPH radical in the order roots > stem > leaves > whole plant with values 76.62%, 63.87%, 58% and 29% at a dose of 1 mg, respectively. All extracts of Sida cordifolia. (SC) have effective reducing power and free-radical scavenging activity. Only the root extract exhibited superoxide-scavenging activity and inhibited lipid peroxidation in rat liver homogenate. All these antioxidant properties were concentration dependent. In addition, total phenolics content of all the extracts of S. cordifolia. were determined as gallic acid equivalents. **[121]**

Different extracts extract different amounts

This report has also revealed that the solvents used for extraction plays a very Important role in it level of activity. **[102]**

Successive isolation of botanical compounds from plant material is largely dependent on the type of solvent used in the extraction procedure. The traditional healers use primarily water as the solvent but we found in this study the plant extracts by methanol provided more consistent antimicrobial activity compared to those extracted by water... None of the aqueous extracts produced zones of inhibition in the Kirby-Bauer analysis. This might have resulted from the lack of solubility of the active constituents in aqueous solutions while methanol extract showed some degree of antibacterial activity. **[446]**

The activity spectrum of any plant materials depends of the solvent of extraction used. 62.5% of the broader spectrum of antimicrobial activity of plant material was obtained with methanol extract. Based on these results, it is possible to conclude that methanol extract has stronger and broader spectrum of antimicrobial activity as compared to hexane, water or ethanol extract. This observation confirmed the evidence of the previous study which reported that methanol is the better solvent for extraction of antimicrobial substances from medicinal plants than water, ethanol, ethyl acetate or hexane. **[106]**

The methanolic and aquueous extracts of Sida cordifolia exhibited more in-hibitory activity on gram negative bacteria than gram positive. Better anti-fungal activity was observed with aqueous extract even at low temperatures. **[125]**   Phytochemicals are known to possess antimicrobial activity and better extracted using methanol and acqueous based solvents. This may be the reason for the strong antimicrobial activity of the methanolic and aqueous extracts compared to acetone extract. **[125]**   The antibacterial activity was found to increase in the different fruits extracts in order of petroleum ether extracts (2.02% yield W/W), chloroform extracts (1.03% yield W/W), and methanol extracts (6.13% yield W/W). **[51]**   Sida acuta-The zone of inhibition was highest with ethanol extract followed methanol, ethyl acetate and aqueous extracts for all the microorganisms used. Aqueous extract was effective only on P. vulgaris. **[523]**

In the present study different extracts of leaves and stem of Sida cordata were evaluated for its anthelmintic activity against Pheretima posthuma (Indian earth worm) and compared with standard Albendazole. Various concentrations of the leaves and stem extracts (5, 25, 50,100 mg/ml) respectively were screened for their anthelmintic activity which involved the determination of time of paralysis and time of death of the test worms. It was found out the petroleum ether extract(100mg/ml) showed 62.33 and 78 minutes, water extract (100mg/ml) showed 72.33 and 59.33 minutes, ethanol(100mg/ml) showed 79.66 and 90 minutes and chloroform with 83and 78 minutes for paralysis and death respectively comparable to the Albendazole at the given experimental concentrations. The aqueous extract of stem exhibited a significant anthelmintic activity effect over other extracts at the given experimental concentrations. Dose dependent activity was observed in both leaf and stem extracts but leaves extract showed more significant activity than stem extracts. **[497]**

The aqueous extract was found to be moderately effective against bacteria and exhibited high antifungal activity at a concentration of 2mg/disc. The methanolic extract was effective on bacteria and did not show any antifungal activity. Acetone fraction did not contain any antimicrobial activity-Phytochemical including alkaloids, flavonoids, triterpenoids, saponins, thymol and other compounds of phenolic nature were known to possess antimicrobial activity and better extracted using methanol and aqueous-based solvents. This may be the reason for the strong antimicrobial activity of the methanolic and aqueous extracts compared to acetone extract. [125]

The results of phytochemical screening of S. acuta -- **petroleum ether extract** = alkaloids, steroids, carbohydrates, flavones, anthocynins and fatty acids -- **chloroform extract** = carbohydrates and fatty acids -- **ethanol extract** = alkaloids, steroids, carbohydrates, glycosides, amino acids and proteins, saponins, flavones, anthocynins, fatty acids and phenolic compounds. [96]

Total phenolic and flavonoid content of various fractions

Fraction	Phenol content (mg GAE/g)	Flavonoid content (mg RE/g)
Mother extract of fruit	18± 1.2	15 ± 0.4
Petroleum ether fraction	14 ± 1.4	11 ± 0.6
Chloroform fraction	56 ± 0.7	20 ± 0.2
Ethyl acetate fraction	86 ± 1.3	30 ± 0.5
Butanol fraction	32 ± 1.1	18 ± 0.8
Aqueous fraction	16 ± 0.8	11 ± 0.3

[677- Sida indica]

Percentage Yield of Different Extracts of Sida indica

Solvent	Percentage of yield (%)
Pet ether	2.18
Chloroform	2.04
Ethyl acetate	1.38
n-Butanol	3.84
Ethanol	5.81
Water	6.12

Sida acuta-invitro-leaf-45 clinical isolates isolated from nasal cavity of HIV/AIDS patients of S aureus-The killing rate study showed that ethanol and hot water extracts killed the test isolates faster than the cold water extract. Generally, ethanol proved to be the best solvent for the extraction of the active ingredients from the plant material... the hot water extract produced higher inhibitory activity than the cold water in this research. [273]

Comparison of documented and obtained values of Extractive values in various solvents of Atibala (*Sida indica*)

Solvent for Extract	%Obtained Value	Values in AFI
1. Water	8.2	Less than 9
2. Ethanol	0.6	Less than 3
3. Methanol	1.2	Not available
4. Chloroform	1.6	Not available
5. Petroleum ether	2.0	Not available
6. Acetone	0.4	Not available

Each test is performed with 5 gm of the drug sample as per the procedures mentioned in Ayurvedic Pharmacopeia of India (API). [447]

Antioxidant activity of Sida Acuta plant extracts by DPPH assay.

Plant extracts	IC50 (µg/mL)
1. Pet ether(PE)	321 ± 4.00
2. Toluene(TU)	78 ± 2.00
3. Chloroform(CL)	142.33 ± 2.51
4. Ethyl acetate(EA)	113 ± 3.60
5. Acetone(AC)	194.33 ± 4.04
6. Hydro alcohol(HA)	402 ± 2.51
7. Rutin	21.66 ± 2.08

Values expressed as Mean ± SEM. One way ANOVA followed by Dunnet's post hoc test. [647]

Inhibition zone diameters of different S. rhombifolia extracts

Bacteria species	Diameters of inhibition (mm)				
	A	B	C	D	Gent
E. coli	11.5	11.5	10.2	9.6	23.0
P. vulgaris	9. 5	15.1	12.2	N	26.2
M. morganii	11.2	11.4	N	N	19.4
S. typhi	12.5	15.8	13.3	10.3	26.5
S. enteritidis	14.1	8.7	N	15.6	22.2
S. dysenteriae	11.5	23.6	21.2	14.3	22.5
K. pneumoniae	18.5	19.3	19.2	N	26.5

A: MeOH; B: water/ MeOH (1v:4v); C: water /MeOH (1v:1v); D: water/MeOH (3v:2v); Gent: Gentamycin; N: diameter < 8 mm; Values are expressed as mean SD, (n = 3). [47]

Side effects and interactions

Sida cordifolia-rats-leaves-80% ethanolic extract-showed lower percentage of ulcers compared to indomethacin, but sill at 200mg/kg produced twice as many ulcers as control. **[537]**

Major Interactions   Medications that can cause an irregular heartbeat (QT interval-prolonging drugs) interacts with SIDA CORDIFOLIA. Country mallow can increase the speed of your heartbeat. Taking country mallow along with medications that can cause an irregular heartbeat might cause serious side effects including heart attack.... Taking country mallow with methylxanthines might cause side effects such as jitteriness, nervousness, a fast heartbeat, high blood pressure, and anxiety. Methylxanthines include aminophylline, caffeine, and theophylline... Taking country mallow along with stimulant drugs might cause serious problems including increased heart rate and high blood pressure. **[533]**

Moderate Interaction   Dexamethasone (Decadron) interacts with SIDA CORDIFOLIA... Ergot Derivatives interacts with SIDA CORDIFOLIA... Taking country mallow with ergot derivatives might increase blood pressure too much... Medications for depression (MAOIs) interacts with SIDA CORDIFOLIA. Taking country mallow with these medications used for depression might cause too much stimulation. This could cause serious side effects including fast heartbeat, high blood pressure, seizures, nervousness, and others.   Medications for diabetes (Antidiabetes drugs) interacts with SIDA CORDIFOLIA. **[533]**

Bala {Sida cordifolia} may cause headache, heart attack, insomnia, irregular heartbeat, irritability, memory loss, nervousness, psychosis, seizure, slow or rapid heart rate, stroke, or tremor.

Bala may cause CNS (central nervous system) depressant effects. Drowsiness or sedation may occur. Use caution if driving or operating heavy machinery.

Use cautiously in individuals younger than 18 years of age, due to a lack of safety information.

Use cautiously if taken for prolonged periods, due to a lack of scientific evidence.

Use cautiously in patients with heart disease, including arrhythmia, coronary artery disease, cerebrovascular disease, and a history of stroke or transient ischemic attack, due to potential side effects from the ephedrine constituent in bala.

Bala may cause changes in blood pressure. Caution is advised in patients taking drugs, herbs, or supplements that affect blood pressure.

Use cautiously in patients with depression and anxiety, in patients sensitive to stimulants such as caffeine, or in patients with insomnia or tremor, due to potential side effects from the ephedrine constituent of bala.

Use cautiously in patients using stimulants, including those that potentially contain ephedrine, due to the potential for additive negative effects.

Bala may lower blood sugar levels. Caution is advised in patients with diabetes or hypoglycemia, and in those taking drugs, herbs, or supplements that affect blood sugar. Blood glucose levels may need to be monitored by a qualified healthcare professional, including a pharmacist. Medication adjustments may be necessary.

Use cautiously in patients with previous monoamine oxidase inhibitor (MAOI) use due to potential side effects from the ephedrine in bala.

Use cautiously in patients using other energizing and diet supplements that may contain ephedrine, due to the potential for additive negative effects.

Avoid use in patients taking ergot alkaloids and cardiac glycosides, due to the risk of irregular heart beat.

Avoid in pregnant or breastfeeding women, due to a lack of available scientific evidence.

Avoid with known allergy or hypersensitivity to bala (Sida cordifolia), its constituents, or members of the Malvaceae family.

Pregnancy and Breastfeeding Avoid in pregnant or breastfeeding women, due to a lack of available scientific evidence. [378]

Sida acuta var. carpinfolia
{full information in **Sida as Weed** chapter}

625-Sida carpinifolia-invivo/invitro- fallow deer (Dama dama)- a neurological syndrome characterized by muscular weakness, intention tremors, visual and standing-up deficits, falls, and abnormal behavior and posture, **626**- Sida carpinifolia-invivo/invitro-pony horses-fatal-included multiple cytoplasmatic vacuoles in swollen neurons in the brain, cerebellum, spinal cord, autonomic ganglia (trigeminal and celiac ganglia), and submucosal and myenteric plexus of the intestines. In the kidneys, there was marked vacuolation of the proximal convoluted tubular cells, **627**- Sida carpinifolia-invitro-The indolizidine alkaloid swainsonine has been identified as the toxic constituent-the swainsonine concentration was 0.006% on a dry weight basis, **628**- Sida carpinifolia- Saanen goats- Abnormal excretion of oligosaccharides was observed from the 2nd day of S. carpinifolia ingestion until one day after withdrawal of the plant from the diet-were typical of poisoning caused by plants of this group and were seen from the 37th day on S. carpinifolia diet until seven days after withdrawal of the plant, when signs gradually became scarce and less evident, **629**-Sida carpinifolia-invivo/invitro-cattle-poisoning-marching gait, alert gaze, head tremors, and poor growth. Histologic and ultrastructural lesions consisted of vacuolization and distension of neuronal perikarya, mainly from Purkinje cells, and of the cytoplasm of acinar pancreatic and thyroid follicular cells-no complete recovery,

Sida rodrigoi Monteiro-invivo-goats-toxic levels of swansonine were identified in the plant-poisoning as a plant induced α-mannosidosis animals showed weight loss, indifference to the environment, unsteady gait and ataxia. **[620]**

Side effects: There are no known side effects with Sida indica. Seek medical advice for its use during pregnancy. **[444-Ayurveda]**

Interactions with medicines

To the best of our knowledge, this is the first comprehensive report dealing with the interaction between alkaloid compounds with the {pharmaceutical} antimicrobial drugs currently in use. Synergy research in phytomedicine has established as a new key activity in recent years. It is one main aim of this research to find a scientific rational for the therapeutic superiority of herbal drugs derived from traditional medicine as compared with single constituents thereof. Synergy effects of the mixture of bioactive constituents and their byproducts contained in plant extracts are claimed to be responsible for the improved effectiveness of many extracts and conventional antimicrobial drugs. Such properties can be partly attributed to the diverse array of secondary metabolite such as alkaloids which are known to be essential for plants' defense against microbial attack or insect and animal predation. **[211]**

In short according our results, polyphenol-rich fractions from Sida alba L. were found to possess promising antimicrobial activities when applied alone or in combination with conventional antimicrobial drugs to treat infectious diseases due to multi-resistant bacterial strains. **[11]**

A synergistic effect between alkaloid compounds and the antifungal references such as Nystatin and Clotrimazole- alkaloid compounds in combination with antifungal references (Nystatin and Clotrimazole) exhibited antimicrobial effects against candida strains tested-- MIC 10.42±3.61 (μg/ml)-MFC 29.17±19.09 (μg/ml)--Nystatin MIC=4.17±1.80 (μg/ml)-MFC 12.5±0.00 (μg/ml)--Clotrimazole MIC= 6.25±0.00 (μg/ml)-MFC 14.58±9.55 (μg/ml)--S. cordifolia+Nystatin-MIC 1.04±0.45 (μg/ml)--S. cordifolia+Clotrimazole-MIC 1.56±0.00 (μg/ml). **[27]**

Had bacteriocidal and baceriostatic effect on all bacteria- these effects were stronger in all cases than the control (Cotrimoxazol)-when combined with Co-trimoxazol killed all bacteria (both gram positive and negative) within 5 hours (no mention of how long it took to kill them without the Co-trimoxazol). **[11]**

Actions comparable to medicines

Sida acuta

98-invitro-whole plant- All the flavonoid extracts showed varying degrees of antifungal activity on *C. albicans*. Three extracts (free flavonoids of stem, bound flavonoids of root and leaf) were more effective than traditional antibiotic terbinafine to combat the pathogenic fungi,   **102**-invitro-leaf-1000 mg/ml-100% ethanolic extract-at 1000 mg/ml has better ZI (zone of inhibition) (22) than gentamicin (18) against B. subtilis-has better ZI (44) than gentamicin (34) against Staph aureus,   **186**-invitro-whole plant-methanol extract-400 mg/kg caused significant inhibition of acetic acid induced writhing (p>0.05). The maximum inhibition was at 400mg/kg bw(83.78%). The effects were comparable with that of reference standard, indomethacin that showed 78.97% inhibition of writhing,   **273**-invitro-leaf-45 clinical isolates isolated from nasal cavity of HIV/AIDS patients of S aureus-ethanol extract antimicrobial activity 86%-MIC .96-1.8 ug/ml--lincomycin antimicrobial activity 80%-lincomycin MIC 7.8-31.2 ug/ml {This is quite encouraging, since crude ethanol extract was used in this study.} **572**-Analgesic-(writhing) maximum inhibition was noted for MESA 400mg/kg (83.78%). The effects were comparable with that of reference standard, indomethacin that showed 78.97% inhibition of writhing,   **572**-Analgesic-hot plate analgesia) 400 mg/kg showed significant (P<0.01-0.001) increase in reaction time but the dose of 100 mg/kg did not produce any effect compared to control (P>0.05). The effects very much comparable with pentazocin 10 mg/kg.,

Sida cordifolia

26-rats-water extract-100 mg/kg bw-Rotenone induced oxidative damage was attenuated by the water extract- The maximum effect in all the above activities was observed in the water extract (100mg/kg) treated group, which was comparable to l-deprenyl treated group,   **31**-rats-root-ethanolic extract- In short, the study revealed that 50% ethanolic extract of Sida cordifolia has got potent antioxidant and antiinflammatory activity and the activity is comparable with the standard drug deprenyl,   **45**-The ethyl acetate extract of Sida cordifolia root showed comparable antiinflammatory activity with indomethacin,   **67**-rats-neurotoxicity-ethanolic extract of root-50 mg/100 g bw/day comparable with the standard drug deprenyl,   **68**-Sida cordifolia-rats-neurotoxicity-ethanolic extract of root-50 mg/100 g bw/day comparable with the standard drug deprenyl, **125**-leaf-acqueous extract-2 mg acqueous as powerful as Fluconazole 25 mcg,   **133**-rats-the inhibition of the writhing reflex in mice by the plant extracts (p.o. at a dose of 100 and 200 mg/kg, body weight) were compared against the standard analgesic, aminopyrine 50 mg/kg, p.o.,   **133**-the activities of the extracts were comparable to the standard drug, phenylbutazone,   **152**-invitro-seed-petroleum ether>cold distilled water extract>petroleum ether (40-600C), chloroform, alcohol and aqueous extracts-at 300µg/ml the activity was comparable to that of standard drug norfloxacin, except the chloroform extract of seed which was resistant,

152-invitro-seed oil-petroleum ether (40-600C) extract-ZI 26-28mm (300 µg)-ZI no activity at 100 µg -- chloroform extract ZI 22-26mm (300 µg)-ZI no activity at 100 µg--Griseofulvin ZI 25mm (50 µg/ml)-Against C. albicans seed extracts were resistant at 100µg/ml concentration, whereas the same extracts at 300µg/ml concentration showed promising activity and comparable to standard drug griseofulvin,   **182**-invitro-root-50% ethanol extract-Fumaric acid isolated from S. cordifolia also showed hepatoprotectiveactivity, which was comparable with silymarin-it significantly protects the liver cells and reduces the severity of damage caused by alcohol intoxication- Fumaric acid isolated from S. cordifolia showed hepatoprotective activity comparable with silymarin,   **182**-invitro-root-50% ethanol extract-The studies conducted in our laboratory showed that 50 % ethanolic extract of S. cordifolia has potent anti-oxidant and anti-inflammatory activity. It has a protective effect on quinolinic acid-induced neurotoxicity, which was comparable with the standard drug deprenyl,   **285**-The present study revealed that *Sida cordifolia* has mild to moderate antiinflammatory activity. The activity of the ethyl acetate (EA) extract of root at a dose of 600 mg/kg is equivalent to that of indomethacin and exhibited no ulcerogenicity indicating its safety on the gastrointestinal tract (data not shown). A drug having good antiinflammatory activity with lesser or negligible ulcerogenicity is preferable for treating chronic disease related to inflammation. Interestingly the extracts showed very good peripheral and central analgesic activity as evident from the writhing and hot plate tests. [285]   **403**-The powder and different extracts of the whole plant of S. cordifolia were tested for antihepatotoxic activity against CCl4-, paracetamol-, and rifampicin-induced hepatotoxicities in rats. The methanolic, aqueous and total aqueous extracts showed significant antihepatotoxic activity comparable to that of silymarin,   **408**-the ethyl acetate (EA) extract of root (SCR-E) showed comparable anti-inflammatory activity with indomethacin and possessed significantly higher activity when compared with that of the methanol extract of the root part (SCR-M),   **534**-invivo-roots-acqueous extract- Present preliminary studies confirm better cardiotonic activity of Sida cordifolia Linn than digoxin,   **537**-rats-leaves-80% ethanolic extract-showed acute anti inflammatory activity higher than control group, but it did not show so strong effect as Indomethacin, which produced significant inhibition (58.13%) (P<0.05) .It was found that reduction in the inflammation was 48.83 % (P<0.05) with 100mg/kg Sida cordifolia Linn and 53.48 % (P<0.05) with 200 mg/kg Sida cordifolia Linn. Similarly the extract administered at 200 mg/kg, p.o. had a greater anti-granulation (56 %) effect but less than indomethacin (60.2 %). (since cordifolia seems dose dependent, does it match control at 300 mg/kg?],

Sida rhombifolia

136-rats-roots-water and ethanol extracts-200/400/600 mg/kg bw-produced significant (P< 0.05) and a dose dependent anti-inflammatory activity-ethanolic best-extracts were 80-100% of effect of Indomethacin (5 mg/ kg bw),   **278**-invitro-root-50 mg/ml-petroleum ether extract ZI=16.5 ± 0.5 mm-chloroform extract ZI=14.5 ± 1.5 mm- methanol extracts ZI= 17.5 ± 2 mm-Ciprofloxacin ZI=30 mm--the results showed that antibacterial activities were comparable to each other. But their activities were relatively weaker as compared to that of the reference compound (ciprofloxacin),   **541**-In all categories (LPO: lipid peroxides; SOD: superoxide dismutase; GPX: glutathione peroxidase; TRG: total reduced glutathione; ASA: ascorbic acid) except GPX, treatment resulted in lower values than the control, and generally close to the standard drug Diclofenac 0.3 mg/kg),   **545**-rats-aerial parts-80% ethanol extract-produced about 43.84% and 69.95% writhing inhibition at the dose of 250 and 500 mg/kg of body weight respectively, which were comparable to the standard drug diclofenac sodium where the inhibition was about 82.27% at the dose of 25 mg/kg of body weight (dose dependent),

Sida indica

448-the analgesic activity of the acqueous and ethanolic extracts (400 mg/kg bw) was found to be more or less similar when compared positive control pentazocin (4 mg/kg bw)... The anti-inflammatory activity of various extracts (400 mg/kg bw) were greater than the positive control Diclofenac (10 mg/kg bw),   **453**-whole plant-100mg/kg bw-zone of inhibition (mm)-Acqueous extract 19mm-ethanolic extract 20mm-Hexane extract 0 mm-chloroform extract 0 mm-streptomycin (1mg 22.6mm) 19.6mm- Ampicillin (1 mg/ml) 34.60±0.50,   **454**-rats,invitro-leaves-400 mg/kg bw-extracts reduced blood glucose levels: ether 35%-benzene 46%-ethanolic 30%, acqueous 54%-comparable to tolbutamide 40 mg/kg bw 55%,

Sida rhomboidea

185-invitro-leaf- Percentage inhibition of edema by butanolic extract (33.05, P<0.001) is comparable to that of phenylbutazone, 100 mg/kg inhibition (38.83%),

Sida cardifolia

177-rats-whole plant?-50% ethanol extract- potent anti-antioxidant and anti-inflammatory activity when compared with standard drug deprenyl,   **499**-mice-Acetic acid-induced writhing test-The analgesic activity study revealed that polyphenol rich fractions showed good activity compared with that of standard drug paracetamol,

Cryptolepine   (S. acuta, cordifolia, rhombifolia, spinosa, and ?)
Indoquinoline alkaloid

381-was found to have similar activity to that of chloroquine,   **386**-rats-10–40 mg/kg i.p.- produced significant dose-dependent inhibition of the carrageenan-induced rat paw edema, and carrageenan-induced pleurisy in rats. These effects were compared with those of the non-steroidal anti-inflammatory drug indomethacin (10 mg/kg),   **388**-results showed that negatively charged cryptolepine liposomes were at least 2-4 times more active than free cryptolepine whereas positively charged liposomes were comparable to the activity of free cryptolepine. However, none of the liposome preparations were superior to amphotericin B in their antifungal activity, produced a 20% maximal effect at 2 mg/kg,   **389**-is of about the same potency as phentolamine (pA2 of = 7.5 ± 0.40, pA2 of cryptolepine = 6.6 ± 0.35). We here report a potential effect of small doses of cryptolepine (3.0 ×

10-7-10-6M) on the effect of noradrenaline, an effect which has not been obtained with phentolamine, and methoxamine - induced contractions of the vas deferens, **391**-mouse-mouse model of arterial thrombosis-produced 25% maximal protection at 1 mg/kg while381-Cryptolepine was found to have similar activity to that of chloroquine,

Vasicine   Quinazoline alkaloid, phenolic acid

315-Its uterotonic activity was found to be similar to that of oxytocin and methyl ergometrine [313] - showed bronchodilatory activity in both in vitro and in vivo, its activity being comparable to that of theophylline-Vasicine also exhibited marked respiratory and uterine stimulant activity and moderate degree of hypotensive activity not reported earlier.

Silver and Nanoparticles

When Sida is combined with metallic nanoparticles (silver, gold, zinc) the result is more powerful medicine. The technology is not that difficult – it is possible to make Sida nanoparticles in a home lab.

58-Silver nanoparticles possess unique properties which find myriad applications such as antimicrobial, anticancer, larvicidal, catalytic, and wound healing activities. Biogenic syntheses of silver nanoparticles using plants and their pharmacological and other potential applications are gaining momentum owing to its assured rewards, **77**- The field of nanotechnology is one of the most active areas of research in modern materials science. Nanotechnology is concerned with the development of experimental processes for the synthesis of nanoparticles of different sizes, shapes and controlled disparity. .. The use of environmentally benign materials like plant leaf extract, bacteria and fungi for the synthesis of nanoparticles offers copious benefits of eco-friendliness and compatibility for pharmaceutical and biomedical applications as they do not use toxic chemicals in the synthesis protocols. Chemical synthesis methods lead to the presence of some toxic chemicals absorbed on the surface that may have adverse effect in the medical applications. Green synthesis provides advancement over chemical and physical methods as it is cost effective, environment friendly, easily scaled up for large scale synthesis and in this method there is no need to use high pressure, energy, temperature and toxic chemicals, **77**- Sida acuta-Silver nanoparticles were synthesized by a rapid, cost effective and environmentally benign technique using ground leaves extract of Artemisia annua and Sida acuta as reducing as well as capping agent. Silver nanoparticles (AgNps) were formed within 10-15 minutes by sunlight irradiation of aqueous solution (0.1M) of silver nitrate ($AgNO_3$) with leaves extract of Artemisia annua and Sida acuta. The synthesized AgNp's of both extracts were characterized using UV-visible spectrophotometer. The reaction mixtures showed absorbance at 450nm which is characteristic of silver nanoparticles due to the surface plasmon resonance absorption band, **354**-invivo-leaf-?extract-synthesized silver nanoparticles-larvicidal-the use of S. acuta synthesized silver nanoparticles can be a rapid, environmentally safer biopesticide which can form a novel approach to develop effective biocides for controlling the target

308

vector mosquitoes. This is the first report on the mosquito larvicidal activity of the plant aqueous extract and synthesized nanoparticles,   **705**-Green synthesis of silver nanoparticles using biological entities is gaining interest because of their potential applications in nano-medicine. Herein, we report the biological synthesis of Sida indica silver nanoparticles (AIAgNPs) using aqueous Sida indica leaf extract (AILE) and evaluation of their biological applications... The mode of action through the induction apoptosis by AIAgNPs in COLO 205 cells is exciting with promising application of nano-materials in biomedical research. **[705]**

Synthesis of Zn Nanoparticles

Zinc acetate dihydrate and sodium hydroxide were used as the precursor material. The dried aqueous extract was dissolved in respective solvent, approximately 3 ml was prepared. Three sets of conical flasks with 50 ml distilled water each were prepared and labeled as 0.25 ml, 0.5 ml and 1 ml respectively. 0.02 M aqueous Zinc acetate dihydrate (0.219 gm) was added to each of the three flasks under vigorous stirring. After 10 min stirring aqueous leaf extract of S. indica were introduced into the above solution with the concentration of 0.25 ml,0.5 ml,1 ml to the three labeled flasks followed by the addition of aqueous 2.0M NaOH resulted in a white aqueous solution at pH 12. The pH meter was used for adjusting of pH. pH of the medium influence the size of Zn nanoparticles at great concern, which were then positioned in a magnetic stirrer for 2 hr. The precipitate were then taken out and washed repetitively with distilled water followed by ethanol to remove the impurities of the final product. Then a white powder of Zn nanoparticles was obtained after drying at 60°C in vacuum oven overnight. **[683]**

Medicinal comparisons between Sida species

Sida acuta is an effective anti-cancer agent, whereas S. cordifolia and S. rhombifolia were marginal in this. Acuta has antiproliferative activity against HepG-2 liver cancer cells and reduced their viability to about 30% after 72 hours. **[141]**

Polyphenol contents, antioxidant and anti-inflammatory activities from six species of Malvaceae (Sida acuta Burm, Sida alba L., Sida cordifolia L., Sida rhombifolia L., Sida urens L. and Cienfuegosia digitata Cav.) extracts were investigated in this study in order to provide a scientific basis for the traditional use of plants to treat hepatitis B in Burkina Faso... the extracts of Cienfuegosia digitata and those of Sida alba exhibited the best and significant results in polyphenol contents, antioxidants properties and anti-inflammatory activity. **[593]**

The number of leaves, leaf area, quantity of epicuticular wax and dry matter vary with the stage of development of each species of Sida spp. evaluated. Sida spinosa presented greater values than Sida rhombifolia and Sida urens of specific leaf area at the vegetative stage and of wax at the reproductive stage, which can be related to its competitive ability and lower susceptibility to some herbicides. **[509]**

The drug plant 'Bala' (=Sida cordifolia L.) is often adulterated with Sida retusa L. (Kerala), Sida indica (L.) Sweet. and Urena lobata L **[612]** Sida indica-Its medicinal qualities are quite similar to those of the plant – Bala – Sida cordifolia. **[444]**

The four plants, S. acuta, S. cordifolia, S. alnifolia and S. mysorensis showed the presence of DEHP at considerably high concentration... The present study has shown that the whole plant of some Sida species contain DEHP and the compound is a potent inhibitor of LOX. The enzyme inhibition may partially impart the anti-inflammatory property of the plant. The highest LOX inhibitory effect was exhibited by S. cordifolia methanolic extract followed by S. alnifolia, S. acuta and S. mysorensis. **[292]**

S. acuta is an effective anti-cancer agent, whereas S. cordifolia and S. rhombifolia were marginal in this. Acuta has antiproliferative activity against HepG-2 liver cancer cells and reduced their viability to about 30% after 72 hours. **[141]**

In the ABTS test, the ethanolic extracts of the plants showed antioxidant activity in the following order: S. cordifolia>E. alsinoides>C. dactylon. However, a different order of activity was observed when the same test was performed with the corresponding water infusions (E. alsinoides>C. dactylon>S. cordifolia), indicating the differential solubility of active principles. **[123-S. cordifolia]**

Ayurveda-During a survey of Indian herbal drug markets it was observed that the roots and whole plants of other species of Sida , viz. S. acuta, S. cordata and S. rhombifolia , were being sold under the same vernacular name... Four varieties of bala namely common Bala (S. cordifolia Linn, and S. acuta Burm.), Atibala (S. spinosa Lina), Nagabala (S. veronicaefolia Lam.) and Mahabala (Sida rhombifolia Linn. Mast. var. rhomboidea Mast), are mentioned in Bhavaprakasa Nighantu, which constitute the group Balacatustayam. Of these four types, Bala is the most widely used. This has been equated with Sida cordifolia. There are some other plants which also are used as Bala in various parts of the country. They are S. rhombifolia Linn. Mast. var. retusa Linn, S. spinosa Linn,), Sida indica (Linn.) Sweet, A. hirtum (Lam.) Sweet. (A. graveolens Roxb.), Abutilon glaucum (Cav.) Sweet. (A. muticum Sweet), Urena lobata Linn, U. sinuata Linn., Pavonia zeylanica cav., Grewia tenax(Forsk) Aschers. (G. populifolia Vahl.) and G. hirsuta Vahl. (including G. helicterifolia Wall., G. polygama Mast.). **[548]**

Four varieties of bala namely common Bala (S. cordifolia Linn, and S. acuta Burm.), Atibala (S. spinosa Lina), Nagabala (S. veronicaefolia Lam.) and Mahabala (Sida rhombifolia Linn. Mast. var. rhomboidea Mast), are mentioned in Bhavaprakasa Nighantu, which constitute the group Balacatustayam. Of these four types, Bala is the most widely used. This has been equated with Sida cordifolia. There are some other plants which also are used as Bala in various parts of the country. They are S. rhombifolia Linn. Mast. var. retusa Linn, S. spinosa Linn,), Sida indica (Linn.) Sweet, A. hirtum (Lam.) Sweet. (A. graveolens Roxb.), Abutilon glaucum (Cav.) Sweet. (A. muticum Sweet), Urena lobata Linn, U. sinuata Linn., Pavonia zeylanica cav.,

Grewia tenax(Forsk) Aschers. (G. populifolia Vahl.) and G. hirsuta Vahl. (including G. helicterifolia Wall., G. polygama Mast.)... The present investigation proved conclusively that all the 14 plants can be used as Bala because most of them contained biologically active compounds such as alkaloids, mucilages, flavonoids, phenolic acids. Of the 14 species used as bala, the roots of 11 plants have been screened and ten of them were found to contain ephedrine which is considered as the active principle of bala. Of these ten plants only S. cordifolia was found to yield ephedrine earlier. Therefore nine new source plants were found to yield ephedrine. In 6 plants ephedrine occurred along with other alkaloids. Only in S. rhombifolia var. rhomboidea, some alkaloids other than ephedrine were found as the active principles. [561]

Traditional Uses of Sida

Folkloric use of Sida is as diverse as there are people in the tropics. I avoided research on Sida preparations involving other plants for this first edition - did not want to muddy the results. Hot water tea and ethanolic tinctures are your two basic preparation methods. There are not many sites that carry significant amounts of information on traditional uses of Sidas, except for Ayurveda, though I have listed a few. I was fortunate in the timing of my research; some of the best sites for traditional uses of Sida have now closed or require membership.

I want to reiterate once again that nothing in this book is meant to be medical advice. In this section we give historical uses for educational and informational purposes only.

Many traditional uses are individually listed in both the **Pathogens** and **Benefits** chapters under the appropriate topics. This section on traditional uses of the Sidas comprises two parts. The first part is a sample listing of some "recipes," that is, examples of how Sida has traditionally been applied to some health needs. There is no attempt to be complete or exhaustive, but a sample number of preparations are given. The hope is that the combined traditional references in this book give a general guide to how Sida has been employed time out of mind. Note also that for the most part only six species of Sida are represented – it is unfortunate that Sida's traditional uses have been under-investigated as much as the scientific uses. On the other hand, the known medicinal species of Sida all have, more or less, the same constituents and actions, so research on one species most likely applies to the others. In India, "Bala" may effectively be one of several Sidas.

Some dooryard gardens are specialized in the production of certain food crops for household or local demand or as cash crops. In others, plants are grown strictly for medicinal use. Dooryard gardens owned by shamans have a species composition distinct from those owned by midwives and the general populace **[9]**

The second part is on Ayurveda (as well as Siddah, the counterpart in South India) and how Sidas are an essential part of Ayurvedic medicine. Ayurveda has thousands of years of practice on hundreds of millions of people. Five of the top Ayurvedic herbs are Sidas, including the famous "Bala." It is beyond my competence to give a treatise on Ayurveda, but by capturing the words of Ayurvedic practitioners I hope to give some meaning to a very complex subject.

Who Said What in this Book

- Any comments I make are personal observations and are in this font,
- My comments will not have a citation number.
- The peer-review research is always in this font and will have a citation number at its beginning (**279-**) or end (**[279]**). Traditional and Ayurvedic citations are preceded by a **Tr**, are also bracketed, but are not in bold (**Tr** 279-]. {Short comments I make in the text will be in these brackets}

Sites with information on traditional use

PROTA Plant Resources of Tropical Africa – Your guide to the use of African plants   https://www.prota4u.org/

A surprising number of plants are considered African. An excellent resource that lists all the traditional uses is Plant Resources of Tropical Africa. This database lists a number of Sidas in great detail, including medicinal and other uses. It also connects with other databases, under medical uses there are 20 other sources.

PROTA is a full listing of plants containing everything from their names, chromosome number, to cultivation and ecology. While this listing is supposedly only African plants, that seems to be native and acquired, since the Sidas are not native to Africa. They are desperately trying to keep this amazing resource open, so when you visit, give them a donation. **[358]**

Philippian Medicinal Plants website http://www. stuartxchange.com

Choose the button, "Philipean Alternative Medicine". Then at the top click on, "Search". Once there click on the big illustration. Look up by Latin name, has a selection of traditional uses. Dr. Godofredo Umali-Stuart **[524-528]**

Ayurhelp website   http://www.ayurhelp.com

An site dedicated to propagate Ayurveda knowledge. Home Remedies and Ayurvedic Plants. **[730]**

efloraofindia Google group

https://sites. google.com/site/ efloraofindia/

I am deeply indebted to the efloraofindia Google group who have allowed me to use some of their magnificent photographs of Sida plants. They are a kind and welcoming group and I heartily recommend any of my readers joining them. They are non-commercial and have one of the largest Indian Flora databases on the net with more than 12,000 species, including some species from around the world. **[796]**

Traditional uses of Sida

Plants have been used as medicines for thousands of years. People depend on plants for several purposes like for wood, timber, non-timber forest products, food, medicine, etc. They have always been used as a rich source of biologically active drugs and have numerous traditional uses to serve mankind for many thousand years. Nowdays, they are used widely because of growing awareness of people towards unwanted side effects and high cost of the allopathic medicines which makes them beyond the reach of common people. According to WHO (World Health Organization) report, about 80% of the population, mostly in developing countries, still depends on traditional medicinal system for their primary health care. India is one of the twelve mega-biodiversity centers with 4 hot-spots of biodiversity. Ethnobotanical knowledge has been reported from its several parts. The different systems of medicinal usage like Ayurveda, homeopathy and Unani which are the local health traditions, focus on the use of plant products for the treatment of human and animal diseases. Medicinal plants contain numerous biologically active compounds which are helpful in the treatment of various diseases and improving the life. The presence of various life sustaining constituents in plants made scientists to investigate them for their uses in treating certain infectious diseases and management of chronic wounds. In addition to being a good source of anti-infective agents, they are also cost-effective and have fewer side effects... The information on medicinal plants has been accumulated in the course of several centuries based on various systems of medicine. India has very rich plant diversity and houses about 47,000 plant species but traditional healers' use only 2500 plant species out of which about 100 species of plants serve as the natural principle source of medicine. [712]

Traditional healers claim that their medicine is cheaper and more effective than modem medicine... plant-derived medicines have been part of traditional health care in most parts of the world and the antimicrobial properties of plant-derived compounds are well documented and there is increasing interest in plants as sources of antimicrobial agents. Medicinal plants have been used for centuries as remedies for human diseases because they contain components of therapeutic value. Recently, some higher plant products have attracted the attention of microbiologists to search for some phytochemicals for their exploitation as antimicrobials, such plant products would be biodegradable and safe to human health [55]

The results of this study indicate that medicinal plants are used frequently by local people in the region. Some of the plants are already under threat because of overexploitation, including clearing land for agriculture, encroachment and abrupt change in environmental conditions. The majority bulk of the inhabitants seem to be unaware of the great threat to medicinal plants growing in the wild. [241]

Sida in General

Sida is one of ethno-medicinally important genus of plants. The plants from genus Sida are used in India over 2000 years. The most medicinally important species of Sida like Sida acuta, Sida cordifolia, S. rhombifolia, S. spinosa, S. car-penifolia, S. humilis, S. veronicaefolia - are used in Ayurvedic system. [107]

The genus Sida of the family Malvaceae is profusely represented in India. It has a wide range of tolerance and its distribution extends from the sub-temperate regions of the Himalayas to the plains. Though only six species are recorded from the plains of Bengal and nine from all over India, a wide range of form variations is frequent in this genus. Of the different species, in S. rhombifolia and S. acuta, the maximum phenotypic variations occur. A study of such variations is of special interest, not only from the academic viewpoint, but also due to the high medicinal importance of species of Sida. Almost all the species, occurring in India and specially in Bengal, contain medicinal principles which are obtained differentially from different plant parts, namely roots, stems, leaves, flowers, fruits and seeds. [216]

An Ethnobotanical investigation in the central region of Burkina Faso has shown that many species are traditionally used to treat various kinds of pain diseases. Among such plants, S. acuta Burn f. and S. cordifolia L. (Malvaceae) are the most frequently and widely used. [75]

314

Sida acuta

CONCLUSION: S. acuta is a plant of wide usage in traditional medicine. In traditional medicine, the part is often assumed to treat diseases such as fever, head ache, skin diseases, diarrhea and dysentery. Following these traditional usages many studies have been conducted in laboratories for the efficacy of the plant; in addition the plant may have many other properties since it has not been tested for all desired pharmacological activities. Since the global scenario is now changing towards the use of non toxic plant product having traditional medicine use, development of modern drugs from S.acuta should be emphasized for the control of various diseases. The plant S.acuta holds tremendous potential for pharmaceutical products of commercial values. [270-2015]

Folkloric Uses:

- Poultices made from boiled leaves are applied to ulcers and sores.

- Decoction of roots and leaves are emollient; taken internally for hemorrhoids, fever, impotency and as a tonic.

- Decoction also used as demulcent; for gonorrhea and rheumatism.

- Roots use as stomachic and antipyretic.

- Decoction or infusion used for fevers, dyspepsia and debility.

- An infusion with ginger added is given in intermittent fevers and chronic bowel complaints, a teacupful twice a day.

- Root juice, sugared or mixed with honey, used to expel worms.

- Juice of leaves, mixed with honey, given for dysentery and chest pains.

- Fresh juice of roots applied to wounds and ulcers to promote healing.

- In Nicaragua, whole plant used for asthma, colds, fever, worms, and renal inflammations. In India, used for fever, bronchitis, ulcers, diarrhea, skin diseases; paste of leaves mixed with coconut oil used for dandruff and hair strengthening. In Nigeria, used for malaria, ulcer, fever, breast cancer, poisoning, inducing abortion. In Sri Lanka, roots and leaves used for hemorrhoids, fever, impotency, gonorrhea, and rheumatism.

- In the Yucatan, decoction of roots used for vomiting of blood; decoction of leaves used for fever.

- In India, seeds are given for enlarged glands and for inflammatory swellings.

- In Togo, West Africa, leaves used for eczema, kidney stones, headache.

- In Indian traditional medicine, used for treating liver disorders, urinary disease and disorders of the blood and bile.

- In the Ivory Coast, used for malaria.

- Fiber from the bark is yellow, delicate, filamentous, soft, very lustrous and silky in appearance, of medium strength. In the Ilocos it is used to make a superior-quality rope, of pleasing color and gloss.

- Stems are used for making brooms and baskets.   [526]

The leaves when bruised are shiny and are put on the hands of midwives when they are about to remove dead children from the womb. **[96]**

Sida is traditionally used to cure diarrhea in Australia. In Mexico, leaves are smoked for its simulative effects and in some parts of India, Sida leaves are used in tea for the same purpose. The plant is traditionally used as an astringent and as antidote for scorpion stings and snake bites... Kuniata and Rapp 2001 reported that it is because of the presence of different chemicals including alkaloids that arrow leaf Sida is not liked by cattle... In the Gold Coast, S. acuta plant is used to cure several diseases. The leaves when bruised are shiny and are put in the hands of midwives when they are about to remove death children from the womb and they are frequently used to procure abortion... Ethnobotanical investigation in some part of Africa has shown that species are traditionally used to treat various kinds of illnesses. Among such plants Sida acuta (Malvaceae) are the most frequently and widely put to use. **[256]**

The alkaloids displayed good antimicrobial activity against several test micro-organisms. The GC-MS analysis of the same alkaloid extract revealed the presence of two major alkaloids; cryptolepine and quindoline. The results of the present study support the traditional medicinal use of S. acuta and suggest that a great attention should be paid to this plant which is found to have many pharmacological properties. **[7-2006]**

S. acuta is a plant of wide usage in traditional medicine... many studies have been conducted in laboratories for the efficiency of the plant, in addition the plant may have many other properties since it has not been tested for all desired pharmacological activities . Since the global scenario is now changing towards the use of non toxic plant product having traditional medicine use, development of modern drug from S. acuta should be emphasized for the control of various diseases. The plant S. acuta holds tremendous potential for pharmaceutical products of commercial values. **[270-2015]**

Sida cordifolia

Folkloric Uses:

- Decoction of leaves used as emollient and a diuretic.

- Pounded in water, juice used for spermatorrhea and gonorrhea.

- Infusion of roots, used for nervous and urinary disease; also for disorders of the blood and bile.

- In China, plant used as diuretic.

- Root juice used for healing wounds.

- Juice of whole plant used for rheumatism and spermatorrhea.

- Decoction of root and ginger used for intermittent fevers with shivering fits.

- Root bark powder in milk and sugar used for frequent micturition and leucorrhea.

- Root, alone or with asafoetida and rock salt, used for neurologic disorders (headaches, paralysis).
- Infusion of root used for delirium.
- Roots also used internally for asthma and as a cardiac tonic.
- Infusion of leaves used as cooling medicine for fevers and to check bloody fluxes.
- Bruised fresh leaves used for boils to promote suppuration.
- Leaves cooked and eaten for bleeding piles.
- Leaves are mucilaginous and used as a demulcent.
- In Konkan, leaves for opthalmia.
- Seeds considered aphrodisiac; used for gonorrhea, cystitis, colds and tenesmus.
- Gujarat folk tribes in India use the herb for coronary manifestations.
- Fiber: Produces a fiber, as valued as jute. **[525]**

For elephantiasis, the juice of the whole plant has been pounded with a little water, made into paste with the juice of the palmyra tree, and applied to the affected area. For eye disease, a paste made from bala leaves has been applied to the affected eye. For general musculoskeletal soreness, bala oil has been used to massage the affected area. For gonorrhea, whole plant juice has been pounded with water and taken by mouth as tea in doses of 1/4 seer (approximately one cup). For wound dressing, a paste made from bala leaves has been applied to the affected area. Children (under 18 years old) - There is no proven safe or effective dose for bala in children. **[378]**

In traditional medicine in Benin the whole plant is used as a cure for cancer and leukemia, the seeds are a cure for infections and the roots cure urinary tract problems and fever. The powdered whole plant is applied to open wounds of horses in Niger. In Senegal, Côte d'Ivoire, Burkina Faso, Burundi, Kenya, Papua New Guinea and the Philippines the leaves are taken as a cure for dysentery. The pounded leaves are applied as a poultice to sprains and swellings and a leaf decoction is drunk for control of intestinal worms. In DR Congo a leaf infusion is given to children in case of rheumatism, lung disorders and fever. In Rwanda the leaf extract is used for curing pneumonia and syphilis. In Mauritius plant sap is diluted and drunk to relieve colic and a leaf decoction is a cure for cystitis, and is used as an astringent and diuretic. To cure eye inflammation a root macerate is applied to the eyelids in Burkina Faso, while in Tanzania a root preparation is applied and in Malaysia the leaves are applied for this purpose. The juice of the whole plant pounded with a little water is given for spermatorrhoea. In the Central African Republic and in Kenya the root extract is drunk to induce abortion. Women chew the bark to encourage menstruation. An infusion of the roots is given for diseases such as hemiplegia and facial paralysis, for asthma as well as for disorders of the blood and bile. Powdered root bark is given with milk and sugar to persons suffering from leucorrhoea. The seeds are considered to have aphrodisiac properties and are used as a cure for gonorrhoea, cystitis, and colic. **[358]**

Part used: Root

Dose: Juice extract – 10 – 20 ml, in divided dose per day.

Powder – 3 – 6 grams in divided dose per day.

Decoction – Kashaya – 50 -100 ml in divided dose epr day.

External application: Its paste is prepared with water and applied externally to relieve joint pain, headache and inflammation. **[444]**

Decoction of the root of bala and ginger is given in intermittent fever attended with cold shivering fits. Root juice is also used to promote healing of wounds. Powder of the root and bark together, is given with milk and sugar for frequent micturition. Oil prepared from the decoction of root bark mixed with milk and sesame oil, finds application in diseases of the nervous system, and is very efficacious in curing facial paralysis and sciatica. Yogaratnakaram a treatise on medicine, written by Yeturi Srinivasa charyulu, describes Bala as 'divine medicine'. He gives two preparations in detail, using Bala for treating various ailments....   Leaves are cooked and eaten in cases of bleeding piles. Juice of the whole plant, pounded with a little water is given in doses of ¼ seer for spermatorrohea, rheumatism, and gonorrhoea. Made into paste with juice of palmyra tree, it is applied locally, in elephantiasis. The herb has rasayana (rejuvenating) properties and assists in convalescence and debility. The oils are used topically to massage the sore muscles, sore joints in arthritis and rheumatism, in sciatica and neuritis of legs. **[377]**

Popularly known as 'bala', the root of Sida cordifolia L. (Malvaceae) is regarded as a valuable drug in the Ayurvedic System of Indian Medicine. It is also used in the traditional medicine systems in China, Brazil and other countries for a wide range of illnesses. **[312]**

Sida cordifolia -- Abortifacient, Alterative, Amebicide, Anticonvulsant, Aphrodisiac, Antipyretic, Astringent, Bechic, Bitter, Cardiotonic, Cerebrotonic, Circulotonic, Curare, Demulcent, Depurative, Digestive, Diuretic, Emollient, Hypotensive, Insecticide, Lipogenic, Pectoral, Protisticide, Sedative, Stomachic, Teratogen, Tonic. **Juice of the plant—** invigorating, spermatopoietic, used in spermatorrhoea. **Seeds—** nervine tonic. **Root—**(official part in Indian medicine) used for the treatment of rheumatism; neurological disorders (hemiplegia, facial paralysis, sciatica); polyuria, dysuria, cystitis, strangury and hematuria; leucorrhoea and other uterine disorders; fevers and general debility. **Leaves—**demulcent, febrifuge; used in dysentery. **Root bark**, pulverized and mixed with oil of sesame and milk, has been said to be effective in cases of facial paralysis and sciatica. Ethnic communities of Ranchi, Hazaribag and Varanasi districts consider the plant useful in venereal diseases. Ethnic communities of Delhi area use seeds in spermatorrhoea and gonorrhoea. In Ayurvedic system root-extract is used in leucorrhoea and menorrhagia. Different parts of the plant are used in many other diseases in Ayurveda and tribal systems. **Whole plant**: Plant is boiled, and the water used as an herbal bath for washing the skin as an anti-pruritic, as an anti-pyretic for chickenpox and measles, by the Guyana Patamona. Leaf: Leaves are boiled, and the water drunk as an anti-pyretic, by the Guyana

318

Patamona. Medicinal Plants of the Guianas (Guyana, Surinam, French Guiana) **[375]**

Sida cordifolia-Leaves are cooked and eaten in cases of bleeding piles. Juice of the whole plant, pounded with a little water is given in doses of ¼ seer for spermatorrhea, rheumatism, and gonorrhea. Made into paste with juice of palmyra tree, it is applied locally, in elephantiasis. The herb has rasayana (rejuvenating) properties and assists in convalescence and debility. It is very effective as medicated oil. The popular Mahanarayana taila, Balati taila, Prabhanjana Vimardhana, Ksheera-bala taila contain this herb. The oils are used topically to massage the sore muscles, sore joints in arthritis and rheumatism, in sciatica and neuritis of legs. Another oil called Dhanvantari tailam (21 and 101 times boiled) which contains Bala along with 47 other substances, and is prepared in milk and given for all disorders produced by the derangement of 'Vata', such as emaciation, weakness, diseases of reproductive organs. The leaves can be used as an infusion in treating fevers and delirium. The root of this plant is astringent, diuretic, and tonic, and its infusion is useful in cystitis, strangury, haematuria, bleeding piles, chronic dysentery, leucorrhoea, and gonorrhea. The seeds contain much larger quantities of alkaloids than the leaves and roots and are used as an aphrodisiac. They are also useful in treating colic, tenesmus and gonorrhea.... Bala has been in use for over 2000 years in treating bronchial asthma, cold and cough, chills, aching joints and bones. The alkaloid ephedrine, which was so far observed in different varieties of Ephedra sp., has been identified in this plant which is responsible for treating asthma. The presence of this sympathomimetic substance also explains its use as a cardiac stimulant in the old Hindu medicine. In the Konkan, the leaves with other cooling leaves are applied in opthalmia. The leaves, mixed with rice, are given to alleviate the bloody flux. The Thongas of Portugal and the East Africans use this plant as a remedy to treat children's ailments. In Cambodia the roots are considered as diuretic and depurative; they are given in the treatment of gonorrhea and ringworm. Decoction of the root of bala and ginger is given in intermittent fever attended with cold shivering fits. Root juice is also used to promote healing of wounds. Powder of the root and bark together is given with milk and sugar for frequent micturition. Oil prepared from the decoction of root bark mixed with milk and sesame oil finds application in diseases of the nervous system, and is very efficacious in curing facial paralysis and sciatica. **[377]**

Among the 33 herbs around Garhwal Himalaya, India, Sida cordifolia was dominant in the tropical and sub-tropical regions. Sida cordifolia is valued 50% more than Sida acuta in the tropics, and is the only Sida cited in sub-tropics, where it is the most valued medicinal of all studied. **[241]** Sida cordifolia has been used in India for over 2,000 years now to treat a variety of health disorders like bronchial asthma, cold & flu, chills, lack of perspiration, headache, nasal congestion, aching joints and bones, and edema. **[161]**

....

S. rhombifolia is one of the most important species among the twenty genus of Sida used as medicinal plant throughout the world. **[47]**

Sida rhombifolia

Folkloric Uses:

- In the Philippines decoction of the roots is used as a gargle for toothaches; internally, as a stomachic.

- Decoction of bitter bark used for fever.

- A decoction from any plant part used for irregular menses.

- Plant used for poulticing ulcers, boils, swellings, broken bone, cuts, herpes.

- Plant poultice used as application for chicken pox.

- Pulped leaves applied externally for stomach aches.

- Pulped leaves with Blumea balsifera (dalapot) applied externally for headaches, and to the gums for toothaches.

- Plant parts with coconut oil applied externally for itches and scurf.

- In Cuba, decoction of roots used for infantile diarrhea.

- The roots when crushed with ginger, held in the mouth, for toothaches.

- The leaves and juice, taken by mouth for stomach cramps.

- Fresh leaves are mucilaginous and emollient and a cataplasm used to promote maturation of abscesses.

- Pulped roots applied to sore breasts.

- In Amboina, crushed roots held in mouth for toothaches; also, chewed with ginger.

- Juice swallowed for abdominal cramps.

- In Borneo, reported use as abortifacient.

- Juice of pounded leaves used for fevers.

- Flowers applied to wasp stings.

- The leaves have been used as tea.

- The flowers are used for wasp stings.

- Mucilage used as emollient and for scorpion stings.

- In India, mucilaginous roots used as demulcent and emollient.

- Root decoction has been used for bronchitis and asthma; also for fevers and various abdominal troubles.

- In Johore medicine, used for rheumatism.

- Australian aborigines use the herb to treat diarrhea.

- Decoction of old root used to relieve constipation.

- Hindus use it for fever, nervous and urinary diseases.

- In Ayurveda, widely used in the treatment of fever; also, as diuretic.

- In Indonesia, a trditional medicinal plant for the treatment of gout.

- Tea: In some parts of Mexico, leaves reportedly used as substitute for tea.

- Fiber: Stem yields a good fiber; considered a good substitute for jute. [524]

Seychelles, Vernacular name: herbe dure - H(003),
contusion, leaves of Sida rhombifolia, to pound, local application + oil of ricin

Popular republic of Congo (Brazzaville) (ex Brazaville Congo) Vernacular name: kili (Akwa) - (fevers, malaria, yellow fever - H(051), leaves of Sida rhombifolia of Bidens pilosa of Quassia africana, decoction, bath

Togo - (stop production of mothers milk) - H(002), barks of the underground part of Rauvolfia vomitora, leaves of Sida rhombifolia, to dry, powder, to dilute in wine, VO.

Comoros, Vernacular name: ifoudouwé (Great Comoros), foundrankoré (Anjouan island) - skin problems - H(013), leaves of Sida rhombifolia, to pound, local application

Equatorial Guinea - (treating a urogential infection) - H(045) + H(038) antiseptic for urinary conduct, leaves juice of Sida rhombifolia, in vagina

Uganda - (diziness, vertigo) - H(036), leaves of Sida rhombifolia, maceration (H2O), to filter, VO.

Burundi (Zaïre-Nil ridge region) - (mouth infection) - H(076) stomatitis, vesicles in the mouth, decoction stem Sida., VO.

Angola (region of Malanje) Vernacular name: nzunzu (Umbundu) - (chemical-driven liver damage) - H(126) hepatitis, roots tea of Sida rhombifolia, VO.

Gabon Vernacular name: kembitchi / bakembitchi - (purification) - H(201) purification of the hunters after transporting a body, leaves maceration, bath

Democratic republic of Congo (Shabunda, Kabare, Walikale) Vernacular name: mudundu (Mashi), kanjunju (Kirega) - (snake bite) - H(020) snake, vaccine made with the decoction of young leaves of Sida rhombifolia

Madagascar (Betsileo country) Vernacular name: tsindaorina - (anxiety/stress) - H(099) nervous breakdown, leaves decoction of Sida rhombifolia

Democratic republic of Congo (ex. Zaïre) (ex. Belgian Congo) (Kisantu region) - (burns) - H(111), leaves, RNS. - (internal parasites) - H(068), vermifuge against amoebas, raw leaves of Sida rhombifolia, VO.

Kenya Bondo district) Vernacular name: anyango nyaywora (Luo) - (diarrhea, stomach ache) - H(008) (chira), diarrhoea, H(104) stomach ache, infusion of leaves of Sida rhombifolia, VO.

Rwanda (Gisenyi district) Vernacular name: umucundura - (lung disease) - H(037) pneumonia, roots pounded, crushed + H2O, extract, VO.

Southern Ethiopia (Maale and Ari ethnic communities) Vernacular name: chuksha (A) -

Cameroon - (anemia) - H(091), whole plant of Sida rhombifolia, maceration (H2O), VO.

Central African Republic - (rib pain) - H(031), leaves of Sida rhombifolia, to pound, maceration (H2O), VO. + local salt

Madagascar Vernacular name: tsindahory - (skin problem) - H(013) rash, roots, leaves, juice, local application

Nigeria (Local markets in Lagos state) Vernacular name: iseketu pupa - (skin wound, diarrhoea, emollient) - H(004) wound; H(008) diarrhoea, H(193) emollient, leaves of Sida rhombifolia , RNS. (Information obtained from herb sellers and traditional medicine practitioners from three popular and largest markets in Lagos)

Madagascar - (cancer) - H(078) tumors, ONS., RNS.

Burundi (Occidental) Vernacular name: umuvumvu (Kirundi) - (labor pain) - H(022, 2), leaves, pressed in H2O, VO., (ocytocic)

Madagascar - (spleen, fevers) - H(051) fever, leaves, decoction, VO. - H(127), leaves, decoction, VO.

Gabon Vernacular name: nnom-nzisim (Fang) - (unidentified disease) - H(000), leaves, RNS., enema

Democratic republic of Congo (ex. Zaïre) (Equator, Lisala) - (veneral disease) - H(100) blen., leaves, infusion, RNS.

Uganda (Sango bay area) Vernacular name: akavuvu - (eye cataracts) - H(001, 5) cataract, application of leaves on eyes 2 x / Day

Cameroun Vernacular name: nsengnebew (Babungo) - (insomnia) - H(098) drowsiness, leaves of Sida rhombifolia are chewed and the juice is swallowed - (anti-inflammatory) - H(113), ONS. of Sida rhombifolia, RNS.

karaaba (Afaan Oromoo) - Burundi (Zaïre-Nil ridge region) [360]

In traditional African medicine decoctions of the roots and leaves are widely used as emollients. The leaves or the leaf sap are applied to the skin as an antiseptic and to treat abscesses, ulcers and wounds, for instance in Equatorial Guinea, Gabon, DR Congo, Tanzania and Madagascar. The roots and leaves (DR Congo) or the leaves alone (Gabon) are used as an abortifacient. In Cameroon a watery maceration of the leaves is drunk as an antihypertensive agent, as a sedative, against sexually transmitted diseases and to cure diarrhea. The same cure for diarrhea is used in DR Congo where it is also thought to help overcome general stomach complaints and dysentery. Leaves and roots are used in Senegal, the Central African Republic and Madagascar for respiratory diseases like asthma, bronchitis, dyspnoea and pneumonia. The flowers are applied to wasp stings or eaten to ease labor pains. In the Philippines and Indonesia a paste of the leaves mixed with coconut oil is applied to scurf and itch. In Malaysia the plant has been used to treat pulmonary tuberculosis. In Fiji and Papua New Guinea the leaves are used to treat strained muscles, labor pains and migraine. Roots are chewed against toothache in Cameroon and Indonesia, and against dysentery in South-East Asia. Cultivated in Australia (Queensland), North and South America, also in Africa as fiber plant. The bark fiber has the quality of jute. In India used as medicine (mucilage). Leaves and young shoots are eaten in Middle and South America as vegetable. The dried leaves are also used as tea. S. rhombifolia is one of the most variable species of the genus Sida. As result of this variation it was described by several authors under different names. A satisfactory analysis of this complex is needed. [358]

The hot aqueous extract of dried aerial parts of Sida rhombifolia is used for snake bite in East Africa. The hot aqueous extract of entire plant of S. rhombifolia in Borneo is used as an abortifacient when it is taken orally by pregnant women. The hot aqueous extract of entire plant is used as an abortifacient on oral administration in pregnant women in Central Africa. In India, the decoction of entire plant of S. rhombifolia when given orally to human adults reduces rheumatic pain. The decoction is also mixed with equal proportion of cow's milk and taken every morning for about a week for the same purpose. The hot aqueous extract of the plant in Malaysia is used for irregular menses when taken orally by adult females. The decoction prepared from entire plant of S. rhombifolia in Mexico is used to treat head cold when applied externally. The hot aqueous extract of the entire plant in Mozambique is used for cough when given orally to both sexes of human adults. The roots and leaves in Honduras are used as poultice when applied externally on boils. The hot aqueous extracts of the entire plant in India is used as an aphrodisiac and in treatment of fever and urinary diseases when given orally to adult humans. The infusion of dried leaf of S. rhombifolia in Central Africa is used for diabetes, chest pain and diarrhea on oral administration. The infusion of this plant is applied locally for the treatment of skin diseases and infected wounds. The leaf juice of the plant in India has been in use for the treatment of spermatorrhea on oral administration. The leaf juice of this plant in Madagascar is applied externally in abscesses and the leaf is useful in treating menstrual pain in Argentina. The leaf and root infusions of the plant in Cameron are given orally in dysentery and diarrhea whereas in Mozambique, these are applied externally as emollient. The decoction of leaf and root of this plant are given orally to facilitate child birth.

The hot aqueous extracts of dried leaf and root of the plant in India are used to treat nervous diseases, heart diseases, burning sensation of the body and as aphrodisiac and tonic. The decoction of leaf and stem of S. rhombifolia in Guatemala is taken orally in urinary inflammation. In India the leaf juice mixed with sesame oil for the treatment of snake bite and the fresh leaf juice is given orally in spermatorrhoea. The fresh leaf juice in New Guinea has been in use for the treatment of diarrhea in children. The fresh plant juice in India, is taken orally to dissolve stones in urinary tract, while in Nepal, the plant juice is applied externally for boils. The plant is eaten by pregnant women during third or fourth month of pregnancy in Borneo for abortion, while the aqueous extract of the root in Central Africa is taken orally to induce abortion. The dried root in Australia is used by traditional people for abdominal upset and in Buka Island it is taken for the treatment of diarrhea. The decoction of root in India is used orally for the treatment of pulmonary tuberculosis and the aqueous extract to treat malaria. The dried root of the plant, in combination with Casuarina equisetifolia, is chewed for 2 days by the local people to treat dysentery in Papua-New Guinea. The decoction of the dried root of the plant along with Cissampelos pareira var. orbiculata in Tanzania is used to treat habitual abortion.

The twig of the plant is used by local people in India as toothbrush to strengthen gums. The leaf paste is applied topically for boil and taken orally with milk in dysentery. The stem of the plant in Rotuma is chewed for dental hygiene and the infusion is used for prevention of miscarriage. The infusion of flower, fruit and leaf are used by adult human externally for loss of hair in Mexico. The decoction of flower is used for cleansing open sores, while the infusion is used as an emollient and for dysentery in Madeira. The S. rhombifolia infusion is taken orally in Guatemela for the treatment of gonorrhoea and the leaf juice in Guinea is applied by traditional healer in vagina as an antiseptic. The leaf paste of the plant is applied externally for cuts and boils by the Tharus of Nainital district in India. In Nicaragua, the decoction of the leaf is taken orally by adult human in the treatment of fever, cough, aches, infections, cold, diarrhea and childbirth. The leaf of S. rhombifolia in Peru is used traditionally in gonorrhoea, tuberculosis, tumors, snake bite, alopecia, lupus, urinary bladder ailments, urethritis and as analgesic, sedative, emenogogue, lactogogue and diuretic. The hot aqueous extract of the dried leaf is used externally in Guatemela for abscesses, furuncles, erysipelas, scrofula, skin eruption, dermatitis, inflammation and conjunctivitis. The decoction of the leaf is taken orally by Garifuna of eastern Nicargua in fever, aches, pain, infections, venereal diseases, respiratory and pulmonary disorder. [522]

This indigenous plant holds a remarkable reputation among the medical practitioners for its anti-rheumatism activity and is an important ingredient in polyherbal formulations. Being a Rasayana drug they are rejuvenating and age-sustaining tonics for promoting vitality and longevity. It is also used for the treatment of asthma and other chest ailments. [464]   Its stems are used as rough cordage, sacking and for making brooms. The stems have a high-quality fiber and were once exported from India and elsewhere as "hemp". [217]

Pounded leaves of the plant are applied as a paste to reduce swelling and rid of boils and headaches. Root decoction is taken as tea to treat diarrhea. In India the plant is used in the treatment of gonorrhea. In Europe it is used as anti-tuber-cular agent. Decoction of the plant is used to treat rheumatic pain, strengthening of cardiac ailments, and biliary problems in children. Fresh plant juice is used as demulcent and diuretic. It is widely used in the traditional medicine practices of different cultures to treat various types of ailments like malaria, chest pain, fever, abdominal pain and as a tonic. [217]

Sida retusa

An infusion made from the roots of this plant is held in great repute by the local ayurvedic physicians in the treatment of rheumatism and a variety of neurological complaints including epilepsy. It is used in calculus troubles as a diuretic and as an antipyretic in fevers attended with shivering and fits. [529]

Stems considered emollient and demulcent, for external and internal use. Leaves used for dressing ulcers. Poultice of leaves used for insect bites. Hindus use the roots for rheumatism. In Ayurveda, used for rheumatism and variety of neurological problems including epilepsy. Used in calculus troubles as diuretic and as febrifuge. [527]

Sida indica

Considered analgesic, anti-inflammatory, anthelmintic, aphrodisiac, astringent, demulcent, digestive, diuretic, expectorant, laxative. Studies have shown hepatoprotective, hypoglycemic, immunomodulatory, antinociceptive, antimicrobial, antimalarial, antifertiity, hepatoprotective, antioxidant, analgesic, anti-malarial, and wound healing properties. Leaves considered stomachic and antiperiodic. [729]

Folkloric Uses:

- In the Philippines, decoction of leaves used for cleansing wounds and ulcers.

- Decoction of leaves also used as enemas or vaginal injections.

- Leaves used as emollient decoction, used by Filipinos as demulcent, diuretic, sedative, and aphrodisiac.

- Plant leaves are demulcent; given as decoction for bronchitis, bilious diarrhea, gonorrhea, bladder inflammation, urethritis and fevers. Decoction also for fomentation over aching body parts for its emollient benefits.

- Bark is astringent and diuretic.

- Seeds are demulcent, laxative, expectorant and aphrodisiac; useful for gonorrhea and cystitis.

- In China, used for tinnitus, deafness, earaches, fevers, hives, tuberculosis, weeping ulcers; as diuretic.

- In India, used for coughs and fevers, body aches, hemorrhoids, gonorrhea, bronchitis, dysuria, diabetes, dysmenorrhea, diarrhea, boils and skin ulcers. Bark and root used as diuretic.

- Infusion of root used to relieve strangury and hematuria; also used for leprosy.

- Infusion of leaves and roots used as cooling medicine in fevers.

- Decoction of leaves used as mouthwash in toothache and tender gums; also used in gonorrhea and bladder inflammation.

- Flowers and leaves applied locally to boils and ulcers.

- Leaf decoction used as eyewash and mouthwash for toothaches and tender gums.

- Decoction of leaves yield a mucilage to hot water and used as fomentation for painful parts.

- Decoction of seeds used for piles and wounds. Also used for gonorrhea, gleet, and chronic cystitis.

- Seeds burnt on charcoal, and the recta of threadworm-affected children are exposed to the smoke.

- In Indo-China, the young flowers and seeds are used as diuretic, emollient, and tonic.

- In Tamil, India, leaf juice and root taken orally for dental problems. [729]

Sida spinosa

(syn. S. alba, S. alnifolia)

It is used as tonic and for the treatment of asthma and other chest ailments. The ethanolic extract of S. alnifolia possesses hypoglycemic activity. It also depressed the normal blood pressure. It is a tonic in wasting diseases, cures ulcer and biliousness, useful in urinary infection, leprosy and skin infection. The leaves possess demulcent and refrigerant properties and useful in gonorrhea, gleet and scalding urine. The roots are used as tonic diaphoretic and useful in treatment of fever, debility, as demulcent, and in irritability of bladder. [217]

It may be concluded from this study that Sida spinosa Linn. leaf extract has antimicrobial activity against certain bacteria and fungi. It is expected that using natural products as therapeutic agents will probably not elicit resistance in microorganisms. This can explain the rationale for the use of the plant in treating infections in traditional medicine. The plant could be a veritable and cheaper substitute for conventional drugs since the plant is easily obtainable and the extract can easily be made via a simple process of maceration or infusion. [55]

Niger	**H(113) whitlow, boiled leaves, local application**
Senegal	H(008), ONS. of Sida alba, RNS., VO.
	H(091), ONS. of Sida alba, RNS., VO.
Burundi	H(097), leaves, decoction (H2O) , enema , (orchitis)
Sudan	H(020), ONS, RNS
Tanzania	H(020) snake, chewed leaves, juice, VO.
Burkina Faso	HH(020) insects, leaves, stems, sap, local application
Ivory Coast	H(051) fever,
	H(103) odontalgia,
	H(137) analgesic,
	H(157) convulsion childs, ONS of Sida carpinifolia., RNS.
	H(091) stimulating, leaves, decoction, VO.
Tanzania	H(002) galactogen, roots extract et of leaves of Sida acuta, VO
	H(014) powder of leaves et roots in an dressing as emollient
	H(193), powder of leaves & roots in an dressing as emollient
Mozambique	H(026), painful menstruation (dysmenorrhoea), infusion of leaves, 1/2 tea cup, 2 X / day
	H(051), leaves, decoction in warm H2O, inhalation of steam

H(187), depressed fontanel, roots, decoction, VO, 1/2 teaspoon, 3x/d

Sierra Leone   H(013) pus formation, a poultice of the leaves with clay is rubbed on a boil to induce pus formation

H(157) inner stem bark of Sida stipulata is peeled off and made into a twine together with a black thread, tied into 3- 4 knots and hung around the neck of a child as a remedy for convulsions

Zimbabwe   H(031), roots of Sida acuta , infusion., VO. **[370]**

Sida veronicaefolia

Sida veronicaefolia is very popular with rural womenfolk, especially in the areas where it grows in its natural habitat, and is used extensively in traditional medicine for shortening and reducing the pain of labour in childbirth. It is believed to render parturition almost painless and leads to shorter period of postpartum bleeding. Soup of this plant is taken in the last days of pregnancy. **[347]**

This herb is good to treat brain complications. It is a nervine tonic and thus helps to strengthen, calm and stimulate the nervous system. It helps to relax the body and is good for managing stress, anxiety or depression. It is quite effective in the treatment of brain complications like loss of memory and nervine debility. It is mainly nadibalya, medhya, snehana amlatanasaka, hardya and rayayana. Supports the good health of the digestive system. Effective in respiratory complications. Aphrodisiac in nature. Resolves urinary tract infections. **[807]**

Ayurveda

The old Indian Systems of Medicine (ISM) are among the most ancient medical traditions known, and derive maximum formulations from plants and plant extracts found in the forests. About 400 plants are used in the regular production of Ayurveda, Unani, Siddha, and tribal medicine. About 75% of these are taken from tropical forests and 25% from temperate forests. Thirty (30) percent of ISM preparations are derived from roots, 14% from bark, 16% from whole plants, 5% from flowers, 10% from fruits, 6% from leaves, 7% from seeds, 3% from wood, 4% from rhizomes, and 6% from stems. Fewer than 20% of the plants used are cultivated **[241]**

The use of herbal medicine can be traced back to 2100 BC in ancient China at the time of Xia dynasty, and in India during the Vedic period. The first written reports are timed to 600 BC with Charaka samhita of India, and in China the same became systematic by 400 BC. The basic concept in these medicinal systems is that the disease is a manifestation of a general imbalance of the dichotomous energies that govern life as a whole and human life in particular, and they focus on medicine that can balance these energies and maintain good health. In Ayurvedha of India, the forces are said to be agni (strength, health and innovation) and ama (weakness, disease and intoxication). In India there are also other systems of traditional medicine besides Ayurvedha and these are called Siddha, which originated almost at the same time as Ayurvedha from southern India, and Unani, which entered India during the Mogul dynasty periods. Like Ayurvedha, practitioners of Siddha medicine believe in a perfect balance of three doshas known as vatha (space and air elements), pitta (fire and water elements) and kapha (water and earth elements). **[495]**

Ayurveda means science of life in Sanskrit (Ayur means life; Veda means science) and aims at the holistic management of health and disease. It remains one of the most ancient medical systems widely practiced in the Indian subcontinent and has a sound philosophical, experiential and experimental basis... An entire section of the Materia Medica of Ayurveda termed Rasayanas is devoted to the enhancement of the body resistance. Interestingly, a somewhat similar role is ascribed to tonics and various herbals in the Chinese and European systems of medicine. Rasayana generally means nourishing and rejuvenating drugs with multiple applications for longevity, memory enhancement, immunomodulation and adaptogenic. Various drugs listed as Rasayana have been researched and have been reported to possess pharmacological activities such as immuno-stimulant, tonic, neurostimulant, antiaging, antibacterial, antiviral, antiseptic, anti-rheumatic, anticancer, anti-inflammatory, adaptogenic, anti-stress etc. Several botanicals from the Rasayana category have been studied for immuno-modulation and have a potential of becoming new scaffolds for safer, synergistic, cocktail immunodrugs. Ayurvedic medicines largely use herbal and herbo-mineral preparations to treat all the diseases encountered in India which include many found in other parts of the world such as cancer, cardiovascular disease, asthma, viral hepatitis and diabetes. Ayurvedic physicians and hospitals have long histories of drugs used: compositions, formulations, dosage regimens, side effects and therapeutic effects. These records are particularly valuable since these medicines have been effectively tested on people for thousands of years **[728]**

Inflammation, although first characterized by Cornelius Celsus, a physician in first Century Rome, it was Rudolf Virchow, a German physician in nineteenth century who suggested a link between inflammation and cancer, cardiovascular diseases, diabetes, pulmonary diseases, neurological diseases and other chronic diseases. Extensive research within last three decades has confirmed these observations and identified the molecular basis for most chronic diseases and for the associated inflammation... In an attempt to identify novel anti-inflammatory agents which are safe and effective, in contrast to high throughput screen, we have turned to "reverse pharmacology" or "bed to benchside" approach. We found that Ayurveda, a science of long life, almost 6000 years old, can serve as a "goldmine" for novel anti-inflammatory agents used for centuries to treat chronic diseases... This "Science of Life" is a holistic healing system, which is designed to promote good health and longevity rather than curing a disease. **[614]**

328

One of the fundamental ideas in Ayurveda is that your body is intelligent and seeks health if you support it through good habits. Additionally, health is defined as a dynamic state – not just the absence of disease as in modern medicine. The idea in Ayurvedic nutrition is that health can be increased not just maintained through right lifestyle and diet. Thus, an Ayurvedic diet is an individualized approach that brings a dynamic state of being. The goal of Ayurveda is to correct the conscious, intelligent function of the body and mind. Chemicals are also attributes of any substance; however, they are not dynamic in an isolated state. Each Dravya or substance in nature has its own unique quality and group of attributes. Isolating one or two of these attributes, or chemicals, is very much like removing the liver from the body to obtain more enzymes. The "donor" of the liver of course dies and its unique grouping of attributes also is dissipated at death along with consciousness. When we isolate one part of an herb or mineral we effectively "kill" the greater capacity of the substance to work directly on the conscious, intelligent principle of our body. This is perhaps the most fundamental difference between the "Ayurvedic model" and the modern "biochemical model" of using herbs.... there are too many ingredients, both passive, inactive and active in botanicals to warrant an isolative approach as their interactions and relationships cannot be studied with the biochemical model – there are simply too many possibilities present at once to use this narrow methodology of classification. **[438]**

One of the main strategies in Ayurveda medicine is to increase body's natural resistance to disease or stress-causing agent rather than directly neutralizing the agent itself in practice. This has been achieved by using plant extracts of various plant materials. The medicinal plants are widely used by the traditional medical practitioners for curing various diseases in their day to day practice. Plants are one of the most important sources of medicines. Herbs occupy the important place in the Ayurveda Materia Medica and therapeutics. The important advantages claimed for therapeutic uses of medicinal plants in various ailments are their safety besides being economical, effective and their easy availability. Because of these advantages the medicinal plants have been widely used by the traditional medical practitioners in their day to day practice. In traditional systems of medicine the Indian medicinal plants have been used in successful management of various disease conditions. The medicinal use of plants is very old. The writings indicate that therapeutic use of plants is as old as 4000–5000 B.C. and Chinese used first the natural herbal preparations as medicines. In India, however, earliest references of use of plants as medicine appear in Rigveda which is said to be written between 3500–1600 B.C. Later the properties and therapeutic uses of medicinal plants were studied in detail and recorded empirically by the ancient physicians in Ayurveda which is a basic foundation of ancient medical science in India. Whereas conventional medicine is primarily oriented toward the treatment of disease, Ayurvedic medicine is oriented toward prevention, health maintenance, and treatment. In conventional medicine, drugs are developed based on the concept that the elimination of specific causes of a disease, such as microorganisms, will cure a disease. On the other hand, the belief in Ayurvedic medicine is that a disease is the product of an imbalance in the body and mental elements that reduce the body's resistance to diseases. If the imbalance is corrected and the body's defense mechanisms are strengthened by herbal formulas, lifestyle changes, and diet, then the body will resist a disease with a goal of eliminating it. Herbal and herbo-mineral products regularly used in Ayurveda are believed to strengthen the body's defenses. Scientific evidence is gradually developing in support of the Ayurvedic concept. [10]

The whole plant or its parts like leaves, stem, bark, root, flower, fruits and seed are used as a source of medicine by the folk healers and local community. Large quantity of this raw drug traded in the market as a raw material for herbal drugs industries. Now a day, again the people have started using plants and plant-based drugs in order to avoid the toxicity and health hazards associated with indiscriminate use of synthetic drugs and antibiotics. Although, several of plant species have been tested for their antimicrobial properties but the vast majority of plants have not been adequately evaluated. [639]

Ayurveda exploits the potential of various herbs as drugs and plays an important role in modern health care, particularly where satisfactory treatment is not available. In recent years, the clinical importance of herbal drugs has received considerable attention. There is a need to evaluate the potential of Ayurvedic remedies as adjuvant to counteract side effectiveness of certain modern therapies. [233]

Sida in Ayurveda

Genus Sida L., belonging to family Malvaceae, comprises about 200 species distributed throughout the world and 17 species are reported to occur in India. [1]   Sida is one of the important medicinal plant species used to treat various diseases in Ayurveda and other traditional systems of medicine. Roots of many of the species are valued for their medicinal properties. The plant is also well documented in Ayurveda, ancient Indian system of medicine. [15]

The most medicinally important species of Sida, like S. acuta, S. cordifolia, S. rhombifolia, S. spinosa, S. carpenifolia, S. humilis, S. veronicaefolia, are used in Ayurvedic system. [107]

The compounds identified from stem and leaves add to the value of these plants. The stem and leaves of the fourteen plants used as bala are found to be rich in alkaloids, flavonoids, phenolic acids and mucilages, the same compounds present in the root which is the drug. [673]   The favourable combination of sympathomimetic amines and vasicinone in these species (Sida acuta Burm., S. humilis Willd., S. rhombifolia L., and S. spinosa L.) would account for their major therapeutic uses in the Indian system of medicine. [205]

What is Bala?

Bala is officially Sida cordifolia, but is effectively a number of other Sidas.

Bala is native to tropical regions of India and Sri Lanka. The plant is considered to be one of the most valuable medicinal plants in Ayurveda, the

330

ancient traditional medical system of India. Bala is said to contain five of the six tastes, a rare property, indicating that it provides nourishment from the five mahabhutas (earth, water, fire, air, and space). Bala is associated with Parvathi, the ancient Hindu goddess of beauty and grace. The herb is part of a trio of "beautifying" herbs, together with ashoka and shatavari, associated with women in Indian herbal folk medicine. [2]

The genus Sida is used as 'Bala' in Ayurveda. Sida (Bala) is of great importance in the Indian traditional system of medicine and this is perhaps the most widely used raw drug in the production of different Ayurveda formulations. Root is the officinal part. The drug called 'Bala' in Sanskrit is well reputed as anti-rheumatic and anti-pyretic in the Ayurvedic system of medicine and is also used for curing neurological disorders, headache, leucorrhoea, tuberculosis, diabetes, fever and uterine disorders. It is also reported to possess anti-tumor, anti-HIV, hepatoprotective, abortifacient, antimicrobial and immunostimulant properties. [217]

What does Bala do?

Of all the herbs having absorbent, strength promoting and Vata pacifying action, Bala is the best. It is safe to use during lactation and in children. Seek medical advice for its use during pregnancy. [444]

Bala is a root drug commonly used in Ayurveda as a general tonic and "rasayana" drug. It is reported to be cool, sweet, demulcent, aphrodisiac and tonic. Bala {is effective} in nervous and urinary diseases, disorders of blood, in chronic bowel complaints, tuberculosis and rheumatism. Fresh juice of roots is applied against wounds and ulcers. [561]

According to Ayurveda 'Bala' balances all the doshas – vata, pitta, kapha... Yogaratnakaram, a treatise on medicine written by Yeturi Srinivasa charyulu, describes Bala as 'divine medicine'. Bala has been in use for over 2000 years in treating bronchial asthma, cold and cough, chills, aching joints and bones. [539]

Bala normalizes vata and sooths excited nerves. For this reason the oil prepared using this herb is used to massage patients who suffer from paralysis, cervical spondylosis, facial paralysis etc. Bala controls motility of large intestine. It helps to absorb water and nutrients from intestines. Hence its preparations are widely used in Grahani or Irritable Bowel Syndrome (IBS). This herb is a very good cardiac tonic and reduces petechial hemorrhage. Ayurveda acharyas recommend use of this plant in these conditions. Bala is known for its "shukrala" properties. Shukrala means increasing shukra dhatu. Because of this property bala is used in ayurvedic preparations which increase sperm count and sperm motility. It helps to increase quality and quantity of semen. This herb is mainly used in male and female infertility. Texts of ayurveda praise the herb Bala as Vrishya (aphrodisiac). Hence this herb is used in conditions like erectile dysfunction and premature ejaculation. The herbal preparations which are used in Female infertility contain this herb as main ingredient as it acts as a very good uterine tonic. The diuretic properties of this herb help in cystitis and it rejuvenates urinary system. [730]

Bala cures diarrhea and is invigorating and nutritive. It is also efficacious in diseases caused by deranged kapha. The rejuvenating action of this herb extends to the nervous, circulatory, and urinary systems. It has a diuretic effect and is useful in urinary problems, including cystitis. Being cooling and astringent, it is used in inflammations and bleeding disorders also. [377]

Rasayana

The part of the Ayurveda system that provides an approach to prevention and treatment of degenerative diseases is known as Rasayana, and plants used for this purpose are classed as rejuvenators. This group of plants generally possesses strong antioxidant activity. [42]   Ayurveda has a special class of botanicals known as Rasayana with immunomodulatory and adaptogenic activities. [728]   Bala is a very good rasayana herb. Hence it is widely used in convalescing patients as it supplies essential nutrients. It helps to build a healthy body and strengthens body immune system. [730]

Sida cordifolia as Bala

(Sida cordifolia) the whole plant is being used by Ayurvedic physicians for treatment of different diseases. The raw drug also forms a chief ingredient of several important formulations and preparations, as for e.g. 'Ksirabala', 'Dhanvantaram', 'Balaristam', 'Asvagandhadileham', 'Balataila' etc. The drug is well reputed in Ayurveda and Siddha system of medicine for ailment of different diseases. [612]

(Sida cordifolia) has a long history of use by Ayurveda and rural area particularly for medicinal properties. It is in use as folk medicine in India since time immemorial. [Agharkar S P. medicinal plants of Bombay presidenc.Pbl. scientific publishers.Jodhpur.India 1991; 194-195] - cited in [118]

The What is Bala controversy

The drug plant 'Bala' (=Sida cordifolia L.) is often adulterated with Sida retusa, S. indica and Urena lobata, [612]   The raw drug material traded under the name 'bala' includes materials (traded in the form of roots, seeds and whole plants) obtained from *Sida rhombifolia, S. acuta, S. cordifolia, S. cordata*, etc. [8]

While the name 'bala' is said to be traditionally correlated to Sida cordifolia (aka North Indian bala), S. alnifolia (also known as South Indian bala) and S. rhombifolia, the name is also shared by several other species of Sida as well as other unrelated taxa. Sida cordifolia was reported as the primary source for bala in Ayurvedic formulations while S. acuta and S. rhombifolia are considered as substitutes or adulterants, on account of similarity of their alkaloid profiles. [312]

The present investigation proved conclusively that all the 14 plants can be used as Bala because most of them contained biologically active compounds such as alkaloids, mucilages, flavonoids, phenolic acids. Of the 14 species used as bala, the roots of 11 plants have been screened and ten of them were found to contain ephedrine which is considered as the active principle of bala:

S. cordifolia Linn

S. acuta Burm

S. spinosa Lina

S. veronicaefolia

S. rhombifolia var. rhomboidea

S. rhombifolia var. retusa

S. indica... [561]

Of these *S. cordifolia* Linn. is considered as the source of raw drug bala in North India while in South India vaidyas prefer *S. rhombifolia*... In markets the drug is commonly adulterated with *Sida acuta* widely seen as a weed in the barren lands and roadsides of Kerala. The availability of *S. retusa* is decreasing day by day and cultivation is meager. [668]

Ayurveda in the greater medical world

To cure the problems caused by infection of such microbes, the current therapy is based on use of synthetic drugs and antibiotics. Although the synthetic drugs have been used in emergency, they possess many side effects. Therefore, it is necessary to introduce an alternative remedial regimen. In the traditional system of India, various indigenous plants are used in the diagnosis, prevention and cure of physical and mental problems of the people. The drugs of herbal origin are used as a medicine in Unani and Ayurveda since ancient times. Medicinal plants are the source of important therapeutic aid for alleviating human and animal ailments. [639]

The nature has provided a complete warehouse of remedies to cure ailments of mankind. The secrets of Ayuervedha individualizing the healing method were preserved in some parts of India. Many medicinal compounds glycosides, Carbohydrates, proteins and amino acids, saponins, flavanoids, glycosides, phytosterols, and phenolic compounds are isolated from these plants. Nature is a best friend of our pharmacy field. Natural drugs are effective in action without side effects. [448]

A beautiful poetic verse from the *Sushruta Samhita* reads, "Life is the dynamic combination of the body, senses, mind, and spirit, or the conscious principle." Ayurveda is the first holistic science defining health as a four-dimensional state of wellbeing of your body, mind, senses, and spirit. If all of Ayurveda were to be summarized in a single word, it would be balance (*santulan*)... Ayurveda, the ancient science of life from India, became the answer to all my ailments. Ayurveda not only fights disease but also teaches people how to become – and remain – healthy. It addresses the root causes of why we manifest health challenges at the levels of the body, mind, spirit, and five senses. Ayurveda gave me the tools I needed to take my health in to my own hands. Ayurveda teaches that health is our birthright, and that it exists at the core of each person, though hidden at times by disease and distress. It views each person as a whole, multi-dimensional being and addresses every aspect of him or her. Finally I discovered a system of healing that didn't judge or label me, or give me a quick-fix solution... And the solution to my problems could be attained right now from the comfort of my own kitchen and garden. Imagine that. Since following Ayurveda's vast health-promoting practice, I can't even remember the last time I needed to visit a doctor. [722]

Ayurveda specifics

Conventional or synthetic drugs used in the treatment of liver diseases are sometimes inadequate and can have serious adverse effects. On the other hand, Ayurveda, an indigenous system of medicine in India, has a long tradition of treating liver disorders with plant drugs. [549]

The present communication reports that an aqueous extract prepared from the roots of Sida retusa can protect against liver damage induced by thioacetamide and allyl alcohol. The hepatoprotective activity is shown by the normalization of various serum enzymes elevated in response to thioacetamide-induced liver damage. The investigation provides biochemical evidence to validate the use of Sida retusa as a component of some hepatotonic preparations used by Ayurvedic physicians. [542]

The Siddha and Ayurvedic systems of treatment are being increasingly recognized as an alternate approach to arthritic treatment. Herbal medicine provides a foundation for various traditional medicine systems worldwide. The Sida species is one of the most important families of medicinal plants in India. Roots of these herbs are held in great repute in treatment of rheumatism. [127]

Siddha

Siddha system of medicine also known as Siddha vaidya in India, considered as the crown of all the traditional arts of the ancient world owing to its richness and simplicity, practiced by siddhars. Siddha medicine uses herbs, metals, minerals as well as animals in preparing highly effective medicines, is the oldest medical system in existence. The hallmark of traditional Siddha system is KAYAKARPAM i.e., imparting immunity to diseases. [405]

Siddha is a comprehensive system that places equal emphasis on the body, mind and spirit and strives to restore the innate harmony of the individual. Treatment is aimed at restoring balance to the mind-body system. Diet and lifestyle play a major role not only in maintaining health but also in curing diseases. This concept of the Siddha medicine is termed as pathiam and apathiam, which is essentially a list of do's and don'ts... According to the Siddha system, the individual is a microcosm of the universe. The human body consists of the five primordial elements: earth, water, fire, air and space; the three humours: vatha, pitta and kapha; and seven physical constituents. Food is the basic building material of the human body and gets processed into humours, tissues and wastes. The equilibrium of humours is considered as health and its disturbance or imbalance leads to a diseased state... Reflecting this theory of cosmic oneness, the five senses are said to correspond with the five elements. Ether (Veli) is responsible for hearing; air (katru) for sense of touch; fire (thee) for sight; water (neer) for taste; and earth (mann) for the sense of smell.... The diagnostic methodology in Siddha treatment is unique as it is made purely on the basis of the clinical acumen of the physician. The pulse, skin, tongue, complexion, speech, eye, stools and urine are examined. This approach is collectively known as "Eight types of examination"; and among the eight, the examination of pulse is very important in confirming the diagnosis. [745]

Siddha system has enormous pharmacopoeia containing vegetable, animal and mineral products and treatment techniques consisting in use of 32 types of internal medicines and 32 types of external medicines, application of heat and cold, ointments, potions and poultice, blood letting, counter irritation, bath, suction, manipulative processes such as thokkanam, varma, yoga and concentration on hygiene and diet (pathiam), periodical use of purgatives and emetics, use of drugs which include, apart from herbs, preparations from metals and minerals such as copper, silver, gold, lead and preparations from products of animal origin such as brain, liver, bones, blood, skull, horns of various animals, tissues of reptiles and also Kayakalpa to prevent or postpone greying of hair, formation of wrinkles and ageing, prevention or treatment of diseases, and postponement of death (to any desired length of time). Some empirical treatment techniques under the guise of magic exorcism, incantation, pilgrimage, peregrinations, mountaineering and similar activities have also been in practice since ages.... There has been a resurgence of traditional medical systems the world over, based on the holistic nature of their approach to healing. The efficacy of indigenous systems has been proved in various contexts. They tend to use locally available, cost effective materials for treatment. Hence, the Siddha system which also has strong cultural and historical bonds with the people of Tamil Nadu is becoming increasingly relevant. [745]

Composition of the Sidas

Medicinal plants are of great importance to the health of individuals and communities. The medicinal value of these plants lies in some chemical substances that produce a definite physiological action on the human body. The most important of these bioactive constituents of plants are alkaloids, tannins, flavonoids, and phenolic compounds. [420]

Flavonoids have been shown to possess antimutagenic and antimalignant effects. Moreover, flavonoids have a chemopreventive role in cancer through

335

their effects on signal transduction in cell proliferation[31] and angiogenesis. Tannins and phenolic compounds are considered to have cancer-preventive properties. These induced cell death in cancer cells by concentration-dependent decrease of ATP and a deterioration of cellular gross morphology. Alkaloids shown to inhibit cell growth without cell death, thus providing enhanced opportunities for DNA repair, immune stimulation, anti-inflammation and cancer prevention. Phytosterols inhibited tumor growth by an alteration of signal transduction pathways. **[348]**

Phytochemicals are secondary metabolites of plants known to exhibit diverse pharmacological and biochemical effects on living organisms. The phytochemicals, tannins, saponins, alkaloids, flavonoids, terpenes and phenolics were found to be present in S. acuta leaves and are in amounts to be of medicinal value. Many plants containing alkaloids and flavonoids have diuretic, antispasmodic, anti-inflammatory and analgesic effects. Alkaloids are capable of reducing headache associated with hypertension. It has been reported that alkaloids can be used in the management of cold, fever and chronic catarrh. Flavonoids are known for their antioxidant activity and hence they help to protect the body against cancer and other degenerative diseases. Flavonoids have been shown to have antibacterial, antinflammatory, antiallergic, antimutagenic, antiviral, antineoplastic, antithrombotic and vasodilatory activity. Tannins are known to exhibit antiviral, antibacterial and antitumor activities. It was also reported that certain tannins are able to inhibit HIV replication selectively and is also used as diuretic. Tannins are well known for their antioxidant and antimicrobial properties as well as for soothing relief, skin regeneration, as anti inflammatory and diuresis. Saponins are expectants, cough depressants and administered for hemolytic activities. In medicine, saponin is used as hyper-cholesterolemia, hyperglycaemia, antioxidant, anticancer, antiinflammatory and weight loss. It has also been reported to have antifungal properties. Saponins exhibit cytotoxic effect and growth inhibition against a variety of all making them have antinflammatory and anticancer properties. Terpenes are very important group of organic compounds that have been reported as potent drugs used in treatment of wide range of ailments. The most rapidly acting anti malarial Artemisin and its derivates are terpenes. Phenols also found present in plant sources are major group of compounds acting as primary antioxidant or free radical scavenger. The efficacy of the utilization of S. acuta leaves in herbal/ traditional/folklore medicine may be attributed to its phytochemical profile. **[223]**

It should be noted that steroidal compounds are of importance and interest in pharmacy due to their relationship with such compounds as sex hormones. The presence of steroidal compounds in the plants is an indication that the plants can be used or expectant mothers or breast feeding mothers to ensure their hormonal balance, since steroidal structure could serve as potent starting material in synthesis of these hormones. **[300]**

Lipids are an important component of living cells. Together with carbohydrates and proteins, lipids are the main constituents of plant and animal cells. Cholesterol and triglycerides are lipids. Lipids are easily stored in the body. They serve as a source of fuel and are an important constituent of the structure of cells. Lipids include fatty acids, neutral fats, waxes and steroids (like cortisone). Compound lipids (lipids complexed with another type of chemical compound) comprise the... phospholipids. **[734]**

What we know about the composition of genus Sida is very incomplete, despite it being a plant that has been used daily forever. Over time billions have used Sida for their health needs. Even the main medicinal species have not had their constituents adequately researched. Be that as it may, what we do know is that this genus is incredibly rich in medicinal constituents. I confess a weakness in my knowledge of biochemistry, so I expect mistakes have been made. The saving grace is that you can use the citation number to go back to the original research. This book is a compilation of known peer-review research and is not to be considered medical advice.

Knowing what the constituents are is of course important, but there has been scant research on how they interact with each other (synergy) and what the plant manifests as a whole. Every part of Sida is medicinal, often with particular strengths. Different extraction methods extract different things in different proportions (see the section on **Sida Actions**). The extraction of the whole plant is called the crude extract and I recommend it. The question is: "is this particular substance in this species of Sida?" It does not matter all that much how it was detected (what extract), so long as we know it is there. How much is a more difficult question.

Both the ethanol extract and the aqueous extract frequently compare well with any other extract, even outperforming them. I have been using an ethanol extract of the leaves regularly for five years now and it has worked well for me, but writing this book has convinced me to extract the whole plant, since they all have their own specialties. The root and leaf are often considered the most medicinal. The leaf tea shows up well in these research studies, and that is how the vast majority of the world uses Sida.

The Constituents

This section contains the compounds known to be present in the various Sidas. I tried to include what is important to an herbalist: what parts of the plant, or what constituents, what extraction method, and measurable results. Unfortunately most listings fail in these respects. There may, or may not, be any further information in the listing about how the sample was prepared. Most of these results just confirm the presence of a compound; few studies give an absolute amount. Usually only one type of sida is tested, and within that, only one extract testing one part of that particular Sida is usually tested. Studies can show up more than once in these listings (such as Alkaloids – Quinazoline - Vasicine – a citation for vasicine can also show up under Quinazoline, or even Alkaloids).

Sample Listing

Magnesium   metal

Magnesium plays an important role in over 300 enzymatic reactions within the body including the metabolism of food, synthesis of fatty acids and proteins, and the transmission of nerve impulses. Magnesium is one of the seven essential macrominerals; these are minerals that need to be consumed in relatively large amounts - at least 100 milligrams per day. **[797]**

Sida acuta

223-invitro-leaves-extract?-24.5 mg/100 gm, **264**-100% ethanolic leaf extract-122.11mg/100 g, **274**-invitro-leaves -14.40 Mg/100g, **415**-invitro-S. acuta had exceptionally high concentrations of minerals,

---

Line by Line Explanation

Magnesium = One of the constituents of Sida

Metal = I may (or may not) say what type of compound here

Magnesium plays an important role... = descriptive information about this constituent that may or may not be there.

[797] = This is the citation number for the research from which this narrative passage was taken. Look it up in the **References** for the author, title of the research, and the journal in which it was published.

Sida acuta = Which Sida or Sidas were tested for Magnesium. If a Sida has more than one result, it has its own paragraph. If it only has one result it usually is bundled under Other Sidas.

223 = The citation number for this research. See above for details.

invitro = the type of research performed. Invitro means it was done in the lab, which is pretty much everything in this section.

leaves = what part of the plant was studied? **Note:** Different parts of the plant can have differences in their constituent makeup.

extract? = the extract used in this study. Often the studies will not tell you the extract - this particular study just said it followed "standard procedures". I usually assume methanol in those cases since it is the preferred extract for researchers – it generally extracts the most of any compound.

24.5 mg/100 gm = In this case they actually gave a quantity – 24.5 milligrams of magnesium was found in 100 grams of leaf. Various methods of measure have been employed in these studies. It was beyond my ability to compare or standardize the various measures.

This section has very condensed information that often leaves out interesting details, so the following section contains tables of results and other information too lengthy for this section. Direct quotes from the researchers are included whenever possible.

(+/-)-syringaresinol   a lignan
This compound inhibits Helicobacter pylori motility [1]

Sida acuta   253-invitro-whole plant-EtOAc-soluble extract,

(S)-(+)-Nb-methyltryptophan methyl ester
indole alkaloid, carboxylated tryptamine [312]

Sida cordifolia   312-invitro-roots,

1- Eicosene
(Cetyl ethylene) sometimes included in medications to treat eczema [1]

Sida cordifolia   217-invitro-whole plant?,

1, 3-dilinoleoyl-2-oleine   triglyceride
mildly antibacterial activity. [150]

Sida rhomboidea   150-invitro-fruit-ether>chloroform>acetone extract -detected,

1-O-β-D-glucopyranosyl-(2S,3S.4R,8Z)-2-[(2'R)-2'-hydroxy palmito-ylamino]-8-octadecene-1,3,4'-triol
Sida cordifolia   217-invitro-whole plant?,

1-O-linoloyl-3-O-β-D-galactopyranosyl-syn-glycerol
Sida cordifolia   217-invitro-whole plant?,

11-methoxy-quindoline   alkaloid
cryptolepine derivative [186]

Sida acuta

220-review, 253-invitro-whole plant-EtOAc-soluble extract, 186-invitro-whole plant-methanol extract-main alkaloid with its derivatives such as quindoline, quindolinone, cryptolepinone and 11-methoxy-quindoline,

132-hydroxy phaeophytin B   porphyrin

Sida rhombifolia   59-invitro-whole plant?,

17^3-ethoxypheophorbide A   porphyrin

Sida rhombifolia   59-invitro-whole plant?,

20-hydroxy ecdysone   phytoecdysteroid

Its purpose is presumably to disrupt the development and reproduction of insect pests [1]

Sida cordifolia   217--invitro--whole plant?--20-hydroxy,24-hydroxymethyl ecdysone,

22-dehydrocampesterol   sterol

Seed germination stimulant [798]

Sida rhomboidea   520-invitro-leaves-boiling distilled water extract,

22-dihydrospinasterol   sterol

Sida rhomboidea   520-invitro-leaves-boiling distilled water extract,

24-methylenecholesterol   sterol

similar to cholesterol [755]

Sida rhomboidea   520-invitro-leaves-boiling distilled water extract.

3β,6α,23ε-trihydroxy-6α-cholest-9(11)-ene

Steroid conjugate

Sida cordifolia   217-invitro-whole plant?,

4-ketopinoresinol   Phenolic compound

protects against oxidative stress-induced cell injury

Sida acuta 186-invitro-whole plant-methanol extract?-detected, 253-invitro-whole plant-EtOAc-soluble extract,

5,10-dimethylquindolin-11-one

inhibited induced preneoplastic lesions 83.3% **[253]**

Sida acuta

93-invitro-leaves-70% aqueous methanol (v/v) acidified to pH 2 253-invitro-whole plant-EtOAc-soluble extract-10 μg/mL induced 83.3% inhibition of preneoplastic lesions.

5,7-dihydroxy-3-isoprenyl flavone

Sida cordifolia 118-review-detected, 571-invitro-chloroform extract-bioactive flavone,

5,7-dihydroxy-4'-methoxyflavone flavone

Sida rhomboidea 59-invitro-whole plant?,

5-hydroxy-3-isoprenyl flavone

Sida cordifolia 118-review-detected, 571-invitro-chloroform extract,

6-phenyl ethyl amine

Sida cordifolia 118-review-aerial parts-detected,

7-o-beta glucopyranoside flavanone

Sida indica 709-flower-review, 710-flower, root-review

7a-methoxy-α-tocopherol tocopherol derivative

Sida acuta 565-invitro-whole plant

9-hydroxy–cis-11-octadecenoic acid fatty acid

(11-octadecenoic acid) the main trans fatty acid isomer present in milk fat [1]

Sida cordifolia   217-invitro-whole plant?,

Abutilin   flavenoid

Sida acuta   709-review-root-detected-abutilin a,   710-Ayurveda-review-flowers-detected,

Acanthoside B

International commercially available compound,   Compounds with a 5-membered ring of four carbons and an oxygen. They are aromatic heterocycles. The reduced form is tetrahydrofuran. **[799]**

Sida acuta   327-invitro,

Alantolactone   isomeric sesquiterpene lactone

Sida indica   710-Ayurveda-review-detected-includes isoalantolactone,

Alkaloids

Sida acuta

6-invitro-leaf-chloroform/95% ethanol extracts both detected,   **11**-invitro-acquesous acetone extract,   **52**-invitro-root-present in pet ether extract, abundant in methanol extract,   **86**-invitro- ethanolic and aqueous extracts,   **96**-invitro-leaf- cold petroleum ether extract-present,   **96**-invitro-leaf- 95% ethanol extract-present,   **102**-invitro-leaf-water and 100% methanolic extracts-moderate amounts,   **106**-invitro-strongly present,   **113**-invitro-whole plant?- ethanolic and aqueous extracts-detected,   **204**-invitro-leaf-cold water extract-1%,   **213**-invitro-leaf-100% methanol/chloroform extracts -detected,   **214**-invitro-whole plant?-70% aqueous methanol extracts-detected,   **221**-invitro-buds=7 mg/gm – leaves=3.35 mg/gm – stem=1.1 mg/gm – roots=0.15 mg/gm,   **223**-invitro-leaves-moderately present-1751.67 mg/100 gm,   **224**-leaf-present in hexane and chloroform extracts, absent in water and methanol extracts,   **230**-leaf-boiled leaves-alkaloids very strongly present,   **237**-invitro-0.076 mg/100g,   **264**-100% ethanolic leaf extract -1500.26 mg/100 g,   **265**-leaf-80% ethanol extract-detected,   **274**-invitro-leaves-523.00 Mg/100g,   **300**-invitro-leaf-ethanol extract-detected,   **420**-invitro-possesses very high levels of alkaloids and flavonoids, and is employed in medicinal uses-1.04%±0.20 by weight,   **460**-rats-ethanolic extract-substance is present, **463**-invitro-leaf-methanolic extract, 500-invitro-hydroalcoholic root extract, **579**-invitro- leaves, stems and roots-hexane and ethanol extracts-detected, **645**-invitro-leaf-cold water extract-detected, **645**-invitro-leaf-acetone extract-detected, **652**-rats-leaf-ethanol extract-detected, **668**-invitro-roots-methanol extract-detected,

Sida cordifolia

24-roots-80% ethanol extract, **32**-invitro-root-40% ethanol extract-detected, **120**-aerial parts-ethanolic extract, **148**-aerial parts-alcoholic extract-detected, **240**-invitro-leaves = 10.5 g/100gm-stem bark = 4.75 g/100 gm, **249**-invitro-10.5 mg/100 gm, alkaloids, **409**-invitro- that maximum accumulation of alkaloids and phenols occurred in summer season in all the three plant species. Peak concentrations of alkaloids and phenols were observed in flowering stage. Interestingly, no alkaloids or phenols accumulated in the seedling stage, **470**-invirto-roots-80% ethanol extract-present, **591**-rats-whole plant-70% ethanol extract-detected, **663**-invitro-seed-water extract=113.52 µg/mg--Acetone extract=96.37 µg/mg --Petroleum Ether extract=85.35µg/mg--chloroform extract=80.59µg/mg, **668**-invitro-roots-methanol extract-detected,

Sida rhombifolia

47-invitro-aqueous methanol extract, **136**-invitro-root-boiling water extract-none detected, **136**-invitro-root-95% ethanol extract-detected, **486**-invitro-whole plant?- water, 70% ethanol extract, **543**-invitro-whole plant-ethanolic and acqueous extract, **544**-leaves and/or roots-chloroform extract-detected, **544**-leaves and/or roots-ethanol extract-detected, **545**-invitro-aerial parts-80% ethanol extract, **578**-invitro-whole plant?-water extract-detected, **668**-invitro-roots-methanol extract-detected,

Sida cordata

293-invitro-leaf-acetone extract-present, **293**-invitro-leaf-methanol extract-present, **498**-invitro-leaves and stems- successive solvent extraction method, **500**-invitro-root- hydroalcoholic extract-detected, **668**-invitro-roots-methanol extract-detected,

Sida indica

443-invitro-leaves-petroleum ether (60-800C) for 8 hr. to remove fatty matter-95% methanol extract-alkaloids, **445**-invitro-leaves, twigs and roots, **446**-invitro-acqueous and methanol extracts-nothing detected, 447-invitro-roots-present, **448**-rats-whole plant-is present-ether/chloro-form/ethanol/acqueous extract (sequential extraction from a marc, extract taken out at each phase for testing. Acqueous extract on the remains after the three previous extractions), **449**-mice/sheeps's blood-leaves- ethanolic extract (200 mg/kg bw) but not acqueous extract (400 mg/kg bw), **451**-rats-leaves, twigs, and roots-acqueous extract-tropane alkaloids, **677**-invitro-fruits-80% ethanol extract/Petroleum ether extract/Chloroform extract/Ethyl acetate extract/Butanol extract/Aqueous extract--not detected, **680**-invitro-whole plant-cold distilled water extract-detected—ethanol extract-

343

detected,   **681**-invitro-whole plant-80% ethanol extract with distilled water-detected,   **683**-invitro-leaves-cold distilled water extract-not detected,   **684**-invitro-leaf--hydro-methanolic extract-very strongly detected,   **687**-whole plant?-acetone extract-detected,   **709**- review-leaf-detected,   **712**-vinvitro-leaf-Petroleum ether extract not detected --Ethyl acetate extract detected--Chloroform extract detected--Methanolic extract detected--Aqueous extract not detected,   **712**-invitro-stem-Hydroalcoholic extract not detected--Methanolic extract not detected--Aqueous extract not detected.

Sida rhomboidea   **185**-invitro-leaf-detected,   **325**-nvitro-detected,

Sida tiagii

551—fruit--n-Hexane Extract and ethyl acetate extract,   **552**-invitro-fruit-ethanolic extract>n-hexane extract/ethyl acetate extract-The filtrate was partitioned with n-hexane (n-hexane extract, HS) and ethyl acetate (ethyl acetate extract-nothing with ethanol,   **607**-mice-fruit-hot 95% ethanol extract>n-hexane/ethyl acetate extracts-detected,

Sida tuberculata   **490**- ethanol extract roots 70%, leaves 40%,   **613**-leaves and roots-aqueous infusion.

Sida veronicaefolia

346-invitro-whole   plant?-ethanolic   extract>water-soluble   fraction-not detected, **348**-mice-leaves-petroleum, ether, chloro-form, ethanol, and aqueous solutions subsequently combined-detected.

Other Sidas

99-Sida   spinosa-invitro-whole   plant-hot   60-80%   ethanolic   extract, **200-Sida cardifolia**-leaf-acetone extract,   **344-S. humilis**-invitro-whole plant?-methanolic extract-minimally present,   **535-Sida urens**-invitro-leaves-95% ethanol extract-detected,   **668-Sida retusa**-invitro-roots-methanol extract-detected,

Amino acids

Sida acuta   **52**-invitro-root-methanol and pet ether extracts,   **96**-invitro-leaf- 95% ethanol extract-present,

Sida cordifolia   **591**-rats-whole plant-70% ethanol extract-detected,

Sida tiagii   **551**-fruit-95% ethanolic extract,   **552**-invitro-fruit-ethanolic extract>n-hexane extract/ethyl acetate extract-The filtrate was partitioned with ethyl acetate extract-ethanolic extract works,

Sida cordata   **293**-invitro-leaf-methanol extract-present,   **498**-invitro-leaves and stems- successive solvent extraction method.

Sida indica

448-rats-whole plant-is present-ether/chloroform/ethanol/acqueous extract (sequential extraction from a marc, extract taken out at each phase for testing. Acqueous extract on the remains after the three previous extractions, **449**-mice/sheeps's blood-leaves-acqueous extract (400 mg/kg bw) and ethanolic extract (200 mg/kg bw), **680**-invitro-whole plant-cold distilled water extract-not detected—ethanol extract-detected, **684**-invitro-leaf--hydro-methanolic extract-not detected, **709**-review-leaf-detected-including free amino acids.

Other Sida

344-Sida humilis-invitro-whole plant?-methanolic extract-detected minimally, **348-S. veronicaefolia**-mice-leaves-petroleum, ether, chloroform, ethanol, and aqueous solutions subsequently combined-detected

Ampesterol   steroid

Sida acuta   **186**-review, **220**-invitro, **581**-invitro-whole plant-methanol extract-major steroid of the plant,

Amyrin   pentacyclic triterpenol
Widely distributed in nature... one source is epicuticular wax [1]

Sida acuta   **217**-invitro-whole plant?,

Anthocynin   water-soluble vacuolar pigments
Water-soluble vacuolar pigments that, depending on their pH, may appear red, purple, or blue. [1]

Sida acuta   **96**-invitro-leaf- cold petroleum ether extract-present, **96**-invitro-leaf- 95% ethanol extract-present, **106**-invitro-detected

Sida indica   **684**-invitro-leaf--hydro-methanolic extract-not detected,

Anthranoid   not detected
Sida acuta   **106**-invitro-not detected,

....

More drought spells will occur in the future climate and the availability of productive land will be reduced. Permanent bioenergy cultures will have to be based on marginal agricultural production systems. The perennial species addressed here are potentially suited candidates because they have high water use efficiency and do not need to be grown under highly intensive conditions. **[475]**

Anthraquinones

Naturally occurring phenolic compounds. [1]

Sida acuta

96-invitro-leaf- cold petroleum ether extract-present, **102**-invitro-leaf-water and 100% methanolic extracts-moderate amount, **106**-invitro-very present, **214**-invitro-whole plant?-70% aqueous methanol extracts-detected, **579**-invitro- leaves, stems and roots-hexane and ethanol extracts-detected,

Sida cordifolia
120-aerial parts, **240**-invitro-leaf and stem bark-methanol extract,

Sida rhombifolia
47-invitro-whole plant?-aqueous methanol extract, **578**-invitro-whole plant?-water extract-none detected,

Sida indica

683-invitro-leaves-cold distilled water extract-detected, **684**-invitro-leaf--hydro-methanolic extract-not detected, **687**-whole plant?-acetone extract-not detected,

Antioxidants

An oxidizing agent, or oxidant, gains electrons and is reduced in a chemical reaction. Also known as the electron acceptor, the oxidizing agent is normally in one of its higher possible oxidation states because it will gain electrons and be reduced. Examples of oxidizing agents include halogens, potassium nitrate, and nitric acid. In sum: A reducing agent reduces other substances and loses electrons; therefore, its oxidation state increases; An oxidizing agent oxidizes other substances and gains electrons; therefore, its oxidation state decreases. **[800]**

Sida acuta

15-invitro-full text gives DPPH, FRAP, and ABTS values, **77**-invitro-leaves-hot distilled water extract-the antioxidant activity of both the extracts and synthesized AgNP's was analyzed by 1,1-diphenyl-2-picrylhydrazzyl (DPPH) radical scavenging assay using ascorbic acid as control and they were all found to exhibit good antioxidant activity especially at lower concentrations, **89**-invitro-whole plant-aqueous acetone extract (70%, v/v)- PMAb (μmolTrolox/μg) 1.20 ± 0.04 6- ABTS assay (μmol Trolox/μg)-.12 ± 1.18, **92**-invitro-whole plant?-methanol extract-cytotoxic concentration (CC50) value=(461.53±0.23_ gmL−1)- the results extracts showed that of S. acuta and U. lobata may be a promising alternative to synthetic substances as natural compound with high antiproliferative and antioxidant activities--it seems that the extracts of S. acuta utilize their antioxidant properties by increasing SOD activity to nearly 1.8–2.2 its normal level in order to protect cells against negative effects of stress produced by the proliferation of HepG-2 cells, **103**-invitro-leaf-ethanolic and methanolic extracts-the antioxidant property of Sida acuta was recently demonstrated, **115**-invitro-leaf-methanol extract-exhibited the potential free radical scavenging activity (antioxidant activity) having IC50 value of 86.34µg/ml. The reducing power of the extract was linearly proportional to the concentration of the sample, **141**-whole plant?-methanol extract-taken together, the results extracts showed that of S. acuta and U. lobata may be a promising alternative to synthetic substances as natural compound with high antiproliferative and antioxidant activities, **254**-invitro-whole plant?-aqueous acetone extract- can be used as an easily accessible source of natural antioxidants, natural lipoxygenase and exnthine oxidase inhibitories -the aqueous acetone extracts of Sida acuta showed a good relation between phenolic compounds contents and the antioxidant activities (R2=.091 with ABTS method, **264** -rats-100% ethanol extract-60 mg/kg bw-possesses an antioxidant property which, in a dose dependent manner, reduces/ameliorates oxidative stress, **433**-invitro-whole plant-80% ethanol extract-The crude ethanolic extract of whole plant of Sida spinosa exhibited significant inhibition of nitric oxide & superoxide scavenging activity, **460**-rats-whole plant-70% ethanol extract-400mg/kg bw-significantly quenched the free radical damage-showed a significant increase in activities of antioxidant enzymes that reduces the oxidative stress induced damage exhibiting a potent antioxidant and anticancer activity, **561**-invitro-leaves-detected, **565**-invitro-whole plant-three compounds showed significant antioxidant effect (EC50 = 86.9, 68.2, and 70.9 µM, respectively) in the DPPH radicals scavenging activity assay, **593**-invitro-whole plant-?extract- Sida spinosa exhibited the best and significant results in polyphenol contents, antioxidants properties and anti-inflammatory activity (over S acuta, S cordifolia, S rhombifolia, S urens), **644**-invitro-whole plant-chloroform extract- in vitro free radical scavenging assays activity, the roots posses moderate antioxidants activities when compared with standard drug of Ascorbic acid. Therefore, based on the results it can be concluded that the chloroform extract of Sida acuta may hold enormous resource of pharmaceutical properties, **647**-rats-whole plant-petroleum ether, toluene, chloroform, acetone, ethyl acetate and hydroalcoholic extracts-all extracts had antioxidant activity, **653**-invitro-leaves-chloroform and ethanolic extracts-exhibits strong free radical scavenging activity in all the tested methods and shows maximum scavenging of DPPH, Nitric oxide, hydroxyl and hydrogen peroxide at 100µg/ml concentration compared to chloroform and ethanol extract of leaves.

Sida cordifolia

15-invitro-full text gives DPPH, FRAP, and ABTS values, **24**-roots-80% ethanol extract- In DPPH scavenging assay the IC50 value was found to be 50 µg/mL which was not comparable to the standard ascorbic acid, **27**-invitro-aerial parts?-80% acetone extract (400 ml acetone + 100 ml water) for 24 h under mechanic agitation at room temperature-The antioxidant activity of the samples was significant using three separate methods-antioxidant capacity noticed that the reduction capacity of DPPH radicals obtained the best result comparatively to the others methods of free radical scavenging (but scored on all three antioxidant tests), **28**-rats?- 50 % ethanolic extract- The activity of antioxidant enzymes and glutathione content, which was lowered due to alcohol toxicity, was increased to a near-normal level,   **31**-rats-root-50% ethanolic extract- has got potent antioxidant and antiinflammatory activity and the activity is comparable with the standard drug deprenyl,   **33**-rats-leaves-hydroalcoholic extract-100 and 500 mg/kg- both doses significantly increased endogenous antioxidants in heart tissue homogenate. Moreover, biochemical findings were supported by histopath-ological observations, **42**-rats- The results from the ABTS assay showed that the ethanolic extract of Sida cordifolia was IC50 16.07 µg/ml- The relative antioxidant capacity for the water infusion was IC50 342.82 µg/ml- results of water infusion on lipid peroxidation were IC50 126.78 µg/ml,   **67**-rats-root-50% ethanolic extract-quinolinic acid induced neurotoxicity- 50 mg/100g bw/day-potent antioxidant and antiinflammatory activity-the activity is comparable to deprenyl,   **120**-aerial parts-aqueous and hydro-alcoholic extracts-test results indicate that S. cordifolia has a rich content of antioxidant compounds, mostly saponins-low correlation between antioxidant activity and saponins content,   **121**-invitro-ethanol extract-all extracts of Sida cordifolia. (SC) have effective reducing power and free-radical scavenging activity-Only the root extract exhibited superoxide-scavenging activity and inhibited lipid peroxidation in rat liver homogenate-All these antioxidant properties were concentration dependent,   **141**-whole plant?-methanol extract-The results of the antioxidant properties showed that theses extracts significantly increased SOD, CAT and GsT activity after 48 h,   **146**-invitro-whole plant-ethanol and acqueous extract (10, 20, 30, 40 mg/ml)- possesses potent antioxidant activity- ethanolic extract almost quantitatively equivalent to the standard ascorbic acid,   **148**-aerial parts-alcoholic extract-Interestingly at 400 mg/kg, a significant increase in antioxidant enzymes such as catalase and superoxide-dismutase-activity was seen in the diabetic rats,   **163**-leaves-petroleum ether extract (60 ∘C for 8 h) (100 and 500 mg/kg) significantly increased endogenous antioxidants in HTH. Moreover, biochemical findings were supported by histopathological observations, **169**-rats-whole plant?-ethanol extract- Oxidative stress was increased in alcohol-treated rats as evidenced by the lowered activities of antioxidant enzymes, decreased level of reduced glutathione (GSH), increased lipid peroxidation products, and decreased expression of γ-glutamyl cysteine synthase in liver. The co-administration of Sida cordifolia with alcohol almost reversed these changes,   **175**-invitro-water extract-200&400 mg/kg bw- The flavonoids and phenols present in Sida cordifolia contribute for antioxidant potentiality that exhibits nephroprotective activity,   **182**-rats-roots-50 % ethanolic extract-has potent anti-oxidant and anti-inflammatory activity-exerts an antioxidant effect by decreasing lipid peroxidation, increasing GSH level and maintaining a normal level of antioxidant enzymes-The activity of antioxidant enzymes and glutathione content, which was lowered due to alcohol toxicity, was increased to a near-normal level,   **470**-invitro-roots-ethanol extract- The antioxidant property of ethanolic extract of S. cordifolia was assessed by DPPH free radical scavenging activity-the IC50 value was found to be 50 µg/mL which was not comparable to the standard ascorbic acid,   **502**-invitro-whole plant?-methanol extract-showed a potent antioxidant activity,   **561**-invitro-leaves-detected,   **593**-invitro-whole plant-?extract-Sida spinosa exhibited the best and significant results in

348

polyphenol contents, antioxidants properties and anti-inflammatory activity (over S acuta, S cordifolia, S rhombifolia, S urens), **641**-seed-cold distilled methanol extract- exhibited a potent anti-oxidant activity in both DPPH and superoxide anion radical scavenging assays (IC50 = 0.005 ± 0.0004, and 0.078 ± 0.002 mg/mL, respectively), **662**-invitro-leaves-cold distilled water extract-the biofunctionalized AgNPs displayed remarkable antioxidant activities-The AgNPs exhibited higher phosphomolybdate reducing power (2127 AEAA) when compared to the aqueous extract (1428AEAA)and standard (742AEAA).The ferric reducing power of AgNPs (1.83AU at a concentration of 1000 mg/ml) was estimated by the reduction of Fe3þ/ferricyanide complex and it was higher than the standard ferulic acid (1.61AU)as well as aqueous extract (1.27AU).The AgNPs exhibited higher superoxide radical scavenging activity (IC50 value46.25 mg/ml) when compared to aqueous extract (IC50 value81.99 mg/ml) and standard (IC50value202.2 mg/ml). The DPPH radical scavenging activity of AgNPs was found to be dose-dependent and higher (IC50 value 50.12 mg/ml) when compared to aqueous extract (IC50 value 77.48 mg/ml) and standard (IC50value 153.4 mg/ml).

Sida rhombifolia

15-invitro-full text gives DPPH, FRAP, and ABTS values, **75**-Sida retusa-invitro-root-only root extract inhibited lipid peroxidation in rat liver, **141**-whole plant?-methanol extract-The results of the antioxidant properties showed that theses extracts significantly increased SOD, CAT and GsT activity after 48 h, **146**-invitro-whole plant-ethanol and acqueous extract (10, 20, 30, 40 mg/ml)- possesses potent antioxidant activity- ethanolic extract almost quantitatively equivalent to the standard ascorbic acid, **170**-invitro-water and methanolic extracts-the methanolic extract of Sida rhombifolia Linn. exhibited better antioxidant activity (IC50: 10.77 & 42 µg/mL) than aqueous extract (IC50: 44.36 and 62.68 µg/mL) in DPPH scavenging assay, **195**-invitro-ethyl acetate extract-had the highest content of phenolic compounds (88.311 ± 2.660 mg•GAE/g) and the best antioxidant activity for the DPPH and TEAC assay (IC50 = 70.503 ±1.629 and 20.580 ± 0.271, respectively), **407**-rats-seed-80% methanol extract-Seed extract possibly due to its free radical scavenging property was capable in augmenting the deficient functioning of impaired enzymes of antioxidant defense system, **536**-rats-whole plant?-ethanol extract- causes myocardial adaptation by augmenting endogenous antioxidants and protects rat hearts from decline in cardiac function and oxidative stress associated with ISP induced myocardial injury, **538**-rats-root-ethanol extract-inorganic mineral analysis of Sida rhombifolia. L root shown that the root contains antioxidant micronutrients such as calcium, sodium, zinc and magnesium in considerable levels, **541**-rats-roots-alcoholic extract- The biological defense system constituting the superoxide dismutase, glutathione peroxidase, ascorbic acid showed a significant increase while the lipid peroxide content was found to decrease to large extent on SRE treatment thereby indicating the extracts free radical scavenging property, **593**-invitro-whole plant-?extract-Sida spinosa exhibited the best and significant results in polyphenol contents, antioxidants properties and anti-inflammatory activity (over S acuta, S cordifolia, S rhombifolia, S urens), **619**-whole plant-ethyl acetate extract- scavenging DPPH radicals and ferrous ions with EC50 of 380.5 and 263.4 μg/mL, respectively, **634**-invitro-whole plant?-cold methanolic extract- Free Radical Scavenging Activity-The IC50 value μg/mL- Sida rhombifolia Upper root= 11.0 ±0.17-- Sida rhombifolia root= 135.80 ±6.16-- positive control Ascorbic acid= IC50 of 2.89.

Sida retusa

15-invitro-full text gives DPPH, FRAP, and ABTS values, **57**-rats-The comparative antioxidant potentials of ethanol extract of roots, stems, leaves, and whole plant were studied-All extracts of this plant showed effective free radical scavenging activity, reducing power, and superoxide scavenging activity. Only root extract inhibited lipid peroxidation in rat liver and brain homogenate. All these antioxidant properties were concentration dependent, **464**-mice/rats-seed-80% methanol extract- We report for the first time that chemopreventive and anti-hepatotoxic potentials of S. rhombifolia ssp. retusa seed extract of is due to free radical scavenging activity and restoration and maintenance of cellular integrity.... Seed extract possibly due to its free radical scavenging property was capable in augmenting the deficient functioning of impaired enzymes of antioxidant defense system.

Sida cordata

15-invitro-roots-methanolic extract-full text gives DPPH, FRAP, and ABTS values, **282**-invitro-leaf-methanol extract-Our observations revealed that the crude extract of Sida cordata show significant antioxidant and cytotoxic properties. According the discussion above on introduction paragraph and on the basis of the results of the research it can be inferred that Sida cordata may be a good source for the further investigation to discover a new drug for cancer treatment, **293**-invitro-leaves-methanol extract-maximum anti-oxidant activity of 81.93% at 500 μg/ml, **494**-rats-whole plant-methanol extract>n-hexane (SCHE)→ethyl acetate (SCEE)→n-butanol (SCBE)- Although the extract and all its derived fractions exhibited good antioxidant activities however, the most distinguished scavenging potential was observed for SCEE, **496**-rats-whole plant-methanolic extract- ethyl acetate fraction- This may be related to its antioxidative properties, **549**-rats-leaf-ether/ 95% ethanol extract-significantly (up to P<0.001) reduced the lipid peroxidation in the liver tissue and restored activities of defense antioxidant enzymes GSH, SOD and CAT towards normal levels, which was confirmed by the histopathological studies.

Sida indica

15-invitro-full text gives DPPH, FRAP, and ABTS values, **561**-invitro-leaves-detected, **593**-invitro-whole plant-?extract- Sida spinosa exhibited the best and significant results in polyphenol contents, antioxidants properties and anti-inflammatory activity (over S acuta, S cordifolia, S rhombifolia, S urens), **638**-invitro-methanol extract- at a minimum concentration (25 μg mL-1), all of the extracts had less than 50% DPPH radical scavenging activity, but when used at a concentration of 50 μg mL-1, the control leaf and NPK root extracts displayed higher radical scavenging activities (60.6 and 52.4%, respectively) than the other extracts. At 100 µg mL-1 and above, all of the leaves extracts, except CAN leaf extracts, exhibited scavenging activities greater than 50% DPPH, **674**-invitro-leaf-boiling distilled water extract- polyphenol stabilized gold nanoparticles displayed good in vitro free radical scavenging activities as indicated in various in vitro antioxidant assays, **677**-invitro-fruits-80% ethanol extract/Petroleum ether extract/Chloroform extract/Ethyl acetate extract/Butanol extract/Aqueous extract--Ethyl acetate fraction has produced highly significant antioxidant activity followed by chloroform extract. The both extracts are rich in total phenol and flavanoid content (and) can be considered as new source of natural antioxidant (the other extracts all have lesser amounts as well), **679**-rats-root-ethanolic extract- Nephro protective action in this study could be due to the antioxidant and other phytochemical of root, **684**-invitro-leaf--hydro-methanolic extract- Due to its cytotoxicity and antioxidant activities, **686**- invitro-leaf and seed-methanol extract-the current findings reconfirmed those of earlier studies that found S. indica to be a reliable natural antioxidant that can safely be used in the pharmaceutical and food industries to prevent the effects of reactive oxygen species and reduce the risks of cardiovascular disease. Thus, the extracts of the roots and leaves of S. indica can play an important role in the prevention of several degenerative diseases, such as hepatic disorders, immune dysfunction, cataracts and macular degeneration, by inhibiting the production of reactive oxygen species, thus reducing the risk of these diseases and promoting proper organ function.

Sida rhomboidea

280-invitro-leaves-boiled distilled water extract-SR treatment to GM treated rats (GM + SR) recorded significant decrement ($p < 0.05$) in plasma and urine urea and creatinine, renal lipid peroxidation along with significant increment ($p < 0.05$) in renal enzymatic and non-enzymatic antioxidants, **288**-rats-leaves-ethanol extract-a potent antioxidant and free radical scavenger-pre-treatment improves cardiac antioxidant status in IP induced Myocardial infarction by effective scavenging of free radicals generated during oxidation of catecholamines thus collectively contributing to its overall antioxidant and anti ischemic activity, **288**-rats-leaves-ethanol extract-a potent antioxidant and free radical scavenger-pre-treatment improves cardiac antioxidant status in IP induced Myocardial infarction by effective scavenging of free radicals generated during oxidation of catecholamines thus collectively contributing to its overall antioxidant and anti ischemic activity, **320**-leaves-methanol extract-It can be concluded from the present study that the methanol extract possesses potent antioxidant and free radical scavenging properties that have been demonstrated using a variety of in vitro experimental models- higher reducing potential ODmax=1.20±0.27), **323**- Sida rhomboidea-invitro-leaf-?extract.

Sida spinosa

11-review- Previous studies performed in our laboratory showed that aqueous acetone extract possesses antioxidant properties, **15**-invitro-full text gives DPPH, FRAP, and ABTS values, **254**-invitro--invitro-whole plant?-

aqueous acetone extract- can be used as an easily accessible source of natural antioxidants, natural lipoxygenase and exnthine oxidase inhibitorie-the antioxidant potential was evaluated using three methods: inhibition of free radical 2,2-diphenyl-1-picrylhydramzyl (DPPH), ABTS radical cation decolorization assay and Iron (III) to iron (II) reduction activity (FRAP), **561**-invitro-leaves-detected, **566**-invitro-whole plant-80% ethanolic extract-The study reveals in-vitro antioxidant activity, **593**-invitro-whole plant-?extract-exhibited the best and significant results in polyphenol contents, antioxidants properties and anti-inflammatory activity (over S acuta, S cordifolia, S rhombifolia, S urens).

Sida cardifolia

177-mice/rats-whole plant-50% ethanolic extract-500mg/kg bw-potent anti-antioxidant and anti-inflammatory activity when compared with standard drug deprenyl, **200**- invitro-leaf-acetone extract-Thus acetone leaf extract of Sida cardifolia had maximum amount of polyphenols and flavonoids which is directly related to their greater antioxidant activity also. Thus active molecules present in the acetone leaf extract of Sida cardifolia has antioxidant property which may be useful in targeting the release of free radical intermediates along with the generation of ROS from various metabolic activities.

Other Sidas

15-Sida mysorensis-invitro-full text gives DPPH, FRAP, and ABTS values461-Sida retusa-rats-roots-methanol extract-The quantity of S. retusa root extract required for 50% inhibition of lipid peroxidation, scavenging hydroxyl radical and superoxide radical was 1130.24 ug/ml respectively, **318-Sida pilosa**-whole plant?-water extract/ethyl acetate-highest antioxidant activity, **490-Sida tuberculata**-invitro-leaves, roots-acqueous extract-ethanolic extract three ethanol concentrations were tested on extraction: 20, 30 and 40% (v/v) for leaves and 50, 70 and 90% (v/v) for roots-Our data showed a protective effect of all extracts of S. tuberculata against oxidative damage by deoxyribose and TBARS assays, **553-Sida tiagii**-rats-fruit-95% ethanol extract-showed antioxidant activity in diabetic rats, **593-Sida urens**--invitro-whole plant-?extract-Sida spinosa exhibited the best and significant results in polyphenol contents, antioxidants properties and anti-inflammatory activity (over S acuta, S cordifolia, S rhombifolia, S urens), **561- Sida veronicaefolia**-invitro-leaves-detected.

Apigenin   flavone

Apigenin is a natural compound found in many fruits and vegetables. It induces autophagy (a kind of cellular waste-recycling system) in leukemia cells, which may support a possible chemopreventive role. [1]

Sida acuta   93-invitro-leaves-70% methanol extract(v/v)-acidified to pH 2- allowed the identification of apigenin,

352

Sida cordata

494-invitro-methanolic extract-detected-Presence of apigenin with some unknown compounds was observed by using thin layer chromatography.

Sida spinosa

593-invitro-whole plant-?extract- Sida spinosa exhibited the best and significant results in polyphenol contents, antioxidants properties and anti-inflammatory activity (over S acuta, S cordifolia, S rhombifolia, S urens).

Sida indica   **709**-review-flowers-detected-includes Apigenin 7-o-beta rhamnopyranosyl,   **710**-Ayurveda-review-flowers-detected,

Sida veronicaefolia   **561**-invitro-detected-methoxy derivative,

Arabinose   Polysaccharide

Foods that contain arabinose are usually designed for pre-diabetic and diabetic patients. These foods are especially popular in Japan and China, where arabinose is legally used as a food additive. [1]

Sida acuta   **217**-invitro-whole plant?,   **561**-PhD dissertation-leaves-detected,

Sida cordifolia / Sida rhombifolia / Sida spinosa / Sida veronicaefolia / Sida rhombifolia var. rhomboidea / Sida rhombifolia var. retusa / Sida indica / Abutilon hirtum (Sida graveolens) / Sida glutinosa / Abutilon hirtum (Sida graveolens)   **561**-PhD dissertation-leaves-detected,

Arachidic acid   Saturated fatty acid

Detergents, photographic materials and lubricants [1]

Sida acuta   **217**-invitro-whole plant?,

Ascorbic acid

An essential nutrient involved in the repair of tissue, used to treat and prevent scurvy. [1]

Sida acuta

52-India-whole plant-hot water extract-Quantitative estimation showed the presence of ascorbic acid 13.0%,   **223**-invitro-leaf-ascorbic acid 22.43± 0.21 mg/100g,   **264**-100% ethanolic leaf extract - 24.27mg/100 g.

Sida rhombifolia

541-rats-roots-90% alcoholic extract-The biological defense system constituting the superoxide dismutase, glutathione peroxidase, ascorbic acid showed a significant increase while the lipid peroxide content was found to decrease to large extent on SRE treatment thereby indicating the extracts free radical scavenging property.

Sida rhomboidea **130**-leaf-water extract-ascorbic acid 1.9 mg/100 mg.

Ash

Sida acuta **52**-invitro-root-3.5%, **223**-invitro-leaves- 6.33 %, **274**-invitro-leaves-7.94% by weight,

Sida cordifolia **158**-invitro-seed-3.80% ± 0.5,

Sida rhombifolia **538**-invitro-roots-95% ethanol extract-total ash 7.8%.

Sida indica

447-invitro-roots-Percentage of Total Ash 5.4, **539**-Ayurveda-contains asparagin and ash **680**-invitro-whole plant-cold distilled water extract-ethanol extract-total ash 40%,

Sida hermaphrodita **475**-invitro-shoot-11%,

Asparagin(e) α-amino acid

An α-amino acid that is used in the biosynthesis of proteins. [1]

Sida cordifolia **217**-invitro-whole plant?

Sida indica 539-review-Ayurveda-contains asparagin and ash

Aspartic acid

An α-amino acid that is used in the biosynthesis of proteins. [1]

Sida indica **570**-invitro-petroleum ether extract then 50% alcohol extract,

Beta-carotene

The leaves of S. acuta possess significant quantities of fat soluble vitamin A precursor, β-Carotene and water soluble vitamins - ascorbic acid, niacin, thiamin and riboflavin as presented in Table 3. Vitamins are a diverse group of organic molecules required in very small quantities in the diet for health, growth and survival. The absence of vitamin from the diet or an inadequate intake results in characteristics deficiency signs and ultimately death... The composition of calcium, iron, phosphorous, sodium and magnesium in S. acuta leaves as obtained in this study indicates that nutritional benefits would be derived in addition to utilization of S. acuta leaves for medicinal purposes. **[223]**

Sida acuta 223-invitro-leaves- 925 mg/100 gm

Benzoic acid

A constituent of Whitfield's ointment which is used for the treatment of fungal skin diseases such as tinea, ringworm, and athlete's foot. As the principal component of gum benzoin, benzoic acid is also a major ingredient in both tincture of benzoin and Friar's balsam. Such products have a long history of use as topical antiseptics and inhalant decongestants. Benzoic acid was used as an expectorant, analgesic, and antiseptic in the early 20th century. **[1]**

Sida acuta / Sida cordifolia / Sida rhombifolia / Sida spinosa / Sida veronicaefolia / Sida rhombifolia var. rhomboidea / Sida rhombifolia var. retusa / Sida indica / Abutilon hirtum (Sida graveolens) / Sida glutinosa / Abutilon hirtum (Sida graveolens) 561-leaves-detected.

Berberine Benzylisoquinoline alkaloid

Berberine is one of the few compounds known to activate adenosine monophosphate-activated protein kinase (AMPK), your metabolic master switch--Berberine may benefit diabetes, metabolic syndrome, obesity, heart health, gut health and more--Berberine has been shown to control blood sugar and lipid metabolism as effectively as the diabetes drug metformin [http://articles.mercola.com /sites /articles/ archive/2015/06/22/ berberine-benefits.aspx]   Tests of the antiseptic action of berberine against bacteria, yeasts, viruses, and amoebas have shown a range of activity levels from apparent potent action to mild suppression-has hypotensive action-lowers cholesterol through a mechanism different than that of the statin drugs, suggesting potential use both as an alternative to the statins and as a complementary therapy that might be used with statins in an attempt to gain better control over cholesterol. **[561]**

Sida acuta 561-doctoral dissertation-important alkaloid, from the leaves of Sida acuta in appreciable amounts,

Betaine

Biologically, betaine is involved in methylation reactions and detoxification of homocysteine [1]   Aerial parts of 26 taxa, distributed in 18 genera and all 5 tribes of the Malvaceae-Glycinebetaine was obtained in high yield (0.5–4.6%, dry weight) from all the plants studied- The same compounds as those found in the aerial parts were usually detected, but the glycinebetaine contents of the roots and flowers were considerably lower. **[481]**

All Sidas

481-Glycinebetaine was obtained in high yield (0.5–4.6%, dry weight) from all the plants studied- The same compounds as those found in the aerial parts were usually detected, but the glycinebetaine contents of the roots and flowers were considerably lower,

Sida acuta   **217**-invitro-whole plant?, **754**-invitro-roots and aerial parts,

Sida humilis, Sida spinosa   **754**-invitro-roots and aerial parts,

Sida cordifolia

217-invitro-whole plant?,   **312**-invitro-roots,   **481**-Glycinebetaine was obtained in high yield (0.5–4.6%, dry weight) from the aerial parts-contents of the roots and flowers were considerably lower,

Sida rhombifolia

544-citing-Dinesh Jabhav, Medicinal plants of India, A Guide to Ayurvedic & Ethnomedicinal uses of plants, Vol 1, Scientific Publishers India, 2008, 213-214,   **754**- invitro-roots and aerial parts,

Sida rhomboidea   **520**-invitro-leaves-boiling distilled water extract,

Cadmium   mineral

Sida hermaprodita

482-invivo-whole plant-mineral excess soils, lowest readings of contamination still rich-1.20-60.41 mg kg dw,   **623** -invitro-absorbed high levels of zinc, lower levels of lead, copper, and nickel, and absorbed cadmium at least,

Caffeic acid   hydroxycinnamic acid

Outperformed other antioxidants, reducing aflatoxin production by more than 95 percent.   Caffeic acid also shows immunomodulatory and anti-inflammatory activity. **[1]**

Sida acuta   **659**-invitro-leaves-methanolic extract-1.16 µg/g dw.

356

Sida indica

570-invitro-petroleum ether extract then 50% alcohol extract, 709-review-whole plant-detected, 712-review.

Calcium mineral

Sida acuta

223-invitro-leaves- 85 mg/100 gm, 264-invitro-leaf-100% ethanol extract -14428 ± 0.02 mg/100 g, 274-invitro-leaves - 44.32 Mg/100g, 415-invitro-S. acuta had exceptionally high concentrations of minerals, 699-invitro-higher in calcium and phosphorus (critical for antler development) than iron clay peas, soybeans or alfalfa.

Sida cordifolia

240-invitro-leaves = 88.72 mg/100gm-stem bark = 95.49 mg/100gm, 290-aerial parts-3.06 g/kg

Sida rhombifolia

504-invitro- cultivated under mineral nutrition standard conditions-63+ days after emergence-337.6 mg Ca per plant, 512-invivo-root-medium-Among weed species the relative concentration of a particular nutrient in the root system dry matter(high, med, low), 538-invitro-roots-95% ethanol extract-.85%,

Sida hermaphrodita

476-invivo/invitro-whole plant-municipal sewage-6.03 g. kg-1 dm.

Sida indica

539-review-Ayurveda-calcium carbonate

Caloric value

Sida acuta

274-invitro-leaves- 360.54 Kcal/100gm.

Sida hermaphrodita

473-invitro-energy productivity level was 219.5 GJ•ha-1, 474-invitro- seed dressing of Virginia fanpetals led to significant increase in biomass yield (2 t/ha) and production of energy per hectare (18.5%), in comparison to the control plot (without dressing)-significantly higher yields (5 t/ha) of dry matter and more production of energy per hectare (30.5%), were obtained from Virginia fanpetals' trials, than that of the tested willow, 475-stems-The calorific value was reduced from 17.4 to 15.8 MJ per kg DM from the early to the late winter, indicating that dead stems may lose energetic value during the winter, 564-invitro-Hot water pre-treatment (HWT) - It could be notice that dipping seeds into boiling water, the HWT method significantly broke seed dormancy.

Campesterol   phytosterol

Sida acuta   217-invitro-whole plant?,

Sida rhomboidea   520-invitro-leaf-boiling distilled water extract,

Capric acid

A saturated fatty acid. Its formula is CH3(CH2)8COOH. May be responsible for the mitochondrial proliferation associated with the ketogenic diet. [1]

Sida indica   709-review-root-detected,

Caprylic acid   Eight-carbon saturated fatty acid

Known by the systematic name octanoic acid, found naturally in the milk of various mammals, and as a minor constituent of coconut oil and palm kernel oil... an antimicrobial pesticide used as a food contact surface sanitizer... used as an algaecide, bactericide, and fungicide in nurseries, greenhouses, garden centers etc. [1]

Sida indica   709-review-root-detected,

Carbohydrate   saccharide [1]

Includes sugars, starch, and cellulose [1]   Carbohydrate provides energy to cells in the body particularly the brain, the only carbohydrate dependent organ on the body [223]

Sida acuta

6-invitro-leaf-chloroform/95% ethanol extracts both detected,   52-invitro-root-5.39%-present in methanol extract, absent in pet ether extract,   96--invitro--leaf--cold petroleum ether extract-present--cold chloroform extract-present-95% ethanol extract-present,   217-invitro-whole plant?,   223-invitro-leaves-a very good source 85.0+0.0mg/100g,   230-leaf-boiled leaves-not present,   274-invitro-leaves- 6.21% By weight,   460-rats-ethanolic extract-substance is present,   645-invitro-leaf-cold water extract-not detected,   645-invitro-leaf-acetone extract-not detected-reducing sugar not present,   646-leaves and stem-detected-relatively high total carbohydrates,

Sida cordifolia

32-invitro-root-40% ethanol extract-detected,   118-review-detected-(94,000 ppm to 475,000ppm),   120-aerial parts-aqueous and hydroalcoholic extracts-Specific chromatographic analysis for carbohydrates showed stains with similar to those from reference standards, and enabled identification of glucose, arabinose, galactose (carbohydrates commonly found associated with saponins), fructose and sorbose (reported as companions of saponins in plants), **591**-rats-whole plant-70% ethanol extract-detected,

Sida rhombifolia   **543**-invitro-whole plant-ethanolic extract,

Sida cordata   **293**-invitro-leaf-acetone extract-present---methanol extract-present, **498**-invitro-leaves and stems- successive solvent extraction method,

Sida indica

447-invitro-roots-not detected, **448**-rats-whole plant-is present-ether/ chloroform/ethanol/acqueous extract (sequential extraction from a marc, extract taken out at each phase for testing. Acqueous extract on the remains after the three previous extractions, **449**-mice/sheeps's blood-leaves-acqueous extract (400 mg/kg bw) and ethanolic extract (200 mg/kg bw), **454**-invitro-leaves-detected, **677**-invitro-fruits-80% ethanol extract-detected, **680**-invitro-whole plant-cold distilled water extract-detected— ethanol extract-detected, **681**-invitro-whole plant-80% ethanol extract with distilled water-detected, **684**-invitro-leaf--hydro-methanolic extract-not detected, **687**-whole plant?-acetone extract-detected-especially the flower, **709**-review-Different parts of plants-detected, **712**-invitro-leaf-Petroleum ether extract not detected --Ethyl acetate extract detected --Chloroform extract detected--Methanolic extract detected--Aqueous extract detected, **712**-invitro-stem-Hydroalcoholic extract detected--Methanolic extract detected--Aqueous extract detected,

Sida tiagii

551-fruit-95% ethanolic extract, **552**-invitro-fruit-ethanolic extract>n-hexane extract/ethyl acetate extract-The filtrate was partitioned with ethyl acetate extract-ethanolic extract works, **607**-mice-fruit-hot 95% ethanol extract>n-hexane/ethyl acetate extracts-detected,

Sida rhomboidea   **185**-invitro-leaf-detected,   **325**-invitro-leaf-detected,

Sida cardifolia   **200**-leaf-acetone extract,

Carbon   element

Sida hermaphrodita   **475**-invitro-shoot-39.2-40.2%,

Carboxylated tryptamines   monoamine alkaloid
Tryptamine is a monoamine alkaloid which is hypothesized to play a role as a neuromodulator or neurotransmitter. [1]   Soma, food of the immortals according to the Bower Manuscript (Kashmir, 6th century A.D.)-3 Sida spp. part of this-rich in tryptamines. [22]

Sida acuta, Sida rhombifolia, Sida spinosa, Sida humilis

754- invitro-roots and aerial parts,

Cardenolides   a type of steroid

Often toxic; specifically, they are heart-arresting... Some plant and animal species use cardenolides as defense mechanisms, notably the milkweed butterflies. Species such as the monarch and the queen ingest the cardenolides contained in the milkweeds (Asclepias) that they mostly feed on as larvae. The cardenolide content in butterflies deters most vertebrate predators. [1]

Sida acuta   213-invitro-chloroform/100% methanol extract-detected,

Carotenoids

Organic pigments that are produced by plants. Humans are mostly incapable of synthesizing carotenoids and must obtain them through their diet. [1]

Sida rhombifolia   578-invitro-whole plant?-water extract-none detected,

Catechin

A natural phenol and antioxidant-part of chemical family of flavonoids. [1]

Sida acuta   659-invitro-leaves-methanolic extract-.18 µg/g dw.

Chlorogenic acid   Antioxidant

May slow the release of glucose into the bloodstream after a meal. [1]

Sida acuta   659-invitro-leaves-methanolic extract-2.22 µg/g dw,

Cholesterol   sterol

An essential structural component of all animal cell membranes; essential to maintain both membrane structural integrity and fluidity. Cholesterol enables animal cells to dispense with a cell wall (to protect membrane integrity and cell viability), thereby allowing animal cells to change shape rapidly and animals to move (unlike bacteria and plant cells, which are restricted by their cell walls) [1]

Sida acuta

103-cholesterol-rats-leaf-ethanolic and methanolic extracts-200 mg/kg bw-Both extracts significantly reduced plasma total cholesterol ($p<0.05$) and triglyceride ($p<0.001$),   217-invitro-whole plant?,

360

Sida retusa
196-cholesterol-rats-leaf-water extract-200 mg/kg bw-a dose of 200 mg/kg of aqueous extract has shown reduction in triglycerides (TG) (16%), cholesterol (4%), and glucose level (10%),

Sida rhomboidea
128-cholesterol-rats-leaf-?extract-200 & 400 mg/kg bw-treatment to Triton WR 1339 treated rats recorded significant decrement in Plasma cholesterol, Triglyceride, while HDL was increased (all three p<0.05), **520**—mice--leaf--boiling distilled water extract--cholesterol,

Choline   water-soluble vitamin-like essential nutrient [1]
A macronutrient that's important for liver function, normal brain development, nerve function, muscle movement, supporting energy levels and maintaining a healthy metabolism. **[801]**

Sida spinosa, Sida humilis   **754**- invitro-roots and aerial parts,

Sida acuta   **217**-invitro-whole plant?, **568**-invitro-roots and aerial parts, **754**- invitro-roots and aerial parts,

Sida cordifolia   **217**-invitro-whole plant?, **312**-invitro-roots,

Sida rhombifolia
544-citing-Dinesh Jabhav, Medicinal plants of India, A Guide to Ayurvedic & Ethnomedicinal uses of plants, Vol 1, Scientific Publishers India, 2008, 213-214, **568**-invitro-roots and aerial parts, **670**-invitro-aerial parts or roots, **754**- invitro-roots and aerial parts.

Sida rhomboidea   **520**-invitro-leaves-boiling distilled water extract,

Chrome   Mineral

Sida cordifolia   **240**-invitro-leaves = 1.45 mg/100gm-stem bark = 1.05 mg/100gm,

Sida indica   **447**-invitro-roots-not present as chromates,

Chrysoenol   Flavone glycoside

Sida indica   **709**-review-flowers-detected-including Chrysoenol-7-o-beta-glucopyranoside, **710**-review-flowers-detected,

Chrysoeriol   A flavone (5,7,3'-OMe,4'-flavone) [1]

Chemically the 3'-methoxy derivative of luteolin... Vasorelaxant and hypotensive activity in vitro and in vivo in a murine model by intravenous infusion. [1]

Sida indica   710-review-review-flowers-detected,

Cinnamic acid   Unsaturated carboxylic acid

Used in flavors, synthetic indigo, and certain pharmaceuticals [1]

Sida acuta / Sida cordifolia / Sida rhombifolia / Sida spinosa / Sida veronicaefolia / Sida rhombifolia var. rhomboidea / Sida rhombifolia var. retusa / Sida indica / Abutilon hirtum (Sida graveolens) / Sida glutinosa / and Abutilon hirtum (Sida graveolens)

561-invitro-leaves-detected,

Copper   Mineral

Sida acuta

210-invitro-had exceptionally high concentrations of copper,   415-invitro-had exceptionally high concentrations of minerals.

Sida cordifolia   240-invitro-leaves = 0.48 mg/100gm-stem bark = 0.69 mg/100gm,

Sida hermaphrodita

482-invivo-whole plant-mineral excess soils, lowest readings of contamination still rich,   623-invitro-absorbed high levels of zinc, lower levels of lead, copper, and nickel, and absorbed cadmium at least.

Coronaric acid

A mono-unsaturated, epoxide derivative of the de-saturated fatty acid, linoleic acid. [1]

Sida cordifolia

118-review-seeds-fatty acids to 0.32 %,   358-invitro-seed-detected,   362-review-seed-a fatty oil containing the cocacinegenic acid coronaric acid (3%), 558-invitro-detected-cis-9,10-epoxy octadec-cis-12-enoic (coronaric) ,

Coumaric acid   polyphenol

Sida cordifolia   659-invitro-leaves-methanolic extract-none detected,

Courmarin   benzopyrone chemical class [1]

Coumarins (1-benzopyran-2-one) are chemical compounds in the benzopyrone class of organic compounds found in many plants. They possess a variety of biological properties, including antimicrobial, antiviral, antiin-flammatory, antidiabetic, antioxidant, and enzyme inhibitory activity. **[802]**

Sida spinosa   11-invitro-acquesous acetone extract

Sida indica   680-invitro-whole plant-cold distilled water extract-not detected—ethanol extract-not detected,   **687**-whole plant?-acetone extract-strongly detected-especially flower and pod,

Cryptolepine   (S. acuta, cordifolia, rhombifolia, spinosa, and ?)
Indoquinoline alkaloid

Antimalarial drug with cytotoxic properties **[1]**   Cryptolepine itself has been found to produce a variety of pharmacological effects, including hypotensive and antipyretic properties, presynamtic alpha-adreno-receptor blocking action, antimuscarinic properties, anti-inflammatory properties and antibacterial effects. Cryptolepine has potent in vitro activity against the malaria parasite and possesses cytotoxic activity, inhibiting DNA synthesis in B16 melanoma cells. **[244]**

Sida acuta

7-aerial parts-chloroform extract,   **17**-invitro-cryptolepine,   **19**-invitro-detected,   **62**-invitro-whole plant-detected,   **186**-invitro,   **220**-invitro, 252-invivo-acqueous extract + ethanolic extract-{mosquitos}FcM29-Cameroon (chloroquine-resistant strain) and a Nigerian chloroquine-sensitive strain-antiplasmodial-IC50 values 3.9 to −5.4 µg/ml,   **253**-invitro-whole plant-EtOAc-soluble extract-detected,   **310**-invitro,   **761**-invitro- leaf, stem, root and seed-detected-The major alkaloid of Sida acuta was shown to be cryptolepine,   **362**-invitro-roots and aerial parts,   **459**-invitro-leaf?-hot water decoction/ethanol extract- The IC50 values obtained for these extracts ranged from 3.9 to −5.4 µg/ml. Purification of this active fraction led to the identification of cryptolepine as the active antiplasmodial constituent of the plant,   **581**-invitro-whole plant-methanol extract-main alkaloid with its derivatives such as quindoline, quindolinone, cryptolepinone and 11-methoxy-quindoline,   **601**-Nigeria-entire plant-contains the alkaloid cryptolepine,   **646**-invitro-detected.

Sida cordifolia

35-invitro-detected,   **164**-cryptolepine-invitro-As an activator of p21WAF1/CIP1 promoter activity, we isolated cryptolepine (CLP: 5-methyl indolo (2,3b)-quiniine), an indoloquinoline alkaloid, from the traditional Ayurvedic medicinal plant Sida cordifolia, **217**-invitro-whole plant?, **312**-invitro-roots?, **378**-invitro, **400**-invitro-root?-cold methanol extract-we isolated cryptolepine (CLP: 5-methyl indolo (2,3b)-quiniine), an indoloquinoline alkaloid, from the traditional Ayurvedic medicinal plant Sida cordifolia.

Sida rhombifolia

59-invitro-aerial parts-95% ethanolic extract, **544**-citing-Dinesh Jabhav, Medicinal plants of India, A Guide to Ayurvedic & Ethnomedicinal uses of plants, Vol 1, Scientific Publishers India, 2008, 213-214., **622**-invitro-salt of cryptolepine.

Cryptolepinone   Indoquinoline alkaloid

Cryptolepine derivative. Inhibited induced preneoplastic lesions 83.3% **[220]**

Sida acuta

220-invitro-potential chemopreventive agent, **253**-mousse-whole plant-EtOAc-soluble extract, **572**-invitro-whole plant-methanol extract, **581**-invitro-whole plant-methanol extract-main alkaloid with its derivatives such as quindoline, quindolinone, cryptolepinone and 11-methoxy-quindoline,

Sida rhombifolia   **59**-invitro-whole plant?,

Cyanidin-3-rutinoside   Anthocyanin

A natural colorant found in blackcurrants and other fruits and flowers **[1]**

Sida indica   **454**-India-aerial parts,

D-galactose   monosaccharide sugar [1]

D-Glucose is a primary source of energy for living organisms. It is naturally occurring and is found in fruits and other parts of plants in its free state. It is used therapeutically in fluid and nutrient replacement. **[803]** Chronic systemic exposure of mice, rats, and Drosophila to D-galactose causes the acceleration of senescence (aging) and has been used as an aging model... The Leloir pathway consists of the latter stage of a two-part process that converts β-D-galactose to UDP-glucose. **[1]**

Sida indica   **709**-review-seed-detected.

Daucosterol   glucoside of β-sitosterol
a strong anti-feedant against adults of the rice weevil **[786]**

Sida acuta   **217**-invitro-whole plant?,

Daucoglycoside   {A poorly understood glycoside}
Sida acuta   **327**-invitro,

Diterpenes   **composed of two terpene units** [1]
Biosynthesized by plants and form the basis for biologically important compounds such as retinol, retinal, and phytol. They are known to be antimicrobial and antiinflammatory. **[1]**

Sida rhombifolia
136-invitro-root-boiling water extract-not detected,   **47**-invitro-aqueous methanol extract,   **51**-invitro-fruit-Methanol extract,   **136**-invitro-root-boiling water extract-detected,   **136**-invitro-root-95% ethanol extract-detected,   **543**-invitro-whole plant-ether extract,   **545**-invitro-aerial parts-80% ethanol extract-nil.

Ecdysteroids (phytoecsysteroids)
triterpenoid
Plants comprise rich sources of ecdysteroids in high concentration and with broad structural diversity. Ecdysteroids have a number of proven beneficial effects on mammals... ecdysteroids exert numerous effects in vertebrates that are similar to those of vertebrate hormonal steroids, and they may serve as effective anabolic, hepatoprotective, immunoprotective, antioxidant and hypoglycemic agents... The application of phytoecdysteroids is a promising alternative to the use of anabolic-androgenic steroids because of the apparent lack of adverse effects. The prospective use of phytoecdysteroids may extend to treatments of pathological conditions where anabolic steroids are routinely applied. **[191]**

Sida acuta **56**-invitro-seed-methanolic, hexane extract-found to contain significant amounts of ecdysteroids,   **217**-invitro-whole plant?

Sida cordifolia   **56**-invitro-seed-methanolic, hexane extract-no detectable amount,   **217**-invitro-whole plant?,   **312**-invitro-seeds-4 phytoecdysteroids detected in small amounts.

Sida rhombifolia
56-invitro-seed-methanolic, hexane extract-found to contain significant amounts of ecdysteroids,   **312**-invitro-seeds-4 phytoecdysteroids detected

in small amounts,   **436**-invitro-detected,   **492**-invitro-total of nine naturally occurring ecdysteroids were identified, of these two are identified for the first time in S. rhombifolia,   **573**-invitro-seven ecdysteroids were isolated.

Sida cordata   56-invitro-seed-methanolic, hexane extract-no detectable amount,   **312**-invitro-seeds-4 phytoecdysteroids detected in small amounts,

Sida spinosa

56-invitro-seed-methanolic, hexane extract-no detectable amount,   **312**-invitro-seeds-4 phytoecdysteroids detected in small amounts,   **493**-invitro-aerial parts-two ecdysteriods identified,   **573**-invitro-aerial parts,

Other Sidas

56-Sida filicaulis-invitro-seed-methanolic, hexane extract-found to contain significant amounts of ecdysteroids,   **56-Most other sidas**-Taken together, it appears that the majority of *Sida* species are either devoid or contain only low levels of ecdysteroids in their seeds-**no detectable amount**,   **490- Sida tuberculata**-leaves and roots-water and ethanol extracts-a considerable source of ecdysteroids.

Ephedrine   Sympathomimetic amine/substituted amphetamine

It is on the World Health Organization's List of Essential Medicines, the most effective and safe medicines needed in a health system... increases blood pressure and acts as a bronchodilator. **[1]**   One of the most significant results of the present study is the discovery of ephedrine as the major component of all the plants screened except one. This compound was seen distributed in almost all the parts like roots, leaves and or stem. **[561]**

Sida acuta

71-invitro-root-detected,   **217**-invitro-whole plant?-also Ψ- ephedrine,   **761**-invitro- leaf, stem, root and seed,   **362**-roots-ephedrine (0.07 %),   **548**-invitro-whole plant,   **561**-PhD dissertation-root,

Sida cordifolia

53-review,   **71**-invitro-whole plant-0.112%-most of any sida studied,   **118**--review--whole plant--to 0.085 %--stems-0.22 %--roots-0.06 %--leaves-ephedrine and pseudoephridine to 0.28 %,   **217**-invitro-whole plant?- Ψ-ephedrine,   **133**-invitro-whole plant-successively extracted with chloroform (3x72 h), methanol (3x72 h) and 80% ethanol (3x72 h),   **176**-invitro-whole plant?,   **218**-review,   **312**-invitro-roots-not detected,   **761**-invitro- leaf, stem, root and seed,   **358**-review,   **378**-review,   **411**-invitro-root-roots, the parts traditionally used, reportedly accumulate high levels of ephedrine, **413**-The maximum root yield and ephedrine content were recorded at eight months after planting and further delay in harvesting showed a sharp decline in both root yield and ephedrine content. The results indicated Sida cordifolia preferred open condition for higher root yield and ephedrine content,   **521**-

invitro-0.8 % Ephedrine, **533**-review, **562**-review, **612**-Though seed contain the maximum amount of active constituent, 'ephedrine' but root is used extensively.

Sida rhombifolia

71-invitro-root-detected, **544**-citing-Dinesh Jabhav, Medicinal plants of India, A Guide to Ayurvedic & Ethnomedicinal uses of plants, Vol 1, Scientific Publishers India, 2008, 213-214.

Sida cordata **71**-invitro-root-smallest amount measured-0.005%.

Sida rhomboidea

217-invitro-whole plant?, **520**-invitro-leaves-boiling distilled water extract, **561** -invitro-only Sida where some alkaloids other than ephedrine were found as the active principles.

Sida spinosa **561**- invitro –root, leaf and stem,

Sida retusa **561**- invitro -root and stem,

Sida veronicaefolia, Sida indica **561**-invitro-root.

Epicatechin **flavenol** Primary antioxidant in chocolate [1]

Sida acuta **659**-invitro-leaves-methanolic extract-119 µg/g dw.

Escoporone **coumarin**

Sida rhombifolia **622**-invitro,

Eugenol **[4-allyl-2-methoxyphenol]**

Perfumes, flavorings, essential oils. A local antiseptic and anesthetic. **[1]**

Sida indica **442**- mice-eugenol-50 mg/kg bw-significant analgesic activity,

Evofolin-A, Evofolin-B **Phenolic compounds**

Sida acuta **253**-invitro-whole plant-EtOAc-soluble extract, **581**-invitro-whole plant-methanol extract-detected.

....

Sida is one of the important medicinal plant species used to treat various diseases in Ayurveda and other traditional systems of medicine. **[15]**

Fat   triglyceride

Serves both structural and metabolic functions [1]

Sida acuta   223-invitro-leaves-percentage fat composition of 0.67% characterizes it as a low fat source,   **274**-invitro-leaf-crude fat 2.7%,   **652**-rats-leaf-ethanol extract-not detected,

Sida cordifolia   158-invitro-seed-10.56% ± 0.3,   **352**-seeds-Linoleic acid predominated (54.9–69.4%) as the fatty acid of all the oils, and malvalic (1.3–11.4%) and sterculic acids (0.4–1.1%) were significant.

Sida rhombifolia

352-seeds-Linoleic acid predominated (54.9–69.4%) as the fatty acid of all the oils, and malvalic (1.3–11.4%) and sterculic acids (0.4–1.1%) were significant,   **489**-invitro,   **538**-invitro-roots-95% ethanol extract-crude lipids 2.8%,   **543**-invitro-whole plant-ethanolic and acqueous extract-Fixed oils and fats.

Sida hermaphrodita   475-invitro-shoot-2.1-2.5%,   **546**-invitro-whole plant-fat- 3.46 percent of dry matter.

Sida indica   680-invitro-whole plant-cold distilled water extract-detected—ethanol extract-detected,

Fatty acids

Important dietary sources of fuel for animals. [1]

Sida acuta

96-invitro-leaf- cold petroleum ether extract-present--cold chloroform extract-present--95% ethanol extract-present,   **217**-invitro-whole plant?,   **559**-linoleic acid-invitro-seed-a polyunsaturated omega-6 essential fatty acid,   **559**-myristic acid-invitro-seed-acts as a lipid anchor in biomem-branes. Used in soaps and cosmetics,   **559**-oleic acid-invitro-seed-fixed oil,   **559**-plamitoleic acid-invitro-seed-fixed oil,   **559**-stearic acid-invitro-seed-saturated fatty acid-one of the most common saturated fatty acids found in nature.

Sida cordifolia

56-invitro-seed-methanolic, hexane extract-Among 11 species of Sida examined, seed extracts of S. acuta and S. rhombifolia were found to contain significant amounts of ecdysteroids-the remaining species showed no detectable levels of ecdysteroids-S acuta>S rhombifolia>S filicaulis>all other tested Sida no detectable amount,   **118**-palmitic acid-review-detected-the most common saturated fatty acid found in animals, plants and microorganisms,   **118**-stearic acid-review-detected-one of the most common saturated fatty acids found in nature,   **217**-invitro-whole plant?,   **312**-invitro-seeds-epoxy and cyclopropenoid fatty acids detected,   **559**-invitro-seed-studied for its fatty acid composition,   **574**-invitro- a rich source of hydrobromic acid-reactive fatty acids.

Sida rhombifolia

56-see listing under Sida acuta,   **312**-invitro-seeds-4 phytoecdysteroids detected in small amounts,   **436**-invitro-detected,   **492**-invitro- a total of nine naturally occurring ecdysteroids were identified, of these two are identified for the first time in S. rhombifolia,   **573**-invitro-seven ecdy-steroids were isolated.

Sida cordata

56-see listing under Sida acuta,   **312**-invitro-seeds-4 phytoecdysteroids detected in small amounts.

Sida spinosa

56-see listing under Sida acuta,   **493**-invitro-aerial parts-two ecdysteriods identified,   **573**-invitro-aerial parts.

Sida indica

454-**oleic acid**-invitro-leaves-water extract-400 mg/kg bw-(A monoun-saturated omega-9 fatty acid. A component in many foods, in the form of its triglycerides [1]),   **454**-palmitic acid-invitro-leaves-water extract-400 mg/kg bw-the most common saturated fatty acid found in animals, plants and microorganisms,   **454**-stearic acid-seeds-one of the most common satur-ated fatty acids found in nature,   **709**-review-Different parts of plants-detected,

Other Sidas

56-S filicaulis-invitro-seed-methanolic, hexane extract,   **490-Sida tuberculata**-leaves and roots-water and ethanol extracts-a considerable source of ecdysteroids,

Ferulic acid   **Phenolic compound**

May have direct antitumor activity against breast cancer and liver cancer. Ferulic acid may have pro-apoptotic effects in cancer cells, thereby leading to their destruction. **[1]**

Sida acuta   **18**-invitro-root-detected,   **253**-invitro-whole plant-EtOAc-soluble extract,

Sida rhombifolia   **622**-invitro-aerial parts-a ferulic acid derivative, ethoxy-ferulate,

....

The use of plants for healing is as ancient and universal as medicine itself. Plants act generally to stimulate and supplement the body's healing forces, they are the natural food for human beings. **[83]**

Fiber, Dietary   non-starch polysaccharides

Sida acuta   **223**-invitro-leaves- 9.50 %,   **274**-invitro-leaves- 5.30% by weight,   **358**-review,

Other Sidas

118-Sida cordifolia-review-detected-14,000ppm to 71,000ppm,   **358**-**Sida spinosa**-review,   **358-Sida linifolia** Juss. ex Cav.-review,   **358**-**Sida urens** L.-review,   **475-Sida hermaphrodita**-invitro-shoot-20.1-24.3%,   **538-Sida rhombifolia**-invitro-roots-95% ethanol extract-crude fiber 36.7%.

Flavenol   One of the most common flavonoids [673]

Sida acuta, Sida spinosa   **254**-invitro-aqueous acetone extract>n-hexane, dichloromethane, ethyl acetate and n-butanol fractions-determined,

Sida indica   **561**-PhD dissertation-detected,

Flavone   A class of flavonoids [1]

Sida acuta   **645**-invitro-leaf--cold water extract-detected--acetone extract-detected,

Sida indica   **561**-invitro-detected,

Flavonoid   Polyphenol

Most common group of polyphenolic compounds in human diet. Found ubiquitously in plants. Anti-carcinogenic. **[521]**   Flavonoids are known to have medicinal properties and play a major role in the successful medical treatments from ancient times and their use has persevered till date. They are potent water-soluble antioxidants and free radical scavengers, which prevent oxidative cell damage and have strong anticancer activity. They are used to improve aquaresis and as anti-inflammatory, anti-spasmodic, and anti-allergic, anti-microbial agents. **[184]**

Sida acuta

15-invitro-root-Methanolic extract (10% w/v)-.84 mg QE/g {Total flavonoid content is expressed as mg quercetin equivalent (QE)/g of dried plant material},   **52**-invitro-root-methanol extract-abundant,   **86**-invitro-ethanolic and aqueous extracts,   **96**-invitro-leaf- cold petroleum ether extract-present-flavones,   **96**-invitro-leaf- 95% ethanol extract-present-flavones,   **98**-invitro-whole plant- The study showed that flavonoids of S. acuta can be exploited for future anticanadidal drug,   **102**-invitro-leaf-water and 100% methanolic extracts-trace amounts, **106**-invitro-detected, **113**-invitro-whole plant?- ethanolic and aqueous extracts-detected, **84**-invitro-root, stem, leaves and buds-80% ethanol extract- Free flavonoids were found to be more potent than bound flavonoids, **184**-invitro-root, stem, leaves and buds-80% ethanol extract>petroleum ether, ethyl ether and ethyl acetate extracts- All the flavonoid extracts showed varying degrees of antifungal activity on *C. albicans*. Some of these extracts were more effective than traditional antibiotic terbinafine to combat the pathogenic fungi, **204**-invitro-leaf-cold water extract-1%, **213**-invitro-chloroform/100% methanol extract-tested positive for flavonoids, **214**-invitro-whole plant?- 70% aqueous methanol extracts-detected, **223**-invitro-leaves-moderately present-1255 mg/100 gm, **224**-leaf-present in all four extracts-hexane/ chloroform/water/methanol extracts, **230**-leaf-boiled leaves-flavenoids strongly present, **237**-invitro-0.112 mg/100g, **254**--invitro--whole plant?--n-hexane, dichloromethane, ethyl acetate and n-butanol fractions of aqueous acetone extracts--1.79-3.49 mg./100 mg., **264**-100% ethanolic leaf extract -1163.86 mg/100 g, **265**-leaf-80% ethanol extract-detected, **271**-invitro- root, stem, leaf and buds-1 water extract (distilled water)-80% methanol extract followed by standard tests for flavenoids- Total flavonoids were found to be maximum in leaves-(8.5 mg/gm dw). Free flavonoids from roots and bound flavonoid from stems exhibited antibacterial activity against all tested bacteria, **274**-invitro-leaves - 310.00 Mg/100g, **300**-invitro-leaf-ethanol extract-detected, **420**-invitro-leaves and stems-cold water extract-0.98% ±0.10 by weight, this phytochemical was found to be present (no quantity given), **460**-rats-ethanolic extract-substance is present, **463**-invitro-leaf-methanolic extract, **500**-invitro-hydroalcoholic root extract, **579**-invitro- leaves, stems and roots-hexane and ethanol extracts-detected, **645**-invitro-leaf-cold water extract-not detected, **645**-invitro-leaf-acetone extract-not detected, **652**-rats-leaf-ethanol extract-detected, **668**-invitro-roots-methanol extract-detected,

Sida cordifolia

15-invitro-root-Methanolic extract (10% w/v)-1.26 mg QE/g, **59**-invitro-aerial parts-95% ethanolic extract-acacetin, **120**-invitro-aerial parts, **148**-aerial parts-alcoholic extract-detected, **171**-invitro-aerial parts-water extract-551.60 ± 15.53 (mg Quercetin/g of extract), **175**-invitro-water extract-200&400 mg/kg bw- The flavonoids and phenols present in Sida cordifolia contribute for antioxidant potentiality that exhibits nephroprotective activity, **240**-invitro-leaves = 19.3 g/100gm-stem bark = 12.4 g/100gm, **312**-invitro-aerial parts-detected 5 flavones, **521**-invitro-10 % Isoflavones, **561**-PhD dissertation-leaves and stem-detected, **591**-rats-whole plant-70% ethanol extract-detected, **663**-invitro-seed-water extract=0µg/mg--Acetone extract=54.95µg/mg--Petroleum Ether extract =49.63µg/mg--chloroform extract=47.53µg/mg, **668**-invitro-roots- meth-anol extract-detected,

Sida rhombifolia

15-invitro-root-Methanolic extract (10% w/v)-.9 mg QE/g, **47**-invitro-aqueous methanol extract, **51**-invitro-fruit-Methanol extract, **126**-

invitro-water/ethanol extracts, **136**-invitro-root-boiling water extract-detected---95% ethanol extract-detected, **187**-invitro, **195**-invitro, **243**-invitro- The flavonoid crude extract yielded approximately 12% with LC50 of 501 mg l-1 and its inhibitory effect ranged from 48 to 71% (100-800 mg l-1), **486**-invitro-whole plant?- water, 70% ethanol extract, **543**-invitro-whole plant-ethanolic and acqueous extract, **544**-leaves and/or roots-ethyl acetate extract-detected---ethanol extract-detected, **545**-invitro-aerial parts-80% ethanol extract-nil, **578**-invitro-whole plant?-water extract-detected, **668**-invitro-roots-methanol extract-detected,

Sida retusa   **15**-invitro-root-Methanolic extract (10% w/v)-.7mg QE/g, **668**-invitro-roots-methanol extract-detected,

Sida cordata

15-invitro-root-Methanolic extract (10% w/v)-.97 mg QE/g, **282**-invitro-leaf-methanol extract-The total flavonoid concentrations was ranged from 110 to 103.33 mg quercetin/gm., **494**-invitro-whole plant-methanol extract-Considerable amount of flavonoid and phenolic contents were recorded in the methanol extract and its derived fractions, **498**-invitro-leaves and stems-successive solvent extraction method, **500**-invitro-root- hydroalcoholic extract-detected, **668**-invitro-roots-methanol extract-detect-ed,

Sida indica

15-invitro-root-Methanolic extract (10% w/v)-1.03 mg QE/g, **443**-rats-leaves-methanol extract-quercetin, **445**-invitro-leaves, twigs and roots, **446**-invitro-acqueous and methanol extracts-nothing detected, **447**-invitro-roots-not present, **448**-rats-whole plant-is present-ether/chloro-form/ethanol/ acqueous extract (sequential extraction from a marc, extract taken out at each phase for testing. Acqueous extract on the remains after the three previous extractions, **449**-mice/sheeps's blood-leaves-acqueous extract (400 mg/kg bw) and ethanolic extract (200 mg/kg bw), **451**-leaves/twigs/roots-boiling water extract, **453**-whole plant-chloroform and ethanol extracts-detected, **454**-invitro-leaves-detected, **638**-invitro-methanol extract-total flavonoids per mg pyrocatechol g-1 dry extract—leaf 61.7-seed 13.2-root 24.8, **677**-invitro-fruits-80% ethanol extract=15 ± 0.4 (mg RE/g)-- Petroleum ether extract=11 ± 0.6 (mg RE/g)--Chloroform extract=20 ± 0.2 (mg RE/g)--Ethyl acetate extract=30 ± 0.5 (mg RE/g)--Butanol extract=18 ± 0.8 (mg RE/g)--Aqueous extract=11 ± 0.3 (mg RE/g), **680**-invitro-whole plant-cold distilled water extract-detected—ethanol extract-detected, **681**-invitro-whole plant-80% ethanol extract with distilled water-not detected, **683**-invitro-leaves-cold distilled water extract-detected, **684**-invitro-leaf--hydro-methanolic extract-not detect-ed, **687**-whole plant?-acetone extract-detected-especially stem and flower, **709**-review-root or leaf-detected, **710**-Ayurveda-review-leaves/ flowers-large amount detected, **712**-nvitro-leaf-Petroleum ether extract detected --Ethyl acetate extract not detected --Chloroform extract detected--Methanolic extract detected--Aqueous extract not detected, **712**-invitro-stem-Hydro-alcoholic extract detected--Methanolic extract detected--Aqueous extract detected,

Sida rhomboidea

130-leaf-water extract-flavenoids 2.3 mg/100 mg, **185**-invitro-leaf-detected, **320**-whole plant?-methanol extract-(26.94±0.94 mg/ml quercetin equivalent-flavanoids), **325**-invitro-leaf-detected.

Sida spinosa

15-invitro-root-Methanolic extract (10% w/v)-1.09 mg QE/g, **99**-invitro-whole plant-hot 60-80% ethanolic extract, **254**-invitro-whole plant?-n-hexane, dichloromethane, ethyl acetate and n-butanol fractions of aqueous acetone extracts-1.04-3.55 mg./100 mg.

Sidas tiagii

551-fruit-95% ethanolic extract, **552**-invitro-fruit-ethanolic extract>n-hexane extract/ethyl acetate extract-The filtrate was partitioned with ethyl acetate extract-ethanolic extract works, **607**-mice-fruit-hot 95% ethanol extract>n-hexane/ethyl acetate extracts-detected.

Sida veronicaefolia

346-invitro-whole plant?-ethanolic extract >water-soluble fraction-detected, **348**-mice-leaves-petroleum, ether, chloroform, ethanol, and aqueous solutions subsequently combined-detected

Other Sidas

15-**Sida mysorensis**-invitro-root-Methanolic extract (10% w/v)-1.18 mg QE/g, **200-Sida cardifolia**-invitro-leaf-acetone extract-Thus acetone leaf extract of Sida cardifolia had maximum amount of polyphenols and flavonoids which is directly related to their greater antioxidant activity also. Thus active molecules present in the acetone leaf extract of Sida cardifolia has antioxidant property which may be useful in targeting the release of free radical intermediates along with the generation of ROS from various metabolic activities, **344-S. humilis**-invitro-whole plant?-methanolic extract -not detected, **483-Sida hermaphrodita**-invitro-50, 60, and 70% ethanolic extract-rutin, **490-Sida tuberculata**-ethanol extract roots 70%, leaves 40%, **535-Sida urens**-invitro-leaves-Keller-ammonia/H2SO4-none detected,

Fructose   monosaccharide

One of the three dietary monosaccharides, along with glucose and galactose, that are absorbed directly into the bloodstream during digestion. [1]

Sida indica

570-invitro-petroleum ether extract then 50% alcohol extract, **709**-review-leaf-detected,

Sida veronicaefolia

346-invitro-whole plant?-ethanolic extract>water-soluble fraction-detected,

Fumaric acid

Showed hepatoprotective activity comparable with silymarin. **[182]**

Sida cordifolia

181-invitro-aerial parts-hepatoprotective activity of fumaric acid, **182**-invitro-root-50% ethanol extract-Fumaric acid isolated from S. cordifolia also showed hepatoprotective activity, which was comparable with silymarin-it significantly protects the liver cells and reduces the severity of damage caused by alcohol intoxication, **217**-invitro-whole plant?

Sida indica **570**-invitro-petroleum ether extract then 50% alcohol extract, **712**-review,

Galactomannans **polysaccharides**

Polysaccharides consisting of a mannose backbone with galactose side groups... A component of the cell wall of the mold Aspergillus[3] and is released during growth. Detection of galactomannan in blood is used to diagnose invasive aspergillosis infections in humans. **[1]**

Sida indica **709**-review-seed-detected, **710**-review-seed-detected,

Galactose **A monosaccharide sugar, milk sugar**

Component of antigens present on blood cells that determine blood type **[1]**

Sida acuta **217**-invitro-whole plant?, **561**-invitro-leaves-detected,

Sida cordifolia / Sida rhombifolia / Sida spinosa / Sida veronicaefolia / Sida rhombifolia var. rhomboidea / Sida rhombifolia var. retusa **561**-invitro-leaves-detected,

Sida indica **561**-invitro-leaves-detected, **570**-invitro-petroleum ether extract then 50% alcohol extract, **709**-review-leaf-detected,

Galacturic acid

Sida acuta **217**-invitro-whole plant?,

Galacturonic acid **sugar acid**

The main component of pectin, in which it exists as the polymer polygalacturonic acid. **[1]**

Sida indica
570-invitro-petroleum ether extract then 50% alcohol extract.

Gallic acid   phenolic acid
Anti-oxidant. A type of phenolic acid, found in gallnuts, sumac, witch hazel, tea leaves, oak bark, and other plants. [1]

Sida acuta
659-invitro-leaves-methanolic extract-2.9 µg/g dw,

Sida indica
676-invitro-root-95% ethanol extract-detected.

Gelatin
Flavorless food derived from collagen obtained from various animal body parts. Some feel it helps to reduce joint pain associated with osteoarthritis [1]

Sida cordifolia
217-invitro-whole plant?,

Genistein   isoflavone
Influences multiple biochemical functions in living cells. Anti-oxidant. Anti-cancer. Angiogenesis inhibitor. [1]

Sida acuta
93-invitro-leaves-70% aqueous methanol (v/v) acidified to pH 2.

Gentisic acid   benzoic acid derivative

Sida acuta
561-invitro-detected,

Sida indica
709-review-flowers-detected,

Glucose   A simple sugar
Glucose circulates in the blood of animals as blood sugar--the most important source of energy for cellular respiration--Glucose is a ubiquitous fuel in biology--It is used as an energy source in most organisms. [1]

Sida acuta
217-invitro-whole plant?,   561-PhD dissertation-leaves-detected.

Sida cordifolia / Sida rhombifolia / Sida spinosa / Sida veronicaefolia / Sida rhombifolia var. rhomboidea / Sida rhombifolia var. retusa
561-PhD dissertation-leaves-detected.

Sida cardifolia

200-invitro-leaf-acetone extract-5.60 µg glucose equivalent/g.

Sida indica

561-PhD dissertation-leaves-detected, 570-invitro-petroleum ether extract then 50% alcohol extract-also gluco-vanilloyl glucose, 709-review-flowers-detected-also Glycopyronoside

Gluco-vanilloyl glucose   simple sugar

Sida indica   570-invitro-petroleum ether extract then 50% alcohol extract,

Glucuronic acid   uronic acid

Glucuronic acid is a precursor of ascorbic acid (vitamin C)-it is important for the metabolism of microorganisms, plants and animals-From urine [1]

Sida acuta / Sida cordifolia / Sida rhombifolia / Sida spinosa / Sida veronicaefolia / Sida rhombifolia var. rhomboidea / Sida rhombifolia var. retusa / Sida indica   561-PhD dissertation-leaves-detected.

Glutamic acid   excitatory neurotransmitter

A key compound in cellular metabolism, and the most abundant excitatory neurotransmitter in our nervous system. [1]

Sida indica   570-invitro-petroleum ether extract then 50% alcohol extract.

Glyceryl-1- eicosanoate   fat

(Glyceryl behenate) used in cosmetics, foods, and oral pharmaceutical formulations [1]

Sida cordifolia   217-invitro-whole plant?,

Glycine   The simplest possible amino acid [1]

Glycine is one of the proteinogenic amino acids. The principal function of glycine is as a precursor to proteins. [1]

376

Sida veronicaefolia

346-invitro-whole plant?-ethanolic extract>water-soluble fraction-detected,

Glycosides   **sugar bound to another functional group** [1]

Many plant glycosides are used as medications. **[1]**

Sida acuta

17-invitro- two kaempferol glycosides,   **86**-invitro- ethanolic and aqueous extracts,   **96**-invitro-leaf- 95% ethanol extract-present,   **102**-invitro-leaf-water and 100% methanolic extracts-cardiac glycosides in moderate amount,   **106**-invitro-not detected,   **113**-invitro-whole plant?- ethanolic and aqueous extracts-detected,   **204**-invitro-leaf-cold water extract-cardiac glycoside-present,   **213**-invitro-leaf-100% methanol/chloroform extracts-cardenolides,   **214**-invitro-whole plant?-70% aqueous methanol extracts-none detected,   **224**-leaf-not present in all four extracts-hexane/chloroform/water/methanol extracts,   **230**-leaf-boiled leaves-glycosides present,   **264**-100% ethanolic leaf extract-Cardiac glycoside-851.62 mg/100 g,   **265**-leaf-80% ethanol extract-Cardiac glycoside-detected,   **300**-invitro-leaf-ethanol extract-detected,   **327**-invitro- daucoglycoside,   **420**-invitro-leaves and stems-cold water extract-found to be present(no quality given),   **460**-rats-ethanolic extract-substance is present,   **579**-invitro- leaves, stems and roots-hexane and ethanol extracts-detected glycosides and cardiac glycosides, **645**-invitro-leaf-cold water extract-detected cardiac glycosides,   **645**-invitro-leaf-acetone extract-detected cardiac glycosides,   **652**-rats-leaf-ethanol extract-detected cardiac glycosides,

Sida cordifolia   **32**-invitro-root-cold 40% ethanol extract-detected,

148-aerial parts-alcoholic extract-detected,   **240**-invitro-leaf and stem bark-methanol extract,   **591**-rats-whole plant-70% ethanol extract-detected,

Sida rhombifolia

47-invitro- methanolic extracts and water and methanol (1v:4v), (1v:1v), (3v:2v) extracts-detected,   **47**-invitro-seed-Two glycosides (phenyl-Ethyl-D-gluco-pyranoside and Phytoécdysteroide) exhibited different biological activities were isolated from the extract of the seeds of S. rhombifolia respectively,   **51**-invitro-fruit-Methanol extract,   **136**-invitro-root-boiling water or 95% ethanol extract-detected,   **543**-invitro-whole plant-ether, ethanolic, acqueous, ether extracts,   **544**-leaves and/or roots-ethyl acetate or ethanol extract-detected,   **545**-invitro-aerial parts-80% ethanol extract-nil.

Sida tiagii

551-fruit-95% ethanolic extract,   **552**-invitro-fruit-ethanolic extract>n-hexane extract/ethyl acetate extract-The filtrate was partitioned with ethyl acetate extract-ethanolic extract good,   **607**-mice-fruit-hot 95% ethanol extract>n-hexane/ethyl acetate extracts-detected-triterpenoid glycosides,

Sida indica

445-invitro-leaves, twigs and roots,   **446**-invitro-acqueous and methanol extracts-nothing detected (cardio glycosides),   **448**-rats-whole plant-is present-ether/chloroform/ethanol/acqueous extract (sequential extraction from a marc, extract taken out at each phase for testing. Acqueous extract on the remains after the three previous extractions,   **451**-leaves/twigs/roots-boiling water extract,   **677**-invitro-fruits-80% ethanol extract/Petroleum ether extract/Chloroform extract/Ethyl acetate extract/Butanol extract/ Aqueous extract--not detected,   **683**-invitro-leaves-cold distilled water extract-detected,   **680**-invitro-whole plant-cold distilled water extract-detected—ethanol extract-detected,   **684**-invitro-leaf--hydro-meth-anolic extract-detected-cardiac glycosides,   **687**-whole plant?-acetone extract-detected-especially the flower,   **709**-review-root/leaf/flower-detected,   **710**-Ayurveda-review-leaves-large amount detected,   **712**-invitro-leaf-Petroleum ether extract detected--Ethyl acetate extract not detected—Chloroform extract detected--Methanolic extract detected--Aqueous extract detected,   **712**-invitro-stem-Hydroalcoholic extract not detected—Methanolic extract detected--Aqueous extract detected.

Sida rhomboidea   **185**-invitro-leaf-detected-but absence of cardiac glycosides,   **325**-invitro-leaf-detected,

Sida spinosa   **99**-invitro-whole plant-hot 60-80% ethanolic extract,

Other Sidas   **293**-**Sida cordata**-invitro-leaf-methanol extract-present, **535**-**Sida urens**-invitro-leaves-Keller-Killani test-detected,

Gossypetin   A flavonol, a type of flavonoid

(3,5,7,8,3',4'-hexahydroxyflavone) Types of flavonoids that exhibit a strong antibacterial activity. Recently it was shown that gossypetin has radioprotective activity. [1]

Sida indica   **454**--invitro--leaves--400 mg/kg bw--ether/benzene/ ethanol/water extracts--includes Gossypetin-7-glucosides, Gossypetin-8-glu-cosides,   **710**-Ayurveda-review-detected,

Heraclenol   furanocoumarin

{Many furanocoumarins are toxic and are produced by plants as a defense mechanism against various types of predators ranging from insects to mammals}

Sida acuta   **217**-invitro-whole plant?,   **327**-invitro,

Hexacosanoic acid   Long-chain saturated fatty acid [1]

A white crystalline solid, most commonly found in beeswax and carnauba wax [1]

Sida cordifolia   **118**-review-detected,   **217**-invitro-whole plant?,

Histidine   α-amino acid

An α-amino acid that is used in the biosynthesis of proteins. **[1]**

Sida indica   **570**-invitro-petroleum ether extract then 50% alcohol extract.

Sida veronicaefolia

346-invitro-whole plant?-ethanolic extract>water-soluble fraction-detected,

Hydrocyanic acid   Hydrogen cyanide (HCN)

A colorless, extremely poisonous and flammable liquid that has many industrial uses. **[1]**

Sida acuta   **274**-invitro-leaves - 98.25 Mg/100g,   **652**-rats-leaf-ethanol extract-detected.

Hypaphorine   indole alkaloid

Sida actua   **217**-invitro-roots and aerial parts,

Sida cordifolia   **118**-review-aerial parts-detected,   **176**-invitro-whole plant?,   **217**-invitro-whole plant?,   **312**-invitro-roots.

Inulin   polysaccharide [1]

Natural storage carbohydrate present in over 36,000 species of plants. **[1]**

Sida acuta   **645**-invitro-leaf-cold water extract-not detected--acetone extract-not detected,

Iron   metal

Sida acuta

223-invitro-leaves- 4.87 mg/100 gm,   **274**-invitro-leaves - 1.01 Mg/100g.

Sida cordifolia

240-invitro-leaves = 5.74 mg/100gm-stem bark = 5.51 mg/100gm, **249**-invitro- 5.74 mg/100 gm.

Sida hermaphrodita   **546**-leaves-63.5 mg/kg dry matter,

Kaempferol   flavonol

A potent anti-oxidant. May reduce the risk of various cancers. **[1]**

Sida acuta

17-invitro- two kaempferol glycosides, **62**-invitro-detected-two kaempferol glycosides, **93**-invitro-leaves-70% aqueous methanol (v/v) acidified to pH 2, **561**-invitro-Methoxy kaempferol, **659**-invitro-leaves-methanolic extract-763.6 µg/g dw.

Sida rhombifolia

195-invitro-ethyl acetate extract-two isolated flavonoids, kaempferol 3,7-di-O-α-l-rhamnopyranoside (lespedin) and kaempferol 3-O-β-d-(6''-E-p-coumaroil) glucopyranoside (tiliroside) was determined, **622**-invitro-kaempferol and kaempferol-3-O-_-D-glycosyl-60 0-_-D-rhamnose.

Other Sidas   **710-Sida indica**-review-detected, **561-Sida spinosa**-invitro-Methoxy kaempferol.

Lauric acid   Saturated fatty acid [1]

Been characterized as having "a more favorable effect on total HDL cholesterol than any other fatty acid [examined], either saturated or unsaturated" **[1]**

Sida indica   **709**-review-root-detected.

Lead   metal

Sida hermaphrodita   **482**-invivo-whole plant-mineral excess soils, lowest readings of contamination still rich, **623**-invitro-absorbed high levels of zinc, lower levels of lead, copper, and nickel, and absorbed cadmium at least.

Other Sidas

240-Sida cordifolia-invitro-leaves = 0.07 mg/100gm-stem bark = 0.07 mg/100gm, **538-Sida rhombifolia**-invitro-roots-95% ethanol extract-nil.

Leucine   α-amino acid
Used in the biosynthesis of proteins [1]

Sida indica   570-invitro-petroleum ether extract then 50% alcohol extract.

Lignin   Phenolic polymer [1]
Particularly important in the formation of cell walls, especially in wood and bark, because they lend rigidity and do not rot easily. [1]

Sida acuta   645-invitro-leaf-cold water extract-detected--acetone extract-detected,

Sida indica   684-invitro-leaf--hydro-methanolic extract-detected,

Sida humilis   344-invitro-whole plant?-methanolic extract-minimally present.

Linoleic acid
Polyunsaturated omega-6 essential fatty acid
An essential fatty acid that must be consumed for proper health. [1]

Sida acuta   217-invitro-whole plant?,   559-invitro-seed-fixed oil,

Sida rhombifolia   544-citing-Dinesh Jabhav, Medicinal plants of India, A Guide to Ayurvedic & Ethnomedicinal uses of plants, Vol 1, Scientific Publishers India, 2008, 213-214.

Sida indica   454-India-seeds,   709-review-root-detected.

Sida cordifolia/Sida rhomboidea   217-invitro-whole plant?

Loliolide   most common monoterpenoid lactone
Has a variety of biological properties such as anti-cancer, antibacterial, antifungal and antioxidant ones. Moreover, plants containing loliolide are used in alternative medicine in treatment of diabetes and depression. Also has allelopathic activity. [752]

Sida acuta   220-invitro,   253-invitro-whole plant-EtOAc-soluble extract,   581-invitro-whole plant-methanol extract-detected,

Luteolin   flavone [1]
Found in many foods. Health benefits range from possibly preventing cancer to protecting the brain-interferes with nearly all types of cancer cells. [757]

Sida indica   **709**-review-flowers-detected,   **710**-Ayurveda-review-flowers-detected.

Magnesium   metal

Magnesium is an essential element in biological systems. It is an essential mineral nutrient (i.e., element) for life and is present in every cell type in every organism. Magnesium plays a role in the stability of all polyphosphate compounds in the cells. Over 300 enzymes require the presence of magnesium ions for their catalytic action. In plants, magnesium is necessary for synthesis of chlorophyll and photosynthesis. **[1]**

Sida acuta

223-invitro-leaves-24.5 mg/100 gm,   **264**-100% ethanolic leaf extract-122.11mg/100 g,   **274**-invitro-leaves -14.40 Mg/100g,   **415**-invitro- S. acuta had exceptionally high concentrations of minerals.

Sida   cordifolia   **240**-invitro-leaves=128.31   mg/100gm-stem bark=45.29 mg/100gm,   **290**-aerial parts -1.17 g/kg

Sida rhombifolia

504-invitro- cultivated under mineral nutrition standard conditions-63+ days after emergence-71.9 mg per plant,   **512**-invivo-root-medium-Among weed species the relative concentration of a particular nutrient in the root system dry matter(high, med, low),   **538**-invitro-roots-95% ethanol extract-.32%,

Other Sidas

476-Sida hermaphrodita-invivo/invitro-Significantly more phosphorus, magnesium and sulphur was contained by Virginia fanpetals biomass from the objects where municipal sewage sludge compost had been applied, **539-Sida indica**-Ayurveda-magnesium phosphate

Makisterone C   Phytoecdysteroid [789]

Sterols found in insect's cotton seed diet **[789]**

Sida cordifolia   **217**-invitro-whole plant?,

Maltobionic acid   polyhydroxy bionic acid [787]

Topical anti-aging benefits **[787]**

Sida acuta   **217**-invitro-whole plant?,

Maltose   Malt sugar, a disaccharide [1]

A component of malt [1]

Sida acuta   217-invitro-whole plant?,

Malvalic acid   Fatty acid

Animal abnormalities from ingesting cottonseed oil [1]

Sida acuta   217-invitro-whole plant?,   362-review-seeds-malvalic acid (1.7%),   575-invitro-seed-present-2.0%/

Sida cordifolia   118-review-seeds-fatty acids to 0.32 %,   217-invitro-whole plant?

Sida rhombifolia

362-review-seeds-malvalic acid (1.7%),   544-citing-Dinesh Jabhav, Medicinal plants of India, A Guide to Ayurvedic & Ethnomedicinal uses of plants, Vol 1, Scientific Publishers India, 2008, 213-214.,   575-invitro-seed-present-2.0%.

Manganese   metal

Manganese is an important element for human health, essential for development, metabolism, and the antioxidant system. Excessive exposure or intake may lead to a condition known as manganism. [1]

Sida cordifolia   240-invitro-leaves = 0.77 mg/100gm-stem bark = 0.88 mg/100gm,   249-invitro- 0.77 mg/100 gm

Sida hermaphrodita   546-manganese - 348.5 mg/kg dry matter.

Mannose   Polysaccharide

Important in human metabolism, especially in the glycosylation of certain proteins--Preliminary studies indicate that D-mannose may help to prevent recurrent urinary tract infections. [1]

Sida acuta / Sida cordifolia / Sida rhombifolia / Sida spinosa / Sida veronicaefolia / Sida rhombifolia var. rhomboidea / Sida rhombifolia var. retusa / Sida indica / Abutilon hirtum (Sida graveolens) / Sida glutinosa / Abutilon hirtum (Sida graveolens)

561-PhD dissertation-leaves-detected,

Moisture

Sida acuta   52-invitro-root-5%,   223-invitro-leaves-the moisture content value of 9.03% obtained for Sida acuta leaves in this study is low and it suggests that the leaves can be kept for a relatively long time. The moisture content of any food can be used as a measure of its keeping quality,   274-invitro-leaves - 54.82% by weight,

Sida cordifolia   158-invitro-seed-10.00±1.6%-seed powder has very low water absorption capacity,   558-seed-5.1%

Sida rhombifolia   538-invitro-roots-95% ethanol extract-moisture 7.5%

Sida indica   447-invitro-roots-Moisture Content 0.8,   680-invitro-whole plant-cold distilled water extract- ethanol extract-moisture 3.2%

Molybdenum   Metal

In 2008, evidence was reported that a scarcity of molybdenum in the Earth's early oceans was a limiting factor for nearly two billion years in the further evolution of eukaryotic life (which includes all plants and animals). [1]   {is also the most slippery thing in the world}

Sida acuta   415-invitro- S. acuta had exceptionally high concentrations of minerals.

Mucilage

A thick, gluey substance produced by nearly all plants and some microorganisms. Mucilage in plants plays a role in the storage of water and food, seed germination, and thickening membranes [1]   The role of mucilages in *bala* or in general in medicinal plants is never understood properly. It was not considered as a pharmacologically active component in bala. But of late, the mucilages are found to exert a large number of pharmacological actions. They were known laxative agents, demulcents, emollients and anti-diarrhoeal agents. They also check fermentation, bacterial growth and adsorb toxins and wastes helping their elimination from the body. Even cholesterol is being lowered by these mechanisms., as also there are repots in which they cause a blood sugar lowering effects. [561]

Sida acuta   358-review-Leaf mucilage used for getting foreign objects out of the eye,   561-invitro-detected,   668-invitro-roots-methanol extract-detected.

Sida rhombifolia   358-review,   543-invitro-whole plant-ethanolic extract,   545-invitro-aerial parts-80% ethanol extract-gums,   561-invitro -detected,   668-invitro-roots-methanol extract-detected,

384

Sida indica

570-invitro-petroleum ether extract then 50% alcohol extract, **680**-invitro-whole plant-cold distilled water extract-detected—ethanol extract-detected-gum and mucilage, **709**-review-leaf-detected, **710**-Ayurveda-review-leaves-large amount detected,

Sida cordifolia, Sida retusa, Sida cordata   **668**-invitro-roots-methanol extract-detected,

Mucins   heavily glycosylated proteins

Mucins' key characteristic is their ability to form gels; therefore they are a key component in most gel-like secretions, serving functions from lubrication to cell signaling to forming chemical barriers. [1]

Sida acuta   **460**-rats-ethanolic extract-substance is present.

Sida cordifolia   **32**-invitro-root-cold 40% ethanol extract-fixed oils-mucilage, **118**-review-detected, **125**-invitro-leaves-acetone/methanol/water extracts-measurable amount-mucins, **217**-invitro-whole plant?

Other Sidas

561-Sida veronicaefolia-invitro-detected, **561-Sida indica**-invitro-detected, **561-Sida retusa**-invitro-detected, **561-Sida spinosa**-invitro-detected.

Myricetin   flavonoid with antioxidant properties

Sida acuta   **93**-invitro-leaves-70% aqueous methanol (v/v) acidified to pH 2,

Myristic acid   A common saturated fatty acid

lipid anchor in biomembranes [1]

Sida acuta   **559**-invitro-seed-fixed oil.

Sida indica   **709**-review-root-detected.

N-hexacosa-11-enoic acid   omega-9 fatty acid

Monounsaturated omega-9 fatty acid found in a variety of plant oils and nuts [1]   Significantly antibacterial [150]

Sida rhombifolia   **150**-invitro-fruit-ether>chloroform>acetone extract -293mg/1000 g,, **353**-fruit,

N-methyl-β phenethylamine   phenethylamine

A positional isomer of the drug amphetamine, with which it shares some properties [1]

Sida acuta   217--invitro--whole plant?--ß-phenethylamines,

Sida rhomboidea   520-invitro-leaves-boiling distilled water extract,

Niacin   Vitamin B3, a vitamin and essential human nutrient

Sida acuta   223-invitro-leaves- 0.33 mg/100 gm,   **264**-100% ethanolic leaf extract - 0.19 mg/100 g

Nickel   transition metal [1]

An essential nutrient for bacteria residing in the large intestine, in effect functioning as a prebiotic [1]

Sida cordifolia   240-invitro-leaves=3.99 mg/100gm-stem bark=3.26 mg/100gm,

Sida hermaphrodita   482-invivo-whole plant-mineral excess soils, lowest readings of contamination still rich,   **623**-invitro-absorbed high levels of zinc, lower levels of lead, copper, and nickel, and absorbed cadmium at least,

Ninhydrin   lab test chemical

Used to detect ammonia or primary and secondary amines... commonly used to detect fingerprints [1]

Sida acuta   645-invitro-leaf-cold water extract or acetone extract-detected,

Nitrogen   element, gas [1]

Dissolves in the blood and body fats [1]

Sida cordifolia   158-invitro-seed-non protein nitrogen-11.20% ± 0.4, **290**-aerial parts-2.31%.

Sida rhombifolia

504-invitro-low-cultivated under mineral nutrition standard conditions-63+ days after emergence-402.6 mg N per plant,   **512**-invivo-root-Among weed species the relative concentration of a particular nutrient in the root system dry matter(high, med, low)

Sida hermaphrodita
475-invitro-shoot-1.2-1.4%, **476**-invivo/invitro-municipal sewage-3.72 g. kg-1 dm)

N-methyl tryptophan
chemical compound

Serves as an enzyme substrate... A (2017) phase I trial studies the best dose of 1-methyl-D-tryptophan in treating metastatic or refractory solid tumors that cannot be removed by surgery. [1]

Sida cordifolia
133-invitro--whole plant--water extract--successively extracted with chloroform (3x72 h), methanol (3x72 h) and 80% ethanol (3x72 h)-detected--1-methyl tryptophan, **217**-invitro-whole plant?

Norpseudoephedrine
amphetamine

A psychostimulant drug of the amphetamine family. [1]

Sida cordifolia
218-review,

N- hentriacontane
paraffin of leaf surface lipids

Sida acuta
217-invitro-whole plant?

N- nonacosane
paraffin of leaf surface lipids

Sida acuta
217-invitro-whole plant?,

N-trans-feruloyltyramine

Melanin biosynthesis inhibitor... Showed high anti-nitric oxide activity. [1] Inhibited induced preneoplastic lesions 75.0%. [253]

Sida acuta
253-invitro-whole plant-EtOAc extract-10 µg/mL-exhibits 75% inhibition of 7,12-dimethylbenz[a]anthracene-induced preneoplastic lesions,

Oil
triglyceride

A mixture of water-fearing and fat-loving chemicals... oil refers to an overall mixture of chemicals [1]   Herbal oils have time-tested health and healing properties [759]

Sida acuta

6-invitro-leaf-chloroform/95% ethanol extracts both detected fixed oil, **83**-invitro-whole plant?-oil content=0.333%, **230**-leaf-boiled leaves-oil not there, **359**-review-seed Oil Content 16.8 (%), **362**-invitro-seed-fatty oil-3%, **559**-seed-The saponifiable fraction was found to have oleic, linoleic, palmitic, stearic, myristic and plamitoleic acids, whereas the unsaponifiable fraction contained β-amyrin, β-sitosterol and an unknown waxy nonsteroidal substance, **575**-invitro-seed-present, **652**-rats-leaf-ethanol extract-not detected.

Sida cordifolia

72-invitro, **118**-review-detected, **125**-invitro-leaves-acetone/methanol/water extracts-measurable amount, **148**-aerial parts-alcoholic extract-fixed oil-detected, **152**-invitro-seed-petroleum ether>cold distilled water extract>petroleum ether (40-600C), chloroform, alcohol and aqueous extracts-very present, **312**-invitro-seeds-30.7%, **352**-seeds-11.5%, **358**-review-seed-30%, **558**-invitro-seed-petroleum ether extract, % on dry wt: 11.5 to 30.7, **574**-invitro-seed-very present, **611**- seed-11.5%-Linoleic acid predominated (54.9–69.4%) as the fatty acid of all the oils, and malvalic (1.3–11.4%) and sterculic acids (0.4–1.1%) were significant.

Sida rhombifolia

352-seeds-20.2%, **358**-review-seed-16%, **575**-invitro-seed-present, **611**-seed-20.2%-Linoleic acid predominated (54.9–69.4%) as the fatty acid of all the oils, and malvalic (1.3–11.4%) and sterculic acids (0.4–1.1%) were significant.

Sida indica

611-seed-12.5%-Linoleic acid predominated (54.9–69.4%) as the fatty acid of all the oils, and malvalic (1.3–11.4%) and sterculic acids (0.4–1.1%) were significant, **638**-invitro-seed-methanol extract-crude oil content 13.6± 0.1%, **680**-invitro-whole plant-cold distilled water extract-detected—ethanol extract-detected-fixed oil, **709**-review-Different parts of plants-detected-essential oil, **712**-review-α-pinene, caryophyllene, caryophyllene oxide, etc.

Sida veroniciflora

558-Sida veroniciflora Lam-seed-15.5% dry, **611**-Sida veronicifolia Linn. syn. S. humilis cav.-seed-15.5%-Linoleic acid predominated (54.9–69.4%) as the fatty acid of all the oils, and malvalic (1.3–11.4%) and sterculic acids (0.4–1.1%) were significant.

Other Sidas

558-**Sida linifolia**-invitro-seed-oil-14.0–17.0% on dry wt, **611**-**Sida ovata** Forsk-seed-12.1%-Linoleic acid predominated (54.9–69.4%) as the fatty acid of all the oils, and malvalic (1.3–11.4%) and sterculic acids (0.4–1.1%) were significant, **611**-**Sida mysorensis** W & A. syn. S. urticaefolia W & A -seed-13.2%-Linoleic acid predominated (54.9–69.4%) as the fatty

388

acid of all the oils, and malvalic (1.3–11.4%) and sterculic acids (0.4–1.1%) were significant.

Oleic acid   omega-9 fatty acid [1]
A common monounsaturated fat in human diet [1]

Sida acuta   217-invitro-whole plant?,   559-invitro-seed-fixed oil,

Sida indica   454-invitro-leaves-water extract-400 mg/kg bw,

Oligosaccharides   saccharide polymer [1]
A saccharide polymer containing a small number of monosaccharides (simple sugars). Oligosaccharides can have many functions including cell recognition and cell binding. [1]

Sida veronicaefolia

346-invitro-whole plant?-ethanolic extract>water-soluble fraction-detected,

Organic acid
Organic compound with acidic properties [1]
Antibacterial...used in food preservation... an improvement in performance similar to or better than that of antibiotic growth promoters, without the public health concern. [1]

Sida indica   709-review-leaf-detected,   710-Ayurveda-review-leaves-large amount detected,

Oxalate   salts of oxalic acid [1]
An excellent ligand for metal ions. It usually binds as a bidentate ligand forming a 5-membered MO2C2 ring. [1]

Sida acuta   274-invitro-leaves-140.80 Mg/100g,

Sida rhombifolia   576-invitro-very present,

Sida veronicaefolia

346-invitro-whole plant?-ethanolic extract>water-soluble fraction-detected-oxalic acid,

P-b-D-Glucosyloxybenzoic acid
{No information found}

Sida indica   709-review-whole plant-detected,

P–coumaric acid   A hydroxycinnamic acid
A major component of lignin. [1]

Sida indica   570-invitro-petroleum ether extract then 50% alcohol extract,   712-review,

P-hydroxybenzoic acid
A popular antioxidant. Phenolic derivative of benzoic acid [1]

Sida indica   570-invitro-petroleum ether extract then 50% alcohol extract,   709-review-whole plant-detected,

P-hydroxy phenethyl trans ferulate
Found in herbs and spices... Serotonergic activity explored [756]

Sida cordifolia   217-invitro-whole plant?,

Palmitic acid   Saturated fatty acid [1]
The most common saturated fatty acid found in animals, plants and microorganisms. [1]

Sida acuta   217-invitro-whole plant?,   559-invitro-seed-fixed oil,

Sida cordifolia   118-review-detected,   217-invitro-whole plant?,

Sida indica   454-seeds,   709-review-root-detected,

Peptide   amino acid monomers [1]
Peptides are distinguished from proteins on the basis of size. Some peptides are anti-microbial. [1]

Sida veronicaefolia
346-invitro-whole plant?-ethanolic extract>water-soluble fraction-detected.

Phaeophytin A   a form of chlorophyll
Pheophytin is a form of chlorophyll a in which the magnesium ion is replaced by two hydrogen ions. It participates in the crucial step of converting light energy to chemical energy. [804]

Sida cordifolia   501-invitro-probably there-slightly unspecific,

Sida rhombifolia   59-phaeophytin A-invitro-whole plant?,

Phenolic compounds   water soluble antioxidants

Phenolic compounds belong to a large heterogeneous group of secondary plant metabolites and are the most important category of water soluble antioxidants...They occur almost in every plant as tannins, lignans and flavonoids. Flavonoids are the most studied compounds (and) represent more than 9000 structurally different compounds...Catechins and other flavanols may act as defense chemicals to protect the plants from predators and insects. They also scavenge ROS formed from the photosynthetic electron transport system in plant cells... Catechin, rutin and quercetin have multiple biological activities such as cardioprotective, antiviral, antibacterial, anti-inflammatory and anticarcinogenic. **[659]**   Phenolic compounds can act as protective agents, inhibitors, natural animal toxicants and pesticides against invading organisms, i.e. herbivores, nematodes, phytophagous insects, and fungal and bacterial pathogens. The scent and pigmentation conferred by other phenolics can attract symbiotic microbes, pollinators and animals that disperse fruits. **[1]**

Sida acuta

11-invitro-acquesous acetone extract, **15**-invitro-root-methanolic extract (10% w/v)-1.45 mg/TAE/g, **18**-invitro-root-detected-ferulic acid, **52**-invitro-root-methanolic extract-8.54%, **63**-invitro-root-detected-ferulic acid, **86**-invitro- ethanolic and aqueous extracts, **89**-invitro-whole plant-aqueous acetone extract (70%, v/v)-detected, **96**-invitro-leaf- 95% ethanol extract-phenolic compounds-present, **93**-invitro-leaves-70% aqueous methanol (v/v) acidified to pH 2-many detected, **106**-invitro-polyphenols-not detected, **113**-invitro-whole plant?- ethanolic and aqueous extracts-detected, **204**-invitro-leaf-cold water extract-0.1%, **213**-invitro-chloroform/100% methanol extract-tested positive for polyphenols, **223**-invitro-leaves-highly present-90 mg/100 gm, **254**-invitro-aqueous acetone extract>n-hexane, dichloro-methane, ethyl acetate and n-butanol fractions-determined, **271**-invitro- root, stem, leaf and buds-Different parts of S. acuta (root, stem, leaf and buds) were subjected for flavonoids extraction, **420**-invitro-0.08% ±0.11 by weight, **460**-rats-ethanolic extract-substance is present, **572**-invitro-whole plant-methanolic extract-Phenolic compounds such as evofolin A and B, scopoletin, vomifoliol, loliolid and 4-Ketopinoresinol have been isolated, **645**-invitro-leaf-cold water extract-detected, **645**-invitro-leaf-acetone extract-detected, **652**-invitro-leaf-ethanol extract-detected, **668**-invitro-roots-methanol extract-detected-polyphenols.

Sida cordifolia

15-invitro-root-methanolic extract (10% w/v)-2.13 mg/TAE/g,   27-invitro, 117-invitro-whole plant?-80% acetone extract-the lack of biologically active antioxidants such as polyphenol compounds,   121-invitro-ethanol extract-detected lots,   171-invitro-aerial parts-water extract-14.90 ± 1.16 (mg of GAE/g of extract),   175-invitro-water extract-200&400 mg/kg bw- The flavonoids and phenols present in Sida cordifolia contribute for antioxidant potentiality that exhibits nephroprotective activity,   211-invitro- aerial parts?- 80% acetone extract (400 ml acetone + 100 ml water) for 24 h under mechanic agitation at room temperature-The phytochemical analysis carried out on Sida cordifolia L., extract show that several polyphenol including flavonoids are found in its extracts,   240-invitro-leaf and stem bark-methanol extract-lots of polyphenols,   409-invitro- that maximum accumulation of alkaloids and phenols occurred in summer season in all the three plant species. Peak concentrations of alkaloids and phenols were observed in flowering stage. Interestingly, no alkaloids or phenols accumulated in the seedling stage,   591-rats-whole plant-70% ethanol extract-detected,   663-invitro-seed-water extract=0μg/mg--Acetone extract = 0μg/mg--Petroleum Ether extract=0μg/mg--chloroform extract=0μg/ mg, 668-invitro-roots-methanol extract-detected-polyphenols.

Sida rhombifolia

15-invitro-root-methanolic extract (10% w/v)-1.27 mg/TAE/g,   47-invitro-methanolic extracts and water and methanol (1v:4v), (1v:1v), (3v:2v) extracts-detected,   51-invitro-fruit-Methanol extract,   57- Sida retusa-rats-root-?extract,   136-invitro-root-boiling water extract-detected,   136-invitro-root-95% ethanol extract-detected,   195-invitro-ethyl acetate extract-had the highest content of phenolic compounds (88.311 ± 2.660 mg•GAE/g) and the best antioxidant activity for the DPPH and TEAC assay (IC50 = 70.503 ±1.629 and 20.580 ± 0.271, respectively),   543-invitro-whole plant-ether extract,   544-leaves and/or roots-chloroform extract-detected,   556-Vietnam- Sida rhombifolia none detected! (in a long list of plants only about a dozen were 2.-4 %, and not that many 1-2% either,   668-invitro-roots-methanol extract-detected-polyphenols.

Sida retusa   15-invitro-root-methanolic extract (10% w/v)-.93 mg/TAE/g,   75- invitro-whole plant-ethanol extract-detected,   668-invitro-roots-methanol extract-detected-polyphenols.

Sida cordata

15-invitro-root-methanolic extract (10% w/v)-1.16 mg/TAE/g,   282-invitro-leaf-methanol extract-The total phenolic content was ranged from 145.45 mg/g to 130mg/gm of dry weight of extract, expressed as gallic acid equivalents,   293-invitro-leaf-acetone extract-present,   494--invitro--methanolic extract--Consider-able amount of flavonoid and phenolic contents were recorded in the methanol extract and its derived fractions,   668-invitro-roots-methanol extract-detected-polyphenols.

Sida indica

15-invitro-root-methanolic extract (10% w/v)-1.45 mg/TAE/g, **442**-invitro-eugenol, **443**-invitro-leaves-petroleum ether (60-800C) for 8 hr. to remove fatty matter-95% methanol extract-phenolic compounds, **447**-invitro-roots-present, **448**-rats-whole plant-is present-ether/chloroform /ethanol/acqueous extract (sequential extraction from a marc, extract taken out at each phase for testing. Acqueous extract on the remains after the three previous extractions, **449**- mice/sheep's blood-leaves- ethanolic extract (200 mg/kg bw) but not acqueous extract (400 mg/kg bw), **452**-invitro-leaf-methanol extract, **556**-Vietnam- 0.1-0.2 % polyphenols by dry weight-(in a long list of plants only about a dozen were 2.-4 %, and not that many 1-2%), **638**-invitro-methanol extract-total phenolics per mg GA g-1 dry extract—Leaf 56.9—seed 14.5-root 33.5, **677**-invitro-fruits-80% ethanol extract=18± 1.2 (mg GAE/g)-- Petroleum ether extract=14 ± 1.4 (mg GAE/g)--Chloroform extract=56 ± 0.7 (mg GAE/g)--Ethyl acetate extract=86 ± 1.3 (mg GAE/g)--Butanol extract=32 ± 1.1 (mg GAE/g)-Aqueous extract=16 ± 0.8 (mg GAE/g), **680**-invitro-whole plant-cold distilled water extract-detected—ethanol extract-detected-phenols, **684**-invitro-leaf--hydro-methanolic extract-not detected, **687**-whole plant?-acetone extract-strongly detected, **712**-invitro-leaf-Petroleum ether extract detected --Ethyl acetate extract detected --Chloroform extract detected--Methanolic extract detected--Aqueous extract not detected, **712**-nvitro-stem-Hydroalcoholic extract detected--Methanolic extract detected--Aqueous extract detected.

Sida rhomboidea

130-leaf-water extract-polyphenols 2.0 mg/100 mg, **320**-whole plant?-methanol extract-(35.60±1.20 mg/ml gallic acid equivalent-polyphenols).

Sida spinosa

11-invitro-aerial parts-aqueous acetone extract (80%, v/v)>hexane wash-polyphenol-rich, **15**-invitro-root-methanolic extract (10% w/v)-1.56 mg/ TAE /g, **254**-invitro-aqueous acetone extract>n-hexane, dichloromethane, ethyl acetate and n-butanol fractions-determined.

Sida mysorensis
15-invitro-root-methanolic extract (10% w/v)-1.87 mg/TAE/g, **556**-Vietnam- 1-2% polyphenols by dry weight.

Sida tiagii

551-fruit-95% ethanolic extract, **552**-invitro-fruit-ethanolic extract>n-hexane extract/ethyl acetate extract-The filtrate was partitioned with ethyl acetate extract-ethanolic extract works.

Sida veronicaefolia

346-invitro-whole plant?-ethanolic extract>water-soluble fraction-detected-phenolic acid, **348**-mice-leaves-petroleum, ether, chloroform, ethanol, and aqueous solutions subsequently combined-detected.

Other Sidas

200-Sida cardifolia-invitro-leaf-acetone extract-Thus acetone leaf extract of Sida cardifolia had maximum amount of polyphenols and flavonoids which is directly related to their greater antioxidant activity also. Thus active molecules present in the acetone leaf extract of Sida cardifolia has antioxidant property which may be useful in targeting the release of free radical intermediates along with the generation of ROS from various metabolic activities, **490- Sida tuberculata**-invitro- leaves, roots-acqueous extract-ethanolic extract three ethanol concentrations were tested on extraction: 20, 30 and 40% (v/v) for leaves and 50, 70 and 90% (v/v) for roots-was also accompanied by significant amounts of another phenolic compound, a kaempferol derivative, **499-Sida urens** -invitro-whole plant?-aqueous acetone extract (80%, v/v)-One noticed that the susceptibility of the bacteria to the polyphenol-rich fractions on the basis of inhibition zone diameters varied according to the microorganism,

Phenylpropanoids

A diverse family of organic compounds that are synthesized by plants from the amino acids phenylalanine and tyrosine. [1]

Sida cordifolia   120-aerial parts-aqueous and hydroalcoholic extracts

Phlobatannin   A fractional part of tannins [1]

Sida acuta

204-invitro-leaf-cold water extract-none present, **265**-leaf-80% ethanol extract-detected, **300**-invitro-leaf-ethanol extract-detected, **415**-invitro -S. acuta had exceptionally high concentrations of minerals, calcium, magnesium and sodium, phosphorous, copper, molybdenum, **420**-invitro - leaves and stems-cold water extraction-none present, **579**-invitro- leaves, stems and roots-hexane and ethanol extracts-detected.

Sida indica   **684**-invitro-leaf--hydro-methanolic extract-not detected, **687**-whole plant?-acetone extract-not detected.

Sida urens   **535**-invitro-leaves-boiled in water with 2% HCl-none detected.

Phosphorous   element

Sida acuta

223-invitro-leaves- 65 mg/100 gm, **274**-invitro-leaves - 1.15 Mg/100g, **415**-invitro- S. acuta had exceptionally high concentrations of minerals, **699**-invitro-higher in calcium and phosphorus (critical for antler development) than iron clay peas, soybeans or alfalfa.

Sida rhombifolia

504-invitro-cultivated under mineral nutrition standard conditions-63+ days after emergence-45.6 mg P per plant, **512**-invivo-root-medium-Among weed species the relative concentration of a particular nutrient in the root system dry matter(high, med, low)

Other Sidas

290- Sida cordifolia-aerial parts-.15 g/kg, **447-Sida indica**-invitro-roots-not present as phosphate, **476-Sida hermaphrodita**-invivo/invitro- Significantly more phosphorus, magnesium and sulphur was contained by Virginia fanpetals biomass from the objects where municipal sewage sludge compost had been applied.

Phytane   diterpenoid alkane [1]

Found many organic molecules of biological importance such as chlorophyll, tocopherol (Vitamin E) and phylloquinone (Vitamin K1). **[1]**

Sida acuta   217-invitro-whole plant?,

Phytate, Phytic acid   perhaps a vitamin

Principal storage form of phosphorus in many plant tissues. Epidemiological correlates of phytate deficiency with disease and reversal of those conditions by adequate intake, and safety-all strongly suggest for phytates inclusion as an essential nutrient. **[1]**

Sida acuta   274-invitro-leaves - 210.07 Mg/100g

Phytosterols   Sterols, Stanols, Phytosteroids

See also: Sitosterol, Steriods, Ecdysteroids and Ecdysterone

Phytosterols, which encompass plant sterols and stanols, are phytosteroids similar to cholesterol which occur in plants. Stanols are saturated sterols, having no double bonds in the sterol ring structure. The European Foods Safety Authority (EFSA) concluded that blood cholesterol can be reduced on average by 7 to 10.5% if a person consumes 1.5 to 2.4 grams of plant sterols and stanols per day, an effect usually established within 2−3 weeks. Longer-term studies extending up to 85 weeks showed that the cholesterol-lowering effect could be sustained. **[1]**

Sida acuta

6-invitro-leaf-chloroform extract did not detect, 95% ethanol extract-detected, **103**-cholesterol-rats-leaf-ethanolic and methanolic extracts-200 mg/kg bw- Both extracts significantly reduced plasma total cholesterol (p<0.05) and triglyceride (p<0.001), **106**-invitro-not detected, **217**-invitro -roots and aerial parts, **220**-stigmasterol, β-sitosterol, ecdysterone -invitro, **260**-invitro- root, stem, leaf and buds- all the parts were rich in sterol content-34.7 mg/g. dw, **327**-β-sitosterol-invitro-detected, **500**-invitro-root- hydroalcoholic extract-detected, **559**-β-sitosterol-invitro-seed-unsaponifiable fraction, **581**-invitro-whole plant-methanol extract-isolation of steroidal compounds- The major steroids of the plant are ecdysterone (major steroid of the plant), β-sitosterol, stigmasterol (major steroid of the plant), ampesterol.

Sida cordifolia
118-β-sitosterol-review-detected, **217**-invitro-whole plant?, **312**-stigmasterol, β-sitosterol-invitro-seeds-USA, **571**-stigmasterol, β-sitosterol-invitro-chloroform extract.

Sida rhombifolia
59-sitosterol-3-O-b-D-glucopyranoside, stigmasterol-invitro-whole plant?, **150**-stigmasterol, β-sitosterol-invitro-root-chloroform extract, **362**-stigmasterol-review-seeds-sterculic acid (11%), **575**-stigmasterol-invitro-seed-present-10.8%.

Sida retusa
196-cholesterol-rats-leaf-water extract-200 mg/kg bw-a dose of 200 mg/kg of aqueous extract has shown reduction in triglycerides (TG) (16%), cholesterol (4%), and glucose level (10%).

Sida indica
441-β-sitosterol-invivo-petroleum ether extract-a potential new mosquito larvicidal compound with LC50 value of 11.49, 3.58 and 26.67 ppm against Aedes aegypti L, Anopheles stephensi Liston and C. quinquefasciatus Say (Diptera: Culicidae), respectively-may be considered as a potent source and β-sitosterol as a new natural mosquito larvicidal agent, **454**-β-sitosterol-India-aerial parts, **520**-sitosterol-Sida rhomboidea-invitro, **570**-β-sitosterol-invitro-petroleum ether extract then 50% alcohol extract-detected, **676**-sitosterol-invitro-root-95% ethanol extract-detected, **680**-invitro-whole plant-cold distilled water extract-detected—ethanol extract-detected, **681**-sterol-invitro-whole plant-80% ethanol extract with distilled water-not detected.

Sida rhomboidea
59-invitro-whole plant?-sitosterol-3-O-b-D-glucopyranoside, **128**-cholesterol-rats-leaf-?extract-200 & 400 mg/kg bw-treatment to Triton WR 1339 treated rats recorded significant decrement in Plasma cholesterol, Triglyceride, while HDL was increased (all three p<0.05), **130**- leaf-water extract-phytosterols 3.0 mg/100 mg, **520**-stigmasterol, sitosterol-invitro -leaves-boiling distilled water extract, **520**—mice--leaf--boiling distilled water extract--cholesterol, spinasterol--24-methylenecholesterol--22-dehydrocampesterol--22-dihydro-spinasterol—campesterol.

Sida veronicaefolia
348-mice-leaves-petroleum, ether, chloroform, ethanol, and aqueous solutions subsequently combined-detected.

Plamitoleic acids   Fatty acid

An omega-7 monounsaturated fatty acid. A common constituent of glycerides of human adipose tissue. It is present in all tissues but, in general, found in higher concentrations in the liver [1]

Sida acuta   559-invitro-seed-fixed oil,

Polyprenol   Natural long-chain isoprenoid alcohol

The interest in polyprenols and dolichols is associated with their wide range of demonstrated biological activity and extremely low toxicity. Polyprenols stimulate the immune system, cellular reparation and spermatogenesis, and have antistress, adaptogenic, antiulcerogenic and wound-healing activity. Dolichols have antioxidant activity and protect cell membranes from peroxidation. Experiments on mice have demonstrated that polyprenols have antiviral activity, in particular against influenza viruses. [1]

Sida rhombifolia   556-invitro- none detected,

Sida indica   556-invitro-0.1-0.2 % polyphenols by dry weight,

Sida mysorensis   556-invitro-1-2% polyphenols by dry weight,

Potassium   element

Potassium ions are necessary for the function of all living cells [1]

Sida acuta   274-invitro-leaves - 117.40 Mg/100g,   415-invitro- S. acuta had exceptionally high concentrations of minerals.

Sida cordifolia   240-invitro-leaves=258.01 mg/100gm - stem bark= 119.82 mg/100gm,   290-aerial parts-4.02 g/kg.

Sida rhombifolia

504-invitro- cultivated under mineral nutrition standard conditions-63+ days after emergence-359.3 mg K per plant,   512-invivo-root-medium- Among weed species the relative concentration of a particular nutrient in the root system dry matter(high, med, low)

Other Sidas

447-**Sida indica**-invitro-roots-not present,   476-**Sida hermaphrodita**-invivo/invitro-municipal sewage-4.39 g. kg-1 dm.

Potassium nitrate (KNO3)

Major uses of potassium nitrate are in fertilizers, tree stump removal, rocket propellants and fireworks. [1]

Sida cordifolia
118-review-detected, 125-invitro-leaves-acetone/methanol/water extracts-measurable amount,

Pristane
saturated terpenoid alkane [1]

Major source is shark liver oil. Induces autoimmune diseases in rodents [1]

Sida acuta
217-invitro-whole plant?,

Protein
essential nutrient

One of the building blocks of body tissue [1] {Surprised that leaves/aerial parts were not tested on all species, considering these are the ingested parts, and leaves test so high in protein with acuta}

Sida acuta

52-invitro-root-methanol and pet ether extracts-9.38%, 96-invitro-leaf-95% ethanol extract-present, 223-invitro-leaf-19.13%- can be termed protein rich and may serve a source of dietary protein supplementation, a nutritional significance, 230-leaf-boiled leaves-proteins very strongly present, 274-invitro-leaf-crude protein 17.85-22% by weight, 359-invitro-seed-23.2%, 415-invitro-Legumes and herbs had higher CP, especially S. acuta, 645-invitro-leaf-cold water extract-detected--acetone extract-detected, 652-rats-leaf-ethanol extract-not detected, 699-invitro-the protein level and digestibility increases dramatically with fertilization and commonly analyses come back at around 40% CP!

Sida cordifolia
118-review-detected-(74,000ppm to 347,000ppm), 158-invitro-seed-22.00% ± 0.9, 352-seeds-14.1%, 611-seed-14.1%

Sida rhombifolia

352-seeds-12.6%, 538-invitro-roots-95% ethanol extract-crude protein 5.7%, 543-invitro-whole plant-acqueous extract, 611-seed-12.6%.

Sida cordata
293-invitro-leaf-methanol extract-present, 498-invitro-leaves and stems-successive solvent extraction method-detected,

Sida indica

447-invitro-roots-not detected, 449-mice/sheeps's blood-leaves-acqueous extract (400 mg/kg bw) and ethanolic extract (200 mg/kg bw), 577- Sida hermaphrodita-invivo-growth enhancers- Molasses supplement caused a substantial increase by about 12 percent of crude protein and decrease by about 17 percent of crude fibre contents, 677-invitro-fruits-80% ethanol extract-detected--water extract not detected,   **680**-invitro-whole plant-cold distilled water extract-not detected—ethanol extract-detected,   **681**-invitro-whole plant-80% ethanol extract with distilled water-detected, **709**-review-root-detected.

Sida hermaphrodita

475-invitro-shoot-7.5-8.1%,   **546**-protein 33.07%,   **577**-invivo-growth enhancers- Molasse supplement caused a substantial increase by about 12 percent of crude protein and decrease by about 17 percent of crude fibre contents,

Sida tiagii

551-fruit-95% ethanolic extract,   **552**-invitro-fruit-ethanolic extract>n-hexane extract/ethyl acetate extract-The filtrate was partitioned with ethyl acetate extract-ethanolic extract works,

Sida veronicifolia

611-seed-15.0%,   **348**-mice-leaves-petroleum, ether, chloroform, ethanol, and aqueous solutions subsequently combined-detected

Other Sidas

611-Sida mysorensis W & A. syn. S. urticaefolia W & A seed-13.6%, **611-Sida ovata Forsk**--seed-17.3%,

Pseudoephedrine

A sympathomimetic drug of the phenethylamine and amphetamine chemical classes. It may be used as a nasal/sinus decongestant, as a stimulant, or as a wakefulness-promoting agent in higher doses. [1]

Sida cordifolia   118-review-leaves-ephedrine and pseudoephridine

to 0.28 %,   **118**-review-aerial parts,   **358**-review, ,   **561**-invitro-root-detected,

Sida rhombifolia   670-invitro-aerial parts or roots,

P–β–D–glucosyloxybenzoic acid

Sida indica   570-invitro-whole plant-petroleum ether extract then

50% ethanol extract.

....

In some cases it is preferable to evaporate the alcohol before taking the tincture or fluid extract. This is advised with babies, children, the elderly and if someone is sensitive to alcohol or recovering from an alcohol addiction. **[379]**

Quercetin plant polyphenol from the flavonoid group [1]
Possible treatment of cancer and various other diseases [1]

Sida acuta
93-invitro-leaves-70% aqueous methanol (v/v) acidified to pH 2, 659-invitro-leaves-methanolic extract-19.62 µg/g dw.

Sida indica
443-invitro-leaves-petroleum ether (60-800C) for 8 hr. to remove fatty matter-95% methanol extract-flavonoids (quercetin), 709-review-flowers-detected-includes Quercetin 7-0-beta glucopyranoside and Quercetin 3-0-alpha, 710-Ayurveda-review-detected.

Quinazolines aromatic heterocycle
The heterocyclic compounds have a great importance in medicinal chemistry. One of the most important heterocycles in medicinal chemistry are quinazolines possessing wide spectrum of biological properties like antibacterial, antifungal, anticonvulsant, anti-inflammatory, anti-HIV, anticancer and analgesic activities. This skeleton is an important pharmacophore considered as a privileged structure. This review highlights the recent advances in the synthesis of quinazolines and quinazolinone derivatives with potent antimicrobial and cytotoxic activities. [805]

Sida acuta, Sida spinosa, Sida humilis 217-invitro-whole plant?, 754- invitro-roots and aerial parts.

Sida cordifolia 118-review-aerial parts-detected, 217—invitro--whole plant?--Ψ- ephedrine.

Sida rhombifolia
544-citing-Dinesh Jabhav, Medicinal plants of India, A Guide to Ayurvedic & Ethnomedicinal uses of plants, Vol 1, Scientific Publishers India, 2008, 213-214., 754- invitro-roots and aerial parts.

Quindoline indoquinoline alkaloid
cryptolepine derivative [186]

Sida acuta
7-aerial parts-chloroform extract, 186-invitro-whole plant-methanol extract-main alkaloid with its derivatives such as quindoline, quindolinone, cryptolepinone and 11-methoxy-quindoline, 253-invitro-whole plant-EtOAc-soluble extract, 572-invitro-whole plant-methanol extract.

Sida rhombifolia 622-invitro-aerial parts-?extract,

400

Quindolinone indoquinoline alkaloid
cryptolepine derivative [186]

Sida acuta
186-invitro-whole plant-methanol extract-main alkaloid with its derivatives such as quindoline, quindolinone, cryptolepinone and 11-methoxy-quindoline, **220**-review, **253**-invitro-whole plant-EtOAc-soluble extract, **572**-invitro-whole plant-methanol extract.

Sida rhombifolia **622**-invitro-aerial parts-?extract.

Quinones oxidized derivatives of aromatic compounds
Natural or synthetic quinones show purgative, antimicrobial, antiparasitic, anti-tumor, anti-cardiovascular disease behavior. [1]

Sida acuta **561**-invitro-detected,

Sida indica **687**- whole plant?-acetone extract-strongly detected,

Sida retusa **561**-invitro-detected,

(R)-N-(1-methoxycarbonyl-2-phenylethyl)-4-hydroxybenzamide

Sida indica **709**-invitro-flowers,

(R)-N-(1'-methoxycarbonyl-2'-phenylethyl)-4-hydroxybenzamide

Sida indica **709**-invitro-flowers,

Reducing agent counterpart of antioxidant
A reducing agent (also called a reductant or reducer) is an element (such as calcium) or compound that loses (or "donates") an electron to another chemical species in a redox chemical reaction. Since the reducing agent is losing electrons, it is said to have been oxidized. If any chemical is an electron donor (reducing agent), another must be an electron recipient (oxidizing agent). A reducing agent is oxidized because it loses electrons in the redox reaction. [1]

Sida acuta

77-Silver nanoparticles were synthesized by a rapid, cost effective and environmentally benign technique using ground leaves extract of Sida acuta as reducing as well as capping agent. Silver nanoparticles (AgNps) were formed within 10-15 minutes by sunlight irradiation of aqueous solution (0.1M) of silver nitrate (AgNO3) with leaves extract, **86**-invitro-ethanolic and aqueous extracts-the phytochemicals detected were reducing compounds, **113**-invitro-whole plant?-ethanolic and aqueous extracts-detected, **115**-invitro-leaf-water extract--reducing activity and absorption both increase with concentration, **307**-invitro-leaves and stems-cold distilled water extract-reduces corrosion rate from 0.0012 to 0.0001 MPY and percentage protection increases from 37.42% to 93.63%, **644**-invitro-whole plant-petroleum ether, chloroform, ethyl acetate, ethanol and water extracts-has rich free radical scavenging activities.

Sida cordifolia

121-invitro-Ethanol extracts were found to be a good scavenger of DPPH radical in the order roots > stem > leaves > whole plant with values 76.62%, 63.87%, 58% and 29% at a dose of 1 mg, respectively. All extracts have effective reducing power and free-radical scavenging activity, **169**-rats-whole plant?-ethanol extract-likely elicits its antioxidant potential by reducing oxidative stress-50 mg/100 g body weight, **182**-rats-roots-50 % ethanolic extract- reduces oxidative stress -has potent anti-oxidant and anti-inflammatory activity, **662**- invitro--leaves--cold distilled water extract-silver nanoparticles (AgNPs)--bio-functionalized AgNPs displayed higher antioxidant activity in terms of reducing power on ferric ion (1.83 AU) and phosphomolybdate (2127 Ascorbic acid Equivalent Antioxidant Activity) and radical scavenging activity against superoxide (IC50 value 46.25 mg/ml) and DPPH radicals (IC50 value 50.12 mg/ml) compared to the standard.

Sida cardifolia

177-mice/rats-whole plant-50% ethanolic extract-500mg/kg bw-by reducing serum biochemical parameters-potent anti-antioxidant and anti-inflammatory activity when compared with standard drug deprenyl, **200**-invitro-leaf-acetone extract- high reducing power activity.

Sida rhomboidea

320-whole plant?-methanol extract-higher reducing potential ODmax= 1.20±0.27), **323**-invitro-leaf-?extract-capable of reducing LDL oxidation and formation of intermediary oxidation products, **547**-invitro-leaf-Results clearly indicated that S rhomboidea was capable of reducing LDL oxidation and formation of intermediary oxidation products.

Other Sidas

57-**Sida retusa**-rats-The comparative antioxidant potentials of ethanol extract of roots, stems, leaves, and whole plant were studied-All extracts of this plant showed effective free radical scavenging activity, reducing power, and superoxide scavenging activity. Only root extract inhibited lipid peroxidation in rat liver and brain homogenate. All these antioxidant properties were concentration dependent, **344-S. humilis**-invitro-whole plant?-methanolic extract-not detected, **634-Sida rhombifolia**-invitro-whole plant?-cold methanolic extract- Total Reducing Power- measured using the potassium ferricyanide method which measures the potential of reducing Fe^{3+} to Fe^{2+} in the presence of the extract-Sida rhombifolia upper root=placed 10th of 15—Sida rhombifolia root=placed 14th of 15, **716-Sida indica**-invitro-whole plant- butanol > ethyl acetate > chloroform > n-hexane and butanol > chloroform >hexane > ethyl acetate fractions- The FRAP assay showed reducing powers-the antioxidant/radical scavenging capacity of the extracts was found to be a dose-dependent activity.

Resins   terpenes and derivatives

The resin produced by most plants is composed mainly of terpenes and derivatives Plants secrete resins and rosins for their protective benefits. They confound a wide range of herbivores, insects, and pathogens. [1]

Sida acuta   **230**-leaf-boiled leaves-resin not there, **652**-rats-leaf-ethanol extract-not detected,

Sida cordifolia

118-review-detected, **125**-invitro-leaves-acetone/methanol/water extracts-measurable amount-also resins acids (protectant and wood preservatives), **148**-aerial parts-alcoholic extract-detected.

Sida indica   **680**-invitro-whole plant-cold distilled water extract-detected—ethanol extract-detected, **709**-review-root-detected.

Rhamnopyranosyl(1-6)-beta glucopyranoside

Sida indica   **709**-review-flowers-detected.

Riboflavin   vitamin B2

Sida acuta   **223**-invitro-leaves- 0.02 mg/100 gm, **264**-100% ethanolic leaf extract - 0.12 mg/100 gm.

Ribose   Simple sugar

The term usually indicates D-ribose, which occurs widely in nature. D-ribose is commonly used in congestive heart failure (as well as other forms of heart disease) and for chronic fatigue syndrome (CFS), also called myalgic encephalomyelitis (ME) [1]

Sida acuta / Sida cordifolia / Sida rhombifolia / Sida spinosa / Sida veronicaefolia / Sida rhombifolia var. rhomboidea / Sida rhombifolia var. retusa / Sida indica
561-PhD dissertation-leaves-detected.

(R)-N-(1-methoxycarbonyl-2-phenylethyl)-4-hydroxybenzamide

Sida indica   709-review-flowers-detected.

(R)-N-(1'-methoxy carbonyl-2'-phenylethyl)-4-hydroxybenzamide

Sida indica   709-review-root-detected.

Rutin   citrus flavenoid

Prevents highly reactive free radicals that may damage cells. It is also an antioxidant [1]

Sida acuta   659-invitro-leaves-methanolic extract-.19 µg/g dw.

Sida cordifolia   217-invitro-whole plant?

Sida hermaphrodita

483-invitro-50, 60, and 70% ethanolic extract-It has been established that the highest yield of rutin can be obtained from raw material ground to 2.5–3.0 mm with the use of 70% ethanol and a time of maceration of 12 h.

S-(+)-N b-methyltryptophan methylester

Sida acuta   217-invitro-roots and aerial parts,

Sida cordifolia   217-invitro-roots and aerial parts,

Sida rhomboidea   520-invitro-leaves-boiling distilled water extract,

S-(+)- Nb,Nb dimethyl tryptophan methyl ester

Sida acuta   217-invitro-roots and aerial parts,

Sapogenins   non-saccharide saponins [1]

Sapogenins are non-saccharide portions of the family of natural products known as saponins. Sapogenins contain steroid or other triterpene frameworks as their key organic feature. [1]

Sida indica   454-invitro-leaves-detected,

Saponins   amphipathic glycosides

Can be used to enhance penetration of macromolecules such as proteins through cell membranes [1]

Sida acuta

6-invitro-leaf-chloroform/95% ethanol extracts both detected,   11-invitro-acquesous acetone extract,   52-invitro-root-none detected,   86-invitro-ethanolic and aqueous extracts,   96-invitro-leaf- 95% ethanol extract-present,   102-invitro-leaf-water and 100% methanolic extracts-moderate amount,   106-invitro-not detected,   113-invitro-whole plant?- ethanolic and aqueous extracts-detected,   204-invitro-leaf-cold water extract-none present,   213-invitro-chloroform/100% methanol extract-detected,   214-invitro-whole plant?-70% aqueous methanol extracts-none detected,   223-invitro-leaves-moderately present-06.67 mg/100 gm,   224-leaf-present in all four extracts-hexane/chloroform/water/methanol extracts,   230-leaf-boiled leaves-saponins present,   237-invitro-has a remarkable concentration of saponins-0.772 mg/100g,   264-100% ethanolic leaf extract-530.27 mg/100 g,   265-leaf-80% ethanol extract-not detected,   274-invitro-leaves - 650.00 Mg/100g,   300-invitro-leaf-ethanol extract-not detected,   420-invitro-leaves and stems-cold water extraction-none present,   460-rats-ethanolic extract-substance is present,   579-invitro- leaves, stems and roots-hexane and ethanol extracts-detected,   652-rats-leaf-ethanol extract-detected,   668-invitro-roots-methanol extract-not detected.

Sida cordifolia

24-roots-80% ethanol extract,   120-aerial parts-aqueous and hydro-alcoholic extracts-good source of saponins with diverse chemical structures, mainly of steroidal nature, some of which may be hecogenin, diosgenin or a homologue... test results indicate that S. cordifolia has a rich content of antioxidant compounds, mostly saponins-low correlation between antioxidant activity and saponins content,   148-aerial parts-alcoholic extract-detected,   240-invitro-leaves = 8.1 g/100gm-stem bark = 4.4 g/100 gm,   470-invirto-roots-80% ethanol extract-present,   591-rats-whole plant-70% ethanol extract-detected,   663-invitro-seed-water extract= 0µg/mg--Acetone extract=0µg/mg--Petroleum Ether extract=0µg/mg—chlor-oform extract=20.39µg/mg,   668-invitro-roots-methanol extract -not detected,

Sida rhombifolia

47-invitro-aqueous methanol extract-detected, 51-invitro-fruit-Methanol extract, 136-invitro-root-boiling water extract-not detected--95% ethanol extract-not detected, 543-invitro-whole plant-ether extract, 545-invitro-aerial parts-80% ethanol extract-detected—water extract-nil, 543-invitro-whole plant-ethanolic and acqueous extract, 544-leaves and/or roots-ethyl acetate extract-detected, 544-leaves and/or roots-ethanol extract-detected, 545-invitro-aerial parts-80% ethanol extract-nil, 668-invitro-roots-methanol extract-not detected.

Sida cordata
293-invitro-leaf-petroleum ether and chloroform extract-present, 668-invitro-roots-methanol extract-not detected.

Sida indica

443-invitro-leaves-petroleum ether (60-800C) for 8 hr. to remove fatty matter-95% methanol extract-saponins, 445- invitro-leaves, twigs and roots, 446-invitro-acqueous and methanol extracts-nothing detected, 447-invitro-roots-present, 448-rats-whole plant-is present-ether/chloroform/ethanol/acqueous extract (sequential extraction from a marc, extract taken out at each phase for testing. Acqueous extract on the remains after the three previous extractions, 449- mice/sheep's blood-leaves- ethanolic extract (200 mg/kg bw) but not acqueous extract (400 mg/kg bw), 451-leaves/twigs/roots-boiling water extract, 454-invitro-leaves-detected-sapogenins (non-saccharide portions of saponins that contain steroid or other triterpene frameworks as their key organic feature), 677-invitro-fruits-80% ethanol extract/Petroleum ether extract/Chloroform extract/Ethyl acetate extract/Butanol extract/Aqueous extract--detected, 680-invitro-whole plant-cold distilled water extract-detected—ethanol extract-detected, 681-invitro-whole plant-80% ethanol extract with distilled water-detected, 683-invitro-leaves-cold distilled water extract-detected, 684-invitro-leaf--hydro-methanolic extract-detected, 687-whole plant?-acetone extract-strongly detected-leaf weaker, flower very strong, 709-review-root or leaf-detected, 712-invitro-leaf-Petroleum ether extract detected--Ethyl acetate extract not detected--Chloroform ex-tract not detected--Methanolic extract detected--Aqueous extract detected, 712-invitro-stem-Hydroalcoholic extract not detected--Methanolic extract not detected--Aqueous extract not detected.

Sida tiagii
551-fruit-95% ethanolic extract-nil, 552-invitro-fruit-ethanolic extract>n-hexane extract/ethyl acetate extract-nil,

Sida veronicaefolia

346-invitro-whole plant?-ethanolic extract>water-solu-ble fraction-not detected, 348-mice-leaves-petroleum, ether, chloroform, ethanol, and aqueous solutions subsequently combined-detected.

Other Sidas

99-Sida spinosa-invitro-whole plant-hot 60-80% ethanolic extract, **130-Sida rhomboidea**-leaf-water extract-saponin 4.5 mg/100 mg, **200-Sida cardifolia**-leaf-acetone extract-none detected, **535-Sida urens**-leaves, **668-Sida retusa**-invitro-roots-methanol extract-not detected,

Scopoletin   A coumarin (6-methoxy-7-hydroxycoumarin)

Exhibits both cytostatic and a cytotoxic effect- associated to the induction of apoptosis. **[79]**

Sida acuta

79-invitro-isolated from Sida acuta-Scopoletin was found to exert a dual action on tumoral lymphocytes exhibiting both a cytostatic and a cytotoxic effect- associated to the induction of apoptosis-These results indicate that scopoletin could be a potential antitumoral compound to be used for cancer treatment... Scopoletin constitutes an active compound that inhibits proliferation of Hepa 1c1c7 mouse hepatoma cells-These effects varied with the concentrations analyzed, **79**-invitro-isolated from Sida acuta-Scopol-etin induced cell proliferation on normal T lymphocytes (Proliferation stimulation index: 1 µg/ml scopoletin: 1.26 ± 0.1; 10 µg/ml scopoletin: 3 ± 0.25; 100 µg/ml scopoletin: 1.86 ± 0.08)-a stimulatory action, **220**-review-scopoletin vomifoliol, **253**-invitro-whole plant-EtOAc-soluble extract, **581**-invitro-whole plant-methanol extract-detected.

Sida rhombifolia   622-invitro.

Cultivation of Sida rhombifolia as a fibre crop has been taken up in several countries, few details have been published. Along the river Niger it is cultivated after retreat of flood-waters. In the Central African Republic it is a border crop in arable fields. The crop cycle is 4.5–5 months. **[358]**

Serine   a-amino acid

Used in the biosynthesis of proteins. Participates in the biosynthesis of purines and pyrimidines. It is the precursor to several amino acids including glycine and cysteine. **[1]**

Sida indica   570-invitro-petroleum ether extract then 50% alcohol extract,

Sesquiterpenes   terpene

Found naturally in plants and insects, as defensive agents or pheromones **[1]**

Sida indica   709-review-Different parts of plants-detected,   712-review--alantolactone and isoalanto-lactone.

Siephedrine   alkaloid

Sida rhombifolia   **544**-citing-Dinesh Jabhav, Medicinal plants of India, A Guide to Ayurvedic & Ethnomedicinal uses of plants, Vol 1, Scientific Publishers India, 2008, 213-214.

Sigmasterol   phytosterol

Sida rhomboidea   **520**-invitro-leaves-boiling distilled water extract,

Sinapic acid   hydroxycinnamic acid
Anti-inflammatory **[756]**

Sida acuta   **253**-invitro-whole plant-EtOAc-soluble extract,

Sitoindosides X   glycowithanolide

Significant anti-stress activity and augmented learning acquisition and memory retention in rats. These findings are consistent with the use of W. somnifera, in Ayurveda, to attenuate cerebral function deficits in the geriatric population and to provide non-specific host defence--50–200 mg/kg **[790]**

Sida cordifolia   **217**-invitro-whole plant?,

Sitosterol, β-sitosterol   Phytosterol (plant sterol)
Has a chemical structure similar to that of cholesterol. **[1]**

Sida acuta   **220**-review,   **327**-invitro-detected,   **559**-invitro-seed-unsaponifiable fraction,   **581**-invitro-whole plant-methanol extract-major steroid of the plant.

Sida cordifolia   **118**-β-sitosterol-review-detected,   **312**-stigmasterol, β-sitosterol-invitro-seeds-USA,   **571**-stigmasterol, β-sitosterol-invitro-chloroform extract.

Sida rhombifolia   **59**-invitro-whole plant?-sitosterol,   **150**-invitro-root-chloroform extract-detected.

Sida rhomboidea   **520**-invitro-leaves-boiling distilled water extract.

Sida indica

441-invivo-petroleum ether extract-a potential new mosquito larvicidal compound with LC50 value of 11.49, 3.58 and 26.67 ppm against Aedes aegypti L, Anopheles stephensi Liston and C. quinquefasciatus Say (Diptera:

Culicidae), respectively-may be considered as a potent source and β-sitosterol as a new natural mosquito larvicidal agent, **454**-India-aerial parts, **570**-invitro-petroleum ether extract then 50% alcohol extract-detected, **676**-sitosterol-invitro-root-95% ethanol extract-detected, **680**- invitro-whole plant-cold distilled water extract-detected—ethanol extract-detected, **681**-sterol-invitro-whole plant-80% ethanol extract with distill-ed water-not detected, **709**-review-Results of this study demon-strated that β-sitosterol as a new natural mosquito larvicidal agent, **710**-Ayurveda-review-detected-β-sitosterol, **712**-review-β-sitosterol.

Sodium   an alkali metal
an essential element for all animals [1]

Sida acuta   **223**-invitro-leaves- 110 mg/100 gm,   **274**-invitro-leaves - 81.90 Mg/100g,   **415**-invitro- S. acuta had exceptionally high concen-trations of minerals,   **530**-rats-leaf-ethanol extract->100 mg/kg bw,

Sida cordifolia   **240**-invitro-leaves = 349.88 mg/100gm-stem bark = 273.16 mg/100gm,   **249**-invitro- 349.88 mg/100 gm

Other Sidas   **447**- **Sida indica**-invitro- roots-present,   **538-Sida rhombifolia**-invitro-roots-95% ethanol extract-.28%

Spinasterol   phytosterol
Sida rhomboidea   **520**-invitro-leaves-boiling distilled water extract,

Starch   polysaccharide
Most common carbohydrate in human diets. Content in copy paper may be as high as 8% [1]

Sida acuta, Sida cordifolia, Sida retusa, Sida cordata
668-invitro-roots-methanol extract-detected.

Sida indica   **683**-invitro-leaves-cold distilled water extract,   **684**-invitro-leaf--hydro-methanolic extract-not detected,

Sida humilis   **344**-invitro-whole plant?-methanolic extract-detected moderate amount,

Stearic acid   Saturated fatty acid
One of the most common saturated fatty acids found in nature. [1]

Sida acuta   **217**-invitro-whole plant?,   **559**-invitro-seed-fixed oil,

Sida cordifolia   118-review-detected,   217-invitro-whole plant?,

Sida indica   454-India-seeds,   709-review-root-detected,

Sterculic acid   Cyclopropane fatty acid

One of the most common saturated fatty acids found in nature. [1]

Sida acuta   217-invitro-whole plant?,   362-review-seeds-sterculic acid (11%),   575-invitro-seed-present-11.0%,

Sida cordifolia   118-review-seeds-fatty acids to 0.32 %,   217-invitro-whole plant?,   558-Sida linifolia-invitro-seed

Sida rhombifolia

362-review-seeds-sterculic acid (11%),   544-citing-Dinesh Jabhav, Medicinal plants of India, A Guide to Ayurvedic & Ethnomedicinal uses of plants, Vol 1, Scientific Publishers India, 2008, 213-214.,   575-invitro-seed-present-10.8%

Other Sida   217-invitro-whole plant?,   558- Sida veroniciflora-invitro-seed-1.1%.

Steriods   organic compound

See also: Phytosterols, ecdysteroids (phytoecsysteroids)

Steroids (such as cholesterol) are important components of cell membranes which alter membrane fluidity, and many steroids are signaling molecules which activate steroid hormone receptors. Steroids play critical roles in a number of disorders. [1]

Sida acuta

96-invitro-leaf-cold petroleum ether extract-present--95% ethanol extract-present,   106-invitro-not detected,   204-invitro-leaf-cold water extract-none present,   224-leaf-not present in all four extracts-hexane/chloroform/ water/ methanol extracts,   230-leaf-boiled leaves-steroids present,   263-seed-significant amounts,   264-100% ethanolic leaf extract-1454.50 mg/100 g,   265-leaf-80% ethanol extract-detected,   300-invitro-leaf-ethanol extract-detected,   420-invitro-leaves and stems-cold water extraction-none present,   500-invitro-hydroalcoholic root extract-sterol,   579-invitro- leaves, stems and roots-hexane and ethanol extracts-detected,   581-invitro-whole plant-methanol extract-The major steroids of the plant are ecdysterone, beta-sitosterol, stigmasterol, ampesterol,   645-invitro-leaf-cold water extract-detected-acetone extract-detected,   652-rats-leaf-ethanol extract-detected,   668-invitro-roots-methanol extract-detected.

Sida cordifolia

24-roots-80% ethanol extract, **32**-invitro-root-40% ethanol extract-detected, **120**-aerial parts- good source of saponins with diverse chemical structures, mainly of steroidal nature, some of which may be hecogenin, diosgenin or a homologue, **148**-aerial parts-alcoholic extract-sterols-detected, **409**-invitro- that maximum accumulation of alkaloids and phenols occurred in summer season in all the three plant species. Peak concentrations of alkaloids and phenols were observed in flowering stage. Interestingly, no alkaloids or phenols accumulated in the seedling stage, **470**-invirto-roots-80% ethanol extract-present, **591**-rats-whole plant-70% ethanol extract-detected, **663**-invitro-seed-water extract=92.26µg /mg--Acetone extract=0µg/mg--Petroleum Ether extract=58.76µg/mg—chloroform extract=0µg/mg, **668**-invitro-roots-methanol extract-detected.

Sida rhombifolia

136-invitro-root-boiling water extract-none detected--95% ethanol extract-detected, **544**-leaves and/or roots-petroleum ether extract-detected, **545** -invitro-aerial parts-80% ethanol extract, **668**-invitro-roots-methanol extract-detected.

Sida cordata **293**-invitro-leaf-petroleum ether extract-present, **500**-invitro-root- hydroalcoholic extract-sterol detected, **668**-invitro-roots-methanol extract-detected,

Sida indica

446-invitro-acqueous and methanol extracts-detected presence, **447**-invitro-roots-present, **448**-rats-whole plant-is present-ether/chloroform /ethanol/ acqueous extract (sequential extraction from a marc, extract taken out at each phase for testing. Acqueous extract on the remains after the three previous extractions, **454**-invitro-leaves-detected, **677**-invitro-fruits-80% ethanol extract/Petroleum ether extract/Chloroform extract/Ethyl acetate extract/Butanol extract-detected--Aqueous extract-not detected, **680**-invitro-whole plant-cold distilled water extract-detected—ethanol extract-detected, **681**-invitro-whole plant-80% ethanol extract with distilled water-not detected, **683**-invitro-leaves-cold distilled water extrac t-detected, **684**-invitro-leaf--hydro-methanolic extract-not detected, **687**-whole plant?-acetone extract-strongly detected-leaf strongly detected, **712**-invitro-leaf-Petroleum ether extract detected --Ethyl acetate extract not detected --Chloroform extract not detected--Methanolic extract detected--Aqueous extract detected, **712**-invitro-stem-Hydroalcoholic extract detected--Methanolic extract not detected--Aqueous extract detected.

Sida rhomboidea **185**-invitro-leaf-detected, **325**-invitro-detected,

Sida spinosa **11**-invitro-acquesous acetone extract, **9**-invitro-whole plant-hot 60-80% ethanolic extract,

Sida tiagii

551-fruit-95% ethanolic extract-sterols, **552**-invitro-fruit-ethanolic extract >n-hexane extract/ethyl acetate extract-The filtrate was partitioned with ethyl acetate extract-ethanolic extract works-sterols, **607**-mice-fruit-hot 95% ethanol extract>n-hexane/ethyl acetate extracts-detected,

Other Sidas
200-Sida cardifolia-leaf-acetone extract, **535-Sida urens**-invitro-leaves-mixed acetic anhydride and HxSO4-none detected, **668-Sida retusa**-invitro-roots-methanol extract-detected,

Sterol   Phytosterols
See also steroid, cholesterol, stigmasterol and β-sitosterol. Cellular membrane &communication, general metabolism [1]

Sida acuta

106-invitro-not detected, **260**-invitro-root, stem, leaf and buds- all the parts were rich in sterol content-34.7 mg/g. dw, **500**-invitro-root-hydroalcoholic extract-detected, **581**-invitro-whole plant-methanol extract-isolation of steroidal compounds- The major steroids of the plant are ecdysterone, beta-sitosterol, stigmasterol, ampesterol.

Sida cordifolia   **312**-review-USA,

Sida indica

681-invitro-whole plant-80% ethanol extract with distilled water-not detected, **709**-review-root or leaf-detected, **710**-Ayurveda- review-leaves-large amount detected, **712**-invitro-leaf-Petroleum ether extract detected --Ethyl acetate extract not detected --Chloroform extract detected--Methanolic extract detected--Aqueous extract detected, **712**-invitro-stem-Hydroalcoholic extract not detected--Methanolic extract not detected--Aqueous extract not detected.

Stigmasterol   A plant sterol, or phytosterol
May prevent cancers, including ovarian, prostate, breast, and colon cancers [1]

Sida acuta

186-review, **217**-invitro-whole plant?, **220**-review, **581**-invitro-whole plant-methanol extract-major steroid of the plant.

Sida cordifolia   **312**-invitro-seeds, **571**-invitro-chloroform extract.

Sida rhombifolia

59-invitro-whole plant?-stigmasterol-3-O-• -Dglucopyranoside, **150**-invitro-root-chloroform extract, **362**-review-seeds-sterculic acid (11%), **575**-invitro-seed-present-10.8%

Other Sidas

520-Sida rhomboidea-invitro-leaves-boiling distilled water extract, **709-Sida indica**-review-flowers-detected-Methylstigmasterol,

Sugar   **monosaccharide**

Refined or in excess can lead to addiction and other health problems **[1]**

Sida acuta   **52**-invitro-root-methanol extract-detected,   **230**-leaf-boiled leaves-reducing sugar not present,   **652**-rats-leaf-ethanol extract-reducing sugar not present,   **668**-invitro-roots-methanol extract-detected,

Sida cordifolia   **24**-roots-80% ethanol extract-reducing sugar, **470**-invirto-roots-80% ethanol extract-reducing sugar present, **668**-invitro-roots-methanol extract-detected,

Sida rhombifolia   **51**-invitro-detected- reducing sugars,   **545**-invitro-aerial parts-80% ethanol extract-reducing sugars,   **668**-invitro-roots-methanol extract-detected,

Sida indica   **447**-invitro-roots-not detected,   **683**-invitro-leaves-cold distilled water extract- reducing sugars-detected,

Other Sidas   **668-Sida retusa**-invitro-roots-methanol extract-detected,   **668-Sida cordata**-invitro-roots-methanol extract-detected,

Sulfur   **chemical element**

Essential element for all life-3 amino acids and 2 vitamins are organosulfur compounds **[1]**

Sida cordifolia   **290**-aerial parts-.12 g/kg

Swainsonine   **indolizidine alkaloid**

Toxic - a glycoside inhibitor responsible for Sida carpinifolia poisoning and death among horses and goats. As a toxin it is a significant cause of economic losses in livestock industries, particularly in North America. Also a potential chemotherapy drug. **[1]**   {Sidas are singularly plastic in their adaptability. I believe that S. carpinfolia is a rogue variety of S. acuta that has never appeared outside of South America. My acuta is preferred long-term deer forage, and I have taken acuta ethanol extract nearly every day for the past 5 years, and my biochemicals readings are optimal.}

Sida carpinifolia

242-aerial parts-poisonous to goats, **621**-invivo-goats-swainsonine toxicosis and inherited mannosidosis-A neurologic disease characterized by ataxia, hypermetria, hyperesthesia, and muscle tremors of the head and neck, **624**-invivo/invitro-sambar deer- The poisoning was characterized by emaciation and neurologic signs followed by unexpected death in some of the animals. Animals presented abnormal consciousness, posterior paresis, and musculoskeletal weakness; less evident were vestibulo-cerebellar signs. Histologically, there was vacuolation of neurons and epithelial cells of the pancreatic acines, thyroid follicules, and renal tubules. Furthermore, in the central nervous system were axonal degeneration, necrosis, and loss of neurons, **625**-invivo/invitro- fallow deer (Dama dama)- a neurological syndrome characterized by muscular weakness, intention tremors, visual and standing-up deficits, falls, and abnormal behavior and posture, **626**-invivo /invitro-pony horses-fatal-included multiple cytoplasmatic vacuoles in swollen neurons in the brain, cerebellum, spinal cord, autonomic ganglia (trigeminal and celiac ganglia), and submucosal and myenteric plexus of the intestines. In the kidneys, there was marked vacuolation of the proximal convoluted tubular cells, **627**-invitro-aerial parts-The indolizidine alkaloid swainsonine has been identified as the toxic constituent-the swainsonine concentration was 0.006% on a dry weight basis, **628**-Saanen goats-Abnormal excretion of oligosaccharides was observed from the 2nd day of S. carpinifolia ingestion until one day after withdrawal of the plant from the diet-were typical of poisoning caused by plants of this group and were seen from the 37th day on S. carpinifolia diet until seven days after withdrawal of the plant, when signs gradually became scarce and less evident, **629**-invivo/invitro-cattle-poisoning-marching gait, alert gaze, head tremors, and poor growth. Histologic and ultrastructural lesions consisted of vacuolization and distension of neuronal perikarya, mainly from Purkinje cells, and of the cytoplasm of acinar pancreatic and thyroid follicular cells-no complete recovery.

Sida rodrigoi monteiro

{This Sida has only appeared around Bolivia, and is adjacent to Sida carpinfolia's range.}

620-invivo-goats-toxic levels of swansonine were identified in the plant-poisoning as a plant induced α-mannosidosis animals showed weight loss, indifference to the environment, unsteady gait and ataxia,

Syringic acid   O-methylated trihydroxybenzoic acid

May have beneficial effects in diabetes mellitus **[763]**

Sida cordifolia / Sida rhombifolia / Sida spinosa / Sida veronicaefolia / Sida rhombifolia var. rhomboidea / Sida rhombifolia var. retusa / Sida indica

561-PhD dissertation-leaves-detected.

414

Sida acuta

253-invitro-whole plant-EtOAc-soluble extract-also has (+/-)-syringaresinol, **561**-PhD dissertation-leaves-detected, **763**-rats-50 mg/kg bw-hypoglycemic -syringic acid tended to bring blood glucose and plasma insulin towards near normal levels in alloxan induced diabetic rats. Oral administration of syringic acid to diabetic rats resulted in significant (P<0.05) reduction of glycoproteins and significant (P<0.05) increase of C-peptide in the plasma when compared to diabetic untreated rats.

Syringin   glucoside of sinapyl alcohol [1]

Found in Eleutherococcus senticosus (Siberian ginseng) [1]

Sida acuta   217-invitro-whole plant?,

Tannin   astringent, polyphenolic biomolecule [1]

Found in plants, seeds, bark, wood, leaves, and fruit skins. Abut 50% of the dry weight of plant leaves are tannins. Traditionally been considered antinutritional, but their beneficial or antinutritional properties depend upon their chemical structure and dosage. Plays a role in protection from predation, and perhaps also as pesticides, and in plant growth regulation. [1]

Sida acuta

15-roots-methanolic extract-total phenols (tannic acid equivalent)=1.24 mg/gm, **52**-invitro-root-0.1%, **86**-invitro- ethanolic and aqueous extracts, **102**-invitro-leaf-water and 100% methanolic extracts-present in high amount, **106**-invitro-not detected, **113**-invitro-whole plant?-ethanolic and aqueous extracts-detected, **204**-invitro-leaf-cold water extract-6%, **214**-invitro-whole plant?-70% aqueous methanol extracts-none detected, **223**-invitro-leaves-higly present-125 mg/100 gm, **224**-leaf-present in all four extracts-hexane/chloroform/water/methanol extracts, **230**-leaf-boiled leaves-tannins present, **237**-invitro-0.054 mg/100g, **254**-invitro-aqueous acetone extract>n-hexane, dichloromethane, ethyl acetate and n-butanol fractions-determined, **264**-100% ethanolic leaf extract-91.46 mg/100 g, **265**-leaf-80% ethanol extract-detected, **265**-leaf-80% ethanol extract-detected, **274**-invitro-leaves - 603.68 Mg/100g, **300**-invitro-leaf-ethanol extract-detected, **420**-invitro-leaves and stems-cold water extract-6.08% ±0.23 by weight, this phytochemical was elsewhere listed as not present, **500**-invitro-hydroalcoholic root extract, **579**-invitro- leaves, stems and roots-hexane and ethanol extracts-detected, **645**-invitro-leaf-cold water extract-detected, **645**-invitro-leaf-acetone extract-detected, **652**-rats-leaf-ethanol extract-not detected.

Sida cordifolia

15-roots-methanolic extract-total phenols (tannic acid equivalent)=1.92 mg/gm, **118**-review-none detected, **120**-aerial parts, **171**-invitro-aerial parts-water extract-11.53 ± 0.78 (mg of GAE/g of extract), **240**-

invitro-leaves = 4.8 g/100gm-stem bark = 5.9 g/100gm, **591**-rats-whole plant-70% ethanol extract-detected, **663**-invitro-seed-water extract= 0μg/mg--Acetone extract=77.93μg/mg--Petroleum Ether extract=80μg/mg—chloroform extract= 0μg/mg.

Sida rhombifolia

47-invitro-aqueous methanol extract-detected, **51**-invitro-fruit-Methanol extract, **136**-invitro-root-boiling water extract-detected--95% ethanol extract-detected, **543**-invitro-whole plant-ether extract, **544**-leaves and/or roots-ethyl acetate extract-detected---ethanol extract-detected, **545**-invitro-aerial parts-80% ethanol extract-nil, **578**-invitro-whole plant?-water extract-detected.

Sida cordata   **498**-invitro-leaves and stems- successive solvent extraction method,   **500**-invitro-root- hydroalcoholic extract-detected,

Sida indica

443-invitro-leaves-petroleum ether (60-800C) for 8 hr. to remove fatty matter-95% methanol extract-tannins,. **445**- invitro-leaves, twigs and roots, **446**-invitro-acqueous and methanol extracts-nothing detected, **447**-invitro-roots-present, **448**-rats-whole plant-is present-ether/chloroform/ethanol/acqueous extract (sequential extraction from a marc, extract taken out at each phase for testing. Acqueous extract on the remains after the three previous extractions, **449**-mice/sheeps's blood-leaves-ethanolic extract (200 mg/kg bw) but not acqueous extract (400 mg/kg bw), **451**-leaves/twigs/roots-boiling water extract, **680**-invitro-whole plant-cold distilled water extract-detected—ethanol extract-detected, **681**-invitro-whole plant-80% ethanol extract with distilled water-detected, **683**-invitro-leaves-cold distilled water extract-detected, **684**-invitro-leaf--hydro-methanolic extract-detected very strong presence, **687**-whole plant?-acetone extract-detected-especially the stem, **687**-whole plant?-acetone extract-detected, **709**-review-root/leaf/stem-detected.

Sida rhomboidea   **185**-invitro-leaf-detected,   **325**-invitro-leaf-detected,

Sida spinosa   **15**-roots-methanolic extract-total phenols (tannic acid equivalent)=1.56 mg/gm,   **254**-invitro-aqueous acetone extract>n-hexane, dichloromethane, ethyl acetate and n-butanol fractions-determined,

Sida tiagii

551-fruit-95% ethanolic extract, **552**-invitro-fruit-ethanolic extract>n-hexane extract/ethyl acetate extract-The filtrate was partitioned with ethyl acetate extract-ethanolic extract works, **607**-mice-fruit-hot 95% ethanol extract>n-hexane/ethyl acetate extracts-detected,

Sida veronicaefolia

346-invitro-whole plant?-ethanolic extract>water-soluble fraction-detected pseudotannins-tannins not detected,   **348**-mice-leaves-petroleum, ether, chloroform, ethanol, & aqueous solutions subsequently combined-detected.

Other Sidas

200-Sida cardifolia-leaf-acetone extract,   **344-S. humilis**-invitro-whole plant?-methanolic extract-not detected,   **535-Sida urens**-invitro-leaves-boiled in water with FeCl,

Taraxast-1,20(30)-dien-3-one

Taraxastane triterpene. A terpene found in plant gums and resins [1]

Sida acuta   **565**-invitro-whole plant

Taraxasterone   Triterpene

Ψ-taraxasterone-Antitrypanosomal-IC50=115.4 μg/ mL **[764]**

Sida acuta   **565**-invitro-whole plant

Terpene   hydrocarbon

Major component of resin (and turpentine)... may protect plants by deterring herbivores and by attracting predators and parasites of herbivores **[1]**

Sida acuta   **217**-invitro-whole plant?,

Terpenoid   organic chemicals similar to terpenes

Monoterpenoids a starting material for synthesis of vitamin 'A'   **[1]**

Sida acuta

86-invitro- ethanolic and aqueous extracts,   **113**-invitro-whole plant?-ethanolic and aqueous extracts-detected,   **204**-invitro-leaf-cold water extract-none present,   **214**-invitro-whole plant?-70% aqueous methanol extracts-detected,   **223**-invitro-leaves-moderately present-85 mg/100 gm, **230**-leaf-boiled leaves-terpenoids present,   **264**-100% ethanolic leaf extract-115.29 mg/100 g,   **265**-leaf-80% ethanol extract-detected,   **300**-invitro-leaf-ethanol extract-detected,   **420**-invitro-leaves and stems-cold water extract-none present,   **460**-rats-ethanolic extract-substance is present, **463**-invitro-leaf-methanolic extract,   **565**-invitro-whole plant,   **645**-invitro-leaf-cold water extract-detected,   **645**-invitro-leaf-acetone extract-detected,   **652**-rats-leaf-ethanol extract-detected.

Sida cordifolia   **32**-invitro-root-40% ethanol extract-detected-triterpenoids,   **106**-invitro-not detected-triterpenes.

417

Sida rhombifolia

47-invitro-aqueous methanol extract-triterpenes, **51**-invitro-fruit-Methanol extract-triterpenes, **126**-invitro-water/ethanol extracts, **136**-invitro-root-boiling water extract-not detected-triterpenes --95% ethanol extract-detected-triterpenes, **543**-invitro-whole plant-ethanol extract--ether extract -triterpenes, **544**-leaves and/or roots-petroleum ether extract-detected--ethanol extract-detected, **545**-invitro-aerial parts-80% ethanol extract-nil-triterpenes.

Sida indica

447-invitro-Water, Ethyl alcohol, Methanol, Chloroform, Petroleum ether and Acetone extracts—triterpenes-detected, **680**-invitro-whole plant-cold distilled water extract-detected—ethanol extract-detected—triterpenes-detected, **683**-invitro-leaves-cold distilled water extract-detected, **684**-invitro-leaf--hydro-methanolic extract-strongly detected, **687**-whole plant?-acetone extract-leaf and stem very strongly detected.

Sida rhomboidea
185-invitro-leaf-triterpenoids-detected—triterpenes-detected, **325**-invitro-leaf-detected—triterpenes-detected.

Other Sidas

535-**Sida urens**-invitro-leaves-mixed with chloroform and H2SO4, **754**-**Sida humilis**-invitro-detected—triterpenes-detected, **607**-**Sida tiagii**-mice-fruit-hot 95% ethanol extract>n-hexane/ethyl acetate extracts-detected—triterpenes-detected.

Thiamin   vitamin B1
An essential nutrient. [1]

Sida acuta   **223**-invitro-leaves- 0.10 mg/100 g,   **264**-ethanolic leaf extract -0.36 mg/100 g.

Threonine   Essential α-amino acid
Used in the biosynthesis of proteins. Threonine is synthesized from aspartate in bacteria such as E. coli. [1]

Sida indica   **570**-invitro-petroleum ether extract then 50% alcohol extract.

Tocopherol   vitamin E compound
Naturally found in foods. Deficiencies of Vitamin E is implicated in many diseases and conditions. [1]

Sida acuta   264-invitro-100% ethanolic leaf extract - 1.85 mg/100 g, 565-invitro-whole plant-α-tocopherol and β-tocopherol,

Sida indica   454-India-aerial parts-(0.3%)-tocopherol oil,   712-review-tocopherol oil,

Triacontanoic acid   A saturated fatty acid

Abundance in the nectar of the flowers which attract bees. [1]

Sida indica   709-review-flowers-detected,

Triterpenes

A class of chemical compounds composed of three terpene units. Animals, plants and fungi all create triterpenes, with arguably the most important example being squalene as it forms the basis of almost all steroids [1]

Sida cordifolia   32-invitro-root-40% ethanol extract-detected-triterpenoids,   106-invitro-not detected.

Sida indica

447-invitro-Water, Ethyl alcohol, Methanol, Chloroform, Petroleum ether and Acetone extracts,   680-invitro-whole plant-cold distilled water extract-detected—ethanol extract-detected,   709-Triterpenoids-review-leaf-detected, 710-Ayurveda-Triterpenoids-review-leaves-large amount detected.

Sida rhomboidea   185-invitro-leaf-triterpenoids-detected,   325-invitro-leaf-detected.

Other Sidas   754- **Sida humilis**-invitro-detected,   607-**Sida tiagii**-mice-fruit-hot 95% ethanol extract>n-hexane/ethyl acetate extracts-detected.

Tryptamine   Monoamine alkaloid

Found in trace amounts in the brains of mammals and is hypothesized to play a role as a neuromodulator or neurotransmitter... Tryptamine is the common functional group in a set of compounds termed collectively substituted tryptamines. This includes many biologically active compounds, including neurotransmitters and psychedelic drugs. [1]

Sida acuta   754- invitro-detected-carboxylated tryptamine,

Sida cordifolia   118-review-aerial parts-detected-carboxylated tryptamine,

Sida rhombifolia

544-citing-Dinesh Jabhav, Medicinal plants of India, A Guide to Ayurvedic & Ethnomedicinal uses of plants, Vol 1, Scientific Publishers India, 2008, 213-214.,   754- invitro-detected-carboxylated tryptamine,

Sida spinosa   754- invitro-detected-carboxylated tryptamine,

Turkesterone   ecdysteroid [1]
{A natural steroid, similar to testasterone. Used as a natural supplement for athletes and body builders}
Sida cordifolia   217-invitro-whole plant?

Tyrosine   amino acid [1]
A non-essential amino acid used by cells to synthesize proteins. Tyrosine is a precursor to neurotransmitters and increases plasma neurotransmitter levels (particularly dopamine and norepinephrine). A number of studies have found tyrosine to be useful during conditions of stress, cold, fatigue, prolonged work and sleep deprivation. [1]

Sida veronicaefolia
346-invitro-whole plant?-ethanolic extract>water-soluble fraction-detected,

Umbelliferone   Polyphenol
A natural product of the coumarin family. Sunscreen agent. pH indicator for 6.5-8.9 [1]

Sida acuta   659-invitro-leaves-methanolic extract-668.7 μg/g dw,

Uresenol   pentacylic triterpene
Sida indica   709-review-flowers-detected,

Vanillan   Phenolic aldehyde [1]
The primary component of the extract of the vanilla bean [1]

Sida indica   12-review,

Vanillic acid   dihydroxybenzoic acid
Used in the synthesis of drugs [1]

Sida cordifolia / Sida rhombifolia / Sida spinosa / Sida veronicaefolia / Sida rhombifolia var. rhomboidea/Sida rhombifolia var. retusa
561-PhD dissertation-leaves-detected.
420

Sida acuta   253-invitro-whole plant-EtOAc-soluble extract,   561-PhD dissertation-leaves-detected.

Sida indica   561-PhD dissertation-leaves-detected,   570-invitro-petroleum ether extract then 50% alcohol extract.

Vasicine   Quinazoline alkaloid, phenolic acid

Its uterotonic activity was found to be similar to that of oxytocin and methyl ergometrine [313]   Bronchodilating action [314]   Vasicine also exhibited marked respiratory and uterine stimulant activity and moderate degree of hypotensive activity not reported earlier. [315]

Sida acuta

217-invitro-whole plant?,   311-invitro,   316-chloroform extract- significant anti-inflammatory activities,   320-invitro- leaf, stem, root and seed-detected,   761-invitro- leaf, stem, root and seed-detected.

Sida cordifolia

118-review-detected,   160-invitro-leaf-vasicine produce hypotension and bradycardia which appears to be due to the stimulation of cardiac muscarinic receptors (directly and/or indirectly), and by a decrease of the peripheral resistances,   217-invitro-whole plant?,   311-invitro,   312-invitro-roots,   320-invitro- leaf, stem, root and seed-detected,   358-review,   362-invitro-roots and/or aerial parts,   411-invitro-leaf-the quinolizidine alkaloids vasicine, vasicinone and vasicinol,   561-invitro-root-detected,   761-invitro- leaf, stem, root and seed-detected.

Sida rhombifolia   670-invitro-aerial parts or roots.
Tr   544-citing-Dinesh Jabhav, Medicinal plants of India, A Guide to Ayurvedic & Ethnomedicinal uses of plants, Vol 1, Scientific Publishers India, 2008, 213-214.

Other Sidas   217-Sida spinosa-invitro-whole plant?,   520-Sida rhomboidea-invitro-leaves-boiling distilled water extract,

Vascicine   Quinazoline alkaloid

Vasicine with vasicinone (1:1) showed pronounced bronchodilatory activity in vivo and in vitro. Also respiratory stimulants. Uterine stimulant effect [1]

Sida rhombifolia   670-invitro-aerial parts or roots,

Sida rhomboidea   520-invitro-leaves-boiling distilled water extract,

Vascinol   Quinazoline alkaloid
Severe antifertility effects [765]

Sida cordifolia

118-review-aerial parts-detected, **133**-invitro-whole plant-water extract-successively extracted with chloroform (3x72 h), methanol (3x72 h) and 80% ethanol (3x72 h)-detected, **176**-invitro-whole plant?-detected, **312**-invitro-roots, **411**-invitro-leaf-the quinolizidine alkaloids vasicine, vasicinone and vasicinol, **561**-PhD dissertation-root-detected.

Sida rhombifolia   **670**-invitro-aerial parts or roots.

Vasicinone   Quinazoline alkaloid

severe antifertility effects [765]

Sida acuta   **217**-invitro-whole plant?,

Sida cordifolia

118-review-detected, **133**-invitro-whole plant-water extract-successively extracted with chloroform (3x72 h), methanol (3x72 h) and 80% ethanol (3x72 h)-detected, **176**-invitro-whole plant?-detected, **217**-invitro-whole plant?, **312**-invitro-roots, **411**-invitro-leaf-the quinolizidine alkaloids vasicine, vasicinone and vasicinol, **561**-PhD dissertation-root-detected.

Sida rhombifolia   **670**-invitro-aerial parts or roots.

Tr   544-citing-Dinesh Jabhav, Medicinal plants of India, A Guide to Ayurvedic & Ethnomedicinal uses of plants, Vol 1, Scientific Publishers India, 2008, 213-214.

Sida spinosa   **217**-invitro-whole plant?,

Vasicinol   Quinazoline alkaloid

Severe antifertility effects [765]

Sida acuta   **217**-invitro-whole plant?,

Sida cordifolia

118-review-aerial parts-detected, **133**-invitro-whole plant-water extract-successively extracted with chloroform (3x72 h), methanol (3x72 h) and 80% ethanol (3x72 h)-detected, **217**-invitro-whole plant?, **312**-invitro-roots, **176**-invitro-whole plant?-detected, **411**-invitro-leaf-the quinolizidine alkaloids vasicine, vasicinone and vasicinol, **561**-PhD dissertation-root-detected,

Sida rhombifolia   **670**-invitro-aerial parts or roots,

Tr   544-citing-Dinesh Jabhav, Medicinal plants of India, A Guide to Ayurvedic &Ethnomedicinal uses of plants, Vol 1, Scientific Publishers India, 2008, 213-214.

Sida spinosa   **217**-invitro-whole plant?,

Vomifoliol   Fenchane monoterpenoid ($C_{13}H_{20}O_3$)

Sida acuta   186-review,   253-invitro-whole plant-EtOAc-soluble extract,   581-invitro-whole plant-methanol extract-detected,

Wax

Diverse class of organic compounds that are hydrophobic, malleable solids near ambient temperatures.   Candles, finishings, and coatings [1]

Sida rhombifolia / Sida spinosa / Sida urens

509-leaf-chloroform extract--The amount of wax in S. spinosa at the reproductive stage was 6-23 times larger than for Those found for S. urens and S. rhombifolia respectivamente. In general, the amount of wax decreased with plant age.

Xanthones   organic compound

Insecticide and larvacide [1]

Sida rhombifolia   578-invitro-whole plant?-water extract-detected,

Xylan   Polysaccharide (hemicellulose) [1]

Ubiquitous as cellulose in plant cell walls [1]

Sida acuta   217-invitro-whole plant?,

Xylose   monosaccharide of the aldopentose type [1]

Source of xylitol. Animal/human food with 0 calories per gram [1]

Sida acuta / Sida cordifolia / Sida rhombifolia / Sida spinosa / Sida veronicaefolia / Sida rhombifolia var. rhomboidea / Sida rhombifolia var. retusa / Sida indica

561-PhD dissertation-leaves-detected.

Zinc   Elemental metal

Essential trace element for humans. Biological roles are ubiquitous [1]

Sida acuta   264-100% ethanolic leaf extract-325.12 mg/100 g,   274-invitro-leaves - 1.07 Mg/100g.

Sida cordifolia   240-invitro-leaves = 11.04 mg/100gm-stem bark = 18.99 mg/100gm.

Sida rhombifolia
538-invitro-roots-95% ethanol extract-371.1 parts per million.

Sida hermaphrodita
482-invivo-whole plant-mineral excess soils, lowest readings of contamination still rich, 623-invitro-absorbed high levels of zinc, lower levels of lead, copper, and nickel, and absorbed cadmium at least.

α-tocospiro B   α-tocopheroid
Cytotoxic (IC50 values < 4 μg/mL) in P-388 and/or HT-29 cell lines in vitro [766]

Sida acuta   565-invitro-whole plant

β-amyrin   triterpene
Widely distributed in nature-commonly found in medicinal plants-acts against inflammation, microbial, fungal, and viral infections and cancer cells [1]

Sida acuta   559-invitro-seed-unsaponifiable fraction,

Sida indica   710-Ayurveda-review-detected,

β-phenethylamines   Monoamine alkaloid
A neurotransmitter in the human central nervous system. Psychoactive and stimulant effects, similar to amphetamine in its action [1]

Sida acuta, Sida humilis   754- invitro-roots and aerial parts,

Sida cordifolia   118-review-detected,   217-invitro-whole plant?, 312-invitro-roots,

Sida rhombifolia
544-citing-Dinesh Jabhav, Medicinal plants of India, A Guide to Ayurvedic & Ethnomedicinal uses of plants, Vol 1, Scientific Publishers India, 2008, 213-214., 754- invitro-roots and aerial parts, 670-invitro-aerial parts or roots,

Sida spinosa   217-invitro-whole plant?,   754- invitro-roots and aerial parts,

Sida indica   441-invitro-whole plant?-petroleum ether extract,

β-sitosterol   phytosterol similar to cholesterol [1]
May reduce benign prostatic hyperplasia & blood cholesterol [1]   Mosquito larvicidal agent [709]

Sida acuta

186-review, **217**-invitro-whole plant?, **220**-review, **327**-invitro-detected, **559**-invitro-seed-unsaponifiable fraction, **581**-invitro-whole plant-methanol extract-major steroid of the plant,

Sida cordifolia

118-review-detected, **217**-invitro-whole plant?-β-sitosterol-3-O-β-D-glucopyranoside, **312**-invitro-seeds, **571**-invitro-chloroform extract,

Sida rhombifolia   **59**-invitro-whole plant?-sitosterol, **150**-invitro-root-chloroform extract-detected.

Sida indica

441-invivo-petroleum ether extract-a potential new mosquito larvicidal compound with LC50 value of 11.49, 3.58 and 26.67 ppm against Aedes aegypti L, Anopheles stephensi Liston and C. quinquefasciatus Say (Diptera: Culicidae), respectively-may be considered as a potent source and β-sitosterol as a new natural mosquito larvicidal agent, **454**-India-aerial parts, **570**-invitro-petroleum ether extract then 50% alcohol extract-detected, **709**-review-Results of this study demonstrated that β-sitosterol as a new natural mosquito larvicidal agent, **710**-Ayurveda-review-detected, **712**-review.

Sida Composition Tables

This section combines two things: some narrative from the researchers themselves that adds important detail, with composition tables that orient around two specific Sidas. Aside from some multi-Sida studies, nearly all the entries here are about Sida acuta or Sida cordifolia. This reflects the state of the research. I have included only a few of the available tables and charts, but I feel there are enough for you to get a feel for what the Sidas offer. Explore the **References** for more studies on a topic.

There is good evidence that the makeup of all eight major medicinal Sidas is similar and generally medicinally equivalent (with the exception of Sida acuta which alone contains berberine). In the absence of more specific information I suggest that these tables generally describe the medicinal species of all medicinal Sidas.

....

Flavonoids are potent water-soluble antioxidants and free radical scavengers, which prevent oxidative cell damage and have strong anticancer activity. They are used to improve aquaresis and as anti-inflammatory, anti-spasmodic, and anti-allergic, anti-microbial agents. **[184]**

425

Several Sidas

Total phenolic and flavonoid contents of *Sida* species

Species	TPC mg CAE/g	TPC mg TAE/g	TF mg QE/g
S. acuta	1.24±0.06	1.45±0.07	0.84±0.04
S. cordata	0.95±0.05	1.16±0.06	0.97±0.04
S. cordifolia	1.92±0.10	2.13±0.11	1.26±0.06
S. indica	1.24±0.06	1.45±0.07	1.03±0.05
S. mysorensis	1.66±0.08	1.87±0.09	1.18±0.05
S. retusa	0.72±0.04	0.93±0.05	0.70±0.03
S. rhombifolia	1.06±0.05	1.27±0.06	0.90±0.04
S. spinosa	1.35±0.07	1.56±0.08	1.09±0.05

Figures in tables are represented as mean of three readings ±SD. TPC=Total phenolic content, TF=Total flavonoids, TAE=Tannic acid equivalent, CAE=Caffeic acid equivalent, QE=Quercetin equivalent. [15]

Furthermore, on the basis of antioxidant activity, the plants under studies can be classified in to 4 groups as Group I: *Sida cordifolia*: with high activity; Group II: *Sida spinosa*, *S. indica*, and *S. mysorensis*: having moderate activity; Group III: *Sida acuta*, and *S. rhombifolia*: low activity; and Group IV: *Sida cordata* and *S. retusa*: with poor activity.... It is interesting to note that the higher content of total phenolic content and flavonoids in *Sida cordifolia*, *S. mysorensis*, *S. spinosa,* and *S. indica* (arranged high to low) is also associated with higher antioxidant activity. [15]

The seeds of

Sida veronicifolia	oil = 15.5%,	protein = 15%
S. cordifolia,	oil = 11.5%,	protein = 14.1%
S. ovata	oil = 12.1%,	protein = 17.3%
S. mysorensis	oil = 13.2%,	protein = 13.6%
S. rhombifolia	oil = 20.2%,	protein = 12.6%
Abutilon crispum	oil = 12.5%,	protein = 18.4%

Linoleic acid predominated (54.9–69.4%) as the fatty acid of all the oils, and malvalic (1.3–11.4%) and sterculic acids (0.4–1.1%) were significant. [352]

Among 11 species of *Sida* examined, seed extracts of *S. acuta* (=*S. carpinifolia*) and *S. rhombifolia* were found to contain significant amounts of ecdysteroids, seed extracts of *S. filicaulis* contained only moderate levels, whilst the remaining species showed no detectable levels of ecdysteroids. The ecdysteroid profiles of the extracts of the three positive species were significantly different, demon-strating that phytoecdysteroids have chemotaxonomic value in this genus. [263]

The quantitative and qualitative variations of the three types of alkaloids, occurring in the roots and aerial portions of the *Sida* species and at different stages of vegetation are also noteworthy. ß –phenethylamines were found to constitute the major bases in the aerial parts, but occurred as minor components, or were absent in roots. It was further observed that the abundance of quinazoline alkaloids was greater in younger (about 6 months old) species. It was also observed that the roots of 6 months old plants afford quinazoline alkaloids as the major entities, while the carboxylated tryptamines were present only in traces. Older roots (about 2 years old) contained these two types of alkaloids in almost equal proportions. [217]

FRAP Assay: The selected *Sida* species may be arranged on basis of activity (both TEAC and AEAC) from lowest as in *S. retusa<S. cordata<S. acuta<S. rhombifolia<S. spinosa <S. indica<S. mysorensis<S. cordifolia* to highest. FRAPAEAC was better than FRAPTEAC. [15]

ABTS Assay: The selected *Sida* species may be arranged on basis of activity (both TEAC and AEAC) from lowest as in *S. cordata<S. retusa<S. mysorensis <S. acuta<S. cordifolia<S. spinosa<S. rhombifolia<S. indica* to highest. ABTSAEAC was better than ABTSTEAC. [15]

DPPH Radical Scavenging Assay: The selected species may be arranged on basis of % RSA from lowest as in *S. retusa<S. cordata<S. acuta<S. rhombifolia<S. indica<S. spinosa<S. mysorensis<S. cordifolia* to highest. TEAC (• M) values for DPPH activity of the *Sida* species were higher than AEAC in all species. [15]

The results suggest that the studied *Sida* species contained varied range of antioxidant activity in relation to polyphenolic contents. It is also observed that extracts with higher concentrations of polyphenolic contents have strong antioxidant effect. From our study, we note that extract of *S. cordifolia* is high in polyphenolic content and possess good antioxidant activity as compared to other selected species. [15]

Furthermore, on the basis of antioxidant activity, the plants under studies can be classified in to 4 groups as Group I: *Sida cordifolia*: with high activity; Group II: *Sida spinosa, S. indica,* and *S. mysorensis*: having moderate activity; Group III: *Sida acuta,* and *S. rhombifolia*: low activity; and Group IV: *Sida cordata* and *S. retusa*: with poor activity.... It is interesting to note that the higher content of total phenolic content and flavonoids in *Sida cordifolia, S. mysorensis, S. spinosa,* and *S. indica* (arranged high to low) are also associated with higher antioxidant activity. [15]

Plant species, parts, weights of plant material, quantity of methanol used, the extract weights obtained and the percentage yields of the extracts of the plants - weight of plant 50 gm

Species	Amt methanol (ml)	Extract weight (gm)	%Yield
S. acuta whole plant	650	12.55	25.1
S. acuta leaves	600	8.53	17.06
S. rhombifolia stems	700	2.94	5.88

[560]

Sida acuta

Phytochemicals are secondary metabolites of plants known to exhibit diverse pharmacological and biochemical effects on living organisms. These phytochem-icals, tannins, saponins, alkaloids, flavonoids, terpenes and phenolics were found to be present in Sida acuta leaves in amounts to be of medicinal value. [270]

Phytochemical composition of the leaf of Sida acuta.

Tannin	91.46 ± 0.02
Alkaloid	1500.26 ± 0.36
Saponin	530.27 ± 0.03
Flavonoid	1163.86 ± 0.10
Steroid	1454.50 ± 0.85
Terpenoid	115.29 ± 0.05
Cardiac glycoside	851.62 ± 0.01 (mg/100 g) [264]

Composition of vitamins in leaf of Sida acuta

Vitamin	Composition (mg/100 g)
Thiamin	0.36 ± 0.01
Niacin	0.19 ± 0.02
Ascorbic acid	24.27 ± 0.25
Tocopherol	1.85 ± 0.32
Riboflavin	0.12 ± 0.5

Composition of Minerals in Leaves of *Sida acuta*

Mineral	Composition (mg/100 mg)
Calcium	144.28 ± 0.02
Magnesium	122.11 ± 0.01
Zinc	325.12 ± 0.02

[264]

Sample of soil and plant (Sida acuta burm F.) were collected from 30 sites of 24 roads (in Nigeria). ... Levels of Pb, Cd, Zn, Cu and Mn in soil were 15.28–76.92, 1.96–9.80, 41.66–237.96, 1.60–4.88 and 76.00–132.00 mg/kg dry weight, respectively. Results of concentrations in plants ranged were from trace–32.37, 4.88–14.93, 27.78–185.19, 1.67–3.89 and 20.00–110.00 mg/kg dry weight for Pb, Cd, Zn, Cu and Mn, respectively. The soil pH was from 6.22–8.44 while sand and loamy sandy textural classes constitute the soil samples. [421]

Phytochemical & Anti-nutrient Compositions of *S. acuta* Leaves

Parameters	Mg/100g	
Hydrocyanic acid (HCN)	98.25	
Phytate	210.07	
Oxalate	140.80	
Tannin	603.68	
Alkaloids	523.00	
Flavonoids	310.00	
Saponin	650.00	[274]

Proximate composition of Sida acuta %

Moisture content	9.03+0.06	
Protein	19.13+0.15	
Fat	0.67+0.06	
Ash	6.33+0.06	
Fiber	9.50+0.10	
Carbohydrate	55.30+ 0.10	[223]

Qualitative Test for Phytochemicals in Sida acuta

Tannins + + +

Saponins + +

Alkaloids + +

Flavonoids + +

Terpenoids + +

Phenolics + + +

+++ = Highly present; ++ = Moderately present   [223]

Phytochemical composition of Sida acuta (mg/100g)

Tannins	125.00+0.00	
Saponins	406.67+2.89	
Alkaloids	1751.67+2.89	
Flavonoids	1255.00+0.00	
Terpenoids	85.00+0.00	
Phenolics	90.00+0.00	[223]

Vitamin composition of Sida acuta

Ascorbic acid	22.43+0.21(mg/100g)
Niacin	0.33+0.06(mg/100g)
Thiamin	0.10+0.00(mg/100g)
Riboflavin	0.02+0.01(mg/100g)
β-Carotene	925+0.02(µg/100g) **[223]**

Mineral composition of Sida acuta

Calcium	85.0+0.00
Iron	4.87+0.06
Phosphorus	65.0+0.00
Sodium	110.0+0.00
Magnesium	24.5+0.00
	(mg/100mg) **[223]**

Minimum inhibitory concentration (MIC) and Minimum Fungicidal concentration (MFC) of free and bound flavonoids of Sida acuta

Part	Extract	MIC (mg/ml)	MFC (mg/ml)
Root	F	-	-
	B	0.156	0.312
Stem	F	0.078	0.078
	B	0.625	1.25
Leaf	F	0.312	0.625
	B	0.156	0.312
Bud	F	0.312	0.625
	B	0.625	1.25

F=free flavenoids; B=bound flavenoids; (-) no activity   **[184]**

Sida acuta-total flavenoids (mg/gm dw)
Stem 12.25>Leaf 9.25>Bud 12.25>Root 9.25
Sida acuta-total activity of flavenoids (ml/g)
Stem 64.82>Leaf 28.36>Bud 15.94>Root 3.2 **[184]**

Sida acuta: Total flavonoids by plant part (mg/gm dry weight): root = 4.75, stem = 5.45, leaf = 8.5, bud = 5.85   **[271]**

Quantity & Total activity of free & bound flavenoids of S. acuta

Part	Extract	Quantity (mg/g dw)	Total Activity (ml/g)
Root	F	4.25	-
	B	5	3.2
Stem	F	8.15	64.
	B	4.1	0.72
Leaf	F	4.25	26.12
	B	5	2.24
Bud	F	8.15	13.14
	B	4.1	2.8

F=free flavenoids; B=bound flavenoids; (-) no activity: Total Activity=weight of extract (mg/g plant material)/MIC (mg/ml) of extract. **[184]**

It was estimated that < 160 gm dw of genetically transformed hairy root cultures of Sida acuta could provide nearly all tested essential elements catering to per diem requirement of the human body. **[259]**

The investigation into proximate and micronutrients composition of Sida acuta leaves in this study has shown S. acuta to be composed of significant amounts of essential food nutrients. These food nutrients are in amounts comparable to those of leafy vegetables which are commonly consumed for good nutrition. The phytochemical constitution and composition of S. acuta are in amounts to be responsible for diverse medicinal and therapeutic purposes. Sida acuta leaves would provide nutritional benefits and medicinal value... S. acuta is a very good source of carbohydrate given a percentage composition of 55.30%. Carbohydrate provides energy to cells in the body particularly the brain, the only carbohydrate dependent organ on the body... The moisture content value of 9.03% obtained for Sida acuta leaves in this study is low and it suggests that the leaves can be kept for a relatively long time. The moisture content of any food can be used as a measure of its keeping quality. **[223]**

ä-Carbolines and benzo-ä-carbolines1 are very rare in nature, and the best representatives of this family are quindoline2 (1a) and cryptolepine3,4 (2a) (Chart 1), two indoloquinoline alkaloids isolated in 1977 and 1929, respectively, from a West African plant: Cryptolepis sanguinolenta (Periplocaceae). Benzo-ä-carbolines are also found in three other plants: Sida acuta (Malvaceae) from Sri Lanka...Considerable interest in this family (indoloquinoline alkaloids) has been shown by several teams throughout the world due to their various and important biological properties such as: antimuscarinic, antibacterial, antiviral, antiplasmodial, and antihyperglycemic activities. Recently, two reports mentioned the cytotoxicity of cryptolepine and analogues toward B16 melanoma cells20 and M109 Madison lung carcinoma.6 Bonjean et al. also showed that cryptolepine interferes with topoisomerase II and primarily inhibits DNA synthesis. Moreover, some quindoline derivatives have been described as potent antitumor-active compounds. [295]

Phytochemicals are secondary metabolites of plants known to exhibit diverse pharmacological and biochemical effects on living organisms. The phyto-chemicals, tannins, saponins, alkaloids, flavonoids, terpenes and phenolics were found to be present in S. acuta leaves and are in amounts to be of medicinal value. [264]   S. acuta contained the highest percentage crude yield of alkaloids 1.04% (of 10 plants studied), S. acuta possesses very high levels of alkaloids and flavonoids, and is employed in medicinal uses. [420] Leaf- S. acuta is laden with antioxidative compounds with remarkable concentrations of saponins (0.772 mg/100g), flavonoids (0.112 mg/100g), alkaloids (0.076 mg/100g) and tannins (0.0541mg/100g)   [237]

Among the compounds isolated from S. acuta, its alkaloids appeared to be of great interest in pharmacological studies. These alkaloids belong to the family of indoloquinolines. Many investigations have been done on this family of compounds and the results showed that they are new leads in the establishment of drugs against many diseases. [7]   The photochemistry of the plant leaves revealed that S. acuta is laden with antioxidative compounds with remarkable concentrations of saponins (0.772 mg/100g), flavonoids (0.112 mg/100g), alkaloids (0.076 mg/100g) and tannins (0.0541mg/100g) [237]   Alkaloids were extracted from each part of S. acuta. Alkaloid content estimated in each gram of dried plant material was recorded (Table1). Buds of the plant showed maximum amount of alkaloid content (7 mg/gm dw), followed by leaves (3.35 mg/gm dw), stem (1.1mg/gm dw) and roots (0.15 mg/gm dw). [221]

Sida cordifolia

The whole plant of Sida cordifolia is used as medicinal herb, because leaves contain small quantities of both ephedrine and pseudoephidrine1, roots and seeds contain alkaloid ephedrine, vasicinol, vasicinone, and N-methyl tryptophan2,3,4 and is extensively used as a common herbal drug5, ... Because of these important medicinal properties Sida cordifolia L. is under threat due to extensive collection and continuous deforestation. This requires conservation of traditional medicinal plant for the future generation. [151]

....

Flavonoids are known to have medicinal properties and play a major role in the successful medical treatments from ancient times and their use has persevered till date [4]. They are potent water-soluble antioxidants and free radical scavengers, which prevent oxidative cell damage and have strong anticancer activity. They are used to improve aquaresis and as anti-inflammatory, anti-spasmodic, and anti-allergic, anti-microbial agents [98]

Quantitative study of some Phytoconstituents showed a significant difference (p < 0.05) between the leaves contents and that of the stem bark with the exception of tannins.

Quantitative phytochemical constituents of Sida cordifolia	Leaves	Stem bark
Alkaloids (g/100g)	10.5±0.71a	4.75±0.21b
Saponins (g/100g)	8.1±0.35a	4.4±0.28 b
Flavonoids (g/100g)	19.3±0.57a	12.4±1.57 b
Tannins (g/100g)	4.8±0.28a	5.9±0.28 a

[240]

Elemental composition of the leaves and stem bark of Sida cordifolia	Leaves	Stem bark
Copper (mg/100g)	0.48 ± 0.11a	0.69 ± 0.10a
Iron (mg/100g)	5.74 ± 0.17a	5.51 ± 0.25a
anganese (mg/100g)	0.77 ± 0.24a	0.88 ± 0.18b
Lead (mg/100g)	0.07 ± 0.02a	0.11 ± 0.03a
Chromium (mg/100g)	1.45 ± 0.08a	1.05 ± 0.11b
Nickel (mg/100g)	3.99 ± 0.38a	3.26 ± 0.25a
Calcium (mg/100g)	88.72 ± 1.75a	95.49 ± 1.76a
Zinc (mg/100g)	11.04 ± 9.14a	18.99 ± 8.01a
Magnesium (mg/100g)	128.31 ± 0.61a	45.29 ± 0.90b
Sodium (mg/100g)	349.88 ± 87.72a	273.16 ± 87.72b
Potassium (mg/100g)	258.01 ± 19.90a	119.82 ± 4.70b

[240]

Qualitative phytochemical screening of the leaves & stem bark of Sida cordifolia.

Phytochemicals	Leaves	Stem bark
Anthraquinones	+	+
Alkaloids	+	+
Tannins	+	+
Saponins	+	+
Flavonoids	+	+
Polyphenols	+	+
Glycosides	+	+

[240]

Quantitative phytochemical constituents of Sida cordifolia.

	Leaves	Stem bark
Alkaloids (g/100g)	10.5±0.71a	4.75±0.21b
Saponins (g/100g)	8.1±0.35a	4.4±0.28 b
Flavonoids (g/100g)	19.3±0.57a	12.4±1.57 b
Tannins (g/100g)	4.8±0.28a	5.9±0.28 a

[240]

Elemental composition of leaves & stem bark of Sida cordifolia.

Elements	Leaves	Stem bark
Copper (mg/100g)	0.48 ± 0.11a	0.69 ± 0.10a
Iron (mg/100g)	5.74 ± 0.17a	5.51 ± 0.25a
Manganese (mg/100g)	0.77 ± 0.24a	0.88 ± 0.18b
Lead (mg/100g)	0.07 ± 0.02a	0.11 ± 0.03a
Chromium (mg/100g)	1.45 ± 0.08a	1.05 ± 0.11b
Nickel (mg/100g)	3.99 ± 0.38a	3.26 ± 0.25a
Calcium (mg/100g)	88.72 ± 1.75a	95.49 ± 1.76a
Zinc (mg/100g)	11.04 ± 9.14a	18.99 ± 8.01a
Magnesium (mg/100g)	128.31 ± 0.61a	45.29 ± 0.90b
Sodium (mg/100g)	349.88 ± 87.72a	273.16 ± 87.72b
Potassium (mg/100g)	258.01 ± 19.90a	119.82 ± 4.70b

[240]

Lipids, Lipophilic Components and Essential Oils from Sida cordifolia L. Seed

Mass of 100, g: 0.92

Moisture, %: 5.1

Oil (petroleum ether), % on dry wt: 11.5

Acid value, mg KOH: 4.8

Iodine value, % J2: 115.9; 81.2

Oxirane oxygen,: 0.61

Saponification value, mg KOH: 185.8; 197.4

Unsaponifiables, %: 4.3   [558]

....

Tannins are well known for their antioxidant, antimicrobial properties, for soothing relief, skin regeneration, as anti inflammatory and diuresis. [223]

434

Phytoconstituents of different parts of "*Sida cordifolia*" plant

Plant parts	Phytoconstituents	Alkaloids %
Whole parts*	Large amount of ephedrine	Extend of 0.085 %
Seeds	Sterculic, malvalic and coronaric acid and other fatty acids.	0.32 %
Leaves	Ephedrine , pseudoephedrine	0.28 %
Stems	Ephedrine	0.22 %
Roots	Ephedrine, saponine, choline pseudo-ephedrine, betaphenethylamine, vasicine, hypaphorine, ecdysterone and related indole alkaloides.	0.06 %
Aerial parts	Ephedrine, pseudoephedrine, Palmitic, stearic and β – sitosterol, hexacosanoic acids, 6-phenyl ethyl amine, carboxylated tryptomines, qunazoline, hypaphorine, vasicinol	0.31%

* (include leaves ,stems ,seeds and roots)   [118]

Miscellaneous Sida

Sida linifolia Cav. - No abstract available, only the following:

Seed Oil, % on dry wt: 14.0–17.0

Iodine value, % J2: 92.0–109.0 (?)

Full Text in other herbs since nothing found in the PDF [558]

Lipids, Lipophilic Components and Essential Oils from Sida veroniciflora Seed

Seed:	15.5% dry,
Oil, % dry wt:	15.5
n25DnD25:	1.4727
Acid value, mg KOH:	5.8
Iodine value, % J2:	109.5
Saponification value, mg KOH:	182.7
Unsaponifiables, %:	5.1 **[558]**

....

Virginia fanpetals (Sida hermaphrodita) biomass contained on average the most nitrogen (3.72 g·kg-1 dm), calcium (6.03 g·kg-1 dm) and sulphur (1.24 g·kg-1 dm) in 2008, while the most potassium (4.39 g·kg-1 dm) in 2010... The macroelements content in the biomass of Virginia fanpetals under cultivation (mean value of three harvests during three years of its cultivation) can be arranged in the following descending order: Ca > K > N > S > Mg > P [476]

Genetics

Everyone knows about the "double helix" of our genes, but Sida is "multi-helix" otherwise known as polyploid.

Polyploid cells and organisms are those containing more than two paired (homologous) sets of chromosomes. Most species whose cells have nuclei (Eukaryotes) are diploid, meaning they have two sets of chromosomes—one set inherited from each parent. **[1]**   In the later subcultures, chromosomal abnormalities such as chromosomal bridges, multinucleate, multinucleolate, asynchrony and polyploidy cells were evident. The occurrence of polyploidy phenomenon may be due to endo-reduplication. **[722]**

DNA is prone to structural polymorphism and a number of alternative DNA structures have been described to date. DNA conformation may differ from a regular double-helix and may involve the association of more than two strands, leading to the formation of triplexes and quadruplexes. Alternative DNA structures offer significant differences in terms of electrostatics, shape and rigidity compared to single- or double-stranded DNA... The cryptolepine derivatives presented here exhibit a significant preference for triplexes over quadruplexes or duplexes. **[582]**

CONCLUSION: Based on our observations, we therefore concluded that, the basic chromosome number x=7 appears to be dominant in the genus and the other numbers appear to have been derived through uneuploid alterations, secondary polyploidy, hybridization and doubling of chromosomes played a major role in the evolution of the genus....   These findings are highly suggestive that polyploids have played a major role in the evolution of Sida. Further, the chromosome number in Sida are not just multiplies of a single basic number, but are multiplies of different basic numbers of x=7, 8, 9, 11, and 17.....   Similar variation is also seen in S. acuta. Present work and previous work revealed 2n=28, while the diploid chromosome number of 2n=14 is reported. On the other hand a different base number n=18 is found . Thus this species has 7 and 9 base numbers..... Experimental results have confirmed that the chromosome numbers in Sida are not just multiplies of a single basic number. Different basic number of x=7, 8, 9, 11 and 17 occur in the genus.   **[372]**

Sida L. (Malvaceae) has been used for centuries in traditional medicines in different countries for the prevention and treatment of different diseases such as diarrhea, dysentery, gastrointestinal and urinary infections, malarial and other fevers, childbirth and miscarriage problems, skin ailments, cardiac and neural problems, asthma, bronchitis and other respiratory problems, weight loss aid, rheumatic and other inflammations, tuberculosis, etc. {Various researchers have demonstrated that at least seven Sida species are medicinally equivalent}. **[609]**

Sida Cultivation Quick Take

Sida acuta

Habitat   Most soil types, except seasonally flooded clays or soils derived from limestone - a weed of degraded pastures, tree plantations, cereals, root crops, vegetables, planted forests, lawns, roadsides, and waste places. **[698]**

Zone (USDA)   8a **[360]**

pH (soil)   weak acid soils ok, prefers fertile clay **[360]**

Sun Exposure   Sun to partial shade **[360]**

Growth Habit   Small, erect, much branched, perennial shrub **[52]**

Plant Height   Up to 0.7m **[201]**

Soil Environment   Grows well in many soils including heavy clay **[107]**

Soil Temperature for Seed Germination   Generally above 60° **[699]**

How Propagated   Both by seed and stem cuttings **[107, 270]**

Seed Germ %   First year seed=mostly 80% emergence **[306]**

Seed Longevity   {no data. In my experience 1-2 years}

Seed Dormancy   1-3 year old seed could not overcome dormancy **[198]**

Seeds per Gram   400 seeds **[359]**

Seed Depth   {0-1 cm} {0-.4"}

Plant Spacing   12-15" (30-38cm) **[360]**

{or 1-2" centers for vertical growth}

Germination/Light   Highest % of seedlings emerge in shade **[306]**

Water Need   Tolerates dry as well as high rainfall conditions **[107]**

Fertilization   10 lb. 10-10-10 fertilizer per 1,000 sq. ft.

Sidedress in May **[699]**

Harvest   {Continuous pruning once established, pull whole plant at end}

As a Weed   A serious weed species in the tropical world **[278]**

Butterflies, Bees, Birds Host   Among best bee plants in Nigeria **[658]**

Sida cordifolia

Habitat   Grows on drier sandy locations, especially near sea-level [362]

Zone (USDA zone)   8a: to -12.2 °C (10 °F) [703]

pH (soil acidity)   weak   acid soils ok, prefers fertile clay [360]

Sun Exposure   Sunny open position [403]

Growth Habit   Small, erect, downy shrub [118]

Plant Height   Up   to   2 meters [40]

Soil Environment   1   soil+2 humus [488]   well-drained loam [612]

Soil Temperature for Seed Germ   Winter=minimum 17° C. [488]

How Propagated   Stem cuttings flower earlier than seed [20]

Seed Germ Percentage   69% germination in 20 days [665]

Seed Longevity   4% germ after 41 years storage at room temp. [359]

Seed Dormancy   Germination time erratic. Takes 10 days to 3 mo. [722]

Seeds per Gram   250 [359]

Seed Depth   Surface sown [612]

Plant Spacing   15-18 in. (38-45 cm)--18-24 in. (45-60 cm) [726]

Germination/Light Protected from light increases germination [198]

Water Need   Medium to wet [721]

Fertilization   Fertilize during growth=regularly but with spacing [488]

Harvest   Harvest (specifically) at 8 months [413]

As a Weed   Considered an invasive weed around the world [161]

Host For Butterflies, Bees, Birds   Attractive to all three [703]

Sida rhombifolia

Habitat   Commonly
found in dry countries [292]

Zone (USDA zone)   9a: to -6.6
°C (20 °F) [726]

pH (soil acidity)   5.0 to 8.0
[404]

Sun Exposure   In an open,
sunny position [671]

Growth Habit   Evergreen
shrub. Stem is erect and branching [671]

Plant Height   24-36"
[360]

Soil Environment   Prefers light
to medium, well-drained soils [671]

Soil Temp for Seed Germ

35°C optimum, 20-30° C ok, 40° no germ [518]

How Propagated   By seeds or
cuttings [671]

Seed Germ Percentage   62% by hot water pretreatment [358]

Seed Longevity   Oldest collection 17 years; 96 to 99% germination [359]

Seed Dormancy   Majority dormant 12—24 months after maturity [362]

Seeds per Gram   428 [359]

Seed Depth   1-4   cm
depth (.4-1.6 inches) [189]

Plant Spacing   24-36   in
(60-90 cm.) [726]

Germination/Light   Light   did
not influence the germination [518]

Water Need   Drought
tender. Well drained soils [671]

Fertilization   Density
higher in the non-fertilized area [512]

Harvest   Leaves are a dried and stored vegetable in S Africa [358]

As a Weed   Density higher in the non-fertilized area [512]

Host For Butterflies, Bees, Birds   Attractive to all three [703]

439

Cultivation of Sida acuta

The genus Sida comprises more than 170 species and most of them are considered as potential weeds in pastures and annual crops {in the tropics and sub-tropics}. These species are widely distributed, hard to control and adapted to weak and acid soils, although they develop better in fertile clay soils. **[509]**

There is very little cultivation information on the Sidas because they are ubiquitous weeds in the tropics and sub-topics and people just go out and harvest what they need. There is a growing awareness among some herbalists, and Ayurvedic practitioners in particular, that population increases, along with growing interest in herbal solutions, have outstripped the sustainable natural supply. Because Sidas are so important to Ayurveda, India is the only country that is actively researching rapid cloning of Sidas.

The best source of cultivation information on Sidas has been the people who kill it as a weed. They have to know how it is propagated, which gives them clues on how to prevent its propagation. While the various Sidas have differentiated themselves somewhat, I think you can look to other Sidas if there is a gap in cultivation information for the species you are trying to grow. Bottom line: they ARE weeds and very forgiving in their growth.

Sida seeds are tough survivors, and it is very difficult to make Sida seeds sprout when they do not want to sprout. The following cultivation information is spotty and incomplete, but this is everything that my research could uncover. I believe what is in this book is pretty much everything known to peer-review science as of 2017. Much of the information on Ayurveda and traditional uses came from peer-review research as well.

Various Sidas have adapted to a large range of climates - hot and not so hot, wet and dry, fertile and infertile – but they all respond to basic care. Some may be hard to start, but once established they can certainly defend themselves. I have only grown Sida acuta, but feel confident that other varieties will grow for me here in the Northern California coastal mountains. The second edition should have all the major varieties' cultivation figured out.

I divide this chapter into two parts: **Cultivation Categories** and **Cultivation Narrative.** In order to keep the Categories easy to read, most entries are short but hopefully have enough information to lead you deeper. The peer-review researchers, who are the basis of this book, often have interesting and informative things to say about cultivation that is too long for the Categories, hence the Narrative.   This section contains paragraph-length narratives that contain a greater depth of information on appropriate information. Some categories had no information in depth. This narrative section also contains miscellaneous, orphaned listings from the Categories.

As always in this book, all research studies have a citation number. This number leads you to the name of that study, its authors, and the publishing journal in **References**. You can then go to Google Scholar and find the original research, a good percentage of which is the full peer-review study.

Why I grow it as an annual

Until last summer my mantra was, "I want this in every greenhouse in the county." I live in the Emerald Triangle and there are a number of friendly but illegal commercial greenhouses right in my "neighborhood" and hundreds in our county. I was still thinking, "Sida is tropical, so it must be grown in a greenhouse." Then I realized that my best Sida bed by far was one of my first-year beds.

Sida is perennial, in that it re-sprouts every year from its perennial roots in the tropics, but that does not happen in Willits. My experience in four years of over-wintering in Zone 8 is that the roots cannot survive Mendocino's combination of a cold and wet winter. After four growing seasons there has been no re-growth from the old roots.

But I got hundreds of Sida sprouts in my main Sida beds because of all the dropped seeds from last season. I transplanted the 50 best sprouts for my main crop, gave away others, but still had hundreds of small plants jammed into the end of one bed (about 25 square feet). I thought of eating them as high-protein sprouts, but was interested in seeing how such a crowded bed would evolve.

Although Sidas can be grown in Willits like tomatoes, it is also true that tomato production in Willits is marginal - not enough heat! This is a native of Central America – tropical! Even in the summer Willits evenings are cool. But this is also a world-class weed! It is the night before Thanksgiving and my Sidas haven't had a frost yet, so most of the Sidas are still surviving, but a few of the weaker acutas were essentially dead and rotting. It was getting to be my last chance to harvest. Sorry Sida plants, I was distracted by finishing this book (and they require so little care!). Note: I still have a few Sida acutas growing in January, past several mild frosts with the temperatures barely below freezing.

The leaves this year weren't much bigger or lusher than last year's poor soil. We know that fertilizer only marginally enhances the size of a Sida crop [512,473]. I think I made a better planting this year, hopefully with better medicinal results, although I have been quite pleased with previous crops.

After selectively harvesting the aerial parts throughout the growing season, you can get a good final harvest as well (mine was in December). By harvesting the plant at the end of the year (just like tomatoes, but hardier) you get all the first-year roots, rather than struggling to cut second- and later-year roots out of a multi-year Sida -- an incredibly resisting mass.

One caveat: only one study anywhere mentioned time to harvest for any Sida; Sida cordifolia's optimum harvest time is 8 months, with ephedrine content dropping sharply at 7 and 9 months, and worse beyond that. How this translates to other Sida species I do not know. My experience is that first-year Sida acuta leaves are medicinally useful at three months.

The tinctures I made from last year's crop seem to be as potent as usual; I have bounced back and forth between commercial and my own extracts twice. Just to be safe I use 6 droppers of my vodka tincture to approximate the yield from four droppers of a 60% extract. So far this approach seems to be working for me. It helps that it is very difficult to overdose on Sida, and for most cures more is better.

A wonderful bonus comes the following Spring - you should have hundreds of high-protein micro-greens begging for your attention. In Winter grow a cover crop in your Sida bed, or mulch lightly -- the seeds are surface sown and need to hide from hungry varmints.

It will be interesting to know the experience of gardeners in the North near Canada. Sida alba is considered "an herbal waif" in Boston. It is amazing that any tropical Sida could in any way survive Boston, but occasionally it does. So where on the scale are you? If you are fully Boston with your winters, then germination from seeds overwintering outside might be scant. Success will depend on the cold hardiness of some very tough seeds, and enough soil temperature to turn them on.

Once Sida acuta matures, it becomes a woody, prickly shrub that is extremely difficult to eradicate. It will deny you passage. It is called "wireweed" because it is so hard to dig up if mature. I see no reason to maintain a Sida acuta plant past the first year.

My fiber friend is wildly enthusiastic over the strength and quality of the first-year Sida acuta stem fiber, further indication of the maturity of first-year plants. It helps that the bark has its own special medicinal qualities that probably would be easier to extract when it is still young and relatively soft.

If you have a greenhouse and have some room in it, you could grow Sida as a permanent crop; though Sida actua has been grown in two different greenhouses in Willits, and neither crop was successful. I am sure that it can be done; perhaps the best reason for a greenhouse would be to extend a short growing season to 8 months or more which might beneficially affect medicinal production. There is no data on when Sida acuta develops the most medicinal content. There is one study that found that eight months was specifically optimal for Sida cordifolia. Again, I am satisfied with the 40% vodka extracts I have made from first-year Sida acuta plants. Nothing else is known, so far.

This was the most difficult section of the book to sort out. Sidas are dominant weeds in tropical and sub-tropical climates. If there is enough warm/hot weather for them to bear fruit, you should have a perennial plant. There are four species of Sida that have significant cultivation information: S. acuta, S. cordifolia, S. rhombifolia, S. spinosa. Other species of Sida sometimes have their own categories, but are often listed under **Other Sida**.

Cultivation Categories

Habitat

(Sida acuta-but indicative of most Sidas) Found on most soil types, except seasonally flooded clays or soils derived from limestone. It competes vigorously with other plant species, but does best in disturbed habitats in tropical or sub-tropical regions with a distinct wet and dry season. It has a deep taproot and can withstand drought, mowing and shallow tillage. It is a weed of degraded pastures, tree plantations, cereals, root crops, vegetables, planted forests, lawns, roadsides, and waste places. In habitats where it occurs, it tends to flourish in riparian areas near watercourses. It has been reported at up to 1500 m altitude in Indonesia, at medium and higher elevations in Kenya and in the foothills of the Andes in Peru. **[698]**

Sida acuta

52--found in pastures, wastelands, cultivated lands, roadsides, lawns, and in planted forests - appears to do best in disturbed habitats,   **270**--does best in distributed habitats in tropical or sub-tropical regions with distinct wet and dry season,   **275**--widely distributed in the sub-tropical regions, found in bushes, in farms, around habitations. Grows abundantly on cultivated fields, waste areas, roadsides and highways, in damp or dry, between 0 and 1800 meters,   **283**--frequently dominates improved pastures, disturbed areas and roadsides in northern Australia--found on moist refugia near the coast, especially in irrigated gardens and orchards near Darwin, around farm dams and on the fringes of sub-coastal swamps,   **299**-The malvaceous weed Sida acuta frequently dominates improved pastures, disturbed areas and roadsides in northern Australia. This small, erect shrub is native to Mexico and Central America but has spread throughout the tropics and subtropics.

Sida cordifolia   **362**--grows on drier sandy locations, especially near sea-level.

Sida rhombifolia

292--commonly found in dry countries such as India and Ceylon,   **671**-seed company-native of Asia, it prefers light to medium, well drained soils in an open, sunny position, and is drought and frost tender.

Sida alba

722--Habitats include cropland, abandoned fields, gardens, grassy areas along railroads and roadsides, and waste areas where the soil has been recently disturbed.

Zone (USDA zone)

Sida acuta   360--8a

Sida cordifolia

703--Hardiness: USDA Zone 8a: to -12.2 °C (10 °F)--USDA Zone 8b: to -9.4 °C (15 °F)--USDA Zone 9a: to -6.6 °C (20 °F)--USDA Zone 9b: to -3.8 °C (25 °F)--USDA Zone 10a: to -1.1 °C (30 °F)--USDA Zone 10b: to 1.7 °C (35 °F)--USDA Zone 11: above 4.5 °C (40 °F),   **726**--USDA Zone 8a: to -12.2 °C (10 °F), USDA Zone 8b: to -9.4 °C (15 °F), USDA Zone 9a: to -6.6 °C (20 °F), USDA Zone 9b: to -3.8 °C (25 °F), USDA Zone 10a: to -1.1 °C (30 °F), USDA Zone 10b: to 1.7 °C (35 °F), USDA Zone 11: above 4.5 °C (40 °F).

Sida rhombifolia
360-9a,   726-USDA Zone 9a: to -6.6 °C (20 °F), USDA Zone 9b: to -3.8 °C (25 °F), USDA Zone 10a: to -1.1 °C (30 °F), USDA Zone 10b: to 1.7 °C (35 °F)

pH (soil acidity)

S. urens, Sida rhombifolia and Sida spinosa are widely distributed, hard to be controlled and adapted to weak and acid soils, although they develop better in fertile clay soils. [509]

Sida rhombifolia

360—pH 4.5-8.5--pH 5.0 to 8.0-75% germination,   404--pH 5.0 to 8.0-75% germination,   518-more than 75% germination at a range of pH from 5.0 to 8.0,   726—pH 4.5-8.5

Sida alba

404--pH 5.0 to 8.0-75% germination,   518--pH 5.0 to 8.0-75% germination,   673--Soil pH range of 5.0 to 8.0 did not affect prickly sida germination.

Sun Exposure

Sida acuta

65-showed better growth and dry matter production in the sun,   306-had the highest percentage of seedlings emerging under shade in each of the last 3 years,   360-sun to partial shade.

Sida cordifolia

488-sunny,   413-invivo-root-Sida cordifolia-preferred open condition for higher root yield and ephedrine content,   702--The seeds can be sown in pots or directly outdoors in full sun to partial shade,   703--Full Sun, Sun to Partial Shade,   721-full sun,   722--Place the planted seeds in a shady covered location to maintain soil moisture and control rain damage. Can also be germinated in full sun if adequate soil moisture is maintained.

Sida rhombifolia
360-full sun,   671-seed company-in an open, sunny position.

Sida alba
722--full or partial sun

....
A number of patented herbal formulations disclosed composition with S. cordifolia as one of their ingredients, for utility as aphrodisiac. [312]

Growth Habit

Sida acuta

52-small, erect, much branched, perennial shrub or herb - stem and branches flattened at the extremities, fibrous, almost woody at times, **201**-branchlets erect, numerous; obovate, dentate broad, and pubescent, **283**-tough, fibrous stems, **360**--sub-shrub, **699**-very fibrous, tough, almost woody shrub-it starts very slowly and may stay less than an inch tall for a month or more--because of the hot temperatures and moisture though, late summer is an ideal time to plant. Sweet Tea is perennial and will come back from the roots every spring {not in N. Calif. Zone 8} and really grows like wild in hot weather when it is already established. In the establishment year it doesn't grow nearly as fast and requires a little patience.

Sida cordifolia

40-a bush of up to 2 m., **118**-small, erect, downy shrub, **122**-a bush of 2 m in height, **161**-perennial sub-shrub.

Sida rhombifolia   **360**-sub-shrub, **671**-seed company-evergreen shrub-stem is erect and branching; the leaves are narrowly oval to rhomboidal, alternate and 7cm long, with serrate margins and a white undersurface; the flowers are yellow, open and petalled, occurring in the leaf axils.

Sida retusa   **527**-erect, still, branched under shrub.

Sida hermaphrodita   **1**-tall, weedy

Plant Height

Sida acuta

52--30 to 100 cm, **201**--up to 0.7m, **360**--18-24", **699**--Individual plants can easily reach four feet tall and three feet wide in a couple of years.

Sida cordifolia

40--up to 2 m. **118**--to 0.75 – 1.5 meters, **122**-a bush of 2 m in height **703**---18-24 in. (45-60 cm)--24-36 in. (60-90 cm), **721**-3 to 4 feet.

Sida rhombifolia   **360**--24-36", **671**-seed company-height of 2m with a spread of 2m.

Sida retusa   **527**-to 0.5 m

Sida hermaphrodita   **1**-12 feet, can be higher

446

Soil Environment

Adapted to weak and acid soils, they develop better in fertile clay soils. **[509]** If there is any large amount of clay in the soil the Sida roots will clump to it, which will make harvesting roots more difficult. Even a moderate amount of clay ends up as way-too-many blobs snarled in the roots.

Sida acuta

107-the plant grows well in many soils including heavy clay,   **270**- frequently found in pastures, cultivated lands, roadsides and lawns. Sida acuta is found on most soil types, except seasonally flooded clays or soils derived from limestone. It competes vigorously with other plant species, but does best in distributed habitats in tropical or sub-tropical regions with distinct wet and dry season,   **699**-well-drained, well-fertilized. Readily germinates along shady edges of food plots where there is fresh organic matter like leaf litter or pine straw. Adaptive to a wide range of soils except calcareous soils (soils derived from limestone) and seasonally flooded clays. It also does not persist in wet soils for very long.

Sida cordifolia

488-1 soil+2 humus,   **612**—a well-drained sandy-loam to clay-loam soil rich in humus is suitable for cultivation of this plant. The plant grows well in tropical and sub-tropical climate but the growth in tropical region is better. The land is repeatedly ploughed to a fine tilth and weeds, pebbles etc. are removed. For a hectare of land, 20-25 tons FYM for low fertile and 15-18 tons for moderately fertile soil are essential--Green manuring is effective where irrigation facilities are available. Groundnut cake, bone-meal, rapeseed cake and vermi-composting are beneficial for better growth of the plant.   **702**-- often grows in wastelands. It can tolerate poor soils if necessary. Soil should be well-draining—**Pots**--perlite can be added to a commercial potting mix for a suitable medium for growing in containers,   **722**-plant the seeds in a well drained mix such as 3 parts perlite to 1 part sterile potting soil or 3 parts #2 perlite to 1 part Sunshine Mix #4. Keep the medium moist until germination.

Sida rhombifolia

189-As experimental plots were used plastic pots with 5 L capacity, filled with soil collected from the arable layer of an Oxisol with a particle size of 380 g kg -1 clay, 50 g kg -1 silt and 570 g k sand. The land was dried in the shade, and then passed on 5 mm mesh sieve, before being packaged in the pots,   **216**- has a wide occurrence with different varieties adapted to different conditions of the soil and other environmental conditions.   **671**-seed company website-it prefers light to medium, well-drained soils in an open, sunny position. Or start in moist but well-drained seed mix.

Sida alba   **722**-moist to mesic soil that is loamy and fertile,

Soil Temperature for Seed Germination
Sidas germinate when soil temperatures are around 70° F. or better

Sida acuta

699-germinates when night time temperatures are generally above 60°-will tolerate a number of light freezes before eventually going dormant.

Sida cordifolia   **488**-temperature during winter=minimum 17° C.

Sida rhombifolia

404--35°C.,   **188**--S. rhombifolia seeds germinated at higher rates at the constant temperature of 35°C or the alternating ones that included 35°C in the treatment,   **189**--apparently variations in temperature do not influence the germination and seedling emergence as in the emergence period (5 to 15 days) , the temperature ranged between 20 ° C and 25 ° C.,   **198**--seeds were germinated in germination boxes (Gerbox) lined with paper, at 25°C., **358**--The optimum temperature range for germination is 25–35°C.,   **362**— the optimum temperature range for germination is 25–35°C.,   **403**—alternate temperature treatments resulted in 62% germination,   **404**-- maximum germination occurred at 35°C--did not germinate at 40°C--Less than 50% of seed from both species were viable at 45°C after 21 days of exposure,   **516**--apparently variations in temperature do not influence the germination and seedling emergence,   **518**--35°C optimum, 20-30°C ok,40% no germ--Maximum germination occurred at 35°C-germinated better than prickly sida at 20 and 25°C, but did not germinate at 40°C. Less than 50% of seed from both species were viable at 45°C after 21 days of exposure,   **671**- seed company- frost tender-{but also?}-a very hardy and fast-growing plant.

Sida alba

404--35-40°C optimum, 20-35°C OK,   **518**--best germinated at 35 or 40°C.,   **673**--optimum temperatures for prickly sida germination occur from 30 to 40 C.

How Propagated

Specifically for Sida, natural propagation occurs only by seed. **[198]** **Propagation by Seeds:** The small brown to black seeds of Sida cordifolia are contained in pale brown to black capsules. It grows easily from seed. To remove the seeds from the capsule, air dry them at room temperature in a bowl or paper bag. Carefully rub the capsules through a strainer with the appropriate size mesh. The seeds should fall through leaving the debris in the strainer. **[722]**

Sida acuta   **107, 270**-can be propagated both by seed and stem cuttings. I find surface planting, or planting no more than 2 cm deep is needed – deeper sowing results in lower germination. Sida acuta can survive on

really bad soil but if you want a good harvest give it the best soil possible. This year I added a foot of moderately fertile manufactured soil, and fertilized with a double dose of organic 12-12-12 and kelp meal. This did not get significantly better growth, but I suppose the medicinal content has gone up.

Sida cordifolia

19-can be grown both from the seeds and by stem cuttings,   **20**-plants propagated from stem cuttings flower earlier than those propagated by seed. In case of seed propagation, one-year-old dormant seeds are either directly sown in the field in-situ, or in a nursery bed. After emerging, seedlings 7-14 days old are transplanted in a space of 75 x 85cm in the field. In vegetative propagation, the stem cuttings obtained from lateral stems are used. Beside these the propagation is also reported from tissue culture practices. Multiple shoot formation from mature nodal explants of 'Bala' on MS medium supplemented with 2.0 mg 1-1,6- benzyl amino-purine, 0.5 mg 1-1α naphthalene acidic acid, 1.0 mg 1-1 adenine sulfate and10% (v/v) coconut milk are reported,   **612**- can be grown both from the seeds and by stem cuttings,   **703**-Propagation Methods: From seed; direct sow after last frost- Self-sows freely; deadhead if you do not want volunteer seedlings next season,   **720**-prick out into small 3" pots and plant in final position when the plants are established,   **722-Propagation by Cuttings**; Sida fallax can be grown from cuttings. Criley recommends using a rooting hormone of 2,000 parts per million (ppm) indolebutyric acid (IBA) in either a liquid or a talc dust form. He suggests either 1 part coarse perlite to 1 part vermiculite or 100% vermiculite as a rooting medium and rooting the cuttings under 30% shade. He cautions, however, that extremely wet conditions, such as often found when using intermittent misting systems, cause leaf drop and poor rooting. Boche reports 85% success rate using stem and tip cuttings grown in 50% shade using a medium of 3 parts peat moss to 1 part vermiculite. Stratton reports 80 to 90% success rates from cuttings but does not detail the procedures used.

Sida alba

673--germination was enhanced by increasing temperature regimes and by subjecting seeds to wet/dry cycles; increasing temperature proved most effective in promoting germination. Both the number of permeable seeds and rate of germination increased with increasing temperatures. Seeds exposed to higher temperatures following a lower temperature regime germinated at greater percentages than those maintained continuously at the higher temperatures. Also, increasing the length of time the seeds remained at the lower temperature before transfer to higher temperatures increased germination. The lower temperature regime seemed to "precondition" the seed for a rapid increase in water permeability. Egley (1990) reported that in moist soil, viability of prickly sida seed exposed 1 d to 50 C was reduced to 45% and seed did not survive 12 hour at 60 C.,

Sida rhombifolia   **671**-seed company-propagation is by seeds or cuttings.

Seed Germination Percentage

Purchasing commercial seed that is coated with a fungicide, I got close to 100% germination. Using the seeds I grew, dipping them into boiling water for 20 seconds just before planting, got 100% germination. The Sida plants volunteering from seed dropped last year must have had good germ, since I had hundreds of them. The germination difficulties seem to come up when someone wants Sida to sprout at some other time than when they want, and Sida is very stubborn about when it wants to sprout.

Sida acuta

81-freshly harvested seeds exhibited only 4% germination at 35°C in the dark, **306**-over 50% of all seedling emergence occurred in the first year and, for most seed lots, over 80% of emergence. No seedling emergence occurred in the fourth and fifth years in full sunlight whereas there were still low levels of seedling emergence under shade--Table 1: Germination. Sida acuta germ percentage was 2%, soft seed 2%, hard seed 0%, dead seed 9%--Table 2: Germination (1983-88). Total germ = full sun 39%, shade 17%, in sun seed germinated for 3 years, in shade seed germinated all 5 years (1% last year), **362**-review-Seeds from Sida acuta have a germination rate of 54%, a month after harvesting.

Sida cordifolia

411-invitro-we have developed a quick and reliable germination procedure for S. cordifolia seeds that is based on boiling and freezing pre-treatments enabling a 50% germination rate, **665**-best germination procedure for Sida cordifolia=12 hr. Refrigerator (5-7° C) and 12 hr. oven (100° C)= 69% germination in 20 days. Longer in oven and the percentage germination becomes very low.

Sida rhombifolia

358-the majority of the seeds of Sida rhombifolia are dormant for 12–24 months after maturity. Germination was 8% at a temperature of 35°C and was increased to 62% by a hot water (80°C) pretreatment of 10 minutes followed by a cold water (5°C) pretreatment of 10 minutes. Treatment of seed by soaking for 25 minutes in H_2SO_4 resulted in a germination of 100%, **291**-homeopathic dilutions of Cymbopogon winterianus (citronella) improved germination and growth of seedlings of Sida rhombifolia.

Seed Longevity

I have germinated two-year-old S. acuta seed 100% by dipping it in boiling water for 20 seconds and planting immediately. Older seed does not sprout/grow well.

Sida acuta

306-studies showing that a considerable proportion of S. acuta seed could remain viable after a full year's exposure on the soil surface in the Northern Territory (Australia).

Sida cordifolia

359-4% germination after 41 years storage in paper bags at room temperature, **665**-the seeds of Sida cordifolia have a viability period of 21 months...We have found the maximum germination percentage at 40° C. The germination percentage increases with increasing temperature up to 40° C but it decreases when temperature increasing from 40° C. There is no germination at 60° C. Seeds of Sida cordifolia go on losing their germinability with the increasing period of temperature in hours, **722**-seeds of Sida fallax (S. cordifolia) can be stored after being cleaned and air dried. Place them in a paper bag or envelope and put them in an airtight container with desiccant. Stratton suggests storing the dried seeds in a cool place at 25% relative humidity. Yoshinaga's tests indicate that seeds stored at 39° F and 10% humidity retained some viability for 2 years.

Sida rhombifolia

359--oldest collection 17 years; average germination change 96 to 99%, **404**-after 21 days of exposure, less than 50% of seed from both species were viable at 45°C.

Sida alba

359--oldest collection 18 years; average germination change 71 to 90%, **404**--after 21 days of exposure, less than 50% of seed from both species were viable at 45°C., **673**--viability was 21, 4, and less than 1%, after burial for 3.5, 4.5, and 5.5 years, respectively--Depth of burial did not influence prickly sida viability after 30 months, however, viable seed was only found at 8 cm (15%) and 38 cm (1%).

Sida hermaphrodita

564-the average germination for all season varied between 4,67% and 10% without hot water priming. When physically scarified, the oldest seeds showed the best germination percent (46%) after HWT treatment.

Seed Dormancy

I find that it is very difficult and unsatisfying to make a Sida sprout when it is not ready to, but allowing it to re-seed when it is ready seems to work very well.

Seeds of the majority of plant species in the world except tropical rainforest and tropical semi-evergreen forest are dormant at maturity. **[564]** Some seeds have water-impermeable coverings that prevent water entry into seeds and thereby prevent germination until the impermeability breaks down.

Historically, such seeds have been termed "hard" because they do not imbibe water after a day or two and remain hard to the touch whereas non-hard seeds rapidly imbibe and become soft. This type of physical "coat-imposed dormancy" prevents germination even though water is externally available. **[432]** Because of a hard seed coat, entirely preventing absorption of water in desert species of Sida, germination is rendered impossible or difficult under laboratory conditions. This block was eliminated by high temperature pretreatments to ensure better germination. The seeds could tolerate extremely high temperatures for sufficiently longer durations without affecting the germination process. **[402]** A puncture through the seed coat, either over the radicle or cotyledons, permitted water imbibition by all mature seeds, but the puncture over the radicle was significantly more effective in inducing germination. **[431]**

Sida acuta

81--freshly harvested seeds exhibited only 4% germination for S. acuta and 8% germination for S. rhombifolia, respectively, at 35°C in the dark. In preliminary tests, only about 4 and 8% imbibed water prior to germination and the rest of the seeds remained unimbibed, **198**--seeds were sun-dried and stored in perforated plastic bags in 30-40% relative humidity at 28 ± 1°C for 1-3 years could not overcome dormancy in even after 3 years due to the hard seed coat whereas permeability of aged seeds of both species increased, **228**-seeds dormant at seed fall and require high alternating temperatures to remove an after-ripening requirement. In addition S. acuta needs a further period at high temperature to fracture its impermeable seed coat... In S. acuta germination was spread over the first 2 months of the season, **359**--85-100 % germination; pre-sowing treatments = seed scarified (chipped with scalpel); germination medium = 1% agar; germination conditions = 20-30°C germination temperature(s), and 8/16 light hours/dark hours (per 24 hour period).

Sida cordifolia

359--88-100 % germination; pre-sowing treatments = seed scarified (covering structure removed & seed coat chipped); germination medium = 1% agar; germination conditions=10-30°C, 8/16-germination temper-ature(s), light hours/dark hours (per 24 hour period), 76-100 % germination; pre-sowing treatments = seed scarified (covering structure removed & seed coat chipped); germination medium = 1% agar; germination conditions = 21-31°C, 8/16, **411**-boiling and freezing pre-treatments enabling a 50% germination rate, **612**--one year old dormant seeds are either directly sown in the field in-situ or in nursery bed. After emerging out, seeding of 7-14 days old are transplanted in a space of 75 x 85cm in the field, **702**--soil should be well draining--the seeds can be sown in pots or directly outdoors in full sun to partial shade--perlite can be added to a commercial potting mix for a suitable medium for growing in containers--the soil should remain relatively moist-- soak the seeds for twenty-four hours prior to planting--Some growers also recommend scarifying the seeds too--Germination may be irregular and can take from two weeks to three months, **702, 720**-for best results, seeds are best sown directly into the ground where required in the spring. Alternatively,

452

sow in late winter/early spring in heat of 20-25° C.—It can help to scarify the seeds by removing the covering structures and chipping the seed coat with a scalpel. Some people have successfully germinated these using agar, germination paper or sand, at temperatures between 20 and 30° C.   **722**-germination time is erratic and can take from 10 days to 3 months. (Kew gives germination time of 3 to 8 months.) Germination rates are also extremely variable.

Sida rhombifolia

198-seeds were kept in an accelerated aging chamber for different times (0, 24, 48 and 72h), at a temperature of 45C and relative humidity of 100%--Germination obtained at 25 ° C was only 2% and 1% in the dark in the light and was elevated up to 60% with increasing temperature to 35 ° C--The accelerated aging of Sida seeds for up to 72 hours provided an increase in seed quality,   **198**-the emergence of Sida seedlings in pots reached only 35.25% after 40 days of observation,   **358**-the majority of the seeds are dormant for 12–24 months after maturity. Germination was 8% at a temperature of 35°C and was increased to 62% by a hot water (80°C) pretreatment of 10 minutes followed by a cold water (5°C) pretreatment of 10 minutes. Treatment of seed by soaking for 25 minutes in H2SO4 resulted in a germination of 100%,   **359**--92% germination; germination medium = 1% agar; germination conditions = 21°C, 12/12; (RBG Kew, Wakehurst Place)--1-57 % germination; germination medium = 1% agar; germination conditions = 25/35 °C; Data from 4 replicates each with 25 seeds,   **359**--97-98 % germination; pre-sowing treatments = seed scarified (covering structure removed & seed coat chipped); germination medium = 1% agar; germination conditions = 21-31°C, 12/12; (RBG Kew, Wakehurst Place)--85-100 % germination; pre-sowing treatments = seed scarified (covering structure removed & seed coat chipped); germination medium = 1% agar; germination conditions = 15-30°C, 8/16; (RBG Kew, Wakehurst Place),   **362**-the majority of the seeds of Sida rhombifolia are dormant 12—24 months after maturity. The optimum temperature range for germination is 25—35°C.,   **362**-review-Sida rhombifolia-Propagation and planting Sida produces large amounts of seed. The majority of the seeds of Sida rhombifolia are dormant 12—24 months after maturity,   **403**-alternate temperature treatments resulted in 62% germination for S. rhombifolia. H2SO4, pyridine, ethyl alcohol, ethyl acetate and diethyl-ether also increased the percentage of germination or imbibition in S. rhombifolia,   **509**-the germination level for S. rhombifolia seeds soaked in water for 24 h was (30%),   **510**-Recently-picked seeds soaked in water for 24 hours germinated 30%,   **516**-samples were collected a maximum 15 days in advance of the installation of each experiment, aiming to prevent the seeds from entering dormancy process,   **671**-seed company-should germinate within a few days,   **What does not work in dormancy:**   **198**-seeds were sun-dried and stored in perforated plastic bags in 30-40% relative humidity at 28 ± 1°C for 1-3 years could not overcome dormancy in even after 3 years due to the hard seed coat whereas permeability of aged seeds of both species increased.

Sida rhomboidea

359-84 % viability following drying to moisture content in equilibrium with 15 % RH and freezing for 9 weeks at -20C, 84-88 % germination; pre-sowing treatments = seed scarified (chipped with scalpel); germination medium = 1% agar; germination conditions = 20-30°C.

Sida alba

430-shifting seeds from a lower to a higher temperature regime increased germination. Seeds shifted from 15/6, 20/10, 25/15, or 30/15 C to higher regimes of 20/10, 25/15, 30/15, 35/20, or 40/25 C germinated to greater percentages than did seeds kept continuously at the lower thermo periods. With an increase in length of time seeds were at a lower temperature, there was an increase in the percentage that germinated after they were moved to a higher regime -- Treatments such as mechanical scarification, soaking in sulfuric acid, storage at room temperatures for long period of time, exposure to high temperatures (70-100C), sonication, and liquid nitrogen render the seed coat permeable to water and induce imbibition and germination -- embryos of freshly matured seeds were partially dormant. When the seed coat was priced by a pin over the radicle end, seeds germinated to 94%, while those pricked over the cotyledon end germinated to 45%. However, embryo dormancy disappeared during a 12-month storage period at room temperatures; seed coats also become permeable during this time, **430**-regimes of 20/10, 25/15, 30/15, 35/20, or 40/25 C germinated to greater percentages than did seeds kept continuously at the lower thermo-periods. With an increase in length of time seeds were at a lower temperature, there was an increase in the percentage that germinated after they were moved to a higher regime, **431**--43-100 % germination; germination medium = 1% agar; germination conditions = 21/11°C, 12/12; (RBG Kew, Wakehurst Place)-germination temperature(s), light hours/dark hours (per 24 hour period), 78-95 % germination; pre-sowing treatments = seed scarified (covering structure removed & seed coat chipped); germination medium = 1% agar; germination conditions = 20-30°C, 8/16; (RBG Kew, Wakehurst Place)-over 90% of the mature seeds imbibed water and germinated when incubated at 35 C after 4 months dry storage at 25 C. **515**-the seed coats of S. spinosa (prickly sida, Malvaceae) become impermeable to water during seed development on the mother plant. After the seeds have dehydrated during the final maturation stages, piercing of seed coats is necessary to induce imbibition of water and germination. Onset of impermeability occurs during seed coat browning, well in advance of seed dehydration, **What does not work in dormancy: 431**-neither freezing and thawing nor moist chilling at 5 C promoted seed germination. However, increasing the incubation temperature and subjecting seeds to wet-dry cycles enhanced germination; high temperatures were more effective than alternate wetting and drying, Freshly-produced, mature prickly sida (Sida spinosa L.) seeds (18 to 21 days after antithesis, < 20% water content) were dormant and neither imbibed water nor germinated when incubated for up to 4 weeks under several light and temperature conditions.

Sida hermaphrodita

564-dramatically increase the germination percent from 11.3% to 80% by immersing seed into heated water regulated for the following temperatures and time regime-65 and 80 °C, for 2 minutes; 95°C for 30 seconds.   **478**--it was noticed that there were no significant differences between HWT treatment made at 80° C and 95° C--germination percent (46%) by means of HWT method.

Seeds per Gram

Sida acuta   **359**--400 seeds.

Sida cordifolia   **558**--100 seeds-.92 gm,   **359**—250.

Sida rhombifolia   **359**—428,   **466**-Avg. 1000 Seed Wt(g): 2.332

Sida rhomboidea   **359**—478.

Seed Depth

I had hundreds of sprouts from the seeds dropped by the Sida plants throughout the growing season; seeds that worked themselves shallowly into the soil. The seeds that I planted in flats (at the most ¼ inch deep) pretty much germinated 100%. Generally it seems best to plant Sida seeds as shallowly as possible.

Sida acuta

306-a considerable portion of S. acuta seed could remain viable after a full year's exposure on the soil surface in the Northern Territory (of Australia-tropical).

Sida cordifolia

612-one-year-old dormant seeds are either directly {surface sown} in the field in-situ or in nursery bed.

Sida rhombifolia

189- two experiments were conducted in greenhouse conditions during September 2008 and January 2009. Seeds of both species were sown at different depths (0, 1, 2, 3, 4 and 5 cm). Sida rhombifolia was less sensitive to seasonal variations, and the highest percentages of emergence occurred between 1 and 4 cm depths-regardless of the time of sowing-the larger percentages emergence occurred between 0.5 cm and 2.0 cm deep,   **404**-emergence was equivalent at planting depths of 0.5–2.0 cm, with declining emergence below 2.0 cm--no germ from depths exceeding 5.0 cm.,   **505**-the highest percentages of emergence occurred between 1 and 4 cm depths-0.5-2 cm optimal, 1-4 cm ok,   **516**-the highest percentages of emergence occurred between 1 and 4 cm depths--the larger percentages emergency occurred between 0.5 cm and 2.0 cm deep--with increasing depth of seed deposition observed significant reduction in the emergence speed--the biggest emergence percentage occurred between 1 and 4 cm deep, regardless of the time of sowing,   **518**-emergence was equivalent at planting depths of 0.5–2.0 cm, with declining emergence below 2.0 cm. Neither species emerged from depths exceeding 5.0 cm.,   **671**-seed company-sow seed 5mm deep in moist but well-drained seed mix. Should germinate within a few days.

Sida alba

404- Prickly Sida emergence was optimal at a planting depth of 0.5 cm, and declined rapidly at deeper planting depths-Neither species emerged from depths exceeding 5.0 cm.-Light did not influence the germination of prickly sida,   **518**-Prickly sida emergence was optimal at a planting depth of 0.5 cm, and declined rapidly at deeper planting depths-no emergence 5 cm., **673**-Prickly Sida emergence of 80% was noted when seeds were planted at a 0.5 cm depth, while only 60, 50, 40, and 20% emergence was observed at depths of 1 to 1.5, 2.0 to 2.5, 3.0, 5.0 cm, respectively. Prickly sida did not emerge from depths greater than 5.0 cm.

Plant Spacing

I have grown Sida acuta with 12" spacings for the last two years with good success, but next year's planting with be somewhat closer, or interplanted with some other crop. With good fertilization and average soil, this year's crop grew straight up 2-4 feet, before beginning to fall over and add additional side branches. I was unhappy at how exposed the soil was throughout this prolonged spiky stage. If repeating this spacing, I will intercrop something to cover the soil. I have tried Medicinal calendulas and purslane, which I find a bit too aggressive. Will try moth beans next year.

Another alternative is to grow them much closer. My "Sida jungle" had spacings in the ½-2" range (average just under 1") and produced a greater mass of leaves on many smaller plants. The leaves tend to be much lighter in color. The dense planting shaded the soil much better. Purslane found it difficult to get established. One by-product of this approach will be constant production of 4-foot plants with no side-branches, providing some very long useful fiber. I find it easiest to start Sida acuta seeds in flats on 2" centers.

Sida acuta   **360**--12-15",   **699**-1.5 live seeds per square foot.

Sida cordifolia

612-after emerging out, seedlings of 7-14 days old are transplanted in a space of 75 x 85cm in the field,   **703**--15-18 in. (38-45 cm)--18-24 in. (45-60 cm), **726**--15-18 in. (38-45 cm)--18-24 in. (45-60 cm).

Sida rhombifolia   **360**-24-36",   **726**--24-36 in. (60-90 cm).

Sida cordata   703-15-18 in. (38-45 cm) - 18-24 in. (45-60 cm).

Sida hermaphrodita

479--various spacing of plant rows: plot 1 where spacing between rows of plants was 0.75 m and plot 2 where spacing between the rows was 0.5 m.

Germination/Light

I refer you to the Seed Dormancy listing for additional information on germination – it was hard to differentiate these two categories.   Light is strongly attenuated as the depth in the ground increases, and species with small seeds generally require light for germination. **[516]**

Sida acuta

306--of all 50 seed lots, S. acuta had the highest percentage of seedlings emerging under shade in each of the last 3 years. Sida acuta germ percentage was 2%, soft seed 2%, hard seed 0%, dead seed 9%. Total germination (1983-88): full sun 39%, shade 17%-- seed grown in the sun germinated for 3 years- seed grown in the shade germinated all 5 years (1% last year).

Sida cordifolia

488-sunny,   665-best germination procedure for Sida cordifolia=12 hr. Refrigerator (5-7° C) and 12 hr. oven (100° C)= 69% germination in 20 days. Longer in oven and the percentage germination becomes very low,   198-in growing conditions, the seeds buried in the ground and protected from light increase their potential and their germination rate over time.

Sida rhombifolia

188- seeds germinated in higher rates at the constant temperature of 35°C or alternating temperatures of 25-35°C.   198-absence of light favored germination and growth speed index. Seeds buried in the ground and protected from light increase their potential and their germination rate over time,   198-reported average germination of only 22% in light and 20.8% in the dark, with no statistically differ, indicating neutral photoblastism. Germination obtained at 25 ° C was only 2% and 1% in the dark in the light and was elevated up to 60% with increasing temperature to 35 ° C.,   404-light did not influence the germination of arrowleaf sida or prickly sida, 516-brightness is not a limiting factor for germination of S. rhombifolia. (Vieira, 2007),   518-light did not influence the germination,   671-seed company- should germinate within a few days.

Sida alba

404-results show that a 30% shade environment (30% constant shade and 30% shade following 14 days of no shade) would favor both prickly sida biomass accumulation and seed production. The ability of prickly sida to readily tolerate 30% shade would account for its competitiveness with crops early in the growing season and its ability to recover from early season

457

herbicide injury. Prickly sida was also able to reproduce when exposed to 90% shade season long [?] Light did not influence the germination of arrowleaf sida or prickly sida,   **518**-no measurable effect,   **673**-light was not a requirement for germination in this temperature range. However, when scarified prickly sida seeds were maintained at day/night temperature regimes of 15/6 and 20/10 C, germination was greater in the dark than in the light.

Water Need

Sida acuta

107-can tolerate dry as well as high rainfall conditions,   **648**-this study clearly demonstrated significantly increased plant height, leaves and higher biomass under high soil fertility and frequent irrigation interval, and low plant density...maintained fitness at all irrigation regimes.

{I left a six pack of small Sida acuta plants in the office for five days without watering and they were ok}

Sida cordifolia

488-watering during Autumn/Winter=rarely (when substrate is dry), Watering during hot season=regularly but without excess, especially during summer,   **612**-Plenty of water is not required for its cultivation,   **702**-the soil should remain relatively moist,   **703**-drought-tolerant; suitable for xeriscaping,   **721**-Medium to wet.

Sida rhombifolia   671-seed company-drought tender- well drained soils.

Fertilization

My Sida acuta crop last year only received light fertilization in not very good soil; in one bed the leaves were very thin and tiny, in another bed the leaves were much larger. Testing both beds that winter showed no nitrogen left in the soi in either bedl. This year with improved soil in the beds and generous dose of 12-12-12 fertilizer the plants are robust but the leaves are if anything smaller. There is ample evidence that fertilization does not particularly affect growth or harvest, but medicinal production seems to benefit from fertilization.

Sida acuta

648--this study clearly demonstrated that Sida acuta exhibited significantly increased plant height, leaves and higher biomass under high soil fertility and frequent irrigation interval, and low plant density,   **699**-Commercial Sida grower: We recommend using 10 lb. 10-10-10 fertilizer per 1,000 sq. ft. at planting and then side dressing with that much or more every year in May.

458

The protein level and digestibility increases dramatically with fertilization and commonly analyses come back at around 40% CP! Incidentally, it is also higher in calcium and phosphorus (critical for antler development) than iron clay peas, soybeans or alfalfa... do not apply lime where you plan to establish Sweet Tea as it has a serious aversion to limestone.

Sida cordifolia

488--fertilizer during growth=regularly but with spacing...Substrate=1 soil+2 humus,   **612**--for a hectare of land, 20-25 tons FYM for low fertile and 15-18 tons for moderately fertile soil are essential. Green manuring is effective where irrigation facilities are available. Groundnut cake, bone-meal, rapeseed cake and vermi-composting are beneficial for better growth of the plant. Neem oil is recommended to remove mites and nematodes from the fields, **721**-apply any organic fertilizer.

Sida rhombifolia

291-invitro-homeopathic dilutions of Cymbopogon winterianus (citronella) improved germination and growth of seedlings of Sida,   **512**-two levels of fertilization (0 and 150 kg ha-1 of formulation 00-20-20 (N-P-K)). Fertilization did not affect the weed community...Sida rhombifolia being (among) the most prominent at all levels of fertilization....Weed interference reduced peanut productivity between 31 and 34% for both the fertilized area and the area without fertilization, respectively....The density of (S. rhombifolia) was higher in the non-fertilized area, but there was no difference in dry matter accumulation between areas {S. rhombifolia grew better and competed better without fertilization}.

Sida indica

638-as the base fertilizer, NPK (25-15-0) was added at the rate of 60 kg ha-1 during soil preparation, and the different experimental fertilizer applications, 100 kg ha-1 CAN (26% N) and 100 kg ha-1 NPK (10-10-40)--Based on the data obtained from the field trial, there were no significant differences in the plant height of S. indica between fertilizer applications. The highest plant height value was obtained from the CAN application in the first year, while in the second year, it was obtained from NPK.   The growth characteristics are all close to each other. The CAN increased leaf yield and seed yield about 20%, NPK somewhat less. {Obviously it likes N},   **686**-the base fertilizer, NPK (25-15-0) was added at the rate of 60 kg ha-1 during soil preparation, and the different experimental fertilizer applications, 100 kg ha-1 CAN (calcium ammonium nitrate - 26% N) and 100 kg ha-1 NPK (10-10-40), were applied to the plots-the results were compared to a control group in which no fertilizer was used,   **686**-when leaves grown on CAN- and NPK-treated and control soils were compared, the control leaf extract showed the highest DPPH radical scavenging activity at all of the studied concentrations. Among the fertilizer applications, leaves treated with NPK showed higher DPPH scavenging activity than leaves treated with CAN. When roots treated with CAN and NPK and the control were compared, the CAN and NPK root extracts showed higher DPPH scavenging activities than the control root extract.

Sida hermaphrodita

473-nitrogen treatment did not influence density, but it increased height of plants. A larger quantity and height of stems was observed after using a higher dose of Phosphorus. Virginia fanpetal biomass yield was not affected by different amounts of Nitrogen applied, whereas more intensive Phosphorus treatment resulted in increased biomass yield.

Harvest

I must admit to being a bit spooked by the S. cordifolia table below. Since my growing season is about 7 months, and if my Sida acuta acted the same as Sida cordifolia, I would be missing the real harvest by one month. Does this schedule apply to other Sidas? Are their periods of greatest potency as narrow in time? Another study suggests an annual harvest of Sida cordifolia. Sida rhombifolia is133 days to harvest. What I do know is that even my early harvests of Sida acuta, say at 90 days, have had good medicinal properties, but I now intend to compare early and late harvests.

Almost all sources use dried Sida parts for tincturing. I have found good success with tincturing fresh leaves and other parts. I generally leave the roots for separate processing, and often they end up dry by the time I get to them.

A WWF (World Wide Fund for Nature) report estimates that over two thirds of the 50,000 medicinal plants in use today are still harvested from the wild, from which 4,000–10,000 may now be endangered **[468]** Generally, whole plants of Sida are harvested, including the roots. Handling after harvest Sida species are mostly used fresh, but can also be dried for storage. **[362]**

Sida acuta

There is no published information about harvesting Sida acuta. What we do know is that millions of people every day go out into the tropical wild and simply pick a bunch of leaves for a tea. My approach has been to begin harvesting leaves when the plant begins to sprout side branches. There usually are a few very large leaves; I call them the "come browse me" leaves. I always pick those. And then any old looking leaves. After that maybe do a little thinning. This plant is made for heavy browsing. The leaves picked fresh are nicely tasteless and make a good potherb (20%+ protein – mine are at least 30%).

I harvest the seed when the seed capsule turns dark brown to black and opens. I carefully pinch the seed pod and it crumbles the seed into my pinched fingers. If it doesn't then the seeds are not ready. Hold it too loosely and you will lose the seed. Another method that works for me is to take a deep bottle and push a cluster of Sida seed capsules into it and roughly rub them all with your fingers.

The ripe seed will mostly fall into the container, while the green seed is pretty resistant to picking.

The seeds have sharp point so be careful – you might want to consider gloves. I find it best to harvest the seeds separately. The seed pods when wet do not as easily come apart.

Sida cordifolia

358-In tropical Africa Sida cordifolia is nowadays only collected from the wild and usually whole plants are harvested, including the roots.   **413**-the maximum root yield and ephedrine content were recorded at eight months after planting and further delay in harvesting showed a sharp decline in both root yield and ephedrine content. The results indicated Sida cordifolia preferred open condition for higher root yield and ephedrine content and the optimum stage of harvest is eight months after planting,   **612**-after one year of plantation, the crop is ready for harvest.

Effect of harvesting stage of Sida cordifolia on ephedrine content and ephedrine yield. Grown in full sun

Harvest at:	Fresh root yield (kg ha-1)	Ephedrine yield (%)	
6 months	594	0.0006	
7 months	1199	0.0045	
8 months	1528	0.2859	
9 months	899	0.0879	
10 months	814	0.0238	**[413]**

Sida rhombifolia

358-Harvesting of Sida rhombifolia is mostly done from the wild- Extraction of the fiber is difficult, but these problems should be easily overcome through experimentation. In the Central African Republic the stems are left to dry for 10–12 days and retting in water takes another 20 days. In South Africa the leaves are preserved by drying before storing to be consumed later as a vegetable.   **465**-from weed transplantation or emergence to plant harvesting at weed pre-flowering stage: 133 days.

Sida indica

638-the seed extracts grown on CAN and NPK soil had higher phenolic compound contents (15.1 and 20.5 mg GAE g-1 dry extract, respectively) than the control seed extract, and similarly, when the root extracts were compared, the CAN and NPK treatments yielded higher phenolic contents (41.8 and 46.1 mg GAE g-1 dry extract, respectively) than the control root extract. However, among the leaf extracts, the control leaf extract had a higher phenolic content (56.9 mg GAE g-1 dry extract) than the CAN and NPK leaf extracts...(NPK, 10-10-40) and calcium ammonium nitrate (CAN, 26% N)

Sida as Weed

Sida acuta

52-once the plant becomes established, it is very competitive, holding and denying sites to other plants, **65**-showed better growth and DM production in the sun but was very susceptible to competition especially intraspecific competition, **278**-a serious weed species in the Northern Territory is Sida acuta, a perennial weed of improved pastures.

Sida cordifolia

161-considered an invasive weed in Africa, Australia, the southern United States, Hawaiian Islands, New Guinea, and French Polynesia.

Sida rhombifolia

512-the density of weeds was higher in the non-fertilized area, but there was no difference in dry matter accumulation between areas.

Sida indica

698-Most of the information available on S. indica is related to its pharmacological properties, its phytochemistry or the ethnobotanical uses. Although literature reports it as a weed and/or as invasive for some countries or regions, not much information is available about its negative impacts. No information is available on the impacts on the native species or the habitats where it is reported as invasive. On the contrary, it is reported as being threatened because it is over-harvested in some countries. There is also conflicting information about it being native or introduced for some countries, as it is listed as both in different sources for a country. Information about the environmental requirements, reproductive biology, habitats and impacts is scarce or lacking, and needed for a thoughtful evaluation of the invasiveness of the species.

Sida alba

517--competition from 2 weeks after cotton emergence until harvest by prickly sida at 64 plants/12 m, reduced yields. prickly sida competition 4 to 6 weeks after cotton emergence until harvest did not reduce the seed cotton yields, **722**-this is primarily a weed of fields and gardens that is rarely observed in high-quality natural habitats.

....

Cultivation of Sida rhombifolia as a fibre crop has been taken up in several countries, few details have been published. Along the river Niger it is cultivated after retreat of flood-waters. In the Central African Republic it is planted as a border crop in arable fields and the crop cycle is 4.5–5 months. **[358]**

Attracts Butterflies, Bees, Birds

All Sidas

604--Illinois-Sida spp.-invivo-food source-migratory shorebirds-Plants composed 35% of the aggregate weight of food found in spring migrating blue-winged teal.   **654**--however, in all three Sida species (Sida acuta, S. cordata and S. cordifolia), the flowers without perceptible smell are yellow, shed pollen during the forenoon period, provide landing platform and offer traces of nectar that is covered by thin hairs at the base of sepals. With these characteristics, the Sida species attract bees, wasps and butterflies to their flowers as soon as they are open in the morning and the foragers collect the forage with great ease for a brief period due to closure of the petals by noon. The bees use these plants as principal pollen source while wasps and butterflies use them as nectar source during which they contact the anthers and stigmas and pollinate the flowers. Since nectar is produced in traces at flower and even plant level, these insects in a quest for nectar move quickly from flower to flower within and between populations and in effect, promote cross-pollination... Nevertheless, Sida species with their huge population size and profuse flowering during the wet season are potential pollen and nectar sources for all these honey bees. Honey bees also collect Sida pollen voraciously and deposit it in their hives. Ceratina bees, small carpenter bees, also gather pollen for use in brood development. The pollen contains the same amino acids in all three Sida species. The pollen grains are sources of six essential amino acids: threonine, valine, methionine, iso-leucine, lysine, and phenylalanine, and eight non-essential amino acids: alanine, aspartic acid, cysteine, cysteine, glutamic acid, hydroxyproline, proline, and serine. DeGroot (1953) reported that honey bees require ten essential amino acids, six out of which are present in the pollen of these plants, plus some non-essential amino acids. The pollen also has a small amount of protein content. It is thus nutritionally important. Therefore, these bees use Sida species as important pollen sources and their pollen collecting activity.

Sida acuta

360-yes,   **658**-field study-The Simpson diversity index values for both woody and herbaceous plant species are indications of high diversity of forage species for honeybees...Sida acuta ranks high among all bee plants in Nigeria...utilized very frequently (by bees),   **660**-field study-bees-Floral Sucrose Content.-Volume/mm 17.7 (range 3.2-36)--% Mass sucrose concentration=11.7 (range 10.2-33.8),   **697**-India-Nectar and host to butterflies.   {The sharp points on the seeds discourage birds from harvesting, but they seem to hang out around the plants anyhow.}

Sida cordifolia   **703**-this plant is attractive to bees, butterflies and/or birds.

....

Many plants screened for their antimicrobial activities showed interesting results with very low MIC and MBC values. **[215-2007]**

Sida rhombifolia

360-yes, **487**-field observation-aerial parts-several types use the Sida family as hosts, S rhombifolia in particular with Pyrgus oileus, **635**-invivo-bee plant-apifauna, **697**-India-Nectar and host to butterflies.

Sida carpinfolia   **635**-invivo-bee plant-apifauna.

Sida alba

692-field study-aerial parts-the flowers attract various bees, including bumblebees, little carpenter bees, and Halictid bees, as well as small to medium-sized butterflies and skippers...The foliage is not known to be toxic and it may be eaten occasionally by mammalian herbivores.

Cultivation Narrative

This section contains paragraph-length narratives that contain a greater depth of information on a given Sida. Only some Sidas have additional information, and of those, only certain categories had additional information. This section also contains listings from the Categories that were too unique to be included there.

Sida acuta

December, 2015   A vicious cold snap has killed my over-wintering Sida acuta plants! The supposed lowest temperature Sida can take is somewhere between freezing and 20° F. We got down into the mid-20s and the plants seemed to be weathering it until a sharply cold wind and its wind chill dropped the temperature to a killing low. These were all next to a warm rock wall but that was not enough. The only plant that survived was around a corner protected from the wind. Sida survives some freezing but do not expect more than that.

Nov 31, 2016   There have been a few days now that hovered right at freezing. Daytime temps since last week have dropped to the 50s, but the Sida is still doing well. Some plants have added some bigger leaves (what I call the "attract the deer leaves"). The tomato plants are long gone, as well as the squash, basil, and other summer plants, but the Sida has maintained, and even shown some growth in the past week.

May, 2017   The soil has to warm up. There were no Sida sprouts until late May, when we discovered maybe 400 sprouts in one bed. There were only a few sprouts in the other bed and the 5 gallon cans (probably because they had inadequate ground cover to protect the seeds). This bed had much scantier growth and tiny leaves, but produced a zillion sprouts. My guess is that this bed was overgrown with weeds in the Winter that protected the young sprouts from depredation in Spring. Either that or they like fertilizer-starved soil to sprout.

Also this is the third year that there has been no re-growth from any roots. I can only assume that our cold and wet winters rot the young roots.

Protein Content %:   **359**—seed 23.2,   **699**—leaf analyses come back at around 40% CP!

Oil Content of Seeds: 359--16.8%

Perennial?:   **293**- Sida is perennial on moist refugia near the coast, especially in irrigated gardens and orchards near Darwin (topical northern Australia), around farm dams and on the fringes of sub-coastal swamps, **699**-perennial and will come back from the roots every spring,   **299**-usually behaves as an annual in northern Australia, although it is occasionally perennial on moist sites.

Growth Management: **699**-Sida acuta is a very fibrous, tough, almost woody plant, which is one reason why it tolerates browsing so well. This can also make mowing difficult so if you decide to mow, make sure to have a sharp blade, get your RPM's up and take it slow. Afterwards we recommend sweeping off your tires if you don't want to spread the seed. Mowing to 12" will return it to a vegetative state, producing more browse for deer well into the fall.

Miscellaneous Observations

Sida acuta is a taproot and perennial shrub, native of central America but today it is found throughout the tropical world. The plant is frequently found in pastures, cultivated lands, roadsides and lawns. Sida acuta is found on most soil types, except seasonally flooded clays or soils derived from limestone. It competes vigorously with other plant species, but does best in distributed habitats in tropical or sub-tropical regions with distinct wet and dry season. **[270]**

(American South) It is adaptive to a wide range of soils except calcareous soils (soils derived from limestone) and seasonally flooded clays. It also does not persist in wet soils for very long. Generally the soil should be fairly well-drained. Do not apply lime where you plan to establish Sweet Tea as it has a serious aversion to limestone. It readily germinates along shady edges of food plots where there is fresh organic matter like leaf litter or pine straw. In these areas you can just shake it out directly onto the ground and slightly work it through the litter and into the soil with a garden rake. We are getting excellent results by shaking the seeds right into dead grass or weeds. The dead weeds or grass provide a mulching effect and protect the small seedling. Once it emerges through the weeds it will take off. **[699]**

(Sida acuta) exhibited significantly increased plant height, leaves and higher biomass under high soil fertility and frequent irrigation interval, and low plant density, this trend was similar to earlier report. This might be as a result of the availability of nutrients, water and space, and also less competition... irrigation interval. S. acuta maintained fitness at all irrigation regimes... patterns of plasticity in S. acuta could be said to be an example of an idealized scenario: "Master-of-some" better able to increase fitness in favourable environments.. the interactions of soil fertility and plant density showed mean values for both species decreased with increase in plant density. The decreased ratio of height in high soil fertility – low plant density, compared to low soil fertility – low plant density, was 66% for S. acuta. This indicates significant plasticity... biomass allocation pattern of S. acuta allocates more to roots and leaves... In the case of S. acuta increasing plant density from 3 to 5 plants in low-fertility soil and from 5 to 10 plants per pot in high-fertility soil significantly reduced stem height and number of leaves. While stem girth of S. acuta was significantly not influenced by varying plant density regardless of soil fertility status... stem height varied with varying soil fertility status, and recorded significantly higher stem height in high soil fertility and 2-day irrigation interval. [648]

(Sida acuta) Seeds were placed on the soil surface under either full sunlight or artificial shade transmitting 10% sunlight.... In all seed lots, except for Sida acuta under shade, over 50% of all seedling emergence occurred in the first year and, for most seed lots, over 80% of emergence. No seedling emergence occurred in the fourth and fifth years in full sunlight whereas there were still low levels of seedling emergence under shade... The species with the highest emergence under shade in the final year was Sida acuta. This would be expected in view of previous studies showing that a considerable proportion of S. acuta seed could remain viable after a full year's exposure on the soil surface in the Northern Territory (Australia) [306]

Seeds of Sida acuta and S. rhombifolia from West Bengal, India, were sun-dried and stored in perforated plastic bags in 30-40% relative humidity at 28 ± 1°C for 1-3 years to study the dormancy behaviour of both fresh and chronologically aged seeds. Freshly harvested seeds exhibited only 4 and 8% germination, respectively, at 35°C in the dark. In preliminary tests, only about 4 and 8% imbibed water prior to germination and the rest of the seeds remained unimbibed. Seed coat imposed dormancy could be removed through conventional dormancy-breaking methods i.e. scarification of the seed coats with concentrated sulfuric acid and alternate high and low temperature treatment and also partially with pyridine (a nonpolar solvent). Chronological aging (after-ripening) under laboratory conditions could not overcome dormancy in S. acuta and S. rhombifolia even after 3 years due to the hard seed coat whereas permeability of aged seeds of both species increased. Elevated leakage of electrolytes was observed in aged seeds than freshly harvested seeds while aged seed germination did not improve for both species. Microscopic analysis of dry seeds revealed no opening in the chalazal region even after 3 years of aging whereas imbibed seeds, regardless of age, had a distinct opening in the chalazal region prior to germination. [81]

Sida cordifolia

Repot every year if possible. [488]   Roots-5-15 cm long with few lateral roots of smaller size. The tap roots are generally branched at the tip. The outer surface of the root is off-yellow to grayish yellow. [118]   Warm as well as moist conditions throughout the year are also preferable for good growth of the plant. Weed the crop at intervals of 20-30 days. [612]

466

Sunlight: Full sun

Soil: well-drained soil

Water: Medium to wet

Temperature: 25F

Fertilizer: Apply any organic fertilizer

Dependable blooms: six to eight hours of direct sunlight a day. **[721]**

Bloom Characteristics: Attractive to bees, butterflies and/or birds.

Water Requirements: Drought-tolerant; suitable for xeriscaping.

Height: 18-24 in. (45-60 cm) - 24-36 in. (60-90 cm)

Spacing: 15-18 in. (38-45 cm) - 18-24 in. (45-60 cm) **[703]**

Hardiness:

USDA Zone 8a: to -12.2 °C (10 °F)

USDA Zone 8b: to -9.4 °C (15 °F)

USDA Zone 9a: to -6.6 °C (20 °F)

USDA Zone 9b: to -3.8 °C (25 °F)

USDA Zone 10a: to -1.1 °C (30 °F)

USDA Zone 10b: to 1.7 °C (35 °F)

USDA Zone 11: above 4.5 °C (40 °F)

Sun Exposure: Full Sun, Sun to Partial Shade

Propagation Methods: From seed; direct sow after last frost

Self-sows freely;   deadhead to stop volunteer seedlings next season. **[703]**

Harvest (Root)   The optimum stage of harvest is eight months after planting. Under a shaded situation, higher root yield was noticed at fourteen months after planting and the yield was very low compared to that under open situation. The maximum root yield and ephedrine content were recorded at eight months after planting and further delay in harvesting showed a sharp decline in both root yield and ephedrine content. The results indicated Sida cordifolia preferred open condition for higher root yield and ephedrine. **[413]**   After one year of plantation, the crop is ready for harvest. **[612]**

Plant Protection   Neem oil is recommended to remove mites and nematodes from the fields. **[612]**

Sida cordifolia cultivation:

Substrate: 1 soil+2 humus,

Temp during winter: min 17° C,
Lighting=sunny,

Watering during Autumn/Winter: rarely (when substrate is dry),

Hot season watering: egularly, without excess, esp. during summer

Fertilizer during growth: regularly
but with spacing,

Pruning: no pruning,

Repotting: repot every year if possible   **[488]**

Miscellaneous Observations

A well-drained sandy-loam to clay-loam soil rich in humus is suitable for cultivation of this plant. The plant grows well in tropical and sub-tropical climate but the growth in tropical region is better... 'Bala' can be grown both from the seeds and by stem cuttings. The plants propagated from stem cuttings flower earlier than those of seed propagation. In case of seed propagation, one-year-old dormant seeds are either directly sown in the field in-situ or in nursery bed. After emerging out, seedlings 7-14 days old are transplanted into a space of 75 x 85cm in the field. In vegetative propagation, the stem cuttings obtained from lateral stems are used. Beside these the propagation is also reported from tissue culture practices. Multiple shoot formation from mature nodal explants of 'Bala' on MS medium supplemented with 2.0 mg 1-1,6- benzyl amino-purine, 0.5 mg 1-1α naphthalene acidic acid, 1.0 mg 1-1 adenine sulfate and10% (v/v) coconut milk are reported. In this method, multiple shoots are initiated within 21st day and each explant is capable of inducing formation of more than twenty shoots. The regenerated plants are induced for rooting and plantlets are introduced in soil. This material may be useful for germplasm conservation and genetic improvement of 'Bala'. The land is repeatedly ploughed to a fine tilth and weeds, pebbles etc. are removed. For a hectare of land, 20-25 tons FYM for low fertile and 15-18 tons for moderately fertile soil are essential. Green manuring is effective where irrigation facilities are available. Groundnut cake, bone-meal, rapeseed cake and vermi-composting are beneficial for better growth of the plant.... The seedlings should be transplanted in a space of 75 x85 cm in the field. Plenty of water is not required for its cultivation. **[612]**

Sida cordifolia as Sida fallax (Hawaii)

Stratton et al recommends soaking the cleaned seed in hot or room temperature water for 1 to 24 hours. Criley recommends either a 24-hour soak or scarification. Plant the seeds in a well drained mix such as 3 parts perlite to 1 part sterile potting soil or 3 parts #2 perlite to 1 part Sunshine Mix #4. Keep the medium moist until germination. Place them in a shady covered location to maintain soil moisture and control rain damage. Can also be germinated in full sun if adequate soil moisture is maintained. Germination time is erratic and can take from 10 days to 3 months. (Mew gives germination time of 3 to 8 months.) Germination rates are also extremely variable. **[722]**

Propagation by Cuttings: Sida fallax can be grown from cuttings. Criley recommends using a rooting hormone of 2,000 parts per million (ppm) indolebutyric acid (IBA) in either a liquid or a talc dust form. He suggests either 1 part coarse perlite to 1 part vermiculite or 100% vermiculite as a rooting medium and rooting the cuttings under 30% shade. He cautions, however, that extremely wet conditions, such as often found when using intermittent misting systems, causes leaf drop and poor rooting. Boche reports 85% success rate using stem and tip cuttings grown in 50% shade using a medium of 3 parts peat moss to 1 part vermiculite. Stratton reports 80 to 90% success rates from cuttings but does not detail the procedures used. **[722]**

Harvesting seed: The small brown to black seeds of Sida fallax are contained in pale brown to black capsules. Sida fallax grows easily from seed. To remove the seeds from the capsule, air-dry them at room temperature in a bowl or paper bag. Carefully rub the capsules through a strainer with the appropriate size mesh. The seeds should fall through leaving the debris in the strainer. Seeds can be stored after being cleaned and air dried. Place them in a paper bag or envelope and put them in an airtight container with desiccant. Stratton suggests storing the dried seeds in a cool place at 25% relative humidity. Yoshinaga's tests indicate that seeds stored at 39° F and 10% humidity retained some viability for 2 years. **[722]**

Medicinal qualities: The species has been equated with Bala, one of the most celebrated medicines of Ayurveda... During a survey of different drug markets in the country, most commercial samples were found to be a mixture of other species of Sida, viz. *Sida acuta, Sida cordata* and *Sida rhombifolia* and these were being sold under the same vernacular name 'Bala' by many pharmaceutical companies. Sometimes, because of the non-availability of the roots, the whole plant (95% aerial parts) were also being sold and used as 'Bala'. Domestication and commercialization of cultivation is one of the area to secure the medicinal plant supply of the required quantity to the pharmaceutical companies. Due to high demand of the crop in ayurvedic industry, cultivation has to be encouraged to satisfy the demand. The biosynthesis of secondary metabolites although controlled genetically, is affected strongly by environmental influences. Hence it is necessary to study the reaction of *Sida cordifolia* to light intensity and to find out the optimum harvesting stage for maximum root yield and quality. This would help to supply uniform quality roots of *Sida cordifolia* according to market demand. **[413]**

Sida rhombifolia

Flower Color: pale yellow

Ecology: Attracts Butterflies

Foliage Duration: annual

Growth Habit: sub-shrub

Propagation Culture: space 24-36" apart

Size: 24-36" tall

Soil Minimum pH: 4.5

Soil Maximum pH: 8.5

Sun Exposure: full sun

Temperature Cold Hardiness: 9a   **[360]**

Osmotic Stress   404--an osmotic stress of 400 kPa reduced arrowleaf sida germination,   518--germinated from 0 to 800 kPa, and an osmotic stress of 400 kPa was necessary to reduce germination.

Harvest   358-In the Central African Republic it is planted as a border crop in arable fields and the crop cycle is 4.5–5 months,   465-(It takes) 133 days from weed transplantation or emergence to plant harvesting at weed pre-flowering stage.

Miscellaneous Observations

The highest germination levels of seeds soaked in water for 24 hours was 30% **[466]**   A native of Asia, it prefers light to medium, well drained soils in an open, sunny position, and is drought- and frost-tender. A very hardy and fast-growing plant. Propagation is by seeds or cuttings. Sow seed 5mm deep in moist but well-drained seed mix. Should germinate within a few days. **[671]** Absence of light favored germination and germination speed index **[198]** Homeopathic dilutions of Cymbopogon winterianus (citronella) improved germination and growth of seedlings of Sida. **[291]**   Less sensitive to seasonal variations, and the highest percentages of emergence occurred between 1 and 4 cm depths. **[189-live planting in greenhouse]**

The majority of the seeds are dormant for 12–24 months after maturity. Germination was 8% at a temperature of 35°C and was increased to 62% by a hot water (80°C) pretreatment of 10 minutes followed by a cold water (5°C) pretreatment of 10 minutes. Treatment of seed by soaking for 25 minutes in H2SO4 resulted in a germination of 100%. The optimum temperature range for germination is 25–35°C. **[358]**   Seeds germinated in higher rates at the constant temperature of 35°C or alternating ones that included 35°C in the treatment. Daily alternating temperatures of 25-35°C were used in light at a radiating intensity of 40 to 60 μmol.m-2.s-1. **[188]**   Germination occurred at 35°C, but did not germinate at 40°C. Less than 50% of seeds were viable at 45°C after 21 days of exposure. Exhibited more than 75% germination at a range of pH from 5.0 to 8.0. Germinated from 0 to 800 kPa-- emergence was equivalent at planting depths of 0.5–2.0 cm, with declining emergence below 2.0 cm. Did not emerge from depths exceeding 5.0 cm. Light did not influence the germination. **[404]**

Maximum arrowleaf sida (Sida rhombifolia L.) germination occurred at 35°C, whereas prickly sida (Sida spinosa L.) germinated to the same extent at 35 or 40°C. Arrowleaf sida germinated better than prickly sida at 20 and 25°C, but did not germinate at 40°C. Less than 50% of seed from both species were viable at 45°C after 21 days of exposure. Both species exhibited more than 75% germination at a range of pH from 5.0 to 8.0. Arrowleaf sida germinated to a greater extent than prickly sida from 0 to −800 kPa, and an osmotic stress of −200 kPa reduced prickly sida germination, whereas −400 kPa was

470

necessary to reduce arrowleaf sida germination. Prickly sida emergence was optimal at a planting depth of 0.5 cm, and declined rapidly at deeper planting depths. However, arrowleaf sida emergence was equivalent at planting depths of 0.5–2.0 cm, with declining emergence below 2.0 cm. Neither species emerged from depths exceeding 5.0 cm. Light did not influence the germination of arrowleaf sida or prickly sida. [518]

Propagation and planting = The majority of the seeds of Sida rhombifolia are dormant for 12–24 months after maturity. Germination was 8% at a temperature of 35°C and was increased to 62% by a hot water (80°C) pretreatment of 10 minutes followed by a cold water (5°C) pretreatment of 10 minutes. Treatment of seed by soaking for 25 minutes in H2SO4 resulted in a germination of 100%. The optimum temperature range for germination is 25–35°C. [362]

Fertilization (0 and 150 kg ha-1 of formulation 00-20-20 (N-P-K)) had no effect... Sida rhombifolia being (among) the most prominent weeds at all levels of fertilization.... Weed interference reduced peanut productivity between 31 and 34% for both the fertilized area and the area without fertilization, respectively.... The density of (S. rhombifolia) was higher in the non-fertilized area, but there was no difference in dry matter accumulation between areas. [512]

Sida indica

Water Requirements: Needs consistently moist soil; do not let dry out

Where to Grow: Suitable for growing in containers

Height: 4-6 ft. (1.2-1.8 m)

Spacing: 36-48 in. (90-120 cm) - 4-6 ft. (1.2-1.8 m)

Hardiness: USDA Zone 10a to Zone 11

Sun Exposure: Full Sun

Danger: Handling plant may cause skin irritation or allergic reaction

Foliage: Grown for foliage, Velvet/Fuzzy-Textured

Soil pH requirements: 6.6 to 7.5 (neutral)

Propagation Methods: Herbaceous stem cuttings, softwood cuttings

From seed: Sow indoors before last frost

Seed Collecting: Allow pods to dry on plant; break open to collect seeds... Allow seed heads to dry on plants; remove and collect seeds... Properly cleaned, seed can be successfully stored

Distribution: This plant has been said to grow in Mesa, Arizona; Alameda, California; Salina, Kansas   **[727]**

Absolute minimum temperature: 7°C

Mean maximum temperature of hottest month: 43°C

Mean minimum temperature of coldest month: 10°C

Soil drainage: free

Soil reaction:	alkaline, neutral	
Soil texture:	light	
Special soil tolerances:	saline	**[698]**

Miscellaneous Observations

As the base fertilizer, NPK (25-15-0) was added at the rate of 60 kg ha-1 during soil preparation, and the different experimental fertilizer applications, 100 kg ha-1 CAN (26% N) and 100 kg ha-1 NPK (10-10-40), were applied to the plots. In both years, the plants ripened after 90-100 days following the spring sowing and were then harvested twice a week until the end of the season.... Based on the data obtained from the field trial, there were no significant differences in the plant height of S. indica between fertilizer applications. The highest plant height value was obtained from the CAN application in the first year, while in the second year, it was obtained from NPK. {the growth characteristics are all close to each other. The CAN increased leaf yield and seed yield about 20%, NPK somewhat less. Obviously it likes N} **[638]**

Seeds will germinate best if you soak them overnight before you sow them, barely covering them with the seed-starting mix. I've found that they usually sprout within 9 days if they are going to do so... Northern gardeners growing these "maples" as houseplants should keep them sunlit and chilly during the winter, preferably at temperatures in the 50s Fahrenheit. **[726]**

Germinated to the same extent at 35 or 40°C. Less than 50% of seed were viable at 45°C after 21 days of exposure. Exhibited more than 75% germination at a range of pH from 5.0 to 8.0. Emergence was optimal at a planting depth of 0.5 cm, and did not emerge from depths exceeding 5.0 cm. Light did not influence the germination. An osmotic stress of 200 kPa reduced germination. **[404]**

Storage at 35° C for 12 weeks or longer, resulted in greater than 90% germination. Puncturing the seed coat over the radicle or cotyledon allowed for water imbibition of all hard seed, but the puncture over the radicle promoted greater than 90% germination. Has been observed to germinate in the field from April through September in north central Kentucky; suggesting that water permeability of seeds increases throughout the year. Also capable of germination under limited soil moisture. After 96 hours of incubation, germination and radicle length were unaffected by osmotic pressures of 0, -300, and -600 kPa. Some seed germinated at an osmotic pressure of -1000 kPa. Smith et al. (1992) reported significant reduction in prickly sida germination when osmotic stress of -200 kPa was imposed for 2 weeks, and seed germination was inhibited when osmotic stress exceeded -600 kPa. Soil pH range of 5.0 to 8.0 did not affect prickly sida germination. Prickly sida emergence of 80% was noted when seeds were planted at a 0.5 cm depth, while only 60, 50, 40, and 20% emergence was observed at depths of 1 to 1.5, 2.0 to 2.5, 3.0, 5.0 cm, respectively. Prickly sida did not emerge from depths greater than 5.0 cm. Optimum temperatures for prickly sida germination occur from 30 to 40° C. Light was not a requirement for germination in this

472

temperature range. When scarified seeds were maintained at day/night temperature regimes of 15/6 and 20/10° C, germination was greater in the dark than in the light. Germination was not promoted by freezing and thawing or by incubation of seed at 5° C. Germination was enhanced by increasing temperature regimes and by subjecting seeds to wet/dry cycles; increasing temperature proved most effective in promoting germination. Both the number of permeable seeds and rate of germination increased with increasing temperatures. Seeds exposed to higher temperatures following a lower temperature regime germinated at greater percentages than those maintained continuously at the higher temperatures. Also, increasing the length of time the seeds remained at the lower temperature before transfer to higher temperatures increased germination. The lower temperature regime seemed to "precondition" the seed for a rapid increase in water permeability. In moist soil, viability of prickly sida seed exposed 1 d to 50° C was reduced to 45% and the seed did not survive 12 hours at 60° C. Seed viability was 21, 4, and less than 1%, after burial for 3.5, 4.5, and 5.5 years, respectively. Depth of burial did not influence prickly sida viability after 30 months; however, viable seed was only found at 8 cm (15%) and 38 cm (1%). **[673]**

Sida hermaphrodita

Field study--High levels of Nitrogen fertilization applied in experiment-- 200 kg ha-1 -- in comparison to a lower dose by half, did not affect plant density significantly. More intensive Phosphorus fertilization (from 39.28 to 52.38 kg ha-1) caused an increment in development of stems by two per 1m-2 in four-year average, that was counted as 20,000 stems per hectare. **[473]**

Stem density and height grew systematically during consecutive years of production. Nitrogen treatment did not influence density, but it increased height of plants. A larger quantity and height of stems was observed after using a higher dose of Phosphorus. Biomass yield was not affected by different amounts of Nitrogen applied, whereas more intensive Phosphorus treatment resulted in increased biomass yield. In the third and fourth years of production an average yield of dry matter of over 11 t·ha-1 was obtained; energy productivity level was 219.5 GJ·ha-1. **[473]**

In case of water deficiency, plants usually are not able to use nutrient elements delivered in mineral fertilizers....   increasing approximately 12 kg·ha-1 dose of Phosphorus resulted in significant rise of yields averaged from four years of research....   certain tendency of increase in yields might be indicated after broadcast of 200 kg·ha-1 of N and 39.28 kg·ha-1 of P, in comparison with the same level of Phosphorus fertilization and lower doses of Nitrogen. **[473]**

Under Polish conditions, other studies on the biology of flowering of S. hermaphrodita showed that as many as 95% of seeds were set... Dormancy-break by heating and by chemical treatment of Sida seeds may occur through disruption of the seed coats. Immediately after the harvest, only 3% of control seeds germinated whereas after 6 months, their germination increased to 14.5–35.5%, but after 1.5 years it decreased. Fresh seeds had the best germination (73%) after immersing into the boiling water; germination capacity decreased along with the water temperature decrease. Water at 70 to 80 °C temperature had the most positive effects on seeds. 81% to 99% of the seeds collected from 10 populations of S. hermaphrodita in Maryland and Ohio germinated, respectively. The average germination for all 10 populations was 92%. **[478]**

In the first set of experiments, the influence of seed dressing on the height of Virginia fanpetals' yields, from the third to fifth year of research (2005–2007) was examined. Seed dressing of Virginia fanpetals led to significant increase in biomass yield (2 tons/hectare) and production of energy per hectare (18.5%), in comparison to the control plot (without dressing). **[474]**

It turns out that it is better to plant root seedlings (in sewage sludge) than to sow seeds, which is proved by the mean values of stems dry mass yield over 3 years... The results indicated that fresh sewage sludge does not provide good conditions for plant sprouting... only a 10% field sprouting ability of the seeds... The root seedlings managed much better in the sludge. Over half of them (52.6%) entered the sprouting phase. **[472]**

Invitro-maximum seed germination of 80% was observed from MS medium sublimated with GA3 2.0 mg/L-treatment with sulfuric acid showed only 50% germination followed by stratification method (moist treatment) which germination was 45% -- Warm, moist treatment enhances after-ripening of seeds with underdeveloped embryos. Warm, moist treated seeds are kept at temperatures of 72 to 86°F (22 to 30°C) for a period of time, usually in moist peat moss, sawdust, or other substrate. **[631]**

Sida As Weed

A weed, in a general sense, is a plant usually wild or feral that is commonly considered to be a nuisance in a garden, lawn, or other agricultural development... Weeds, however, are also helpful to human beings in several ways among which are food, erosion control, medicine, supply of organic matter and mineral nutrients to soil, among others. Recent developments have revealed the importance of weedy species in traditional medicine. For instance, in Kenya, 75 plant species from 34 families are used to cure 59 ailments in traditional medicine of Central Kenya. **[201]** The Sida is a plant native to the Americas, occurring extensively in South America and, to a lesser degree, in the southern United States. **[75]**

Sida acuta

S. acuta is a vigorous competitor in degraded pastures, tree plantations, groundnuts, cereals, root crops, vegetables, planted forests, lawns, roadsides and waste places... with the most serious infestations seen in pastures and rangeland... Its lack of palatability helps enable S. acuta to produce monospecific stands in pasture settings {although I find the leaves pleasantly tasteless, good in salads and as a potherb}... S. acuta is regarded by Holm et al. (1977) as among the 76 most serious weeds of the world. S. acuta was listed as one of 24 top invasive plant candidates for biological control among Pacific Island Countries and Territories... As a perennial weed S. acuta is most commonly recorded as a problem in perennial crops, where it has ample time for full development. Where weed succession advances to later seral stages, its perennial nature gives S. acuta an advantage. However, it establishes and flowers almost as rapidly as an annual and is able therefore to create problems in many crop situations. S. acuta also provides food, shelter and reproductive sites for insect pests of commercial crop plants. {It goes on to list the topical insects it hosts}. **[698]**

Once the plant becomes established, it is very competitive, holding and denying sites to other plants. **[52]** Showed better growth and DM production in the sun but was very susceptible to competition especially intraspecific competition. **[65]** A serious weed species in the Northern Territory {Australia} is Sida acuta, a perennial weed of improved pastures. **[278]**

It was discovered that *Sida acuta* and *Euphorbia heterophylla* were the most common and most abundant {weeds}; and they were found coexisting in all the areas sampled. **[648-Nigeria]**

S. acuta is a weed of plantation crops, cereals, root crops and vegetables throughout the Pacific and South-East Asia. It is a principal weed of maize in Mexico, sorghum in Australia and Thailand, tomatoes in the Philippines, onions in Brazil, and pastures in Australia, Fiji, Nigeria and Papua New Guinea. It is also a weed of tea in Taiwan and Sri Lanka, groundnuts in Ghana, cassava in Ghana and Nigeria, maize in Ghana, Nigeria and Thailand, coconuts in Trinidad, beans in Brazil, pastures under coconuts in Sri Lanka, pineapples in the Philippines, sugarcane and groundnuts in Australia, El Salvador and Trinidad, coffee in Colombia, rubber in Malaysia, upland rice in the Philippines and Nigeria, cotton in El Salvador and Thailand, and cowpeas and sweet potatoes in Nigeria. {It goes on to list the topical insects it hosts}. **[698]**

S. acuta is a vigorous competitor in degraded pastures, tree plantations, groundnuts, cereals, root crops, vegetables, planted forests, lawns, roadsides and waste places, with the most serious infestations seen in pastures and rangeland. Its lack of palatability help enable *S. acuta* to produce monospecific stands in pasture settings. *S. acuta* is considered amongst the ten most serious weeds in New Caledonia, Solomon Islands and Vanuatu, and is regarded by Holm et al. (1977) as among the 76 most serious weeds of the world. **[698]**

Cultural control and sanitary measures

Due to the tough, fibrous stems, deep taproot, unpalatability to livestock, continuous flowering and copious production of seeds with a degree of dormancy, *S. acuta* is very difficult to control. Single plants can be grubbed out prior to onset of flowering, ensuring the taproot is severed well below the crown to prevent. Larger areas can be controlled by repeated cultivation until the supply of seeds in the soil is depleted. This is expensive and usually impractical. Strict control of grazing is required, as overgrazing encourages reinvasion of the weed. Competitive grasses may be effective in suppressing *S. acuta*, when combined with other control. Spread of *S. acuta* should be controlled by slashing or mowing before it flowers, and by keeping stock away from infested paddocks while it is fruiting. Seeds can be eaten by stock and pass undamaged through the gut, or may attach to the hide by means of the sharp awns on each seed. Seeds can be transported on vehicles or as contaminants in hay or seed. [698]

Biological control

Two species have been released in Australia. The chrysomelid beetle *Calligrapha pantherina* is causing extensive defoliation of *S. acuta* in some areas of northern Australia. Defoliation caused a reduction in seed production in northern Australia by an order of magnitude (8000 to 700 per sq m), but seed dormancy and the inability of beetles to locate isolated plants remain a challenge... *C. pantherina* is also capable of damaging *S. rhombifolia*, but is causing only limited damage to this plant in Australia due to climatic factors (Heard and Gardner, 1994). It is helpful to have *S. rhombifolia* as an alternate host (Forno et al., 1992). *Sida spinosa* is another congeneric introduced species in Australia that may act as an alternate host. [698]

Physical/mechanical control

Tillage can be used to control *S. acuta* in pasture situations by slashing, chipping or cultivation... Sida species may also be controlled by electrical discharges. Burning of grasslands may also impact the level of control. [698]

Chemical Control

Mature plants of *S. acuta* are difficult to control with herbicides. Young plants can be killed with amine 2,4-D or flowable atrazine. Mature plants are best treated by slashing early in the wet season... if slashing is not possible, a spray of amine 2,4-D early in the wet season followed by another application later in the season may be effective. Glyphosate, dicamba or picloram may be effective against mature plants... Dicamba has also shown.. In northern Australia, metsulfuron methyl and fluroxypyr are used to control mature plants. [698]

Sida rhombifolia

The Sida is a plant native to the Americas, occurring extensively in South America and, to a lesser degree, in the southern United States. In Brazil, Sida rhombifolia is the most common species in the southern region, occurring, however, in all regions, infesting being in different cultures, such as pastures and vacant areas, making it difficult to mechanical harvesting annual crops, in very tough stem, in addition to serve as a host of a mycoplasma that causes the disease known as "virtual Mallow". [75]

In September 2005, a single specimen of Sida rhombifolia L. was found in a field {in the Netherlands} used for lily cultivation. In the following four years three other Malvaceae species were found: Sida spinosa L., S. cordifolia L., and Malvastrum coromandelianum (L.) Garcke. These four species are widely distributed in the (sub)tropics; in Europe they occur only rarely as casuals... Lily cultivation seems to provide a suitable habitat for the four Malvaceae species. Possibly, the seeds of these species were mixed in with soybean meal and subsequently spread through manure. From three species viable seeds could be collected, but hitherto naturalization of these species does not appear to have occurred. [414]

Effects of competition by S. rhombifolia against coffee plants were among the lowest, since only a slight decrease in all the characteristics evaluated in coffee plants was observed. The other weed species caused severe decrease in growth, mainly with increasing weed plant densities. [465]   Weed interference reduced peanut productivity between 31 and 34% for both the fertilized area and the area without fertilization, respectively. [512]   The weedy periods, from weed transplantation or emergence to plant harvesting, were 133 days... S. rhombifolia caused the least interference in the relative contents of macro and micro-nutrients in coffee shoot dry matter coffee plants. [513]

Fertilization (0 and 150 kg ha-1 of formulation 00-20-20 (N-P-K)). did not affect... Sida rhombifolia being (among) the most prominent at all levels of fertilization.... Weed interference reduced peanut productivity between 31 and 34% for both the fertilized area and the area without fertilization, respectively.... The density of (S. rhombifolia) was higher in the non fertilized area, but there was no difference in dry matter accumulation between areas {S. rhombifolia grew better and competed better without fertilization} [512]

Root system dry matter of S. rhombifolia linearly Increased with Increasing density.... The dry root weight of the coffee plants is decreased linearly with increasing density of S. rhombifolia. S. rhombifolia reduced N concentration in roots by 26, 38, 60, 56, 32 and 41%; K concentration by 24, 57, 51, 53, 6 and 32%, and Ca concentration by 9, 4, 45, 35, 11 and 4%, respectively, Compared to the weed-free treatment. In general, N and K Concentrations were more affected by weeds than Ca concentration. [513]

Sida indica

(Sida indica) is a common weed, found in open, sunny and warm areas, from sea level to ca. 1600 m altitude. It is listed as an invasive mostly in Asia and Oceania. It is not considered a threat at high elevations. The species is used widely in its native range as a traditional medicinal plant, and was probably introduced for cultivation outside its native range for medicinal purposes. For some of the countries where it is reported as invasive, it is also listed as cultivated, making it probable that the species escaped from cultivation into suitable habitats, as it is listed as found in disturbed areas near dwellings and roadsides. [698]

Sida spinosa (Sida alba)

Prickly sida (Sida spinosa) is a widely distributed and troublesome broadleaf weed in cotton, corn, peanut and soybean in the southern U.S. Prickly sida was reported as the most troublesome weed of cotton in 1974 and second most troublesome in 1983. By 2008 and 2009 prickly sida ranked as the 19th most troublesome weed in corn and soybean and 14th in cotton. A Mississippi survey of weeds conducted by Rankins et al. (2005) found prickly sida present in 40% of soybean fields sampled, making it the most prevalent weed. Prickly sida was present in 45% of soybean fields in the Delta region, compared to 43% of fields in eastern Mississippi. [673]

The amount of wax in S. spinosa at the reproductive stage was 6-23 times larger than for those found for S. urens and S. rhombifolia respectively....(the) difficulty in controlling Sida sp. was due to increased layers of wax. However, the... composition of the epicuticular wax layer is more related to this difficulty in the chemical control of some weeds, than its quantity.... the results of lower susceptibility of S. spinos to some herbicides can be explained by a high wax content compared to other species of the genus Sida... the absorption of herbicides is related to its degree of impermeability which can be attributed to changes in composition or increases in formation of waxes. [509]

Sida diseases and pests

The natural enemies of **Sida acuta** and **S. rhombifolia** in Mexico were surveyed over a period of 3 yr... Twelve species were considered to have potential as biological control agents for these weeds. One, Calligrapha pantherina Stål, has been released in Australia and is causing extensive defoliation of S. acuta. Prospects for biological control of these weeds are favorable. [236]

S. acuta usually behaves as an annual in northern Australia, although it occasionally perennates on moist sites. Seeds germinate at the start of the wet season in November and December (Mott, 1980) and plants senesce following the cessation of rain in about May or June. Adult beetles must then survive until the first rains of the next wet season trigger germination. Forno et al. 1992, have shown that adult beetles can survive in the laboratory without food for three months but the rainless period in northern Australia can last six to seven months.... By 1999 however the *sida* densities had been reduced by between 84% and 99% of the original densities and introduced pastures and native herbs and grasses dominated the sites. [299]

The sites that were monitored between 1992 and 1995 showed a decrease in **S. acuta** density of between 58% and 78% in the year following first defoliation by C. pantherina, although densities rebounded at site 2 in subsequent years to above the initial density. S. acuta can respond to a decrease in density by increasing seed production (Lonsdale et al. 1995). A reduction in grazing pressure by the beetle can then allow a rapid return to high weed densities. By 1999 however the sida densities had been reduced by between 84% and 99% of the original densities and introduced pastures and native herbs and grasses dominated the sites. **[283]**

In Sida spp. plants we found Sida micrantha mosaic virus (SiMMV), Euphorbia yellow mosaic virus (EuYMV), and three isolates that represent new species, for which the following names are proposed: Sida chlorotic mottle virus (SiCMoV), Sida bright yellow mosaic virus (SiBYMV) and Sida golden yellow spot virus (SiGYSV), an Old World-like begomovirus... Two satellite DNA molecules were found: Euphorbia yellow mosaic alphasatellite, for the first time detected infecting plants of the genus Sida, and a new alphasatellite associated with ToYSV in L. sibiricus. These results constitute further evidence of the high species diversity of begomoviruses in non-cultivated hosts, particularly Sida spp. **[785]**

Toxicity - Sida carpinfolia

Most sites, even many taxonomic sites, will tell you that sida carpinfolia is a synonym of Sida acuta. Sida carpinfolia has a bad name due to swainsonine (locoweed) having been detected in its makeup in certain studies. It is presumably the only Sida that contains this alkaloid. There are documented incidents where ingestion by goats, or horses or deer would make them sick and perhaps die, counter-balanced of at least one report of it not being toxic at all to similar wildlife and livestock. The taxonomic people say Sida carpinfolia is a variety of Sida acuta, which I think makes sense. Sida acuta is a very adaptable plant and apparently one time in South America it evolved swainsonine to protect itself from vigorous foraging. Note that all the negative reports but one come from one region in South America.

S. acuta - S. carpinifolia - different

The Sida core includes a group of species with distichous leaf arrangement, including the aggressive tropical weeds S. acuta, S. carpinifolia, S. glomerata, and S. jamaicensis. **[777]** Sida acuta var. carpinfolia and Sida carpinfolia var. acuta **[778]** Numerous synonyms of S. acuta are cited by Borssum Waalkes (1966) and Fryxell (1985). The only one of these still to be used to some extent is S. carpinifolia, e.g. in Brazil (Lorenzi, 1982). **[698]**

The bad – 11 studies

Chronic intoxication with swainsonine causes a variety of neurological disorders in livestock. These plant species are known collectively as locoweeds. Two species of Sida are reported to contain swainsonine: Sida carpinfolia and Sida rodrigoi. Effects of intoxication include reduced appetite and consequent reduced growth in young animals and loss of weight in adults, and cessation of reproduction (loss of libido, loss of fertility, and abortion). **[1]** {Also can result in death. All the bad reports but one were from central South America. S. carpinfolia was centered around SE Brazil. S. rodrigoi was adjacent in NW. Argentina and S. Paraguay. The two are roughly geographically connected. The one exception, a report in Jamaica 1970 on goat poisoning by "Sida spp." had no follow-up of any sort. So presumably Sidas are not toxic in the rest of the world.}

620-goats-NE Argentina- Sida rodrigoi (only mention in literature)

621-goast-SE Brazil

624-deer- a zoo in Brazil

625-deer-SE Brazil

626-horses-SE Brazil

627-goats and ponies-SE Brazil

628-goats-SE Brazil

418-cattle-SE Brazil

629-cattle-SE Brazil

242-goats-SE Brazil

aaa-goats- SE Brazil

aaa-animals-Brazil

The good – 7 studies
{These studies affirm Sida acuta as a valuable animal feed}

643-goats-SE Nigeria

776-goats-Phillipines

779-horses, cattle and sheep poisoned-NE Brazil-not guilty

780-goats-Nigeria

781-goats-Nigeria

782-goats-Nigeria

783-animal feed-NE Brazil

....

Antibiotic resistance evolves naturally via natural selection through random mutation, but it could also be engineered by applying an evolutionary stress on a population. {pharmaceutical antibiotics} Once such a gene is generated, bacteria can then transfer the genetic information in a horizontal fashion (between different species of bacteria) by plasmid exchange. **[499]**

In medicine, saponin is used as hypercholesterolemia, hyperglycaemia, antioxidant, anticancer, anti-inflammatory and weight loss. It has also been reported to have antifungal properties. Saponins exhibit cytotoxic effect and growth inhibition against a variety of all making them have antinflammatory and anticancer properties. **[223]**

Appendix

Sida Species Studied

A=acuta, var. carpinfolia, broomweed, wireweed, Common Fanpetals, Bala, Rajabala

As= asiatica

C=cordifolia, Abutilon ramosum, Country Mallow, Flannel weed, Mahabala

Ca=cardifolia

Cb = corymbosa

Cd=cordata

Cf= carpinifolia

F = Sida filicaulis

G=tiagii

H=hermaphrodita

Hu=humilis

I=indica, Abutilon indicum

J = javensis

K=some extracted part, usually cryptolepine (alkaloid)

L=linfolia

M=mysorensis

O=ovata

P=pilosa

R=rhombifolia

Rh=rhomboidea

Ro = rodrigoi

Rt=retusa

S=alba, spinosa

Sh= schimperiana

T=tuberculata

Ti=Tiagii

U=urens

V= veronicaefolia

Y=most Sidas

Z=all Sidas

Parts of the Plant Studied

A=aerial parts
All=all plant
B=bark
Bd=bud
Bl=blossom
F=fruit
Fl=flower
J=juice
K=alkaloid
L=leaf
Le=leaf essential oil
O=seed oil
P=whole plant oil
Pw=powder
R=root
S=seed
Sh=shoot
T=twig sap
St=stem
W=whole plant

How the Benefit(s) was Extracted

A=acqueous, cold water
Ad=acqueous, distilled water
B=hydro distillation of plant oil
Bz=benzene
Bu=butanolic
C=chloroform
D=distillation
Dr=dried
E=ethanol
F=forage, animals foraging on aerial parts
Fr=fresh plant
H=hot water, steam distillation, decoction

J=fresh juice

K=alkaloid, usually cryptolepine, or other extracted part

M=methanol

N=n-hexane

Na=nano-particles

O=ethyl acetate

P=poultice, paste

Pr=pressing or squashing

Pd=powder

R=ether

T=carbon tetracholoride

W=raw, unprocessed

X=acetone

Y=any/all extracts

Z=other

Outcomes - Effects on Pathogens

These are common scientific terms that essentially tell you how much of a pathogen they can stop or kill. How these terms are used in outcomes can be variable. I have cited one researcher's definition here, but it is only that researcher's definition in the context of their particular research. I recommend going back to any research study to determine the researcher's criteria.

IC_{50} = how much of a particular substance is needed to inhibit a given biological process by half. [609]

LC_{50} = concentration that kills 50% of larvae within 24 h [609]

LD_{50} = dose of extract in g/kg body weight of mice/rat to kill 50% of tested animal [609]

MBC (Minimum bactericidal concentration) = the lowest **concentration** of an antibacterial agent required to kill a particular bacterium. The lowest concentration killing 99.9% of the bacterial inocula after 24 h incubation at 37°C. [499] (see also LD50)

MFC (Minimum Fungicidal Concentration) = the lowest concentration of (an anti-fungal) that killed at least 99.9% of the initial inoculums [809]

MIC = the lowest concentration {of sn antipathogen} where no change was observed, indicating no growth of microorganism. [499] The lowest concentration that inhibited fungal growth. [809]

RAA = remarkable activity against

SAA = significant activity against

ZI (zone of inhibition) = If an antibiotic stops the bacteria from growing or kills the bacteria, there will be an area around the wafer where the bacteria have not grown enough to be visible. This is called a **zone of inhibition**. The size of this zone {typically in mm., bigger is better} depends on how effective the antibiotic is at stopping the growth of the bacterium. [1]

Glossary

This glossary was an internal dictionary to help me keep terms straight. I made no attempt to cross reference this with the rest of the book, some terms used in this book may not be in this list. Most definitions come from Wikipedia. If Wikipedia could not provide a useful definition, I would search the medical websites (such as www.webmd.com or medlineplus.gov) until I found one. Many items are also from dictionary.com. Although I think this glossary is reasonably correct I make no warrenty on the accuracy of these terms.

abdomen = The part of the body containing the digestive organs. The belly. Bounded by the diaphragm and the pelvis.

abortifacient = causing abortion

abscess = a collection of pus that has built up within the tissue of the body

ABTS = 2,2′-azinobis-3-ethylbenzothiazoline-6-sulfonic acid [15]

Abutilon indicum = Sida indica, Atibala

adaptogens = plant derived biologically active substances that improve immunity and physical endurance [405] adaptogen increases the power of resistance against physical, chemical or biological noxious agents. [32]

AEAC = Ascorbic acid equivalent antioxidant capacity [15]

Albendazole =for the treatment of a variety of parasitic worm infestations [1]

alkaloid = any of a group of organic basic substances found in plants, many of which are pharmacologically active, e.g., atropine, caffeine, morphine, nicotine, quinine, and strychnine.

Alexeteric = a substance to counteract infection or poison [http://www.ebbd.info/pharmacological-dictionary.html]

alopecia = hair is lost from some or all areas of the body [1]

ALP = alkaline phosphatase [609]

analgesic (painkiller) = a remedy that relieves or allays pain

anthelmintic = antiparasitic drugs that expel parasitic worms (helminths) and other internal parasites from the body by either stunning or killing them and without causing significant damage to the host.

antiemetic = An antiemetic is a drug that is effective against vomiting and nausea. Antiemetics are typically used to treat motion sickness and the side

484

effects of opioid analgesics, general anaesthetics, and chemotherapy directed against cancer.

analgesic = moderates pain

antiemetic = effective against vomiting and nausea

antiherpetic = Countering herpes

antihistamine = something that neutralize or inhibit the effect of histamine in the body, used chiefly in the treatment of allergic disorders and colds.

anti-implantation = a type of contraceptive

antileishmanial = Acting against Leishmania parasites.

antioncogenic = Inhibiting the formation of tumors.

anthelmintic = expels internal parasites and worms

antihistamine = something that neutralize or inhibit the effect of histamine in the body, used chiefly in the treatment of allergic disorders and colds.

anti-implantation = a type of contraceptive

antileishmanial (Leishmaniasis) = a disease caused by protozoan parasites

antimycotic = any agent that destroys or prevents the growth of fungi

antinociceptive = inhibits the sense of pain

antiplatelet drug (anti-aggregant) = a member of a class of pharmaceuticals that decrease platelet aggregation and inhibit thrombus formation. They are effective in the arterial circulation, where anticoagulants have little effect.

antipyretic = Something that reduces fever or quells it.

antisecretory = reduces acid secretion into the stomach

antiseptic = antimicrobial substances that are applied to living tissue/skin to reduce the possibility of infection, sepsis, or putrefaction.

antischistosomal = parasitic flatworms responsible for a highly significant group of infections in humans termed schistosomiasis. Schistosomiasis is considered by the World Health Organization as the second most socioeconomically devastating parasitic disease, (after malaria), with hundreds of millions infected worldwide [1]

antitrypanosomal = against unicellular parasitic flagellate protozoa causing sleeping sickness and Chagas disease. [1]

anxiolytic = used to reduce anxiety

apigenin = a natural compound found in many fruits and vegetables

arterial thrombosis = a blood clot that develops in an artery. It's very dangerous, because it can obstruct the flow of blood to major organs.

arthritis = any condition causing chronic inflammation and pain in the joints, muscles, cartilage, or fibrous tissue

Asparagine = an α-amino acid that is used in the biosynthesis of proteins

astringent = causing the contraction of body tissues, typically of the skin

Atibala = Sida indica, Abutilon indicum

Ayurveda (Ayurveda) = A type of complementary or alternative medicine, Ayurveda names three elemental substances, the doshas (called Vata, Pitta and Kapha), and states that a balance of the doshas results in health, while imbalance results in disease. Humoral balance is emphasized, and suppressing natural urges is considered unhealthy and claimed to lead to illness [1]

azoospermia = a man not having any measurable level of sperm in his semen

bacteria = single celled microbes

Bala (Sanskrit) = Sida cordifolia (usually, since several other Sidas are often substituted)

bile = a bitter greenish-brown alkaline fluid that aids digestion and is secreted by the liver and stored in the gallbladder.

biliary = blockage of the bile ducts

bilious = excess secretion of bile

Bladder stones (vesical calculus, cystoliths) = caused by a buildup of minerals. They can occur if the bladder is not completely emptied after urination. Eventually, the leftover urine becomes concentrated and minerals within the liquid turn into crystals

Blennorrhea = mucous discharge, especially from the urethra or vagina (that is, mucus vaginal discharge)

boil = a painful, circumscribed inflammation of the skin or a hair follicle, having a dead, suppurating inner core: usually caused by a staphylococcal infection

bowel = the part of the alimentary canal below the stomach; the intestine.

bradycardia = abnormally slow heart action

bronchitis = inflammation of the lining of your bronchial tubes, which carry air to and from your lungs

BSI = blood stream infection

bw = body weight (calculating the dose effect-xxx mg/Kg bw- so many milligrams of herbal preparation per kilogram of body weight of the test animal.

CAE = Caffeic acid equivalent [15]

calculus = also called stones, as in kidney stones (urolithiasis) and gallstones

campesterol = a phytosterol whose chemical structure is similar to that of cholesterol [1]

cardenolide = a type of steroid. Many plants contain derivatives, collectively known as cardenolides, including many in the form of cardenolide glycosides... Cardenolide glycosides are often toxic; specifically, they are heart-arresting. [1]

carminative = relieving flatulence (farts)

carotenoids = organic pigments that are produced by plants

486

cataplasm = A poultice or plaster. A soft moist mass, often warm and medicated, that is spread over the skin to treat an inflamed, aching or painful area, to improve the circulation, etc.

Chronotropic drugs = may change the heart rate and rhythm by affecting the electrical conduction system of the heart and the nerves that influence it, such as by changing the rhythm produced by the sinoatrial node. Positive chronotropes increase heart rate; negative chronotropes decrease heart rate.

coagulase = a bacterial enzyme that brings about the coagulation of blood or plasma and is produced by disease-causing forms of staphylococcus.

colic = pain in the abdomen or bowels.

conjunctivitis = pinkeye,

convulsion = a sudden, violent, irregular movement of a limb or of the body, caused by involuntary contraction of muscles and associated especially with brain disorders such as epilepsy, the presence of certain toxins or other agents in the blood, or fever in children.

coronaric acid = a mono-unsaturated, epoxide derivative of the di-saturated fatty acid, linoleic acid

coryza = catarrhal inflammation of the mucous membrane in the nose, caused especially by a cold or by hay fever.

cystitis = inflammation of the bladder

Cytotoxicity = the quality of being toxic to cells

dandruff = small pieces of dead skin in a person's hair

ddt = dose dependent. Generally the more you take the stronger the effect.

debility = a weakened or enfeebled state; weakness

decoction = liquor resulting from concentrating the essence of a substance by heating or boiling, especially a medicinal preparation made from a plant, ie, tea.

demulcent = relieves irritation of the mucous membranes in the mouth by forming a protective film.

depuratives = herbs that have purifying and detoxifying effects

dermatitis = also known as **eczema**, is a group of diseases that results in inflammation of the skin [1]

diabetes = diseases that result in too much sugar in the blood, or high blood glucose.

diaphoretic = inducing perspiration

diarrhea = an intestinal disorder characterized by abnormal frequency and fluidity of fecal evacuations.

diclofenac (diclofenac sodium) = pharmaceutical drug used to relieve pain, swelling (inflammation), and joint stiffness caused by arthritis

dipyridamole = a medication that inhibits blood clot formation when given chronically

diterpenes = biosynthesized by plants and form the basis for biologically important compounds such as retinol, retinal, and phytol. They are known to be antimicrobial and antiinflammatory.

diuretic = any substance that promotes the production of urine

dm or d.m. = dry matter. What remains after it dries out

dosha = (in Ayurvedic medicine) each of three energies believed to circulate in the body and govern physiological activity.

DPPH = 2,2-diphenyl-1-picrylhydrazyl

dysentery = an inflammation of the intestine causing diarrhea with blood

dyspepsia = indigestion

dystocia = obstructed labor

dysuria = painful or difficult urination

ecdysteroids = Phytoecdysteroids are a class of chemicals that plants synthesize for defense against phytophagous (plant eating) insects. These compounds are mimics of hormones used by arthropods in the molting process known as *ecdysis*. When insects eat the plants with these chemicals they may prematurely molt, lose weight, or suffer other metabolic damage and die. [1]

eczema = also known as dermatitis is a group of diseases that results in inflammation of the skin [1]

edema = an excess of watery fluid collecting in the cavities or tissues of the body

elephantiasis = a symptom of a variety of diseases, where parts of a person's body swell to massive proportions

emaciation = excessive Leanness usually caused by Disease or a lack of nutrition

emollient = having the quality of softening or soothing the skin

enteritis = inflammation of the intestine, especially the small intestine

erysipelas = an <u>acute</u> <u>infection</u> typically with a skin rash [1]

ESBL = These bacteria produce enzymes known as Extended Spectrum Beta-Lactamases or ESBLs for short. The ESBL enzyme breaks down and destroys most antibiotics causing them to be inactive, which is why they are not effective against infections caused by these types of bacteria.

EtOAc = Ethyl acetate [1]

febrifuge = dispels or reduces fever

febrile = having or showing the symptoms of a fever

fibrinolytic = the ability to effectively dissolve blood clots

fibroma = benign tumors that are composed of fibrous or connective tissue. They can grow in all organs

fistula = an abnormal or surgically made passage between a hollow or tubular organ and the body surface, or between two hollow or tubular organs
[738]
488

fixed oil = a natural animal or vegetable oil that is not volatile: a mixture of esters of fatty acids, usually triglycerides. Their major source is seeds of a plant.

flavonoid = any of a group of organic compounds that occur as pigments in fruit and flowers

fomentation = a poultice

FRAP = Ferric reducing antioxidant potential [15]

free radical scavenging = anti-oxidant activity

furuncle = skin abscesses caused by staphylococcal infection, which involve a hair follicle and surrounding tissue

GAE = gallic acid equivalent [609]

Gastritis = inflammation, irritation, or erosion of the lining of the stomach

gastrointestinal = of or relating to the stomach and the intestines. For the purposes of this book, everything from the stomach to the anus.

genotoxicity = the property of chemical agents that damages the genetic information within a cell causing mutations, which may lead to cancer. While genotoxicity is often confused with mutagenicity, all mutagens are genotoxic, whereas not all genotoxic substances are mutagenic

GI50 = the concentration for 50% of maximal inhibition of cell proliferation, and should be used for cytostatic (as opposed to cytotoxic) agents

gleet = a watery discharge from the urethra caused by gonorrheal infection

gout = a kind of arthritis

gram-negative bacteria = more resistant to antibiotics than Gram-positive bacteria because there is an extra outer membrane in their cell wall acting as barrier and protection. [499]

granuloma = a mass of granulation tissue, typically produced in response to infection, inflammation, or the presence of a foreign substance.

haemolysis = the rupture or destruction of red blood cells

haemothermia = a putatively holophyletic assemblage of endothermic homeotherms built around birds and mammals, and assuming common ancestry for the two.

HDL = high density lipoproteins [609]

HeLa cell (Hela or hela cell) = an immortal cell line used in scientific research. It is the oldest and most commonly used human cell line.

helminths = also commonly known as parasitic worms, are large multicellular organisms, which when mature can generally be seen with the naked eye.

hematuria = the presence of blood in urine

hemiplegia = paralysis of one side of the body.

hemorrhage = an escape of blood from a ruptured blood vessel, especially when profuse.

Hemorrhagic septicemia (HS) = an acute, highly fatal form of pasteurellosis that affects mainly water buffalo, cattle, and bison-caused by *Pasteurella multocida* serotypes

hemorrhoids = swollen veins located around the anus or in the lower rectum

hepatoprotective = protective of liver

hepatotonic = improve the tone, vigor and function of the liver

hydrococle = a pathological accumulation of serous fluid in a body cavity.

hyperdiuresis = excessive diuresis (secretion of urine)

hypoglycemic = lowers blood glucose levels

hypotension = abnormally low blood pressure

IC50 = how much of a particular substance is needed to inhibit a given biological process by half. **[609]**

indomethacin = a nonsteroidal anti-inflammatory drug (NSAID) commonly used as a prescription medication to reduce fever, pain, stiffness, and swelling from inflammation.

interferon = named for their ability to "interfere" with viral replication by protecting cells from virus infections.

IP, Intraperitoneal injection or IP injection = the injection of a substance into the peritoneum (body cavity). It is more often applied to animals than to humans.

kg ha-1 = kilograms per hectare = 0.893 pounds per acre **[USDA]**

LC50 = concentration that kills 50% of larvae within 24 h **[609]**

LD50 = dose of extract in g/kg body weight of mice/rat to kill 50% of tested animal **[609]**

l-deprenyl = a selective irreversible <u>MAO-B inhibitor</u>. long history of use as medications prescribed for the treatment of <u>depression</u>. **[1]**

LDL = low density lipoprotein cholesterol **[609]**

Leishmania = parasitic protozoans. Leishmania currently affects 12 million people in 98 countries. About 2 million new cases occur each year, and 21 species are known to cause disease in humans.

leucoderma (vitiligo) = long term skin condition characterized by patches of the skin losing their pigment. **[1]**

leucorrhoea = a whitish or yellowish discharge of mucus from the vagina

life extender = anything that adds to your expected life span

lipids = an important component of living cells. Together with carbohydrates and proteins, lipids are the main constituents of plant and animal cells.

lumbago = lower back pain

lysis = the disintegration of a cell by rupture of the cell wall or membrane.

M? = In extracts. Methanol seems to be the preferred extract by researchers, or can mean an extraction process so standard that it is not delineated.

MBC (Minimum bactericidal concentration) = the lowest **concentration** of an antibacterial agent required to kill a particular bacterium. The lowest concentration killing 99.9% of the bacterial inocula after 24 h incubation at 37°C. **[499]** (see also LD50)

membrane stabilizing activity (MSA) = how local anesthetics produce a nerve block

Menorrhoea = the flow of blood at menstruation

MFC (Minimum Fungicidal Concentration) = the percentage of "killed" cells. the percent reduction in CFU per milliliter from the starting inoculum equal to or greater than 90, 95, 97, and 99.9%. Generally ≥99.9% killing is considered the best measurement. More recent studies have all begun using the broth dilution method for MIC determinations

MIC = the lowest concentration of a chemical which prevents visible growth of a bacterium. **[1]**

microbe = any living organism that spends its life at a size too tiny to be seen with the naked eye. Microbes include bacteria and archaebacteria, protists, some fungi and even some very tiny animals

micturition = the act of passing urine

molluscicides = pesticides against molluscs, specifically slugs and snails which damage crops or other valued plants by feeding on them.

mucin = a glycoprotein constituent of mucus

myocardial infarction (MI) (ie, heart attack) = irreversible death (necrosis) of heart muscle secondary to prolonged lack of oxygen supply (ischemia).

nephroprotective = protects the kidneys from harm

nerve tonic = acts therapeutically upon the nerves

neutrophil = the most abundant type of granulocytes and the most abundant (40% to 75%) type of white blood cells in most mammals. They form an essential part of the innate immune system **[1]**

 nociception = signals arriving in the central nervous system resulting from activation of specialized sensory receptors called nociceptors that provide information about tissue damage. Pain then is the unpleasant emotional experience that usually accompanies nociception.

nutrition = taking in and utilizing food material

edema = a build up of fluid in the body which causes the affected tissue to become swollen

oligospermia = low sperm concentration in the semen

oliguria = the production of abnormally small amounts of urine **[738]**

ophthalmic = of or relating to the eye and its diseases

Osteosarcoma = a cancer that starts in the bones

Otitis Media (OM) = inflammation of the middle ear

oxytocin = a peptide hormone and neuropeptide. Used as a medication to facilitate childbirth [1]

P (statistical likelihood) = P < 0.05 – Slightly significant *; P < 0.01 – Significant **; P < 0.001 – Highly significant [152]

parasitemia = demonstrable presence of parasites in the blood

paralysis = the loss of the ability to move (and sometimes to feel anything) in part or most of the body, typically as a result of illness, poison, or injury.

pathogens = a bacterium, virus, or other microorganism that can cause disease.

pharmacognosy = the branch of knowledge concerned with medicinal drugs obtained from plants or other natural sources.

phenolic compounds = (from medicinal herbs and dietary plants) include phenolic acids, flavonoids, tannins, stilbenes, curcuminoids, coumarins, lignans, quinones, and others. They have been shown to be responsible for antimicrobial activity in plants. Their role is to protect plants against microbial or insect damage [499]

Phentolamine = (Regitine) is a reversible nonselective α-adrenergic antagonist-its primary action is vasodilation due to α1 blockade. The primary application for phentolamine is for the control of hypertensive emergencies, most notably due to pheochromocytoma.

phenylpropanoids = a diverse family of organic compounds that are synthesized by plants from the amino acids phenylalanine and tyrosine

piles = hemorrhoids that become inflamed

phentolamine = increases blood flow to the penis, erection [1]

phthisis = an archaic name for tuberculosis, a progressively wasting or consumptive condition

phytoecdysteroids = plants synthesize these for defense against phytophagous (plant eating) insects. When insects eat them they may prematurely molt, lose weight, or suffer other metabolic damage and die. [193] Ecdysteroids may serve as effective anabolic, hepatoprotective, immunoprotective, antioxidant and hypoglycemic agents... The application of phytoecdysteroids is a promising alternative to the use of anabolic-androgenic steroids because of the apparent lack of adverse effects. [191]

Phytosterols, or plant sterols = a family of molecules related to cholesterol. They are found in the cell membranes of plants, where they play important roles, just like cholesterol in humans.

p.o. administration = Oral administration (taken through the mouth) [132]

Polyploid cells and organisms = containing more than two paired (homologous) sets of chromosomes. Most species whose cells have nuclei (Eukaryotes) are diploid, meaning they have two sets of chromosomes—one set inherited from each parent.

polyuria = production of abnormally large volumes of dilute urine

poultice = a cataplasm, A soft moist mass, often warm and medicated, that is spread over the skin to treat an inflamed, aching or painful area, to improve the circulation, etc.

phthisis = pulmonary tuberculosis or a similar progressive systemic disease.

puerperal = of, relating to, or occurring during childbirth or the period immediately following; of or relating to a woman in childbirth

puerperal disease = any bacterial infection of the female reproductive tract following childbirth or miscarriage.

pyretic = fevered, feverish, or inducing fever

QR = quinone reductase [609]

RAA = remarkable activity against

reducing power = Many biochemical reactions involve oxidation (removal of electrons from a compound) & reduction (addition of electrons to a compound). Organisms will then use this reducing power to build its cellular components (it will reduce other compounds in this process).

renal = of or relating to the kidneys

reproduction = anything to do with sex or sexual reproduction, or associated problems

rheumatism = any condition causing chronic inflammation and pain in the joints, muscles, cartilage, or fibrous tissue. This term has been replaced by arthritis

RSA = Radical scavenging activity [15]

SAA = significant activity against

SBT (Serum bactericidal test) = examines the ability of the patient's serum, drawn at various times during the dosing interval, usually at the beginning and end of the administered antimicrobial agent, to kill the infecting organism

seminal weakness = nocturnal emission of semen during sleep

schistosoma = parasitic flatworms responsible for a highly significant group of infections in humans termed schistosomiasis. Schistosomiasis is considered by the World Health Organization as the second most socioeconomically devastating parasitic disease, (after malaria), with hundreds of millions infected worldwide [1]

Shigella flexneri = highly infectious, requiring as little as 100 cells to cause disease in adult volunteers. Endemic in most developing countries and causes more mortality than any other Shigella species.

shigella spp. = they are a subtype of E. coli

shigellosis = watery diarrhea, severe abdominal pain and cramping, eventuating in the bloody mucoid stool characteristic of bacillary dysentery. In the absence of effective treatments, shigellosis patients may develop secondary complications such as septicaemia, pneumonia and haemolytic uremic syndrome. Shigellosis occurs in an estimated 164.7 million people per year, of which 1.1 million cases result in death.

Siddha = Generally the basic concepts of the Siddha medicine are similar to Ayurveda [1]

Sonication = the act of applying sound energy to agitate particles in a sample, for various purposes. [1]

SOD = superoxide dismutase [609]

spermatorrhea = condition of excessive, involuntary ejaculation

spp. = several species, or all known species

strangury = a condition caused by blockage or irritation at the base of the bladder, resulting in severe pain and a strong desire to urinate

sterols (steroid alcohols) = a subgroup of the steroids and an important class of organic molecules. They occur naturally in plants, animals, and fungi, with the most familiar type of animal **sterol** being cholesterol.

stomachic = a medicine or tonic that promotes the appetite or assists digestion

stomatitis = an inflamed and sore mouth

stress = basically is a reaction of mind and body against change in the homeostasis. Stressors are external, environmental demands placed on us to feel stressed (see Adaptogen) [32]

sudorific = induces sweating

suppuration = the process of pus forming

t·ha-1 = tons per hectare

TAE = Tannic acid equivalent [15]

TEAC = Trolox equivalent antioxidant capacity [15]

TG = triglycerides

thrombolytic = Thrombolysis is the breakdown (*lysis*) of blood clots by pharmacological means. It is colloquially referred to as *clot busting* for this reason. Thrombolytic agents can be differentiated from fibrinolytic agents which only dissolve the fibrin while thrombolysis refers to the dissolution of the entire thrombus.

toxic = pharmacological substances whose whole LD50 is less than 5 mg/kg body weight are classified in the range of highly toxic substances, those with a LD50 between 5 mg/kg body weight and 5000 mg/kg body weight are classified in the range of moderately toxic substances and those with the lethal dose is more than 5000 mg/kg body weight not toxic. [499]

TPC = Total phenolic content [15]

TRAIL = tumor necrosis factor (TNF) related apoptosis inducing ligand

triterpenes = any of a group of terpenes found in plant gums and resins

trypanosome = unicellular parasitic flagellate protozoa causing sleeping sickness and Chagas disease.

Unani = a system of medicine practiced in parts of India, thought to be derived via medieval Muslim physicians from Byzantine Greece. It is sometimes contrasted with the Ayurveda system. [738]

494

urethra = transports urine from the bladder to the outside of the body

urethritis = inflammation of the urethra. The most common symptom is painful or difficult urination. It is usually caused by infection with bacteria. The infection is often a sexually transmitted infection [1]

urinary = the system of organs, structures, and ducts by which urine is produced and discharged, in mammals comprising the kidneys, ureters, bladder, and urethra. [1]

urogenital = relating to, or denoting both the urinary and genital organs.

urolithiasis = The process of forming stones in the kidney, bladder, and/or urethra (urinary tract)

Obstructive **uropathy** = a structural or functional hindrance of normal urine flow, sometimes leading to renal dysfunction (obstructive nephropathy)

uterine fibroma = noncancerous growths of the uterus that often appear during childbearing years

vaginal mycosis = yeast infection

vaginal candidiosis = candida yeast infection

vas deferens = the duct that conveys sperm from the testicle to the urethra. Contractions of the vas deferens (among others) push fluids into the prostatic urethra. The semen is stored here until ejaculation occurs. During ejaculation, the smooth muscle in the walls of the vas deferens contracts reflexively, thus propelling the sperm forward. This is also known as peristalsis. The sperm is transferred from the vas deferens into the urethra, collecting secretions from the male accessory sex glands such as the seminal vesicles, prostate gland and the bulbourethral glands, which form the bulk of semen [1]

vasicine (peganine) = a quinazoline alkaloid.

vitamin = an essential nutrient that organisms cannot synthesize the compound in sufficient quantities, and must obtain it through consumption. [1]

vitiligo = see leucoderma

wound = an injury to living tissue caused by a cut, blow, or other impact, typically one in which the skin is cut or broken.

writhing test (analgesic) = Analgesic activity of the ethanolic extract of S. cordifolia was tested using the model of acetic acid induced writhing in mice. The test consists of injecting 0.7% acetic acid solution and observing the animal for specific contraction of body referred as 'writhing'. [24]

Xanthine oxidase = a type of enzyme that generates reactive oxygen species [1]

xenobiotic = a foreign chemical substance found within an organism that is not normally naturally produced by or expected to be present within. It can also cover substances that are present in much higher concentrations than are usual. Specifically, drugs such as antibiotics are xenobiotics in humans because the human body does not produce them itself, nor are they part of a normal food.

ZI (zone of inhibition) = If an antibiotic stops the bacteria from growing or kills the bacteria, there will be an area around the wafer where the bacteria have not grown enough to be visible. This is called a **zone of inhibition**. The size of this zone {typically in mm., bigger is better} depends on how effective the antibiotic is at stopping the growth of the bacterium. **[1]**

References

There are some duplicate listings, as far as I know they are noted. Frankly, at the end of years of research and being more than ready to publish this book I was scared to eliminate anything from this list, lest something be eliminated that I did not want to eliminate. The bottom line is the each version of multiple citations will still lead you to the original research.

1. Wikipedia (online public encyclopedia)
Wikipedia Foundation
Various articles based on the name of the subject

2.. Bala (Sida cordifolia) information
Cupboard Natural Foods and Café, Denton TX

3.. International Journal of Pharmacology and Biological Sciences 4.2 (Aug 2010): 67-70.
ANTIPYRETIC ACTIVITY OF LEAVES OF SIDA ACUTA ON RAT
Mridha, D; Saha, D; Beura, S.

4.. Asian Pacific Journal of Tropical Medicine
Volume 3, Issue 9, September 2010, Pages 691–695
Larvicidal and repellent activities of Sida acuta Burm. F. (Family: Malvaceae) against three important vector mosquitoes
Marimuthu Govindarajan

5.. Pharmaceutical Biology
2000, Vol. 38. No. 1, pp. 40-45 © Swets & Zeitlinger
INVESTIGATION OF MEDICINAL PLANTS OF TOGO FOR ANTIVIRAL AND ANTIMICROBIAL ACTIVITIES
K. Ananil, J.B. Hudson2 , C. de Souzal, K. Akpaganal, G.H.N. Tower 3 , J.T. Amason4 :- and M. Gbeassor.

6.. ANTIMICROBIAL ACTIVITY OF LEAF EXTRACTS OF Sida acuta Burm.
Akilandeswari .S, R.Senthamarai,, Prema.S,, R.Valarmathi
International Journal of Pharma Sciences and Research. 2010;1(5):248-250

7.. African Journal of Biotechnology Vol. 5 (2), pp. 195-200, 16 January 2006
Antibacterial activity of alkaloids from Sida acuta
Damintoti Karou1*, Aly Savadogo1, Antonella Canini2, Saydou Yameogo1, Carla Montesano2, Jacques Simpore3, Vittorio Colizzi2, Alfred S. Traore1.

8 -- Ethnopharmacol. 19: 233-245. (1987).
Diuretic activity of plants used for the treatment of urinary ailments in Guatemala. J.
Caceres A, Giron LM, Martinez AM

496

9.. Economic Botany 50: 71-107 (1996)
Ethnobotany of the Garifuna of the eastern Nicaragua.
Coee FG, Anderson GJ

10.. J Ethnopharmacol. 2000 Aug;71(3):505-11.
Snakebites and ethnobotany in the northwest region of Colombia: Part II: neutralization of lethal and
enzymatic effects of Bothrops atrox venom.
Otero R1, Núñez V, Jiménez SL, Fonnegra R, Osorio RG, García ME, Díaz A.

11.. Annals of Clinical Microbiology and Antimicrobials 2012,11:5
Antimicrobial activity of polyphenol-rich fractions from Sida alba L. (Malvaceae) against co-trimoxazol-
resistant bacteria strains
Kiessoun Konaté1*, Adama Hilou1, Jacques F Mavoungou2,Alexis N Lepengué3, Alain Souza4, Nicolas
Barro5, Jacques Y Datté6, Bertrand M'Batchi3 and Odile G Nacoulma1

12.. Journal of Ethnopharmacology
Volume 89, Issues 2–3, December 2003, Pages 291–294
Antimalarial activity of Sida acuta Burm. f. (Malvaceae) and Pterocarpus erinaceus oir. (Fabaceae)
Damintoti Karoua, Mamoudou H. Dickoa, , , Souleymane Sanona, Jacques Simporeb, Alfred S. Traorea

13.. International Journal of Pharmacognosy, Volume 33, Issue 2, 1995
Screening for antitumor and anti-HIV activities of nine medicinal plants from Zaire
D. N. Muanzaa, K. L. Eulera, L. Williams & D. J. Newman

14.. Afr J Med Med Sci. 2014 Mar;43(1):11-6.
Central nervous system activity of the ethanol leaf extract of Sida acuta in rats.
Ibironke GF, Umukoro AS, Ajonijebu DC.

15.. J Ayurveda Integr Med. 2015 Jan-Mar; 6(1): 24–28.
Total polyphenolic contents and in vitro antioxidant properties of eight Sida species from Western Ghats,
India
M. D. Subramanya, Sandeep R. Pai,1 Vinayak Upadhya,2 Gireesh M. Ankad,2 Shalini S. Bhagwat, and
Harsha V. Hegde1,2

15.. BMC Complement Altern Med. 2012 Aug 11;12:120. doi: 10.1186/1472-6882-12-120.
Toxicity assessment and analgesic activity investigation of aqueous acetone extracts of Sida acuta Burn f .
and Sidacordifolia L. (Malvaceae), medicinal plants of Burkina Faso.
Konaté K1, Bassolé IH, Hilou A, Aworet-Samseny RR, Souza A, Barro N, Dicko MH, Datté JY, M'Batchi
B.

16.. J Ethnopharmacol. 2012 Oct 31;144(1):1-10. doi: 10.1016/j.jep.2012.07.018. Epub 2012 Sep 10.
Ethnobotanical study of plants used in treating hypertension in Edo State of Nigeria.
Gbolade A1.

17.. Phytother Res. 2011 Jan;25(1):147-50. doi: 10.1002/ptr.3219.
Cryptolepine, isolated from Sida acuta, sensitizes human gastric adenocarcinoma cells to TRAIL-induced
apoptosis.
Ahmed F1, Toume K, Ohtsuki T, Rahman M, Sadhu SK, Ishibashi M.

18.. J Ethnopharmacol. 2009 Jul 15;124(2):171-5. doi: 10.1016/j.jep.2009.04.055. Epub 2009 May 5.
Hepatoprotective studies on Sida acuta Burm. f.   xxx 63 and 111 are dupes
Sreedevi CD1, Latha PG, Ancy P, Suja SR, Shyamal S, Shine VJ, Sini S, Anuja GI,Rajasekharan S.

19.. Phytomedicine. 2004;11(4):338-41.
Studies on medicinal plants of Ivory Coast: investigation ofSida acuta for in vitro antiplasmodial activities
and identification of an active constituent.
Banzouzi JT1, Prado R, Menan H, Valentin A, Roumestan C, Mallié M, Pelissier Y, Blache Y.

20.. J Ethnopharmacol. 2003 Dec;89(2-3):291-4.
Antimalarial activity of Sida acuta Burm. f. (Malvaceae) and Pterocarpus erinaceus Poir. (Fabaceae).
Karou D1, Dicko MH, Sanon S, Simpore J, Traore AS.

21.. Anc Sci Life. 2002 Jul;22(1):57-66.
PHARMACOGNOSTIC STUDIES ON Sida acuta Burm.f.
Mohideen S1, Sasikala E, Gopal V.

22.. J Ethnopharmacol. 2014 Aug 8;155(1):373-86. doi: 10.1016/j.jep.2014.05.029. Epub 2014 Jun 5.
Soma, food of the immortals according to the Bower Manuscript (Kashmir, 6th century A.D.).
Leonti M1, Casu L2.

23.. Am J Chin Med. 2013;41(6):1407-25. doi: 10.1142/S0192415X13500948.
Influence of six medicinal herbs on collagenase-induced osteoarthritis in rats.
Nirmal P1, Koppikar S, Bhondave P, Narkhede A, Nagarkar B, Kulkarni V, Wagh N,Kulkarni O,
Harsulkar A, Jagtap S.

24.. Asian Pac J Trop Biomed. 2014 Jan;4(1):18-24. doi: 10.1016/S2221-1691(14)60202-1.
Phytopharmacological evaluation of ethanol extract of Sidacordifolia L. roots.
Momin MA1, Bellah SF, Rahman SM, Rahman AA, Murshid GM, Emran TB.

25.. Indian J Pharmacol. 2013 Sep-Oct;45(5):474-8. doi: 10.4103/0253-7613.117759.
Wound healing activity of Sida cordifolia Linn. in rats.
Pawar RS1, Chaurasiya PK, Rajak H, Singour PK, Toppo FA, Jain A.

26.. Neurotoxicology. 2013 Dec;39:57-64. doi: 10.1016/j.neuro.2013.08.005. Epub 2013 Aug 28.
Ameliorative effect of Sida cordifolia in rotenone induced oxidative stress model of Parkinson's disease.
Khurana N1, Gajbhiye A.

27.. Ann Clin Microbiol Antimicrob. 2012 Dec 26;11:33. doi: 10.1186/1476-0711-11-33. 117 and 211 are
dup
Free radical scavenging capacity, anticandicidal effect of bioactive compounds from Sida cordifolia L., in
combination with nystatin and clotrimazole and their effect on specific immune response in rats.
Ouédraogo M1, Konaté K, Lepengué AN, Souza A, M'Batchi B, Sawadogo LL.

28.. Br J Nutr. 2012 Oct;108(7):1256-63. Epub 2012 Jan 31.
Amelioration of alcohol-induced hepatotoxicity by the administration of ethanolic extract of Sida
cordifolia Linn.
Rejitha S1, Prathibha P, Indira M.

29.. J Ethnobiol Ethnomed. 2011 Oct 19;7:32. doi: 10.1186/1746-4269-7-32.
Ethnomedicinal and ecological status of plants in Garhwal Himalaya, India.
Kumar M1, Sheikh MA, Bussmann RW.

30.. Phytother Res. 2011 Aug;25(8):1236-41. doi: 10.1002/ptr.3550. Epub 2011 Jun 14.
Sida cordifolia leaf extract reduces the orofacial nociceptive response in mice.
Bonjardim LR1, Silva AM, Oliveira MG, Guimarães AG, Antoniolli AR, Santana MF,Serafini MR, Santos
RC, Araújo AA, Estevam CS, Santos MR, Lyra A, Carvalho R,Quintans-Júnior LJ, Azevedo EG, Botelho
MA.

31.. Neurochem Res. 2010 Sep;35(9):1361-7. doi: 10.1007/s11064-010-0192-5. Epub 2010 May 25.
Antiperoxidative and antiinflammatory effect of Sida cordifoliaLinn. on quinolinic acid induced
neurotoxicity.
Swathy SS1, Panicker S, Nithya RS, Anuja MM, Rejitha S, Indira M.

32.. Indian J Pharm Sci. 2009 May;71(3):323-4. doi: 10.4103/0250-474X.56027.
Antistress, Adoptogenic Activity of Sida cordifolia Roots in Mice.
Sumanth M1, Mustafa SS.

33.. J Ethnopharmacol. 2009 Jul 6;124(1):162-5. doi: 10.1016/j.jep.2009.04.004. Epub 2009 Apr 10.
Role of Sida cordifolia L. leaves on biochemical and antioxidant profile during myocardial injury.
Kubavat JB1, Asdaq SM.   xxx dupes 69 and 163

34.. Fitoterapia. 2008 Apr;79(3):229-31. doi: 10.1016/j.fitote.2008.01.001. Epub 2008 Feb 9.
Preliminary evaluation of anti-pyretic and anti-ulcerogenic activities of Sida cordifolia methanolic extract.

498

Philip BK1, Muralidharan A, Natarajan B, Varadamurthy S, Venkataraman S.

35.. Int J Oncol. 2007 Oct;31(4):915-22.
The plant alkaloid cryptolepine induces p21WAF1/CIP1 and cell cycle arrest in a human osteosarcoma cell line.
Matsui TA1, Sowa Y, Murata H, Takagi K, Nakanishi R, Aoki S, Yoshikawa M, Kobayashi M, Sakabe T, Kubo T, Sakai T.

36.. Pak J Pharm Sci. 2007 Jul;20(3):185-8.
Anti-inflammatory and analgesic alkaloid from Sida cordifolialinn.
Sutradhar RK1, Rahman AM, Ahmad M, Bachar SC, Saha A, Roy TG.

37.. Acta Cir Bras. 2006;21 Suppl 1:37-9.
Effect of the aqueous extract of Sida cordifolia on liver regeneration after partial hepatectomy.
Silva RL1, Melo GB, Melo VA, Antoniolli AR, Michellone PR, Zucoloto S, Picinato MA,Franco CF, Mota Gde A, Silva Ode C.

38.. Anc Sci Life. 2006 Jul;26(1-2):65-72.
A comparative study on the effect of plant extracts with the antibiotics on organisms of hospital origin.
Thangavel M1, Raveendran M, Kathirvel M.

39.. Pharmazie. 2006 May;61(5):466-9.
Endothelium-derived factors and k+ channels are involved in the vasorelaxation induced by Sida cordifolia L. in the rat superior mesenteric artery.
Santos MR1, Nascimento NM, Antoniolli AR, Medeiros IA.

40.. Fitoterapia. 2006 Jan;77(1):19-27. Epub 2005 Oct 28.
Cardiovascular effects of Sida cordifolia leaves extract in rats.
Medeiros IA1, Santos MR, Nascimento NM, Duarte JC.

41.. J Ethnopharmacol. 2005 Apr 26;98(3):275-9.
CNS pharmacological effects of the hydroalcoholic extract ofSida cordifolia L. leaves.
Franco CI1, Morais LC, Quintans-Júnior LJ, Almeida RN, Antoniolli AR.

42.. J Ethnopharmacol. 2003 Feb;84(2-3):131-8.   xxx 123 is a dup
Screening of antioxidant activity of three Indian medicinal plants, traditionally used for the management of neurodegenerative diseases.
Auddy B1, Ferreira M, Blasina F, Lafon L, Arredondo F, Dajas F, Tripathi PC, Seal T,Mukherjee B.

43.. J Ethnopharmacol. 2000 Sep;72(1-2):273-7.
Anti-inflammatory, analgesic activity and acute toxicity of Sidacordifolia L. (Malva-branca).
Franzotti EM1, Santos CV, Rodrigues HM, Mourão RH, Andrade MR, Antoniolli AR.

44.. J Neurol Sci. 2000 Jun 15;176(2):124-7.
Association of L-DOPA with recovery following Ayurveda medication in Parkinson's disease.
Nagashayana N1, Sankarankutty P, Nampoothiri MR, Mohan PK, Mohanakumar KP.

45.. Phytother Res. 1999 Feb;13(1):75-7.
Analgesic, antiinflammatory and hypoglycaemic activities ofSida cordifolia.
Kanth VR1, Diwan PV.

46.. Immunopharmacol Immunotoxicol. 2012 Apr;34(2):326-36.
Anti-inflammatory and anti-oxidant properties of Sidarhombifolia stems and roots in adjuvant induced arthritic rats.
Narendhirakannan RT1, Limmy TP.

47.. BMC Complement Altern Med. 2010 Jul 27;10:40. doi: 10.1186/1472-6882-10-40.
In vitro antibacterial activity and acute toxicity studies of aqueous-methanol extract of Sida rhombifolia Linn. (Malvaceae).
Assam AJ1, Dzoyem JP, Pieme CA, Penlap VB.

48.. J Med Sci 2002, 2(3):134-136.
In vitro Antibacterial Activity of the Extractsand a Glycoside from Sida rhombifolia Linn
ME Islam, NA Khatune, ME Haque

49.. Asian Pac J Cancer Prev. 2009;10(6):1107-12.   xxx dup of 464 (407 also a dup)
Sida rhombifolia ssp. retusa seed extract inhibits DEN induced murine hepatic preneoplasia and carbon
tetrachloride hepatotoxicity.
Poojari R1, Gupta S, Maru G, Khade B, Bhagwat S.

50.. Indian Journal of Experimental Biology Vol. 48, September 2010, pp. 865-878
Herbs and herbal constituents active against snake bite
Antony Gomes1*, Rinku Das1, Sumana Sarkhel1, Roshnara Mishra1, Sanghamitra Mukherjee1,Shamik
Bhattacharya2 & Aparna Gomes2

51.. International Journal of PharmTech Research   Vol.2, No.2, pp 1241-1245, April-June 2010
Comparative In vitro Antimicrobial Activity Studies of Sida rhombifolia Linn Fruit Extracts
Rashmi Ranjan Sarangi* , Uma Shankar Mishra, Prasanta Kumar Choudhury

52.. IntRJPharmSci.2012; 03(01); 0026
Phytochemical screening of the root of Sida acuta Burm. F.
D. K. Pradhan1*, M. R. Mishra1*, A. Mishra1, A. K. Panda2, R. K. Behera3, S. Jha4.

53.. Ethnobotanical Leaflets 10: 336-341. 2006.
Bala (Sida cordifolia L.)- Is It Safe Herbal Drug?
Dr. Amrit Pal Singh, BAMS; PGDMB; MD (Alternative Medicine), Herbal Consultant, Ind–Swift Ltd,
Chandigarh.

54.. International Journal of Pharmacy and Pharmaceutical Sciences Vol 6, Issue 11, 2014
AN OVERVIEW ON THE BIOLOGICAL PERSPECTIVES OF SIDA CORDIFOLIA LINN
SRINITHYA B, MEENAKSHI SUNDARAM MUTHURAMAN*
Department of Biotechnology, School of Chemical & Biotechnology, SASTRA University,
Thirumalaisamudram, Thanjavur 613401, India.

55.. Asian Journal of Plant Science and Research, 2011, 1 (3): 65-67
Antimicrobial activity of ethanolic leaf extract of Sida spinosa linn. (Malvaceae)
S. Navaneethakrishnan, P. Suresh Kumar, T. Satyanarayana, S. Mohideen and G. Kiran Kumar

56.. Phytochem Anal. 2001 Mar-Apr;12(2):110-9.   xxx 263 and 491 are dupes
Phytoecdysteroid profiles in seeds of Sida spp. (Malvaceae).
Dinan L1, Bourne P, Whiting P.

57.. J Med Food. 2007 Dec;10(4):683-8.   75 is a dup
Evaluation of in vitro antioxidant activity of Sida rhombifolia(L.) ssp. retusa (L.).
Dhalwal K1, Deshpande YS, Purohit AP.

58.. Journal of Nanotechnology Volume 2015, Article ID 829526, 18 pages
Biosynthesis of Silver Nanoparticles and Its Applications
M. Jannathul Firdhouse and P. Lalitha

59.. Molecules. 2013 Mar 1;18(3):2769-77. doi: 10.3390/molecules18032769.
Secondary metabolites from Sida rhombifolia L. (Malvaceae) and the vasorelaxant activity of
cryptolepinone.
Chaves OS1, Gomes RA, Tomaz AC, Fernandes MG, das Graças Mendes L Jr, de Fátima Agra M, Braga
VA, de Fátima Vanderlei de Souza M.

60.. Small Ruminant Research Volume 42, Issue 2, November 2001, Pages 161–166
Forage species availability, food preference and grazing behaviour of goats in southeastern Nigeria
B.I Odoa, , , F.U Omejeb, J.N Okwora

61.. J Ethnopharmacol. 2000 Sep;72(1-2):273-7.   xxx 119 is a dup
Anti-inflammatory, analgesic activity and acute toxicity of Sida cordifolia L. (Malva-branca).
Franzotti EM, Santos CV, Rodrigues HM, Mourão RH, Andrade MR, Antoniolli AR.

500

62.. Phytother Res. 2011 Jan;25(1):147-50. doi: 10.1002/ptr.3219.
Cryptolepine, isolated from Sida acuta, sensitizes human gastric adenocarcinoma cells to TRAIL-induced apoptosis.
Ahmed F, Toume K, Ohtsuki T, Rahman M, Sadhu SK, Ishibashi M.

63.. J Ethnopharmacol. 2009 Jul 15;124(2):171-5. Epub 2009 May 5.   xxx dup of 18, 111 also dup
Hepatoprotective studies on Sida acuta Burm. f.
Sreedevi CD, Latha PG, Ancy P, Suja SR, Shyamal S, Shine VJ, Sini S, Anuja GI, Rajasekharan S.

64.. Front Pharmacol, 2010
Cameroonian medicinal plants: pharmacology and derived natural products
V Kuete, T Efferth

65.. Journal of Tropical Ecology 1976 Vol. 17 No. 1 pp. 23-30
Seasonal variation, dry matter production, and competitive efficiency of Sida acuta Burm., under exposed and shaded conditions.
Chaudhary, R. L.

66.. Phytother Res. 2011 Aug;25(8):1236-41. doi: 10.1002/ptr.3550. Epub 2011 Jun 14.
Sida cordifolia leaf extract reduces the orofacial nociceptive response in mice.
Bonjardim LR, Silva AM, Oliveira MG, Guimarães AG, Antoniolli AR, Santana MF, Serafini MR, Santos RC,Araújo AA, Estevam CS, Santos MR, Lyra A, Carvalho R, Quintans-Júnior LJ, Azevedo EG, Botelho MA.

67.. Neurochem Res. 2010 Sep;35(9):1361-7. Epub 2010 May 25.
Antiperoxidative and antiinflammatory effect of Sida cordifolia Linn. on quinolinic acid induced neurotoxicity.
Swathy SS, Panicker S, Nithya RS, Anuja MM, Rejitha S, Indira M.

68.. Bioorg Med Chem Lett. 2010 Mar 15;20(6):1837-9. Epub 2010 Feb 6.
Unprecedented NES non-antagonistic inhibitor for nuclear export of Rev from Sida cordifolia.
Tamura S, Kaneko M, Shiomi A, Yang GM, Yamaura T, Murakami N.

69.. J Ethnopharmacol. 2009 Jul 6;124(1):162-5. Epub 2009 Apr 10.   xxx dup of 33 (and 163)
Role of Sida cordifolia L. leaves on biochemical and antioxidant profile during myocardial injury.
Kubavat JB, Asdaq SM.

70.. Fitoterapia. 2008 Apr;79(3):229-31. Epub 2008 Feb 9.   xxx dup of 34
Preliminary evaluation of anti-pyretic and anti-ulcerogenic activities ofSida cordifolia methanolic extract.
Philip BK, Muralidharan A, Natarajan B, Varadamurthy S, Venkataraman S.

71.. Journal of Planar Chromatography- Modern TLC (2005) 18(105) : 364-367   548 dup
HPTL JouC method for chemical standardization of Sida species & estimation of alkaloid Ephedrine,
Sayyada Khatoon, Manjoosha Srivastava, AKS Rawai & Shanta Mehrotra

72.. Ethnobotanical Leaflets 13: 1069-1087, 2009.
Ethnobotanical Studies from Amaravathy Range of Indira Gandhi Wildlife Sanctuary, Western Ghats, Coimbatore District, Southern India
V.S. Ramachandran1 , Shijo Joseph2 and R. Aruna3

73.. Anti-cancer Drug Design [2000, 15(3):191-201]
DNA intercalation, topoisomerase II inhibition and cytotoxic activity of the plant alkaloid neocryptolepine.
Bailly C , Laine W , Baldeyrou B , De Pauw-Gillet MC , Colson P , Houssier C , Cimanga K , Van Miert S , Vlietinck AJ , Pieters L

74.. Pakist J Biol Sci, 2000
Larvicidal Activity of a New Glycoside, Phenyl Ethyl bD Glucopyranoside from the Stem of the Plant Sida rhombifolia
IM Ekramul, KA Naznin, WM Islam, HM Ekramul

75.. J Med Food. 2007 Dec;10(4):683-8.   dup of 57
Evaluation of in vitro antioxidant activity of Sida rhombifolia (L.) ssp. retusa (L.).
Dhalwal K, Deshpande YS, Purohit AP.

76.. BMC Complementary and Alternative Medicine 2012, 12:120
http://www.biomedcentral.com/1472-6882/12/120
Toxicity assessment and analgesic activity investigation of aqueous acetone extracts of Sida acuta Burn f.
and Sida cordifolia L. (Malvaceae), medicinal plants of Burkina Faso
Kiessoun Konaté1,4*, Imaël Henri Nestor Bassolé2, Adama Hilou1, Raïssa RR Aworet-Samseny3, Alain
Souza4, Nicolas Barro5, Mamoudou H Dicko2, Jacques Y Datté6 and Bertrand M'Batchi4

77.. J. Mater. Environ. Sci. 5(3) (2014) 899-906 Johnson et al.
Green synthesis of silver nanoparticles using Artemisia annua and Sida acuta leaves extract and their
antimicrobial, antioxidant and corrosion inhibition potentials
A.S. Johnsona, I.B. Obota,b*, U. S. Ukponga a

78.. Plant Soil Environ., 56, 2010 (5): 244–251
Metal levels in some refuse dump soils and plants in Ghana
K. Agyarko1, E. Darteh1, B. Berlinger2

79.. Life Sciences Volume 79, Issue 21, 19 October 2006, Pages 2043–2048
Comparative immunomodulatory effect of scopoletin on tumoral and normal lymphocytes
María Gabriela Manuelea, Graciela Ferraroa, c, Maria Laura Barreiro Arcosb, Paula Lópezc, Graciela
Cremaschib, Claudia Anesinia

80.. Molecular Biotechnology September 2011, Volume 49, Issue 1, pp 77-81
Genetic and Chemical Diversity of High Mucilaginous Plants of Sida Complex by ISSR Markers and
Chemical Fingerprinting
Sanjog T. Thul , Ankit K. Srivastava, Subhash C. Singh, Karuna Shanker

81.. Journal of Medicinal and Aromatic Plant Sciences 2000 Vol. 22 No. 2/3 pp. 200-205
Chalazal regulation of seed coat imposed dormancy in Sida species.
Seal, S.; Gupta, K.

82.. Natural Product Sciences, (12)3: 150-152 2006
Anti-Ulcer Activity of Sida acuta Burm
P Malairajan, Gopalakrishnan, Narasimhan, Jessi Kala Veni

83.. World Applied Sciences Journal 3 (1): 79-81, 2008
Antimicrobial screening of the essential oil of some herbal plants from Western Nigeria
I.A. Ajayi, S.G. Jonathan, A. Adewuyi and R.A. Oderinde 12 1 1

84.. Nigerian Journal of Natural Products and Medicine Vol. 9 2005: 19-21
Analgesic, anti-inflammatory and anti-ulcer activities of Sida acuta in mice and rat
IE Oboh, DN Onwukaeme

85.. Indian Journal Of Traditional Knowledge Vol. 9 (1), January 2010, pp. 158-162
Ethno-medico-botanical knowledge of rural folk in Bhadravathi taluk of Shimoga district, Karnataka
MB Shivanna* & N Rajakumar

86.. Journal of Applied Phytotechnology in Environmental Sanitation Apr2012, Vol. 1 Issue 3, p113-119.
PHYTOCHEMICAL SCREENING AND ANTIBACTERIAL ACTIVITY OF SIDA ACUTA AND
EUPHORBIA HIRTA.
Author(s): T. A., Ibrahim; F. O., Adetuyi; Lola, Ajala

87. Healing plants of Peninsular India (book)
Parrotta ,J. A.
CABI Publishin g1,4inllingfon tU,K. pp.483-486

88.. Golden Res Thoughts, 2011 - aygrt.isrj.org
Genus Sida–The plants with ethno medicinal & therapeutic potential
R Wake, N Patil, UK Halde
502

89.. African Journal of Biotechnology Vol. 4 (8), pp. 823-828, August 2005
Antioxidant and antibacterial activities of polyphenols from ethnomedicinal plants of Burkina Faso
Damintoti Karou1, Mamoudou H. Dicko1, 2*, Jacques Simpore3, and Alfred S. Traore1

90.. J. Res. Educ. Indian Med., Jan. - March, 2012 Vol. XVIII (1) : 21-26
Inhibitory effect of the root of Sida acuta Burm. f. on calcium oxalate crystal growth
T Vimala, S Gopalakrishnan

91.. Int J Pharmacog. 1997;35:179-184
ANTI-INFLAMMATORY AND ANALGESIC ACTIVITY OF METHANOLIC EXTRACT OF WHOLE
PLANT OF SIDA ACUTA (LINN.F.ND)
Virendra Sharma, Pooja Sinoriya, Sunil Sharma

92.. Environmental Toxicology and Pharmacology
In vitro cytotoxicity and antioxidant activities of five medicinal plants of Malvaceae family from
Cameroon
C.A. Piemea,c,*, V.N. Penlapb, J. Ngoganga, M. Costachec

93.. CARYOLOGIA Vol. 60, no. 1-2: 90-95, 2007
Identification of phenolic compounds from medicinal and melliferous plants and their cytotoxic activity in
cancer cells
A Daniela, E Pichichero, L Canuti, R Cicconi, D Karou

94.. Bioresource Technology Volume 98, Issue 9, July 2007, Pages 1788–1794
Phytoextraction capacity of the plants growing on tannery sludge dumping sites
Amit K. Gupta, Sarita Sinha,

95.. BMC Complementary and Alternative Medicine 2013 13:79
In vitro anticancer screening of 24 locally used Nigerian medicinal plants
Saudat Adamson Fadeyi, Olugbeminiyi O Fadeyi, Adedeji A Adejumo, Cosmas Okoro and Elbert Lewis
Myles

96.. International Journal of PharmTech Research Vol.1, No.4, pp 1260-1266, Oct-Dec 2009
PHYTOCHEMICAL AND CONTRACEPTIVE PROPERTY OF SIDA ACUTA BURM FI. IIN. IN
ALBIO RATS
Ramesh L. Londonkar1, Sharangouda J. Patil2 * and Saraswati B. Patil3

97.. Journal of Biological Sciences 6 (3) 2006
Suitability of some local bast fiber plants in pulp and papermaking
Olotuah, OF

98.. Int. J. Drug Dev. & Res.,July-September 2012, 4(3): 92-96   xxx 184 is a dup
Antifungal activity of flavonoids of Sida acuta Burm f. against Candida albicans
Jindal Alka*, Kumar Padma, Jain Chitra

99.. J. Nat. Prod. Plant Resour., 2011, 1 (2): 36-40
Anitimicrobial activity of ethanolic extract of the whole plant of Sida Spinosa Linn. (Malvaceae)
S. Selvadurai**, R. Senthamarai, T. Sri Vijaya Kirubha, K. Vasuki

100.. International Journal of Phytomedicine 4 (2012) 40-47
Pharmacological and Toxicological Effects of Aqueous Acetone Extract of Sida alba L. (Malvaceae) in
Animals Model
K.Konaté1 , M.Ouédraogo2 , J. F. Mavoungou3 , A.N.Lepengué4 , A.Souza5 O.G.Nacoulma

101.. Tropical Journal of Pharmaceutical Research, December 2007; 6 (4): 809-813
Antimicrobial activity of the ethanol extract of the aerial parts of Sida acuta burm. f.(malvaceae)
IE Obah, JO Akerele, O Obasuyi

102.. Journal of Medicinal Plants Research Vol. 3(9), pp. 621-624, September, 2009
Antimicrobial activity of ethanolic and aqueous extracts of Sida acuta on microorganisms from skin
infections

103.. Journal of Pharmacology and Toxicology 2010 Vol. 5 No. 1 pp. 1-12
Comparative evaluation of the protective effect of the ethanolic and methanolic leaf extracts of Sida acuta against hyperglycaemia and alterations of biochemical and haematological indices in alloxan diabetic rats.
Ekor, M.; Odewabi, A. O.; Bakre, A. G.; Oritogun, K. S.; Ajayi, T. E.; Sanwo, O. V.

104.. International Journal of PharmTech Research Vol.2, No.1, pp 585-587, Jan-Mar 2010
Wound Healing Actvity of Sida acuta in Rats
S.Akilandeswari*, R.Senthamarai, R.Valarmathi and S.Prema1

105.. Fitoterapia 77 (2006) 19 – 27
Cardiovascular effects of Sida cordifolia leaves extract in rats
I.A. Medeiros *, M.R.V. Santos, N.M.S. Nascimento, J.C. Duarte

106.. International Journal of Biology Vol 3, No 4 (2011)
Screening of Some Plants Used in the Cameroonian Folk Medicine for the Treatment of Infectious Diseases
Laure Brigitte Kouitcheu Mabeku, Kuiate Jules Roger, Oyono Essame Jean Louis

107.. International Research Journal of Pharmacy. 2013;4(1):88-92
ETHNO MEDICINAL AND THERAPEUTIC POTENTIAL OF SIDA ACUTA BURM.F.
Pradhan Dusmanta Kumar, Panda Ashok Kumar, Behera Rajani Kanta, Jha Shivesh, Mishra Manas Ranjan, Mishra Ashutosh, Choudhary Sanjay

108.. Phytotherapy Research Volume 9, Issue 5, pages 359–363, August 1995   xxx 251 is a dup
In vitro and in vivo antimalarial activity of cryptolepine, a plant-derived indoloquinoline
G. C. Kirby1,*, A. Paine1,2, D. C. Warhurst1, B. K. Noamese2 andJ. D. Phillipson3

109.. International Journal of PharmTech Research Vol.2, No.2, pp 1644-1648, April-June 2010
Screening of Gastric Antiulcer Activity of Sida acuta Burm
S.Akilandeswari*, R.Senthamarai, R.Valarmathi, S.Shanthi and S.Prema1

110.. Research Journal of Pharmaceutical, Biological and Chemical 3.2 (2012): 515-518.
Antipyretic efficacy of Various Extracts of Sida acuta leaves.
Shrama, R., D. Sharma, and S. Kumar.

111.. Journal of Ethnopharmacology Volume 124, Issue 2, 15 July 2009, Pages 171–175
Hepatoprotective studies on Sida acuta Burm. f.
C.D. Sreedevia, P.G. Lathab, P. Ancya, S.R. Sujab, S. Shyamalb, V.J. Shineb, S. Sinib, G.I. Anujab, S. Rajasekharanb
xxx dup of 18, 63 dup

112.. Albanian Journal of Agricultural Sciences. 2014;13(1):71-80
Assessing the Heavy Metal Transfer and Translocation by Sida Acuta and Pennisetum Purpureum for Phytoremediation Purposes
CLEMENT O. OGUNKUNLE, PAUL O. FATOBA, AYODELE O. OYEDEJI, OLUSEGUN O. AWOTOYE

113.. Journal of Applied Phytotechnology in Environmental Sanitation. 2012;1(3):113-119
PHYTOCHEMICAL SCREENING AND ANTIBACTERIAL ACTIVITY OF SIDA ACUTA AND EUPHORBIA HIRTA
IBRAHIM T.A., ADETUYI F.O., AJALA LOLA

114.. Pakistan Journal of Biological Sciences. 2010;13(22):1092-1098   xxx dup of 254 corrected
In vitro Antioxidant, Lipoxygenase and Xanthine Oxidase Inhibitory Activities of Fractions from Cienfuegosia digitata Cav., Sida alba L. and Sida acuta Burn f. (Malvaceae)
J. Millogo-Rasolodimby, A. Lamien-Meda, M. Kiendrebeogo, N.T.R. Meda, A.Y. Coulibaly, A. Souza, K. Konate, M. Lamidi, O.G. Nacoulma

115.. Journal of Pharmacognosy and Phytochemistry. 2013;2(2):125-133
In-vitro Antioxidant and Thrombolytic activity of Methanol extract of Sida acuta.

504

Entaz Bahar, Joushan Ara, Mahbubul Alam, Bashutosh Nath, Unmesh Bhowmik, Nazmunnahar Runi

116.. Journal of Biological Sciences. 2006;6(1):160-163
Analgesic and Anti-inflammatory Principle from Sida cordifolia Linn
Ranajit Kumar Sutradhar, AKM Matior Rahman, Mesbahuddin Ahmad, Sitesh Chandra Bachar, Achinto Saha.

117.. Annals of Clinical Microbiology and Antimicrobials. 2012;11(1):33   xxx 211 is a dup
Free radical scavenging capacity, anticandicidal effect of bioactive compounds from Sida Cordifolia L., in combination with nystatin and clotrimazole and their effect on specific immune response in rats
Ouédraogo Maurice, Konaté Kiessoun, Lepengué Alexis Nicaise, Souza Alain, M'Batchi Bertrand, Sawadogo Laya L

118.. Journal of Applied Pharmaceutical Science 01 (02); 2011: 23-31
Sida cordifolia (Linn) – An overview
Ankit Jain, Shreya Choubey, P.K.Singour, H. Rajak and R.S. Pawar

119.. Journal of Ethnopharmacology Volume 72, Issues 1–2, 1 September 2000, Pages 273–277   Anti-inflammatory, analgesic activity and acute toxicity of Sida cordifolia L. (Malva-branca)
Franzotti, Em; Santos, Cv; Rodrigues, Hm; Mourão, Rh; Andrade, Mr; Antoniolli
xxx dup of 18, 63 dup

120.. Revista Cubana de Plantas Medicinales. 2013;18(2):298-314
Quantification, chemical and biological characterization of the saponosides material from Sida cordifolia L. (escobilla)
Oscar Julián Velásquez Ballesteros, Elizabeth Murillo Perea, John Jairo Méndez, Walter Murillo Arango, Diana Alexandra Noreña

121.. Pharmaceutical Biology Volume 43, Issue 9, 2005
Evaluation of the Antioxidant Activity of Sida cordifolia
K. Dhalwala, Y.S. Deshpandea, A.P. Purohita & S.S. Kadama

122.. JOURNAL OF NATURAL REMEDIES Vol. 7/2 (2007) 289 - 293
Comparative Food Intake Inhibitory activity of Sida cordifolia L. and Withania somnifera L. in rats
Purnima Ashok1*, S. Arulmozhi1, B. P. Bhaskara1, R. Rajendran2, B.G. Desai1

123.. J Ethnopharmacol. 2003;84:131-8   xxx dup of 42
Screening of antioxidant activity of three Indian medicinal plants, traditionally used for the management of neurodegenerative diseases.
Auddy B, Ferreira M, Blasina F, Lafon L, Arredondo F, Dajas F, et al.

124.. Indian Journal of Pharmaceutical and Biological Research. 2013;1(4):71-75
Ethnomedicinal plants of Jodhpur District, Rajasthan used in herbal and folk remedies
B.B.S.Kapoor, Swati Lakhera

125.. International Research Journal of Pharmacy. 2012;3(9):309-311
ANTIMICROBIAL ACTIVITY OF LEAF EXTRACTS OF SIDA CORDIFOLIA
Serasanambati Mamatha Reddy, Challa Krishna Kumari, Chilakapati Shanmuga Reddy, Yakkanti Raja Ratna Reddy, Chilakapati Damodar Reddy

126.. Revista Colombiana de Biotecnología. 2007;9(1):5-13
Preliminary evaluation of Sida rhombifolia L. toxicity, genotoxicity and antimicrobial activity
Brugés Keile, Reguero Reza María Teresa

127.. Immunopharmacology and Immunotoxicology Volume 34, Issue 2, 2012 pages 326-336
Anti-inflammatory and anti-oxidant properties of Sida rhombifolia stems and roots in adjuvant induced arthritic rats
R.T. Narendhirakannan*a & T.P. Limmya

128.. Japan J Pharmacol 1971, 21: 136-138
Central nervous system effects of Sida retusa root.
Thangam J, Shanthakumari G.

129.. Phytotherapy Research Volume 17, Issue 8, pages 973–975, September 2003
Cytotoxicity and antibacterial activity of Sida rhombifolia (Malvaceae) grown in Bangladesh
M. Ekramul Islam1, M. Ekramul Haque1 andM. A. Mosaddik2,*

130.. Journal of Health Science 55(3) 2009
Dysregulation of lipid and cholesterol metabolism in high fat diet fed hyperlipidemic rats: Protective effect
of Sida rhomboidea. Roxb leaf extract
M Thounaojam, R Jadeja, R Devkar

131.. International Journal of Phytomedicine 2 (2010) 160-165   xxx dup 196
Hypoglycemic and Hypolipidemic Effect of Sida rhombifolia ssp. retusa in Diabetic Induced Animals
Kamlesh Dhalwal1, Vaibhav M. Shinde1*, Bhagat Singh2, Kakasaheb R. Mahadik1

132.. Journal of Ethnopharmacology 98 (2005) 275–279
CNS pharmacological effects of the hydroalcoholic extract of Sida cordifolia L. leaves
C.I.F. Franco a, L.C.S.L. Morais a,L.J. Quintans-Junior ´ a, R.N. Almeida a,*, A.R. Antoniolli b

133.. Indian Journal of Pharmacology Year 2006   Volume 38   Issue 3 Page 207-208
 Analgesic and antiinflammatory activities of Sida cordifolia Linn
RK Sutradhar1, AKM Matior Rahman1, MU Ahmad2, BK Datta3, SC Bachar3, A Saha3

134.. Journal of Health Science Vol. 56 (2010) No. 1 P 92-98
Prevention of High Fat Diet Induced Insulin Resistance in C57BL/6J Mice by Sida rhomboidea ROXB.
Extract
Menaka Chanu Thounaojam1), Ravirajsinh Navalsinh Jadeja1), Ansarullah1), Ranjitsinh Vijaysinh
Devkar1), A. V. Ramachandran1)

135.. Fitoterapia 1998, vol. 69, no 1, pp. 7-12 (12 ref.), pp. 20-23
Antihepatotoxic activity of Sida cordifolia whole plant
KS Rao, SH Mishra

136.. INTERNATIONAL JOURNAL OF PHARMACEUTICAL SCIENCES AND RESEARCH 2013;
Vol. 4(1): 316-321
IN-VIVO ANTI-INFLAMMATORY EFFECT OF AQUEOUS AND ETHANOLIC EXTRACT OF SIDA
RHOMBIFOLIA L. ROOT
P. Logeswari*1, V. Dineshkumar 1, S.M. Prathap Kumar 2 and P.T.A. Usha 1

137.. J. Ethnopharmacol. 19: 233-245
Diuretic activity of plants used for the treatment of urinary ailments in Guatemala.
Caceres A, Giron LM, Martinez AM (1987).

138.. Indian J Exp Biol 1978; 16: 696-698
Antifertility activities of indigenous plants, Sida carpinifolia and Podocarpus brevifolius, in female rats.
Kholkute SD, Munshi SR, Naik SD and Jathar V S.

139.. International Journal of Research in Pharmacy & Science . Apr-Jun2012, Vol. 2 Issue 2
Nephroprotective Effect of Fresh Leaves Extracts of Sida Cordifolia Linn in Gentamicin Induced
Nephrotoxicity in Rats.
Bhatia, Lovkesh; Bhatia, Vivek; Grover, Manav

140.. International Journal of Pharmaceutical Science Invention Volume 2 Issue 9 (September2013)
PP.07-10
Neurohistological Study of the Effect of Ethanolic Leaf Extract of Sida Acuta on the Cerebral Astrocytes
of Adult Wistar Rats.
1,Mokutima A. Eluwa,2,Chidiebere O. Ubah , 3,Amabe O. Akpantah ,4,Olaitan, R. Asuquo ,5,Theresa B.
Ekanem , 6,Ekaette P. Akpan,7,Theresa E. Isamoh.

141.. Environmental Toxicology and Pharmacology 29 (2010) 223–228
In vitro cytotoxicity and antioxidant activities of five medicinal plants of Malvaceae family from
Cameroon
C.A. Piemea,c,*, V.N. Penlapb, J. Ngoganga, M. Costachec

506

142.. Asian Journal of Chemistry Vol. 19, No. 6 (2007), 4459-4462
Diuretic Activity of Sida cordifolia Linn. of Nilgiris
T. PRABHAKAR*, K. RAMESH, P.K.M. NAGARATHNA, T. SREENIVASA RAO, K. LAKSHMAN†
and B. SURESH

143.. Asian Journal of Chemistry Vol. 19, No. 6 (2007), 4649-4652
Antibacterial and Antifungal Activity of Sida cordifolia Linn.
T. PRABHAKAR*, P.K.M. NAGARATHNA†, T. SRINIVAS RAO‡, BENY BABY††,K. RAMESH††
and B. SURESH‡‡

144.. Research Journal of Pharmacology, 2 (2). pp. 13-16, (2008)
Antinociceptive and anti-inflammatory effects of Sida rhombifolia L. in various animal models.
Sulaiman, Mohd Roslan and Moin, Saidi and Alias, Ashraf S. and Zakaria, Zainul Amiruddin

145.. J. Ethnobiol. Ethnomed. 2: 25.
Ethnobotanical investigations among tribes in Madurai District of Tamil Nadu (India).
Ignacimuthu S, Ayyanar M, Sankara-Sivaramann K (2006).

146.. Chinese Medicine 2.2 (Jun 2011): 47-52.
In Vitro Studies on Sida cordifolia Linn for Anthelmintic and Antioxidant Properties
Pawa, Rajesh Singh; Jain, Ankit; Sharma, Preeti; Chaurasiya, Pradeep Kumar; Singour, Pradeep Kumar.

147.. Songklanakarin J. Sci. Technol. 30 (6), 729-737, Nov. - Dec. 2008
Acute and subchronic toxicity study of the water extract from root of Sida rhombifolia Linn. in rats
Seewaboon Sireeratawong1,3*, Nirush Lertprasertsuke,Umarat Srisawat1, Amornat Thuppia1Anongnad
Ngamjariyawat1, Nadthaganya Suwanlikhid1 and Kanjana Jaijoy31

148.. Proceedings of the National Academy of Sciences, India Section B: Biological Sciences June 2014,
Volume 84, Issue 2, pp 397-405
Anti-Hyperglycemic, Anti-Hyperlipidemic and Antioxidant Potential of Alcoholic-Extract of Sida
cordifolia (Areal Part) in Streptozotocin-Induced-Diabetes in Wistar-Rats
Mahrukh Ahmad, Shahid Prawez , Mudasir Sultana, Rajinder Raina, Nrip Kishore Pankaj, Pawan Kumar
Verma, Shafiqur Rahman

149.. Research Journal of Pharmacology, 2 (2). pp. 13-16. (2008)
Antinociceptive and anti-inflammatory effects of Sida rhombifolia L. in various animal models.
Sulaiman, Mohd Roslan and Moin, Saidi and Alias, Ashraf S. and Zakaria, Zainul Amiruddin

150.. Nat Prod Chem Res 1:101   xxx 278 is a dup
Evaluation of Antibacterial Activities of Compounds Isolated From Sida rhombifolia Linn. (Malvaceae)
Sileshi Woldeyes1, Legesse Adane1*, Yinebeb Tariku1, Diriba Muleta2 and Tadesse Begashaw2

151.. International Journal of Pharmacy and Pharmaceutical Sciences, Vol 4, Issue 1, 2012
PHARMACOGNOSTIC AND PHYTOCHEMICAL INVESTIGATION OF SIDA CORDIFOLIA L.-A
THREATENED MEDICINAL HERB
PRAMOD V. PATTAR.* AND M. JAYARAJ.

152.. Journal of Cell and Tissue Research Vol. 10(3) 2385-2388 (2010)
EVALUATION OF ANTIMICROBIAL AND ACUTE ANTIINFLAMMATORY ACTIVITY OF SIDA
CORDIFOLIA LINN SEED OIL
TERNIKAR, S. G., 1 ALAGAWADI, K. R., 1 ISMAILPASHA,2 DWIVEDI, S., 3M AHAMMED RAFI3
AND SHARMA, T.4

153.. Acta Cir. Bras. vol.18 suppl.5 São Paulo 2003
Proliferative effect of medicinal plants and laser on liver regeneration. A considerable experimental model:
from an experimental model to clinical applications1
Orlando de Castro e Silva Jrl; Renata Lemos SilvaII; Gustavo Barreto de MeloII; Valdinaldo Aragão de
MeloIII; Sônia Oliveira LimaII; Ângelo Roberto AntoniolIV; Vanderlei S BagnatoV

154.. Journal of Ethnopharmacology Volume 72, Issues 1–2, 1 September 2000, Pages 273–277
Antiinflammatory, analgesic activity and acute toxicity of Sida cordifolia L (Malva-branca)

155.. Experimental and Toxicologic Pathology Volume 63, Issue 4, May 2011, Pages 351–356
Cardioprotective effect of Sida rhomboidea. Roxb extract against isoproterenol induced myocardial necrosis in rats
Menaka C. Thounaojam, Ravirajsinh N. Jadeja, Ansarullah, Sanjay S. Karn, Jigar D. Shah, Dipak K. Patel, Sunita P. Salunke, Geeta S. Padate, Ranjitsinh V. Devkar, , A.V. Ramachandran

156.. Biologia Geral e Experimental VOLUME 5, NÚMERO 2, 2004/2005, pages 5-9
Cardiovascular effects on rats induced by the total alkaloid fraction of Sida cordifolia.
Márcio Roberto Viana Santos, Murilo Marchioro, Aletéia Lacerda Silveira, José Maria Barbosa Filho, Isac Almeida Medeiros

157.. International Journal of Pharmacy and Pharmaceutical Sciences Vol 4, Issue 2, 2012
EVALUATION OF ANTIFERTILITY POTENTIAL OF AQUEOUS EXTRACT OF SIDA CARDIFOLIA LINN. PLANT IN SWISS ALBINO MICE
SWATI POKALE*1, KALA KULKARNI2

158.. Indian Journal of Weed Science 46(3): 256–260, 2014
Physico-chemical and biological properties of seed powder of flannel weed (Sida cordifolia)
Manish Kumar, Aradhita Ray, Akshma Berwal and Ashok K. Pathera*

159.. Pharmacologyonline 3: 227-239 (2008)
EFFECT OF HYDROALCOHOLIC EXTRACTS OF SIDA CORDIFOLIA L. LEAVES ON LIPID PROFILE IN RATS
Syed Mohammed Basheeruddin Asdaq1*, Niara Nayeem2 and Amit Kumar Das2*1

160.. Revista Brasileira de Farmacognosia, 2003   xxx 311 is a dup
Evaluation of the cardiovascular effects of vasicine, an alkaloid isolated from the leaves of Sida cordifolia L. (Malvaceae)
Silveira, A.L.; Gomes, M.A.S.; Silva Filho, R.N.; Santos, M.R.V.; Medeiros, I.A.*; Barbosa Filho, J.M.

161.. WORLD JOURNAL OF PHARMACY AND PHARMACEUTICAL SCIENCES Volume 3, Issue 10, 1342-1348
BALA RASAYAN (Sida corfolia) AND OSTEO-ARTHRITIS: A CLINICAL REVIEW
Chaubey PK, Singh AK, Singh OP

162.. Pharmazie 61: 466–469 (2006)
Endothelium-derived factors and Kþ channels are involved in the vasorelaxation induced by Sida cordifolia L. in the rat superior mesenteric artery
M. R. V. Santos2, N. M. S. Nascimento1, A. R. Antoniolli2, I. A. Medeiros1

163.. Journal of Ethnopharmacology Volume 124, Issue 1, 6 July 2009, Pages 162–165   xxx dup of 33&69
Role of Sida cordifolia L. leaves on biochemical and antioxidant profile during myocardial injury
J.B. Kubavat, S.M.B. Asdaq

164.. Intern. J. Oncol., 31:915-922 (2007)
The plant alkaloid cryptolepine induces p21WAF1/CIP1 and cell cycle arrest in a human osteosarcoma cell line
Taka-aki, M., Yoshihiro, S., Hiroaki, M., Koichi, T, Ryoko, N.S., Masayuki, Y., Motomasa, K., Tomoya,S., Toshikazu, K. and Toshiyuki, S

165.. European Journal of Pharmacology Volume 409, Issue 1, 1 December 2000, Pages 9–18
Cytotoxicity and cell cycle effects of the plant alkaloids cryptolepine and neocryptolepine: relation to drug-induced apoptosis
Laurent Dassonnevillea, Amélie Lansiauxa, Aurélie Watteleta, Nicole Watteza, Christine Mahieua, Sabine Van Miertb, Luc Pietersb, Christian Baillya

508

166.. Biochemistry, 1998, 37 (15), pp 5136–5146
The DNA Intercalating Alkaloid Cryptolepine Interferes with Topoisomerase II and Inhibits Primarily
DNA Synthesis in B16 Melanoma Cells†
K. Bonjean ,*‡ M. C. De Pauw-Gillet ,‡ M. P. Defresne ,‡ P. Colson ,§ C. Houssier ,§ L. Dassonneville ,?
C. Bailly ,*? R. Greimers ,? C. Wright ,# J. Quetin-Leclercq ,¶+ M. Tits ,¶ and L. Angenot ¶

167.. INTERNATIONAL JOURNAL OF PHARMACEUTICAL AND CHEMICAL SCIENCES Vol. 2
(3) Jul-Sep 2013
Screening of Gastric Antiulcer Activity of Sida cordifolia
S. Akilandeswari,* R. Valarmathi, VN. Indulatha and R. Senthamarai

168.. Tropical Journal of Pharmaceutical Research, December 2007; 6 (4): 809-813
Antimicrobial activity of the ethanol extract of the aerial parts of sida acuta burm.f. (malvaceae)
IE Oboh1, JO Akerele2* and O Obasuyi2

169.. Redox Report: Communications in Free Radical Research Volume 20, Issue 2, 2015, pages 75-80
Nrf2-mediated antioxidant response by ethanolic extract of Sida cordifolia provides protection against
alcohol-induced oxidative stress in liver by upregulation of glutathione metabolism

170.. Asian Journal of Chemistry23.1 (2011): 141-144.
Antihyperglycemic Activity of Root Bark of Polyalthia longifolia Var. pendula and Aerial Parts of Sida
rhombifolia Linn. and Its Relationship with Antioxidant Property
Ghosh, G; Subudhi, B B; Mishra, S K.

171.. International Journal of Pharmaceutical Research and Innovation, Vol. 8, 2015, 11-22
ANTIDIABETIC EFFECT OF SIDA CORDIFOLIA (AQUEOUS EXTRACT) ON DIABETES
INDUCED IN WISTAR RATS USING STREPTOZOTOCIN AND ITS PHYTOCHEMISTRY
Mahrukh Ahmad1, Shahid Prawez2,*, Mudasir Sultana1, Rajinder Raina1, Pawan Kumar Verma1, Azad
Ahmad Ahanger3 and Nrip Kishore Pankaj1

172.. European Journal of Pharmacology Volume 409, Issue 1, 1 December 2000, Pages 9–18
Cytotoxicity and cell cycle effects of the plant alkaloids cryptolepine and neocryptolepine: relation to
drug-induced apoptosis
Laurent Dassonnevillea, Amélie Lansiauxa, Aurélie Watteleta, Nicole Wattezа, Christine Mahieua, Sabine
Van Miertb, Luc Pietersb, Christian Baillya

173.. World Journal of Agricultural Sciences 4 (S): 839-843, 2008
Antimicrobial Activity of Some Important Medicinal Plant Against Plant and Human Pathogens
B. Mahesh and S. Satish 1 2

174.. Natural Product Sciences, 2006
Antiulcer Activity of Sida acuta Burm
P Malairajan, G Gopalakrishnan

175.. Scholars Res Library 2012;4(1):175-80.
Assessment of nephroprotective potential of Sida cordifolia Linn. In experimental animals.
Mehul V, Makwana, Nilesh M, Pandya, Dharmesh, Darji N, Sarav A Desai, et al.

176.. Int J Biol Med Res 2011;2(4):1038-42
Effect of bioactive compounds and its pharmaceutical activities of sida cordifolia (Linn.).
Baby Joseph, Ajisha AU, Satheesna Kumari, Sujatha S.

177.. INTERNATIONAL JOURNAL OF SCIENTIFIC & TECHNOLOGY RESEARCH VOLUME 4,
ISSUE 11, NOVEMBER 2015
Evaluation Of Anti-Arthritic Activity Of Ethanolic Extract Of Sida-Cardifolia
Divya Mani Polireddy

178.. Indian J. Exp. Biol. 16, 696.
Anti fertility activity of indigenous plants Sida carpinifolia and Podocarpus brevifolius stapf in female rats.
Kholkute, S. D., Munshi, S. R., Naik, S. D. and Jathar, V. S. (1978).

179.. International Journal of Pharmacognosy Volume 35, Issue 3, 1997 pages 179-184
Antibacterial Activity Observed in the Seeds of Some Coprophilous Plants
Sushil Kumara, G.D. Bagchia & M.P. Darokara

180.. Indian Journal of Natural Products and Resources Vol. 2(4), December 2011, pp. 428-434
Antidiabetic and anti-hypercholesterolemic effects of aerial parts of Sida cordifolia Linn. on
Streptozotocin-induced diabetic rats
Gagandeep Kaur, Pradeep Kamboj and A N Kalia*

181.. Indian Drugs 1997;34(12):702-6
Isolation and assessment of hepatoprotective activity of fumaric acid obtained for the first time from Sida
cordifolia Linn.
Kumar S Rao, Mishra SH.

182.. Br J Nutr 2012;108:1256–63.
Amelioration of alcohol-induced hepatotoxicity by the administration of ethanolic extract of Sida
cordifolia Linn
Rejitha S, Prathibha P, Indira M.

183.. Iran J Pharmacol Ther 2006;5:175-8.
Bioactive Alkaloid from Sida cordifolia Linn with analgesic and anti-inflammatory activities.
Ranajit Kumar Sutradhar, AKM Matior Rahman, Mesbahuddin Ahmad, Sitesh Chandra Bachar, Achinto
Saha, Samar Kumar Guha.

184.. Int. J. Drug Dev. & Res., July-September 2012, 4 (3): 92-96   xxx dup of 98
Antifungal activity of flavonoids of Sida acuta Burm f. against Candida albicans
Jindal Alka*, Kumar Padma, Jain Chitra

185.. J Ethnopharmacol 1999, 67(2):229-232.
Antinociceptive and anti-inflammatory activity of Sida rhombifolia leaves.
Venkatesh S, Reddy SY, Suresh B, Madhava RB, Ramesh M

186.. Int J Pharmacog. 1997;35:179-184
ANTI-INFLAMMATORY AND ANALGESIC ACTIVITY OF METHANOLIC EXTRACT OF WHOLE
PLANT OF SIDA ACUTA (LINN.F.ND)
Virendra Sharma, Pooja Sinoriya, Sunil Sharma

187.. Journal of Biological Sciences 2009 Vol. 9 No. 5 pp. 504-508
Indonesian Sidaguri (Sida rhombifolia L.) as antigout and inhibition kinetics of flavonoids crude extract
on the activity of xanthine oxidase.
Iswantini, D.; Darusman, L.K.; Hidayat, R. Indonesian Sidaguri

188.. Acta Botanica Brasilica. 2001;15(2):147-154
Seed germination of medicinal woody plants
Shirley G.T.da Rosa, Alfredo Gui Ferreira

189.. Revista Ceres. 2011;58(6):749-754
Effects of seasonal variations on the emergence of Solanum viarum and Sida rhombifolia under different
sowing depths
Marcelo Claro Souza, Mariana Casari Parreira, Carita Liberato do Amaral, Pedro Luís da Costa Aguiar
Alves

190.. Journal of Pharmacognosy and Phytochemistry. 2013;2(3):1-4
Pharmacognostical Study of the Whole Plant of Sida rhombifolia
Pooja Sinoriya, SC Mehta, Virendra Sharma

191.. Curr Med Chem. 2008;15(1):75-91.
Phytoecdysteroids and anabolic-androgenic steroids--structure and effects on humans.
Báthori M1, Tóth N, Hunyadi A, Márki A, Zádor E.

192.. British Journal of Pharmacology and Toxicology. 2013;4(1):18-24
Effect of Long-term use of Sida rhombifolia L. Extract on Haemato-biochemical Parameters of
Experimental Animals
M. Ouédraogo, P. Zerbo, K. Konaté, N. Barro, Laya L. Sawadogo

193.. Wikipedia, https://en.wikipedia.org/wiki/Phytoecdysteroid

194.. International Journal of Pharmaceutical Sciences and Research. 2012;3(9):3136-3145
PRELIMINARY TOXICITY STUDY, ANTI-NOCICEPTIVE AND ANTI-INFLAMMATORY
PROPERTIES OF EXTRACTS FROM SIDA RHOMBIFOLIA L. (MALVACEAE)
Kiessoun Konate*1, Jacques Francois Mavoungou 2, Maurice Ouédraogo 3, Alexis Nicaise Lepengue 4,
Alain Souza 1, Nicolas Barro 6 and Bertrand M'Batchi 1, 4

195.. Antioxidants. 2012;1(1):33-43
Total Phenolic Content and Antioxidant Activity of Some Malvaceae Family Species
Adriana Maria Fernandes de Oliveira, Lilian Sousa Pinheiro, Charlane Kelly Souto Pereira, Wemerson
Neves Matias, Roosevelt Albuquerque Gomes, Otemberg Souza Chaves, Maria de Fátima Vanderlei de
Souza, Reinaldo Nóbrega de Almeida, Temilce Simões de Assis

196.. International Journal of Phytomedicine. 2011;2(2)   xx dup of 131
Hypoglycemic and Hypolipidemic Effect of Sida rhombifolia ssp. retusa in Diabetic Induced Animals
Kamlesh Dhalwal, Vaibhav M. Shinde, Bhagat Singh, Kakasaheb R. Mahadik

197.. Pharmacologyonline 3: 259-266 (2006)
Hepatoprotective Activity of Sida rhombifolia ssp. retusa Against Thioacetamide and Allyl Alcohol
Intoxication in Rats
Kamlesh Dhalwal*, Vaibhav Shinde, K.R. Mahadik and S.S. Kadam

198.. Acta Scientiarum : Agronomy. 2009;31(3):489-494
Influence of accelerated aging and light on the physiological quality of arrowleaf sida seeds
Denise Bruginski de Carvalho, Ruy Inacio Neiva de Carvalho

199.. International Research Journal of Pharmacy. 2011;2(9):157-160
EVALUATION OF ANTIDIARRHOEAL ACTIVITY OF SIDA RHOMBIFOLIA LINN. ROOT
Sarangi Rashmi Ranjan, Mishra Uma Shankar, Panda Susanta Kumar, Behera Saiprasanna

200.. IJPSR, 2015; Vol. 6(4): 1609-1615.
A COMPARITIVE STUDY OF PHYTOCHEMICALS AND ANTIOXIDANT ACTIVITY AMONG
TRADITIONAL MEDICINAL PLANTS
Belakere Lakshmeesh Nanda* and Thulasi T Radhakrishnan

201.. Journal of Applied Pharmaceutical Science Vol. 4 (10), pp. 097-104, October, 2014
Anti-diabetic and hypolipidaemic effect of botanicals: a review of medicinal weeds on KNUST campus,
Kumasi
Christopher Larbie*, Dennis Torkornoo and Jeffrey Dadson

202.. Pharmaceutical Biology.1994; 32(4):337-345
Antibacterial and antifungal Activities of nine medicinal plants from Zaire.
Muanza DN, Kim BW, Euler KL and Williams L: Alam M, Joy S and Ali US

203.. BMC Complement Altern Med. 2012 Aug 11;12:120. doi: 10.1186/1472-6882-12-120.
Toxicity assessment and analgesic activity investigation of aqueous acetone extracts of Sida acuta Burn f .
and Sidacordifolia L. (Malvaceae), medicinal plants of Burkina Faso.
Konaté K1, Bassolé IH, Hilou A, Aworet-Samseny RR, Souza A, Barro N, Dicko MH, Datté JY, M'Batchi
B.

204.. Anc Sci Life. 2008 Apr;27(4):1-8.
Phytochemical constituents of some Indian medicinal plants.
Dhandapani R1, Sabna B.

205.. Journai qf Heaith Science,54(5) 544-550 (200S)
Anxiolytic and Antiseizure Effects of Sida tiagii

511

Bhandri Ashok Kumar Datusalia,""Pankaj Kalra,"Balasubramanian Narasimhan, SunilSharma," and Ramesh Kumar Goyal

206.. J Ethnopharmacol. 2000 Nov;73(1-2):233-41.
Snakebites and ethnobotany in the northwest region of Colombia. Part III: neutralization of the haemorrhagic effect of Bothrops atrox venom.
Otero R1, Núñez V, Barona J, Fonnegra R, Jiménez SL, Osorio RG, Saldarriaga M, Díaz A.

207.. Bioorg Med Chem Lett. 2010 Mar 15;20(6):1837-9. doi: 10.1016/j.bmcl.2010.01.165. Epub 2010 Feb 6.
Unprecedented NES non-antagonistic inhibitor for nuclear export of Rev from Sida cordifolia.
Tamura S1, Kaneko M, Shiomi A, Yang GM, Yamaura T, Murakami N.
208.. J Clin Periodontol. 1992 May;19(5):305-10.
Inhibition of peptidase and glycosidase activities of Porphyromonas gingivalis, Bacteroides intermedius and Treponema denticola by plant extracts.
Homer KA1, Manji F, Beighton D.

210.. Asian-Australasian Journal of Animal Sciences 1997 Vol. 10 No. 1 pp. 28-34   xxx dup of 415
Variability in ash, crude protein, detergent fiber and mineral content of some minor plant species collected from pastures grazed by goats.
Serra, A. B.; Serra, S. D.; Orden, E. A.; Cruz, L. C.; Nakamura, K.; Fujihara, T.

211.. Annals of Clinical Microbiology and Antimicrobials 2012, 11:33   xxx dup of 27 and 117
Free radical scavenging capacity, anticandicidal effect of bioactive compounds from Sida Cordifolia L., in combination with nystatin and clotrimazole and their effect on specific immune response in rats
Maurice Ouédraogo1*, Kiessoun Konaté2,4, Alexis Nicaise Lepengué3 , Alain Souza4 , Bertrand M'Batchi3,4 and Laya L Sawadogo1

212.. Indian Journal of Traditional Knowledge vol 7(1), January 2008. pp.162-165
Plants used in traditional handicrafts in north eastern Andhra Pradesh
KN Reddy, C Pattanaik, CS Reddy

213.. African Journal of Food Agriculture Nutrition and Development, Vol. 5, No. 1 , 2005
POTENTIAL TOXICITY OF SOME TRADITIONAL LEAFY VEGETABLES CONSUMED IN NYANG'OMA DIVISION, WESTERN KENYA
Orech, F. O. 1, T. Akenga2*, J. Ochora3, H. Friis4, J. Aagaard-Hansen5

214.. Journal of Medicinal Plants Research Vol. 7(20), pp. 1452-1460, 25 May, 2013
Antibacterial activity of medicinal plants used as ethnomedicine by the traditional healers of Musiri Thaluk, Trichy District, Tamilnadu, India
Sathya Bama S.1, Sankaranarayanan S.2*, Bama P.2, Ramachandran J.3, Bhuvaneswari N.3 andJayasurya Kingsley S4

215.. Medicinal and Aromatic Plant Science and Biotechnology
African Ethnopharmacology and New Drug Discovery
Damintoti Karou1,3* • Wendyame M. C. Nadembega1,3 • Lassina Ouattara1 • Dénise P.Ilboudo1 • Antonella Canini4 • Jean Baptiste Nikiéma2 • Jacques Simpore1,3 • Vittorio Colizzi4 • Alfred S. Traore1

216.. CYTOLOGIA Vol. 36 (1971) No. 2 P 285-297
Chromosome Studies in Different Species and Varieties of Sida with Special Reference to Accessory Chromosomes
Radharanjan Hazra and Archana Sharma

217.. Int. J. Res. Rev. Pharm. Appl. Sci, 2012 IJRRPAS, 2(2).173-195
Review on the species of Sida used for the preparation of nayopayam kashayam
MD Ajithabai, S Rani, G Jayakumar

218.. Ethnobotanical leaflets, (2006) 10 : 336-341
Bala (Sida cordifolia.L) Is it safe Herbal drug?
Dr.Amrit Pal Singh

512

219.. Research Journal of Pharmacology 3(2): 22-25, 2009   xxx 273 is a dup
Evaluation of the Antibacterial Activity of Extracts of Sida acuta Against Clinical Isolates of
Staphylococcus aureus Isolated from Human Immunodeficiency Virus
IR Iroha, ES Amadi, AC Nwuzo,FN Afiukwa

220.. African Journal of Biotechnology Vol. 6 (25), pp. 2953-2959, 28 December, 2007
Sida acuta Burm. f.: a medicinal plant with numerous potencies
Simplice Damintoti Karou1,3*, Wendyam MC Nadembega1,2, Denise P Ilboudo1,2, Djeneba
Ouermi1,2, Messanvi Gbeassor3, Comlan De Souza3 and Jacques Simpore1,2

221.. Asian Journal of Pharmaceutical and Clinical Research Vol 5, Suppl 1, 2012
ANTIBACTERIAL ACTIVITY OF SIDA ACUTA BURM. F. AGAINST HUMAN PATHOGENS
ALKA JINDAL*, PADMA KUMAR

222.. Science 21 Aug 1992: Vol. 257, Issue 5073, pp. 1050-1055
Epidemiology of Drug Resistance: Implications for a Post—Antimicrobial Era
Mitchell L. Cohen

223.. IOSR Journal of Applied Chemistry Volume 7, Issue 2 Ver. I. (Mar-Apr. 2014), PP 93-98
Proximate, Phytochemical and Micronutrient Composition of Sida acuta
Raimi, Monsurat M. , Oyekanmi, Adeyinka M. , And Adegoke, Bosede M.

224.. African Journal of Clinical and Experimental Microbiology Vol 7, No 2 (2006)
Evaluation of Sida acuta subspecie acuta leaf/flower combination for antimicrobial activity and
phytochemical constituents
Alhaji Saganuwan Saganuwan, Gulumbe Mohammed Lawal

225.. Journal Economic Botany Volume 42, Issue 1 , pp 16-28 October 2008
Herbal medicine among the miskito of Eastern Nicaragua
Philip A. Dennis

226.. Pharmaceutical Biology Volume 42, Issue 1, 2004 pages 13-17
Screening of Antibacterial and Antifungal Activities of Ten Medicinal Plants from Ghana
B.R. Hoffmana, H. DelasAlasa, K. Blancoa, N. Wiederholda, R.E. Lewisa & L. Williamsb*

227.. Arabian Journal of Chemistry Volume 5, Issue 3, July 2012, Pages 325–337
Synergistic inhibition effects between leaves and stem extracts of Sida acuta and iodide ion for mild steel
corrosion in 1 M H2SO4 solutions
U.M. Eduok, S.A. Umoren, , A.P. Udoh

228.. Australian Journal of Experimental Agriculture and Animal Husbandry 20(105) 463 - 469 1980
Germination and establishment of the weeds Sida acuta and Pennisetum pedicellatum in the Northern
Territory
JJ Mott

229.. Online Journal of Animal and Feed Research Volume 2, Issue 2: 182-188 (2012)
USE OF STYLOSANTHES HAMATA AND SIDA ACUTA AS SOLE FEEDS FOR RABBITS
(Oryctolagus cuniculus)
J. NAANDAM*, B.A.Y. PADI, P. BIGOL, R. MENSAH-KUMI

230.. Research in Pharmacy, 1(1): 33-40, 2011
Preliminary Phytochemical Analysis and Conservation of Herbs used by the Tribal people of Bolangir
(Orissa), India as a Remedy against Threatened Miscarriage
Sarada Prasad Mohapatra*

231.. International Journal of Science, Environment and Technology, Vol. 5, No 1, 2016, 17 – 24
THE SURVIVAL OF FOUR TROPICAL PLANTS ON SOILS ARTIFICIALLY POLLUTED WITH
TOXIC LEVELS OF ZINC
U.F. Umeoguaju*1 , C.J. Ononamadu2 , M.C. Okonkwo1 and O.C. Ezeigwe1

232.. Chem. Pharm. Bull. 64, 119–127 (2016) Vol. 64, No. 2
Bio-active Natural Products with TRAIL-Resistance Overcoming Activity

513

Firoj Ahmeda,b and Masami Ishibashi*,

233.. PhD Thesis 2011, DEPARTMENT OF PHARMACY
STUDY OF THE PHARMACOLOGICAL ACTIVITIES OF SUCCESSIVE EXTRACTS OF HERBAL
PLANT - A SYNOPSIS/RESEARCH PROPOSAL SUBMITTED TO THE SHRI JAGDISH PRASAD
JHABARMAL TIBREWALA UNIVERSITY,
MS. NEELAM LAXMAN DASHPUTRE

234.. PhD thesis, UNIVERSITY OF GHANA, LEGON   July 2014
ANTIBACTERIAL ACTIVITIES OF THREE MEDICINAL PLANTS ON ORGANISMS
ASSOCIATED WITH DENTAL PLAQUE
CLEMENT ELESESHIE NYADROH

235.. Pak J Pharm Sci. 2007 Jul;20(3):185-8.
Anti-inflammatory and analgesic alkaloid from Sida cordifolia linn.
Sutradhar RK, Rahman AM, Ahmad M, Bachar SC, Saha A, Roy TG.

236.. Environmental Entomology Volume 20, Issue 3Pp. 882 - 888
Natural Enemies of Sida acuta and S. rhombifolia (Malvaceae) in Mexico and their Potential for Biological
Control of these Weeds in Australia
John D. Gillett, Ken L. S. Harley, Richard C. Kassulke, Hugo J. Miranda

237.. Journal of Applied and Natural Science 1(1):1-7(2009)
Phytochemistry, antibacterial and anticoagulase activities of Sida acuta against clinical isolates of
Staphylococcus aureus
J. P. Essien1, B. S. Antia2 and G. A. Ebong1*

238.. Pharmaceutical Biology 2002, Vol. 40, No. 03, pp. 235–244
Antimicrobial Activity of Plants Collected from Serpentine Outcrops in Sri Lanka
Nishanta Rajakaruna, Cory S. Harris and G.H.N. Towers

239.. Veterinary World. 2008;1(2.000):49-50
Effect of Asparagus racemosus, Sida cordifolia and Levamisole on immunological parameters in
experimentally induced mmunosuppressed broilers.
Tekade S. H., S. G. Mode and S. P. Waghmare

240.. Journal of Science and Arts. 2013;24(3):281-286
CHEMICAL COMPOSITION OF THE LEAVES AND STEM BARK: METHANOL EXTRACT OF
SIDA CORDIFOLIA L.
SAHA DIBYAJYOTI, PAUL SWATI

241.. Journal of Ethnobiology and Ethnomedicine. 2011;7(1):32
Ethnomedicinal and ecological status of plants in Garhwal Himalaya, India
Sheikh Mehraj A, Kumar Munesh, Bussmann Rainer W

242.. Pesquisa Veterinária Brasileira. 2002;22(2):51-57
Aspectos clínicos e patológicos da intoxicação por Sida carpinifolia (Malvaceae) em caprinos no Rio
Grande do Sul
Colodel Edson M., Driemeier David, Loretti Alexandre P., Gimeno Eduardo J., Traverso Sandra D., Seitz
Anderson L., Zlotowski Priscila

243.. Journal of Biological Sciences 2009 Vol. 9 No. 5 pp. 504-508
Indonesian Sidaguri (Sida rhombifolia L.) as antigout and inhibition kinetics of flavonoids crude extract on
the activity of xanthine oxidase.
Iswantini, D.; Darusman, L. K.; Hidayat, R.

244.. Nature Structural Biology 9, 57 - 60 (2001)
The antimalarial and cytotoxic drug cryptolepine intercalates into DNA at cytosine-cytosine sites
John N. Lisgarten1, 2, Miquel Coll1, Jose Portugal1, Colin W. Wright3 & Juan Aymami1, 4

245.. Phytotherapy Research : an international journal devoted to medical and scientific research on plants
and plant products- Vol. 10, no.4, p. 361-363 (1996)

Antimalarial activity of cryptolepine and some other anhydronium bases
Wright, C. W., Philipson, J. D., Awe, S. O., Kirby, G. C., Warhurst, D., Quetin-Leclercq, Joëlle, Angenot, Luc

246.. J Infect Dis. (2001) 184 (6): 770-776.
Chloroquine-Resistant Malaria
Thomas E. Wellems1 and Christopher V. Plowe2

247.. Toxicology Letters 207 (2011) 322–325
Effects of the anti-malarial compound cryptolepine and its analogues in human lymphocytes and sperm in the Comet assay
Rajendran C. Gopalana, Esra Emerce b, Colin W. Wright a, Bensu Karahalil b, Ali E. Karakaya b, Diana Andersona,*

248.. J. Med. Chem., 1998, 41 (6), pp 894–901
Ethnobotanical-Directed Discovery of the Antihyperglycemic Properties of Cryptolepine: Its Isolation from Cryptolepis sanguinolenta, Synthesis, and in Vitro and in Vivo Activities†
Donald E. Bierer ,* Diana M. Fort , Christopher D. Mendez , Jian Luo , Patricia A. Imbach , Larisa G. Dubenko , Shivanand D. Jolad , R. Eric Gerber , Joane Litvak , Qing Lu , Pingsheng Zhang , Michael J. Reed , Nancy Waldeck , Reimar C. Bruening , Ben K. Noamesi ,§ Richard F. Hector , Thomas J. Carlson , and Steven R. King

249.. Letters in Applied Microbiology Volume 40, Issue 1, pages 24–29, January 2005
The killing effect of cryptolepine on Staphylococcus aureus
I.K. Sawer1, M.I. Berry2 andJ.L. Ford2

250.. GHANA MEDICAL JOURNAL March 2010 Volume 44, Number 1
CLINICAL EFFICACY OF A TEA-BAG FORMULATION OF CRYPTOLEPIS SANGUINOLENTA ROOT IN THE TREATMENT OF ACUTE UNCOMPLICATED FALCIPARUM MALARIA
K. A. BUGYEI, G. L. BOYE and M. E. ADDY1

251.. Phytotherapy Research Volume 9, Issue 5, pages 359–363, August 1995   xxx dup of 108
In vitro and in vivo antimalarial activity of cryptolepine, a plant-derived indoloquinoline
G. C. Kirby1,*, A. Paine1,2, D. C. Warhurst1, B. K. Noamese2 andJ. D. Phillipson3

252.. Bioresour Technol. 2007 Jul;98(9):1788-94. Epub 2006 Sep 14.
Phytoextraction capacity of the plants growing on tannery sludge dumping sites.
Gupta AK1, Sinha S.

253.. Arch Pharm Res. 2003 Aug;26(8):585-90.
Compounds obtained from sida acuta with the potential to induce quinone reductase and to inhibit 7,12-dimethylbenz[a]anthracene-induced preneoplastic lesions in a mouse mammary organ culture model.
Jang DS1, Park EJ, Kang YH, Su BN, Hawthorne ME, Vigo JS, Graham JG, Cabieses F,Fong HH, Mehta RG, Pezzuto JM, Kinghorn AD.

254.. Pak J Biol Sci. 2010 Nov 15;13(22):1092-8.   xxx 114 is a dup

In vitro antioxidant, lipoxygenase and xanthine oxidase inhibitory activities of fractions from Cienfuegosia digitata Cav., Sida alba L. andSida acuta Burn f. (Malvaceae).
Konaté K, Souza A, Coulibaly AY, Meda NT, Kiendrebeogo M, Lamien-Meda A, Millogo-Rasolodimby J,Lamidi M, Nacoulma OG.

255.. Ethnobotanical Leaflets 13: 1069-1087, 2009.
Ethnobotanical Studies from Amaravathy Range of Indira Gandhi Wildlife Sanctuary, Western Ghats, Coimbatore District, Southern India
V.S. Ramachandran1 , Shijo Joseph2 and R. Aruna3

256.. The evaluation of the effect of Sida acuta leaf extract on the microanatomy and some biochemical parameters on the liver of Wistar rats
KE Obeten, KC Uruakpa, V Isaac   xxx dup of 572

515

257.. Indian Journal of Traditional Knowledge Vol. 10(2), April 2011, pp. 227-238
Ethnomedical knowledge of plants and healthcare practices among the Kalanguya tribe in Tinoc, Ifugao, Luzon, Philippines
TD Balangcod, AKD Balangcod

258.. Economic Botany January 1991, Volume 45, Issue 1, pp 103-113
Food Plants of the Luo of Siaya District, Kenya 1
TIMOTHY JOHNS 2 AND JOHN O. KOKWARO 3

259.. Journal of Radioanalytical and Nuclear Chemistry March 2015, Volume 303, Issue 3, pp 2101-2112
PIXE-based quantification of health-proactive trace elements in genetically transformed roots of a multi-medicinal plant, Sida acuta Burm.f.
Somanatha Jena, Lopamudra Sahu, Dinesh K. Ray, Sagar K. Mishra, Pradeep K. Chand

260.. International Journal of Current Pharmaceutical Research ISSN- 0975-7066 Vol 5, Issue 2, 2013
EXTRACTION AND QUANTIFICATION OF STEROLS FROM TRIBULUS TERRESTRIS L., SIDA ACUTA BURM F. AND TRIDAX PROCUMBENS L.
ALKA JINDAL, PADMA KUMAR

261.. Am J Infect Control. 2015 Jan;43(1):35-7. doi: 10.1016/j.ajic.2014.09.015.
Staphylococcus aureus and the oral cavity: an overlooked source of carriage and infection?
McCormack MG1, Smith AJ2, Akram AN3, Jackson M1, Robertson D1, Edwards G4.

262.. The International Union for Conservation of Nature and Natural Resources (IUCN), Gland, Switzerland, in partnership with The World Health Organization (WHO), Geneva, Switzerland, and WWF – World Wide Fund for Nature, Gland, Switzerland, 1993.
Guidelines on the Conservation of Medicinal Plants

263.. Phytochemical Analysis Volume 12, Issue 2, pages 110–119, March/April 2001   xxx dup of 56, 491 also dup
Phytoecdysteroid profiles in seeds of Sida spp. (Malvaceae)
Laurence Dinan*, Pauline Bourne andPensri Whiting

264.. African Journal of Biotechnology Vol. 14(49), pp. 3264-3269, 9 December, 2015
Phyto-nutrient composition and antioxidative potential of ethanolic leaf extract of Sida acuta in wistar albino rats
Nwankpa P.1*, Chukwuemeka O. G.2, Uloneme G. C.3, Etteh C. C.1, Ugwuezumba P.4, Nwosu D.5

265.. International Journal of the Physical Sciences Vol. 5(6), pp. 753-762, June 2010   xxx 300 is a dup
Preliminary phytochemical analysis and insecticidalactivity of ethanolic extracts of four tropical plants (Vernonia amygdalina, Sida acuta, Ocimum gratissimum and Telfaria occidentalis) against beans weevil (Acanthscelides obtectus)
S. A. Adeniyi1*, C. L. Orjiekwe1, J. E. Ehiagbonare2and B. D. Arimah3

266.. IOSR Journal of Dental and Medical Sciences (IOSR-JDMS) Volume 8, Issue 5 (Jul.- Aug. 2013), PP 60-63
Histological Study of the Effect of Ethanolic Leaf Extract of Sida Acuta on the Cerebral Cortex of Adult Wistar Rats
M .A Eluwa, P. S Ofem, O. R Asuquo*, A. O. Akpantah, T. B. Ekanem,

267.. J Res Indian Med Yoga Homeopathy 13.3 (1978): 50-66.
Experimental studies on the immunological aspects of Atibala (A. indicum Linn Sw.), Mahabala (Sida rhombifolia Linn.), Bala (Sida cordifolia Linn.) and Bhumibala (Sida veronicaefolia Lam).
Dixit, S. P., P. V. Tewari, and R. M. Gupta.
cited by [239] - 'as well as medicinal plant like Sida cordifolia have immune enhancing properties"

268.. Wikipedia, "Traditional Medicine", https://en.wikipedia.org/wiki/Traditional_medicine

269.. Wikipedia,"Herbalism", https://en.wikipedia.org/wiki/Herbalism#India

270.. International Journal of Universal Pharmacy and Bio Sciences 4(1): January-February 2015
A REVIEW ON SIDA ACUTA

C. Pooja*1 , I.J Kuppast2, J.H Virupaksha3,M.C Ravi4

271.. International Journal of Green Pharmacy6.3 (Jul 2012): 208-211
Extraction and pharmacological evaluation of flavonoids of sida acuta Burm. f.
Jindal, Alka; Kumar, Padma; Singh, Geeta.

272.. Electron. J. Biotechnol. v.2 n.2 Valparaíso ago. 1999
Medicinal plants: a re-emerging health aid
Lucy Hoareau, Assistant Programme Officer, Division of Life Sciences UNESCO
Edgar J. DaSilva, Director, Division of Life Sciences UNESCO

273.. Research Journal of Pharmacology 3 (2): 22-25,2009   xxx dup of 219
Evaluation of the Antibacterial Activity of Extracts of Sida acuta Against Clinical Isolates of
Staphylococcus aureus Isolated from Human Immunodeficiency Virus/Acquired Immunodeficiency
Syndrome Patients
Iroha I R, Amadi E S, Nwuzo A C, Afiukwa F N,

274.. Elixir Org. Chem. 71 (2014) 24654-24660
Chemical assessement of the proximate, minerals, and anti-nutrients composition of Sida acuta leaves
G. N. Enin, B. S. Antia and F. G. Enin

275.. Revista Brasileira de Farmacognosia Volume 26, Issue 2, March–April 2016, Pages 209–215
Neuropharmacological effects of the ethanolic extract of Sida acuta
Dora M. Benjumeaa, , , Isabel C. Gómez-Betancura, Julieta Vásqueza, Fernando Alzateb, Andrea García-
Silvac, José A. Fontenlac

275.. Revista Brasileira de Farmacognosia Volume 26, Issue 2, March–April 2016, Pages 209–215
Neuropharmacological effects of the ethanolic extract of Sida acuta
Dora M. Benjumeaa, , , Isabel C. Gómez-Betancura, Julieta Vásqueza, Fernando Alzateb, Andrea García-
Silvac, José A. Fontenlac

276.. Journal of Animal Production. 2009;11(2):103-108
Addition of Medicinal Weeds in The Ration on Broiler Chicken Performance
Nurhayati, Nelwida, H Handoko

277.. Natural Product Radiance, Vol 3(4) July-Auguest 2004
Plants used for tissue healing of animals
S Jaiswal, SV Singh, B Singh, HN Singh

278.. Nat Prod Chem Res 2012, 1:1   xxx dup of 150
Evaluation of Antibacterial Activities of Compounds Isolated From Sida rhombifolia Linn. (Malvaceae)
Sileshi Woldeyes1, Legesse Adane1*, Yinebeb Tariku1, Diriba Muleta2 and Tadesse Begashaw2

279.. Acta Bot. Bras. vol.24 no.2 São Paulo Apr./June 2010
Local knowledge of medicinal plants in three artisanal fishing communities (Itapoá, Southern Brazil),
according to gender, age, and urbanization
Adriana Heindrickson Cunha MerétikaI,II; Nivaldo PeroniII; Natalia HanazakiI,*

280.. Journal of Ethnopharmacology 132 (2010) 365–367
Sida rhomboidea.Roxb leaf extract ameliorates gentamicin induced nephrotoxicity and renal dysfunction in
rats
Menaka C. Thounaojam, Ravirajsinh N. Jadeja, Ranjitsinh V. Devkar *, A.V. Ramachandran

281.. Acta Farm. Bonaerense 25 (2): 260 -1 (2006)
Anti-inflammatory activity of the hydroalcoholyc extract of leaves of Sida rhombifolia L. (Malvaceae)
Najeh Maissar KHALIL 1*, Joceana Soares SPEROTTO 2 & Melania Palermo MANFRON 2

282.. International Journal of Biological & Pharmaceutical Research. 2014; 5(2): 196-200.
EVALUATION OF IN VITRO ANTIOXIDANT ACTIVITY AND CYTOTOXICITY OF
METHANOLIC EXTRACT OF Sida cordata LEAVES
Md. Rabiul Islam*1 , A.S.M Ali Reza1 , Kazi Ashfak Ahamed Chawdhury1 , Md. Josim Uddin1 , Mst.
Kaniz Farhana2

517

283.. Proceedings of the X International Symposium on Biological Control of Weeds 4-14 July 1999, Montana State University, Bozeman, Montana, USA Neal R. Spencer [ed.]. pp. 35-41 (2000)
The Successful Biological Control of Spinyhead Sida, Sida Acuta [Malvaceae], by Calligrapha pantherina (Col: Chrysomelidae) in Australia's Northern Territory
GRANT J. FLANAGAN1, LESLEE A. HILLS1, and COLIN G. WILSON2

284.. CLINICAL MICROBIOLOGY REVIEWS, Oct. 1999, p. 564–582
Plant products as antimicrobial agents.
Cowan MM.

285.. Phytother. Res. 13, 75–77 (1999)
Analgesic, Antiinflammatory and Hypoglycaemic Activities of Sida cordifolia
V. Ravi Kanth and P. V. Diwan*

286.. Journal of Complementary and Integrative Medicine: Vol. 7: Iss. 1, Article 1. (2010)
Acute and Sub Chronic Oral Toxicity of Sida rhomboidea.Roxb Leaf Extract
Thounaojam, Menaka C.; Jadeja, Ravirajsinh N.; Patel, Dipak K.; Devkar, Ranjitsinh V.; Ramachandran, A V.

287.. Phcog Res 2009;1:208-12
Potential of Sida rhomboidea.Roxb Leaf Extract in Controlling Hypertriglyceridemia in Experimental Models.
Thounaojam M C, Jadeja R N, Ansarullah, Patel V B, Devkar R V, Ramachandran A V.

288.. Experimental and Toxicologic Pathology 63 (2011) 351–356
Cardioprotective effect of Sida rhomboidea. Roxb extract against isoproterenol induced myocardial necrosis in rats
Menaka C. Thounaojam, Ravirajsinh N. Jadeja, Ansarullah, Sanjay S. Karn, Jigar D. Shah, Dipak K. Patel, Sunita P. Salunke, Geeta S. Padate, Ranjitsinh V. Devkar n, A.V. Ramachandran

289.. Planta medica, 1988
Chemistry and bioactivity of sitoindosides IX and X
S Ghosal, R Kaur, SK Bhattacharya

290.. Planta Daninha. 1999;17(1):163-167
Contents of macronutrients and micronutrients and CN relation of several weed species
Luciano S. Souza, Edivaldo D. Velini, Rita C. S. Maimoni-Rodella, Dagoberto Martins

291.. International Journal of High Dilution Research. 2008;7(22):31-35
Effects of high dilutions of Cymbopogon winterianus Jowitt (citronella) on the germination and growth of seedlings of Sida rhombifolia
Giuliani Grazyella Marques-Silva, Carlos Moacir Bonato, Rosimar Maria Marques

292.. J Intercult Ethnopharmacol. 2015 Apr-Jun; 4(2): 147–179.
Medicinal plants with potential anti-arthritic activity
Manjusha Choudhary,1 Vipin Kumar,2 Hitesh Malhotra,1 and Surender Singh3

293.. INTERNATIONAL JOURNAL OF PHARMACEUTICAL SCIENCES AND RESEARCH January, 2014
MEMBRANE STABILIZING ACTIVITY AND ANTIOXIDANT EFFECT OF SIDA CORDATA
Deepak Kumar*, Shefali Arora , Manoj Kumar , Manoj Kumar Thakur and Abhay Pratap Singh

294.. Journal of Ethnopharmacology Volume 133, Issue 2, 27 January 2011, Pages 289–302
Potential antimalarials from Nigerian plants: A review
J.O. Adebayoa, A.U. Krettlia

295.. J. Med. Chem. 2001, 44, 949-960
New Synthesis of Benzo-d-carbolines, Cryptolepines, and Their Salts: In Vitro Cytotoxic, Antiplasmodial, and Antitrypanosomal Activities of d-Carbolines, Benzo-d-carbolines, and Cryptolepines

518

Erwan Arzel,§ Patrick Rocca,*,§ Philippe Grellier,|,† Mehdi Labaeïd,| Franc¸ois Frappier,⊥ Francoise
Gue´ritte, Christiane Gaspard, Francis Marsais,§ Alain Godard,§ and Guy que´guiner

296.. Journal of Horticultural Science & Biotechnology (2012) 87 (1) 36–40
Rapid in vitro multiplication of Sida cordifolia L. – a threatened medicinal plant
By V. P. PRAMOD* and M. JAYARAJ

297.. Toxicol. Sci. (2002) 70 (2): 245-251.
The Popular Herbal Antimalarial, Extract of Cryptolepis sanguinolenta, Is Potently Cytotoxic
Charles Ansah and Nigel J. Gooderham1

298.. Journal of Science and Technology (Ghana), 2005
Reactive oxygen species is associated with cryptolepine cytotoxicity
C Ansah, NJ Gooderham

299.. Proceedings of the X International Symposium on Biological Control of Weeds
4-14 July 1999, Montana State University, Bozeman, Montana, USA
Neal R. Spencer [ed.]. pp. 35-41 (2000)
The Successful Biological Control of Spinyhead Sida, Sida Acuta [Malvaceae], by Calligrapha pantherina
(Col: Chrysomelidae) in Australia's Northern Territory
GRANT J. FLANAGAN1, LESLEE A. HILLS1, and COLIN G. WILSON2

300.. International Journal of the Physical Sciences Vol. 5(6), pp. 753-762, June 2010   xxx dup of 265
Preliminary phytochemical analysis and insecticidal activity of ethanolic extracts of four tropical plants
(Vernonia amygdalina, Sida acuta, Ocimum gratissimum and Telfaria occidentalis) against beans weevil
(Acanthscelides obtectus)
S. A. Adeniyi1*, C. L. Orjiekwe1, J. E. Ehiagbonare2 and B. D. Arimah3

301.. Phytomedicine Volume 5, Issue 3, May 1998, Pages 209-214
Antibacterial and antifungal activities of neocryptolepine, biscryptolepine and cryptoquindoline, alkaloids
isolated from Cryptolepis sanguinolenta
K. Cimanga 1, T. De Bruyne 1, L. Pieters 1, J. Totte 1, L. Tona 2, K. Kambu 2, D. Vanden Berghe 1, A.J.
Vlietinck 1, a

302.. J. Med. Chem., 1998, 41 (15), pp 2754–2764
Antihyperglycemic Activities of Cryptolepine Analogues:? An Ethnobotanical Lead Structure Isolated
from Cryptolepis sanguinolenta†
Donald E. Bierer ,* Larisa G. Dubenko , Pingsheng Zhang , Qing Lu , Patricia A. Imbach , Albert W.
Garofalo , Puay-Wah Phuan , Diana M. Fort , Joane Litvak , R. Eric Gerber , Barbara Sloan , Jian Luo ,
Raymond Cooper , and Gerald M. Reaven

303.. G.J.B.A.H.S.,Vol.4(1):52-55 (January-March, 2015)
THE EFFECT OF Sida acuta ON GLYCOGEN PROFILE OF ADULT WISTAR RAT
*Kebe, E. Obeten; Gabriel Udo-Affah; Kelechi C. Uruakpa; & Anozeng O. Igiri

304.. CRC Press LLC (New York, London), 2004
Scientific Basis for Ayurvedic Therapies
edited by Lakshmi chandra Mishra

305.. Scientific Research and Essay Vol. 4 (3), pp. 120-130, March, 2009
Plants used for female reproductive health care in Oredo local government area, Nigeria
Folu M. Dania Ogbe, Oyomoare L. Eruogun* and Marilyn Uwagboe

306.. Tropical Grasslands (2001) Volume 35, 218–225
Patterns of seedling emergence over 5 years from seed of 38 species placed on the soil surface under shade
and full sunlight in the seasonally dry tropics
THE LATE C.J. GARDENER1,L.V. WHITEMAN1ANDR.M. JONES2

307.. Journal of Minerals and Materials Characterization and Engineering, 2014, 2, 286-291
Investigation of Sida acuta (Wire Weed) Plant Extract as Corrosion Inhibitor for Aluminium-Copper-
Magnessium Alloy in Acidic Medium

Fatai Afolabi Ayeni1*, Saheed Alawode1, Dorcas Joseph1, Patrick Sukop1, Victoria Olawuyi1, Temitope Emmanuel Alonge1, Oladuuni Oyelola Alabi1, Oluwakayode Oluwabunmi2, Francis Ireti Alo3

308.. Biochemistry, 1999, 38 (24), pp 7719–7726
Stimulation of Topoisomerase II-Mediated DNA Cleavage by Three DNA-Intercalating Plant Alkaloids:?
Cryptolepine, Matadine, and Serpentine
Laurent Dassonneville ,‡ Karine Bonjean ,§ Marie-Claire De Pauw-Gillet ,§ Pierre Colson ,? Claude Houssier ,? Joëlle Quetin-Leclercq ,?@ Luc Angenot ,? and Christian Bailly *‡

309.. Current Topics in Medicinal Chemistry, Volume 15, Number 17, September 2015, pp. 1683-1707(25)
Neocryptolepine: A Promising Indoloisoquinoline Alkaloid with Interesting Biological Activity.
Evaluation of the Drug and its Most Relevant Analogs
L. Larghi, Enrique; B. J. Bracca, Andrea; A. Arroyo Aguilar, Abel; A. Heredia, Daniel; L. Pergomet, Jorgelina; O. Simonetti, Sebastian; S. Kaufman, Teodoro

310.. Mini Rev Med Chem. 2008 June ; 8(6): 538–554.
Indolo[3,2-b]quinolines: Synthesis, Biological Evaluation and Structure Activity-Relationships
Eyunni V.K. Suresh Kumar, Jagan R. Etukala, and Seth Y. Ablordeppey*

311.. Rev. Bras. Farmacogn., v. 13 supl 2, p. 37-39, 2003.   xxx dup of 160
Evaluation of the cardiovascular effects of vasicine, an alkaloid isolated from the leaves of Sida cordifolia L. (Malvaceae)
Silveira, A.L.; Gomes, M.A.S.; Silva Filho, R.N.; Santos, M.R.V. Medeiros, I.A.*; Barbosa Filho, J.M.

312.. Current Traditional Medicine, 2015, 1, 5-17
Sida cordifolia, a Traditional Herb in Modern Perspective-A Review
Ahmed Galal1, Vijayasankar Raman1 and Ikhlas A. Khan1,2,*1

313.. The Indian Journal of Medical Research 66(5):865-71 • November 1977
Potent uterine activity of alkaloid vasicine
Om Parkash Gupta, M L Sharma, B.J.R. Ghatak, C.K. Atal

314.. Nature 196(4860):1217 • December 1962
Bronchodilating Action of Vasicinone and Related Compounds
G W CAMBRIDGE, A. B. A. Jansen, D A JARMAN

315.. The Indian Journal of Medical Research 66(4):680-91 • October 1977
Pharmacological investigations of vasicine and vasicinone the alkaloids of Adhatoda vasica
Om Parkash Gupta, M L Sharma, B.J.R. Ghatak,

316.. Phytomedicine: international journal of phytotherapy and phytopharmacology 20(5) • January 2013
Anti-inflammatory and antimicrobial properties of pyrroloquinazoline alkaloids from Adhatoda vasica
Nees Bharat Singh, Ram Avtar Sharma

317.. The American Journal of Chinese Medicine 41(6):1407-1425 • November 2013
Influence of Six Medicinal Herbs on Collagenase-Induced Osteoarthritis in Rats
Pallavi Nirmal,*Soumya Koppikar,*Prashant Bhondave,†Aarti Narkhede,*Bhagyashri Nagarkar,*Vinayak Kulkarni,‡Narendrakumar Wagh,§Omkar Kulkarni,*Abhay Harsulkar†and Suresh Jagtap**

318.. Pharmacology & Pharmacy6.8 (Aug 2015): 380-390.
In Vitro Evaluation of Sida pilosa Retz (Malvaceae) Aqueous Extract and Derived Fractions on Schistosoma mansoni
Jatsa, Hermine Boukeng; Pereira, Cintia Aparecida de Jesus; Pereira, Ana Bárbara Dias; Negrão-Corrêa, Deborah Aparecida; Braga, Fernão Castro; et al.

319.. J Young Pharm. 2009;1(3):233-238
Assessment of lipid lowering effpesticides against molluscs, which are usually used in agriculture or gardening, in order to control gastropod pests specifically slugs and snails which damage crops or other valued plants by feeding on them.ect of Sida rhomboidea. Roxb methanolic extract in experimentally induced hyperlipidemia

520

Patel DK, Patel KA, Patel UK, Thounaojam MC, Jadeja RN, Ansarullah, Padate GS, Salunke SP, Devkar RV, Ramachandran AV

320.. Boletín Latinoamericano y del Caribe de Plantas Medicinales y Aromáticas Vol.9 (3) 2010
Antioxidant and free radical scavenging activity of Sida rhomboidea. Roxb methanolic extract determined using different in vitro models
Menaka C THOUNAOJAM, Ravirajsinh N JADEJA, Ranjitsinh V DEVKAR*, AV RAMACHANDRAN

321.. Immunopharmacology and Immunotoxicology Volume 34, Issue 5, pages 832-843 2012
Sida rhomboidea.Roxb aqueous extract down-regulates in vivo expression of vascular cell adhesion molecules in atherogenic rats and inhibits in vitro macrophage differentiation and foam cell formation
Menaka C. Thounaojama, Ravirajsinh N. Jadejaa, Sunita P. Salunkea, Ranjitsinh V. Devkar*a & A. V. Ramachandrana

322.. SIDA, Contributions to Botany Vol. 16, No. 1 (AUGUST, 1994), pp. 63-78
TAXONOMY OF THE SIDA RHOMBIFOLIA (MALVACEAE) COMPLEX IN INDIA
V.V. SIVARAJAN and A.K. PRADEEP

323.. Cardiovascular Toxicology June 2011, Volume 11, Issue 2, pp 168-179
In Vitro Evidence for the Protective role of Sida rhomboidea. Roxb Extract Against LDL Oxidation and Oxidized LDL-Induced Apoptosis in Human Monocyte–Derived Macrophages
Menaka C. Thounaojam, Ravirajsinh N. Jadeja, Ranjisinh V. Devkar , A. V. Ramachandran

324.. IndianJPharmacol 1997 Volume : 29 Issue : 2 Page : 110-116
Anti-inflammatory and hepatoprotectivea ctivities of Sida rhombifolia Linn
Rao KS,MishraSH.

325.. Journal of Ethnopharmacology Volume 67, Issue 2, November 1999, Pages 229–232
Antinociceptive and anti-inflammatory activity of Sida rhomboidea leaves
S Venkatesh1, a, Y.Siva Rami Reddya, B Suresha, B.Madhava Reddyb, M Rameshb

326.. book Doctorate Thesis, University of Bayreuth GermanyB (1991).
Materia Medica of Ayurveda Based on Madanapala's Nighantu.
B. Jain Publishers, New Delhi, p. 780.
African Traditional Plant Knowledge Today: An Ethnobotanical Study of the Digo at the Kenya Coast.
Pakia, Mohamed (2005).

327.. Zhongguo Zhong Yao Za Zhi. 1993 Nov;18(11):681-2, 703.
[Studies on the chemical constituents of the herb huanghuaren (Sida acutá Burm. f.)].
[Article in Chinese]
Cao JH1, Qi YP.

328.. International Journal of Infectious Diseases Volume 11, Issue 5, September 2007, Pages 423–429
Chronic nasal infection caused by Klebsiella rhinoscleromatis or Klebsiella ozaenae: two forgotten infectious diseases
E. Botelho-Neversa, F. Gourieta, H. Lepidia, A. Couvreta, B. Amphouxa, P. Dessib, D. Raoulta, ,

329.. JMM Case Reports (2014)
First case of Listeria innocua meningitis in a patient on steroids and eternecept
Marco Favaro,1 Loredana Sarmati,2 Giuseppe Sancesario2 and Carla Fontana1,2

330.. Journal of Clinical Microbiology p. 3937–3943 December 2013 Volume 51 Number 12
Scopulariopsis, a Poorly Known Opportunistic Fungus: Spectrum of Species in Clinical Samples and In Vitro Responses to Antifungal Drugs
Marcelo Sandoval-Denis, a Deanna A. Sutton, b Annette W. Fothergill, b Josep Cano-Lira, a Josepa Gené, a C. A. Decock, c G. S. de Hoog, Josep Guarroa

331.. FEMS Microbiol Rev. 2004 Feb;28(1):43-58
Shigella flexneri infection: pathogenesis and vaccine development.
Jennison AV1, Verma NK.

332.. Clin Infect Dis. (2002) 35 (11): 1360-1367   **not relevant**
Trichoderma Species: Report of 2 Cases, Findings of In Vitro Susceptibility Testing, and Review of the
Literature
T. Chouaki1, V. Lavarde2, L. Lachaud3, C. P. Raccurt1, and C. Hennequin1

333.. Infect. Immun. August 1999 vol. 67 no. 8 4208-4215
Citrobacter freundii Invades and Replicates in Human Brain Microvascular Endothelial Cells
Julie L. Badger1, Monique F. Stins1 and Kwang Sik Kim1,2,*

334.. American heart journal, 1962
Antibiotic therapy of bacterial endocarditis: A Review
Philip A. Tumulty, M.D.*

335.. J. Clin. Microbiol. October 2006 vol. 44 no. 10 3551-3556
Candida guilliermondii, an Opportunistic Fungal Pathogen with Decreased Susceptibility to Fluconazole:
Geographic and Temporal Trends from the ARTEMIS DISK Antifungal Surveillance Program
M. A. Pfaller1,*, D. J. Diekema1, M. Mendez2, C. Kibbler3, P. Erzsebet4, S.-C. Chang5, D. L. Gibbs6, V.
A. Newell6 and the Global Antifungal Surveillance Group

336.. Clin Microbiol Rev. 2008 Oct; 21(4): 606–625
Candida parapsilosis, an Emerging Fungal Pathogen
David Trofa,1 Attila Gácser,2 and Joshua D. Nosanchuk1,*

337.. http://antibiotics.toku-e.com/
The Antimicrobial Index.

338.. Journal of Medical Microbiology (2010), 59, 873–880
Candida tropicalis: its prevalence, pathogenicity and increasing resistance to fluconazole
Rajendra J. Kothavade,1 M. M. Kura,2 Arvind G. Valand3 and M. H. Panthaki4

339.. Appl Environ Microbiolv.69(3); 2003 Mar
Early Events in the Fusarium verticillioides-Maize Interaction Characterized by Using a Green Fluorescent
Protein-Expressing Transgenic Isolate
Liat Oren,1 Smadar Ezrati,1 David Cohen,2 and Amir Sharon1,*

340.. Appl Environ Microbiol. 2003 Mar; 69(3): 1695–1701   dup of 340
Early Events in the Fusarium verticillioides-Maize Interaction Characterized by Using a Green Fluorescent
Protein-Expressing Transgenic Isolate
Liat Oren,1 Smadar Ezrati,1 David Cohen,2 and Amir Sharon1,*

341.. Clin Microbiol Rev. 1998 Oct; 11(4): 589–603.
Klebsiella spp. as Nosocomial Pathogens: Epidemiology, Taxonomy, Typing Methods, and Pathogenicity
Factors
R. Podschun* and U. Ullmann

342.. New Egyptian Journal of Microbiology Vol 34 2015
E coli O 157 and Shigella dysenteriae type 1(Shigella shiga) in hemorrhagic diarrhea syndrome
Amal Saeed, Wafaa A. El shafei, Mosaad Abdel fatah Morgan, Fotouh AM Elsharkawy
Benha University, Banha

343.. Iranian Journal of Health and Environment Volume 5, Number 1 (6 2012)
Comparison of Antiseptics' Efficacy on Pseudomonas Aeruginosa, StaphylococcusEpidermidis and
Enterobacter Aeruginosa in Hospital of Imam Khomeini (Urmia)
Fahim Amini, Masoud Yunesian, Mohammad Hadi Dehghani 1, Nima Hosseni Jazani, Ramin Nabizadeh
Nodehi , Maasoumeh Moghaddam Arjomandi

344.. International Journal of Scientific and Research Publications, Volume 3, Issue 4, April 2013
Phytochemical Analysis of Methanolic Extracts of Leaves of Some Medicinal Plants
Sudipa Nag, Anirban Paul and Rituparna Dutta

345.. Journal of Ethnopharmacology Volume 23, Issue 1, May–June 1988, Pages 27-37
Abortifacient properties of an extract from sida veronicaefolia

G.D. Lutterodt *

346.. Journal of Ethnopharmacology Volume 23, Issues 2–3, July–August 1988, Pages 313-322
Responses of gastrointestinal smooth muscle preparations to a muscarinic principle present in Sida veronicaefolia
George D. Lutterodt *

347.. Phytopharmacology 2012, 3(1) 137-144
Protective effects of Sida veronicaefolia against ethanol induced hepatotoxicity in experimental animals
Ajay Sharma*,1, Balakrishnan Sangameswaran2, Suresh Chandra Mahajan3, Manmeet Singh Saluja1

348.. Journal of Pharmacy Research 2012,5(1),315-319
Antitumor activity of Sida Veronicaefolia against Ehrlich Ascites Carcinoma in mice
B Sangameswaran1, Sunil P Pawar2, Manmeet Singh Saluja3* and Ajay Sharma3

349.. Pharmacological Research Volume 32, Issues 1–2, July–August 1995, Pages 89-94
Interaction between oxytocin and 'sidaverin' on the gravid and non-gravid rat uterus
George D. Lutterodt

350.. Research Journal of Pharmacognosy and Phytochemistry 2010 vol 2 Issue 1
Antioxidant activity of Sida veronicaefolia
Manisha P, etal

351.. Journal of Food Composition and Analysis Volume 24, Issue 7, November 2011, Pages 1043–1048
Comparison of ABTS DPPH assays to measure antioxidant capacity in popular antioxidant-rich US foods
Anna Floegela, 1, , Dae-Ok Kimb, Sang-Jin Chungc, Sung I. Kooa, Ock K. Chuna

352.. J Am Oil Chem Soc (1984) 61: 1345.   xxx 611 is a dup
Characteristics and composition of six Malvaceae seeds and the oils.
Rao, K.S. & Lakshminarayana, G.

353.. Middle-East Journal of Scientific Research 22 (5): 681-689, 2014
Evaluation of Antibacterial Activities of Compounds Isolated From Sida rhombifolia Linn. (Malvaceae)
Adam Biftu, Legesse Adane and Yinebeb Tariku

354.. (was 253) Parasitol Res. 2013 Dec;112(12):4073-85
Green synthesis of silver nanoparticles using Sida acuta (Malvaceae) leaf extract against Culex quinquefasciatus, Anopheles stephensi, and Aedes aegypti (Diptera: Culicidae).
Veerakumar K1, Govindarajan M, Rajeswary M.

355.. (was 253) Bioresour Technol. 2007 Jul;98(9):1788-94. Epub 2006 Sep 14.
Phytoextraction capacity of the plants growing on tannery sludge dumping sites.
Gupta AK1, Sinha S.

356.. Bioresour Technol. 2007 Jul;98(9):1788-94. Epub 2006 Sep 14.
Phytoextraction capacity of the plants growing on tannery sludge dumping sites.
Gupta AK1, Sinha S.

357.. Doctoral thesis, federal University of Rio Grande do Sul, Faculty of Agronomy, Graduate Program in Plant Science
Food plants nonconventional the metropolitan area of Porto Alegre,
RS Kinupp, Valdely Ferreira

358.. [Internet] Record from PROTA4U 2011 https://www.prota4u.org
Sida rhombifolia L.
Bosch, C.H., Brink, M. & Achigan-Dako, E.G. (Editors).
PROTA Plant Resources of Tropical Africa - PROTA is registered as a not-for-profit Foundation in the Netherlands and as an international NGO in Kenya : one programme, two legal entities.

359.. Royal Botanic Gardens, Kew   dup at 466
Seed Information Database
http://www.kew.org/

360.. ZipcodeZoo (zipcodezoo.com) is a free, online natural history encyclopedia.
ZipcodeZoo draws on the Catalogue of Life for its basic species list, Wikipedia and WIkispecies for some of its content, the Global Biodiversity Information Facility for its maps, Flickr and the Wikimedia Commons for many of its photos, YouTube for videos, the Taxonomicon for taxonomic information, and Xeno-canto for some of its sound recordings.

361.. SEPASAL Survey of Economic Plants for Arid and Semi-Arid Lands (SEPASAL) database. Published on the Internet; http://apps.kew.org/sepasalweb/sepaweb [accessed 08 27 16] Royal Botanic Gardens, Kew (1999).
SEPASAL's development has been funded by The Clothworkers' Foundation and its Internet development is funded by The Charles Wolfson Charitable Trust. Nutritional information on African wild foods is funded by Nestlé Charitable Trust.

362.. PROSEA (Plant Resources of South-East Asia) Foundation, Bogor, Indonesia.
http://www.proseanet.org. 2001
Various Sida species [Internet] Record from Proseabase.
Perumal, B., van Valkenburg, J.L.C.H. and Bunyapraphatsara, N. (Editors).
Accessed from Internet: 25 to 28-Aug-2016

363.. The Mansfeld's World Database of Agriculture and Horticultural Crops
https://mansfeld.ipk-gatersleben.de/apex/f?p=185:3::::::
The Mansfeld's World Database of Agriculture and Horticultural Crops is an online database developed at IPK since 1998, as a contribution to the project "Federal Information System on Genetic Resources" (BIG), funded by the Federal Ministry of Education, Science, Research and Technology (BMBF).

364.. African Plant Database (version 3.4.0).
Conservatoire et Jardin botaniques de la Ville de Genève and South African National Biodiversity Institute, Pretoria,
"Retrieved 08 22-28 16", from <http://www.ville-ge.ch/musinfo/bd/cjb/africa/>.

365.. Tropicos.org.<http://www.tropicos.org>
Missouri Botanical Garden.
(accessed 22-27 Aug 2016)

366.. https://npgsweb.ars-grin.gov
GRIN - Germplasm Resource Information Network
USDA.

367.. https://www.prota4u.org
PROTA stands for Plant Resources of Tropical Africa .
It is an international documentation programme on the useful plants of Tropical Africa. It synthesizes dispersed information, makes it readily available in various forms and stimulates its use for extension, education, research, development and governance. PROTA is registered as a not-for-profit Foundation in the Netherlands and as an international NGO in Kenya : one programme, two legal entities.

368.. GBIF http://www.gbif.org/species/3933670/synonyms
The Global Biodiversity Information Facility
GBIF is an international open data infrastructure, funded by governments. It provides a single point of access (through this portal and its web services) to hundreds of millions of records, shared freely by hundreds of institutions worldwide, making it the biggest biodiversity database on the Internet.

369.. Catalogue of Life - Indexing the World's Known Species - http://www.catalogueoflife.org/
The Species 2000 & ITIS
In June 2001 the Species 2000 and ITIS organisations, that had previously worked separately, decided to work together to create the Catalogue of Life, estimated at 1.9 million species.

370.. Prelude Medicinal Plants Database
Royal Museum of Central Africa
http://www.africamuseum.be/collections/external/prelude/

524

371.. Sustentabilidade Comunitária website 1/9/2013
A Guanxuma (Sida rhombifolia) by Adrian Rupp
Conhecimentos e técnicas para comunidades autossustentáveis.

372.. American Journal of Phytomedicine and Clinical Therapeutics
Chromosome Numbers and Karyotype Studies of Few Members of Malvales
K.H. Venkatesh*, B. Dinesh, N. Venu and Munirajappa

373.. Nature Reviews Genetics 6, 836-846 (November 2005)
The advantages and disadvantages of being polyploid
Luca Comai
This article was adapted from Comai, L., The advantages and disadvantages of being polyploid. Nature
Reviews Genetics 6, 838-845 (2005) http://www.nature.com/scitable/topicpage/polyploidy-1552814

374.. Invasive Species Compendium: Datasheets, maps, images, abstracts and full text on invasive species
of the world
http://www.cabi.org/isc/datasheet/49985
Partners include over 40 national agricultural and animal agencies

375.. Medicinal Plants blog - Medicinal Plants with usage, patents and their publications -
http://medplants.blogspot.in/
Medicinal Plants with usage, patents, and their publications
Listing several Sida species: Sida cordata Sida cordifolia Sida retusa Sida spinosa

376.. NATIVE PLANT INFORMATION NETWORK   www.wildflower.org
Native Plant Information Network at the Lady Bird Johnson Wildflower Center
Lady Bird Johnson, our former first lady, and actress Helen Hayes founded an organization in 1982 to
protect and preserve North America's native plants and natural landscapes. Welcome to the Native Plant
Information Network (NPIN). Our goal is to assemble and disseminate information that will encourage the
sustainable use and conservation of native wildflowers, plants and landscapes throughout North America.
The Native Plant Information Network is a database of more than 7,200 native species available online.

377.. Med India -- http://www.medindia.net/alternativemedicine/bala.asp#1
"Bala"
Medindia's Medical Review Team consists of a highly qualified team of medical doctors, specialists,
experts and healthcare professionals. They work closely with our team of editors and writers to ensure that
all medical and health content published on the site is accurate and backed by medical research and
studies, with references and citations provided where relevant.

378.. Natural Medicines Professional Database https://naturalmedicines.therapeuticresearch.com
Sida cordifolia-Bala, information provided by www.chamberlins.com

379.. Indigo Herbs of Glastonbury since 2004 - https://www.indigo-herbs.co.uk/natural-health-
guide/benefits/bala
Sida cordifolia (Bala) They do not carry any other sidas.

380.. Biochemistry, 1998, 37 (15), pp 5136–5146
The DNA Intercalating Alkaloid Cryptolepine Interferes with Topoisomerase II and Inhibits Primarily
DNA Synthesis in B16 Melanoma Cells†
K. Bonjean ,*‡ M. C. De Pauw-Gillet ,‡ M. P. Defresne ,‡ P. Colson ,§ C. Houssier ,§ L. Dassonneville ,?
C. Bailly ,*? R. Greimers ,? C. Wright ,# J. Quetin-Leclercq ,¶+ M. Tits ,¶ and L. Angenot ¶

381.. "Phytotherapy Research : an international journal devoted to medical and scientific research on
plants and plant products" - Vol. 10, no.4, p. 361-363 (1996)
Antimalarial activity of cryptolepine and some other anhydronium bases
Wright, C. W., Philipson, J. D., Awe, S. O., Kirby, G. C., Warhurst, D. C., Quetin-Leclercq, Angenot, Luc

382.. Biochemistry, 1999, 38 (24), pp 7719–7726
Stimulation of Topoisomerase II-Mediated DNA Cleavage by Three DNA-Intercalating Plant Alkaloids:?
Cryptolepine, Matadine, and Serpentine†
Laurent Dassonneville, Karine Bonjean , Marie-Claire De Pauw-Gillet , Pierre Colson , Claude Houssier ,
Joëlle Quetin-Leclercq ,Luc Angenot ,and Christian Bailly

383.. Journal of Pharmaceutical Sciences Volume 68, Issue 12 December 1979 Pages 1510–1514
Cryptolepine hydrochloride effect on Staphylococcus aureus
Kwabena Boakye-Yiadom, Samuel M. Heman-Ackah

383.. Phytotherapy Research Volume 17, Issue 4 April 2003 Pages 434–436
Cryptolepine hydrochloride: a potent antimycobacterial alkaloid derived from Cryptolepis sanguinolenta
Simon Gibbons, Fatemeh Fallah, Colin W. Wright

384.. Phytotherapy Research Volume 17, Issue 4 April 2003 Pages 434–436
Cryptolepine hydrochloride: a potent antimycobacterial alkaloid derived from Cryptolepis sanguinolenta
Simon Gibbons, Fatemeh Fallah, Colin W. Wright

385.. Journal of Applied Bacteriology Volume 79, Issue 3, pages 314–321, September 1995
The effect of cryptolepine on the morphology and survival of Escherichia coli, Candida albicans and Saccharomyces cerevisiae
I.K. Sawer, M.I. Berry, M.W. Brown andJ.L. Ford*

386.. Phytotherapy Research Volume 23, Issue 10, pages 1421–1425, October 2009
Anti-inflammatory properties of cryptolepine
Olumayokun A. Olajide1,*, Abayomi M. Ajayi1,3 andColin W. Wright2

387.. Letters in Applied Microbiology Volume 40, Issue 1, pages 24–29, January 2005
The killing effect of cryptolepine on Staphylococcus aureus
I.K. Sawer1, M.I. Berry2 andJ.L. Ford2

388.. Journal of Drug Development and Industrial Pharmacy Volume 22, 1996 - Issue 4 Page 377-381
In Vitro Studies with Liposomal Cryptolepine
M. Singh, M. P. Singh & S. Ablordeppey

391.. Journal of Ethnopharmacology Volume 27, Issues 1–2, November 1989, Pages 141-148
Effects of cryptolepine alone and in combination with dipyridamole on a mouse model of arterial thrombosis
A.O. Oyekan *, J.P.O. Okapor

392.. Journal of Ethnopharmacology Volume 44, Issue 2, October 1994, Pages 73-77
Cryptolepis sanguinolenta activity against diarrhoeal bacteria
Alexandra Paulo a, Madalena Pimentel b, Silvia Viegas d, Ilda Pires d, Aida Duarte b, José Cabrita c, d, Elsa T. Gomes *, a

393.. Planta Med 1996; 62(1): 22-27
In Vitro Biological Activities of Alkaloids from Cryptolepis sanguinolenta
Kanyanga Cimanga1 , Tess De Bruyne1 , Aleidis Lasure1 , Bart Van Poel1 , Luc Pieters1 , Magda Claeys1 , Dirk Vanden Berghe1 , Kabangu Kambu2 , Lutete Tona2 , Arnold J. Vlietinck1

394.. Journal of Pharmacology and Toxicology, 2008, Volume 3, Issue 4, pp 291-301
The mechanism of cryptolepine-induced cell death
C. Ansah, H. Zhu, N. J. Goderham

395.. Chem. Res. Toxicol., 1991, 4 (5), pp 566–572
A metabolically competent human cell line expressing five cDNAs encoding procarcinogen-activating enzymes: application to mutagenicity testing
Charles L. Crespi, Frank J. Gonzalez, Dorothy T. Steimel, Thomas R. Turner, Harry V. Gelboin, Bruce W. Penman, Robert Langenbach

396.. Toxicology Volume 208, Issue 1, 1 March 2005, Pages 141–147
In vitro genotoxicity of the West African anti-malarial herbal Cryptolepis sanguinolenta and its major alkaloid cryptolepine
Charles Ansah, Ayesha Khan, Nigel J. Gooderham,

397.. Toxicological Sciences, 91(1), 132-139. (2006).
Mechanisms of induction of cell cycle arrest and cell death by cryptolepine in human lung adenocarcinoma a549 cells.
Zhu, H., & Gooderham, N. J.

398.. Cancer Treatment Centers of America
Adenocarcinoma Information page
http://www.cancercenter.com/terms/adenocarcinoma/

399.. Investigational new drugs, Vol. 27, no 5, 402-411 p.
Characterization of the cytotoxic activity of the indoloquinoline alkaloid cryptolepine in human tumour cell lines and primary cultures of tumour cells from patients
Laryea, Daniel, Isaksson, Anders, Wright, Colin Larsson, Rolf

400.. INTERNATIONAL JOURNAL OF ONCOLOGY 31: 915-922, 2007 915
The plant alkaloid cryptolepine induces p21WAF1/CIP1 and cell cycle arrest in a human osteosarcoma cell line
TAKA-AKI MATSUI1,2, YOSHIHIRO SOWA1, HIROAKI MURATA2, KOICHI TAKAGI1, RYOKO NAKANISHI1, SHUNJI AOKI3, MASAYUKI YOSHIKAWA4, MOTOMASA KOBAYASHI3, TOMOYA SAKABE2, TOSHIKAZU KUBO2 and TOSHIYUKI SAKAI1

401.. General Pharmacology: The Vascular System Volume 19, Issue 2, 1988, Pages 233-237
Cryptolepine inhibits platelet aggregation in vitro and in vivo and stimulates fibrinolysis ex vivo
A.O. Oyekan 1, J.H. Botting 1, B.K. Noamesi 2

402.. Oecologia December 1971, Volume 6, Issue 4, pp 343–349
Role of high temperature pretreatments on seed germination of desert species ofSida (Malvaceae)
D. D. Chawan

403.. Indian Journal of Plant Physiology 4.3 (1999): 175-178.
Effect of temperature, concentrated H2SO4 and nonpolar solvents on removal of coat imposed dormancy in S. acuta Burm. F. and S. rhombifolia L.
S. Seal, and K. Gupta

404.. dup of 425

405.. Int J Pharm Biomed Res 2012, 3(1), 7-11
Adaptogenic activity of a Siddha medicinal plant: Sida cordata
D. Gnanasekaran1*, C. Umamaheswara Reddy2, B. Jaiprakash3, N. Narayanan4, S. Hannah Elizabeth5,Y. Ravi Kiran1

407.. Asian Pacific J Cancer Prev, 10, 1107-1112   xxx   dup of 464 (and 49)
Sida rhombifolia ssp. retusa Seed Extract Inhibits DEN Induced Murine Hepatic Preneoplasia and Carbon Tetrachloride Hepatotoxicity
Radhika Poojari1*, Sanjay Gupta2, Girish Maru2, Bharat Khade2, Sanjay Bhagwat1

408.. PHYTOTHERAPY RESEARCH Phyther. Res. 13, 75–77 (1999)
Analgesic, Antiinflammatory and Hypoglycaemic Activities of Sida cordifolia
V. Ravi Kanth and P. V. Diwan*

409.. Indian journal of plant physiology 2007, vol. 12, no2, pp. 203-206 (article)
VARIATIONS IN SECONDARY METABOLITES IN SOME ARID ZONE MEDICINAL PLANTS IN RELATION TO SEASON AND PLANT GROWTH
VERMA Vandana ; KASERA Pawan K.

410.. Indian Journal of Fisheries Volume: 51 Issue: 4 Pages: 501-504 October-December 2004
Use of herb, bala (Sida cordifolia Linn.) as growth promoter in the supplementary feed of Cirrhinus mrigala (Ham.).
Author(s): Kour Dalveer; Sharma L.L.; Sharma B.K.

411.. Acta Horticulturae Issue: 860 Pages: 219-222 Published: 2010
Germination of bala (Sida cordifolia L., Malvaceae), an Ayurvedic plant.
Krizevski R.; Lewinsohn E.

412.. Asian Journal of Chemistry19.6 (2007): 4459-4462.
Diuretic Activity of Sida cordifolia Linn. of Nilgiris
T. PRABHAKAR*, K. RAMESH, P.K.M. NAGARATHNA, T. SREENIVASA RAO, K. LAKSHMAN†
and B. SURESH‡

413.. Journal of Tropical Agriculture 53 (1) : 42-47, 2015
Variation in root yield and ephedrine content of Bala (Sida cordifolia Linn.) at differential harvesting
under open and shaded situation
A. Latha* and V.V. Radhakrishnan

414.. GORTERIA Volume: 34 Issue: 5 Pages: 121-136 Published: APR 16 2010
Sida spinosa L., S. rhombifolia L., S. cordifolia L. en Malvastrum coromandelianum (L.) Garcke as
casuals in lily fields
Reijerse A. I.; Verrijdt A. L. A. I.

415.. Asian-Australasian Journal of Animal Sciences 1997 10 1 28-34   xxx 210 is a dup
Variability in ash, crude protein, detergent fiber and mineral content of some minor plant species collected
from pastures grazed by goats.
Serra, A. B.; Serra, S. D.; Orden, E. A.; Cruz, L. C.; Nakamura, K.; Fujihara, T.

416.. Journal of Stored Products Research 1994 30 4 297-301
The ability of powders and slurries from ten plant species to protect stored grain from attack by
Prostephanus truncatus Horn (Coleoptera: Bostrichidae) and Sitophilus oryzae L. (Coleoptera:
Curculionidae).
Niber, B. T.

417.. Nematropica Vol. 43, No. 1 (June 2013)
WEED HOSTS OF THE ROOT-LESION NEMATODE, PRATYLENCHUS SPEIJERI IN
REPLANTING SITES CLEARED FROM NEMATODE-INFESTED PLANTAIN CV. APANTU-PA
(MUSA SPP., AAB-GROUP) FIELDS IN GHANA
Francis C. Brentu, C. Amoatey, E. Oppong, L. W. Duncan

418.. Pesquisa Veterinária Brasileira 2008 28 1 57-62
Experimental poisoning by Sida carpinifolia (Malvaceae) in cattle.
Furlan, F. H.; Lucioli, J.; Veronezi, L. O.; Traverso, S. D.; Gava, A.

419.. Indian Journal of Forestry 2001 24 1 21-28
Analysis of biodiversity and improvement in soil quality under plantations on degraded land.
Verma, R. K.; Shadangi, D. K.; Totey, N. G.

420.. Afr J Biotech. 2005; 4: 685-688.
Phytochemical constituents of some Nigerian medicinal plants.
Edeoga HO, Okwu DE, Mbaebie BO.

421.. African Journal of Biotechnology Vol. 6 (14), pp. 1703-1709, 18 July 2007
Levels of trace metals in soil and vegetation along major and minor roads in metropolitan city of Kaduna,
Nigeria
Okunola, O. J.*, Uzairu, A. and Ndukwe, G.

422.. Journal of Insect Science 1993 6 1 100-101
Feeding deterrent and toxic activity in the leaves of Sida acuta L. (Malvaceae) against the larvae of Earias
vittella.
Dongre, T. K.; Rahalkar, G. W.

423.. Australian Entomological Magazine 1990 17 1 7-15
The phytophagous insect fauna of the introduced shrubs Sida acuta Burm.F. and Sida cordifolia L. in the
Northern Territory, Australia.
Wilson, C. G.; Flanagan, G. J.

424.. Environmental Entomology 1991 20 3 882-888
Natural enemies of Sida acuta and S. rhombifolia (Malvaceae) in Mexico and their potential for biological control of these weeds in Australia.
Gillett, J. D.; Harley, K. L. S.; Kassulke, R. C.; Miranda, H. J.

425.. Indian J. Weed Sci. 40 (1 & 2) : 6-10 (2008)   xxx 404 is a duplicate
Dormancy, Germination and Emergence of Sida rhombifolia L.
B. S. Chauhan and D. E. Johnson
International Rice Research Institute, Los Baños, Philippines

426.. Biological Conservation 1993 65 1 35-41
Trampling resistance, stem flexibility and leaf strength in nine Australian grasses and herbs
Sun, D.; Liddle, M. J.

427.. Agronomy Journal, 1983, 75, 3, pp 566-569
Nutritive value of seven tropical weed species during the dry season
Nuwanyakpa, M. Y.; Bolsen, K. K.; Posler, G. L.; Diaz, M. Q.; Rivera, F. R.

428.. Agricultural Science Digest 2001 21 4 273-274
Common rice weeds used for first aid by Chhattisgarh farmers.
Oudhia, P.

429.. Physiologia Plantarum, 1986. 67(2): p. 320-327.
SEED COAT IMPOSED DORMANCY - HISTOCHEMISTRY OF THE REGION CONTROLLING ONSET OF WATER ENTRY INTO SIDA-SPINOSA SEEDS
Egley, G.H., R.N. Paul, and A.R. Lax,

430.. Weed Science, 1984. 32(6): p. 786-791.
ENVIRONMENTAL-CONDITIONS REQUIRED FOR GERMINATION OF PRICKLY SIDA (SIDA-SPINOSA)
Baskin, J.M. and C.C. Baskin,

431.. Weed Science Vol. 24, No. 2 (Mar., 1976), pp. 239-243
Germination of Developing Prickly Sida Seeds
G. H. Egley

432.. Volume 187 of the series NATO ASI Series pp 207-223
Chapter - Recent Advances in the Development and Germination of Seeds
Water-Impermeable Seed Coverings as Barriers to Germination
G. H. Egley

433.. Journal of Natural Product and Plant Resources, 2011. 1(4): p. 35-39.
In-vitro antioxidant activity of Sida spinosa Linn
Jayasri P*1 , A. Elumalai2, Narendra Naik D1 and Kalugonda Murali Krishna1

434.. International Journal of Phytomedicine, 2011. 3(3): p. 338-345.
Hypoglycemic activity of Sida spinosa Linn. root extract in normoglycemic rats
Ibrahim Shaikh1*, Preeti Kulkarni1, Ankur Patel1, Venkatrao Kulkarni1

435.. JAPANESE JOURNAL OF PHARMACOLOGY Volume: 21 Issue: 1 Pages: 136-&
CENTRAL NERVOUS SYSTEM EFFECTS OF SIDA-RETUSA ROOT (S rhombifolia)
JOSEPH, T; SHANTHAK.   xxx 529 is a dup

436.. APJLS (2011) Volume 4, Number 3 pp. 201-214
PHYTOCHEMICAL FINGERPRINTING, CYTOTOXIC, ANTIMICROBIAL, ANTITUBERCULAR, ANTIMYCOTIC POTENTIALS OF SIDA RHOMBIFOLIA SUBSP. RETUSA AND EMBELIA TSJERIAM-COTTAM
Radhika Poojari

437.. Pharmacognosy Journal - an official journal of phcog.net
Pharmacological Potential of Atibala of Ayurveda : A Review (S. indica)

Dhiman Anil Kumar1 and Kumar Amit2

438.. http://www.ayurvedicnutrition.com/course
Ayurvedic Nutrition & Ayurveda Clinical Study Program European Institute of Vedic Studies

439.. Fitoterapia Volume 73, Issue 2, April 2002, Pages 156–159
Hypoglycemic activity of Abutilon indicum (Sida indica) leaf extracts in rats
Y.N. Seetharama, Gururaj Chalageria, S.Ramachandra Settyb, Bheemacharb

440.. Phytomedicine Volume 12, Issues 1–2, 10 January 2005, Pages 62–64
Hepatoprotective activity of Abutilon indicum on experimental liver damage in rats
E. Porchezhiana, , S.H. Ansarib

441.. Parasitol Res (2008) 102: 981.
Isolation and identification of mosquito larvicidal compound from Abutilon indicum (Linn.) Sweet
Abdul Rahuman, A., Gopalakrishnan, G., Venkatesan, P. et al.

442.. Die Pharmazie [2000, 55(4):314-316]
Analgesic principle from Abutilon indicum
Ahmed M , Amin S , Islam M , Takahashi M , Okuyama E , Hossain CF

443.. International Journal of Pharmaceutical Sciences and Drug Research 2011; 3(2): 97-100
Evaluation of Anti-Ulcer Activity of Methanolic Extract of Abutilon indicum Linn Leaves in Experimental
Rats
N. L. Dashputre1*, N. S. Naikwade2

444.. Easy Ayurvedic website - http://easyayurveda.com/
(Searching on Google for "Atibala" this site came up first)
Abutilon indicum – Atibala – Ayurveda Details, Usage, Health Benefits
Dr Janardhana V Hebbar B.A.M.S., MD (Ayu), PGDPSM, an Indian Ayurvedic doctor and a professional
Ayurveda, health and lifestyle blogger. Has written 5 books on Ayurveda. Worked as Associate Professor
in Alva's Ayurveda Medical College, Moodbidri.

445.. Evidence-Based Complementary and Alternative Medicine Volume 2011 (2011), Article ID 167684,
9 pages   http://dx.doi.org/10.1093/ecam/neq004
Antidiabetic Activities of Abutilon indicum (L.) Sweet Are Mediated by Enhancement of Adipocyte
Differentiation and Activation of the GLUT1 Promoter
Chutwadee Krisanapun,1,2 Seong-Ho Lee,1 Penchom Peungvicha,2 Rungravi Temsiririrkkul,3 and Seung
Joon Baek1

446.. African Journal of Biomedical Research, Vol. 10: 175 - 181
Antibacterial and phytochemical studies on twelve species of Indian medicinal plants
Jigna Parekh, and Sumitra Chanda*

447.. UNIQUE JOURNAL OF AYURVEDIC AND HERBAL MEDICINES 2014, 02 (05): Page 23-2
QUALITATIVE ANALYSIS OF HERBAL MEDICINES W.R.T. ATIBALA (ABUTILON INDICUM
(L.) SWEET.)
Mahesh TS1*, Shreevidya M2

448.. International Journal of Pharmacy and Pharmaceutical Sciences ISSN- 0975-1491 Vol 3, Suppl 2,
2011
PHYTO CHEMICAL INVESTIGATION, ANALGESIC AND ANTI INFLAMMATORY ACTIVITY OF
ABUTILON INDICUM LINN
R.SARASWATHI1, LOKESH UPADHYAY2, R.VENKATAKRISHNAN3, R.MEERA4, P.DEVI5

449.. International Journal of Pharma Sciences and Research (IJPSR) Vol.1(3), 2010, 178-184
Immunomodulatory Activity of Abutilon Indicum linn on Albino Mice
N. L. DASHPUTRE*, N. S. NAIKWADE

450.. Journal of Ethnopharmacology 107 (2006) 182–188
Search for antibacterial and antifungal agents from selected Indian medicinal plants
V. Prashanth Kumar, Neelam S. Chauhan, Harish Padh, M. Rajani *

530

451.. Nutrition Research 29 (2009) 579–587
Aqueous extract of Abutilon indicum Sweet inhibits glucose absorption and stimulates insulin secretion in rodents
Chutwadee Krisanapuna, Penchom Peungvichaa,?,Rungravi Temsiririrkkulb, Yuvadee Wongkrajanga

452.. International Journal of Pharmacognosy and Phytochemical Research 2010; 2(1);1-4
Cytotoxic and Antimicrobial Activity of the Crude Extract of Abutilon Indicum
Muhit Md. Abdul *, Apu Apurba Sarker, Islam Md. Saiful, Ahmed Muniruddin

453.. Pakistan J. Zool., vol. 42(1), pp. 93-97, 2010.
Antibacterial and Irritant Activities of Organic Solvent Extracts of Agave americana Linn., Albizzia lebbek
Benth. Achyranthes aspera Linn. and Abutilon indicum Linn - A Preliminary Investigation
M.T.J. Khan*, K. Ahmad, M.N. Alvi, Noor-ulAmin, B. Mansoor, M. Asif Saeed, F.Z. Khan and M. Jamshaid

454.. Indian Journal of Traditional Knowledge (IJTK) IJTK Vol.02 [2003]
Phytochemical and pharmacological evaluation of leaves of Abutilon indicum
Lakshmayya; Nelluri, Narasimha Rao; Kumar, Pramod; Agarwal, Nanda Kishor; Gouda, T Shivaraj; Setty, S Ramachandra

455.. J Antimicrob Chemother 2011; 66: 1939–1940
The urgent need for new antibacterial agents
Richard Wise* on behalf of the BSAC Working Party on The Urgent Need: Regenerating Antibacterial Drug
Discovery and Development† British Society for Antimicrobial Chemotherapy

456.. Clinical Infectious Diseases 2009; 48:1–12
IDSA Report on Development Pipeline from the Infectious Diseases Society of America
Bad Bugs, No Drugs: No ESKAPE! An Update
Helen W. Boucher,1 George H. Talbot,2 John S. Bradley,3,4 John E. Edwards, Jr,5,6,7 David Gilbert,8 Louis B. Rice,9,10 Michael Scheld,11 Brad Spellberg,5,6,7 and John Bartlett12

457.. http://www.itis.gov/servlet/SingleRpt/SingleRpt?search_topic=TSN&search_value=21725
ITIS website, Taxonomy and Nomenclature, "Sida L."
The ITIS is the result of a partnership of federal agencies formed to satisfy their mutual needs for scientifically credible taxonomic information. Since its inception, ITIS has gained valuable new partners and undergone a name change; ITIS now stands for the Integrated Taxonomic Information System.

458.. WHO/HSE/PED/AIP/2014.2 World Health Organization, Geneva, 2014
Antimicrobial resistance global report on surveillance : 2014 summary
World Health Organization

459.. Phytomedicine Volume 11, Issue 4, 2004, Pages 338-341
Studies on medicinal plants of Ivory Coast: Investigation of Sida acuta for in vitro antiplasmodial activities and identification of an active constituent
J.-T. Banzouzi a, b, R. Prado c, H. Menan d, A. Valentin d, C. Roumestan c, M. Mallié d, Y. Pelissier b, Y. Blache a, *

460.. IAJPR. 2013; 3(9): 7477-7484
ANTICANCER ACTIVITY OF SIDA ACUTA BURM.F AGAINST NITROSODIETHYLAMINE AND CCL4 INDUCED HEPATOCELLULAR CARCINOMA
Mallikarjuna G*1, Prabhakaran V1, Sarat kumar Reddy B2.

461.. Ancient Science RI/LIH Vol : XXV(3&4) January, February, March, April, May, June 2006
ANTIOXIDANT POTENTIAL OF Sida retusa, Urena lobata AND Triumfetta rhomboidea
K.P.Lissy*, Thara K. Simona and M.S. Lathab

462.. J Radioanal Nucl Chem (2015) 303: 2101.
PIXE-based quantification of health-proactive trace elements in genetically transformed roots of a multi-medicinal plant, Sida acuta Burm.f.
Jena, S., Sahu, L., Ray, D.K. et al.

463.. International Journal of Pure and Applied Zoology Volume 2, Issue 1, pp: 51-60, 2014
STUDIES ON THE EFFECT OF SIDA ACUTA AND VETIVERIA ZIZANIOIDES AGAINST THE
MALARIAL VECTOR, ANOPHELES STEPHENSI AND
MALARIAL PARASITE, PLASMODIUM BERGHEI
Narasimhan Aarthi1, Kadarkarai Murugan1*, Pari Madhiyazhagan1, ThiyagarajanNataraj1, Arjunan
Nareshkumar2, Kandasamy Kalimuthu3, Jiang-Shiou Hwang3, Donald R. Barnard4, Hui Wei5,
R. Chandrasekar6 and A. Amsath7

464.. Asian Pacific Journal of Cancer Prevention, Vol 10, 2009
Sida rhombifolia ssp. retusa Seed Extract Inhibits DEN Induced Murine Hepatic Preneoplasia and Carbon
Tetrachloride Hepatotoxicity
Radhika Poojari1*, Sanjay Gupta2, Girish Maru2, Bharat Khade2, SanjayBhagwat1

465.. Planta daninha vol.24 no.3 Viçosa July/Sept. 2006
Effects of weed species competition on the growth of young coffee plants
Ronchi, C.P.I; Silva. A.A.II

466.. Royal Botanic Gardens website, Kew, Great Britain   xxx dup 359
http://data.kew.org/sid/SidServlet?Source=epic&ID=21313&Num=5oB

467.. PROTA Plant Resources of Tropical Africa - Your guide to the use of African plants
[Internet] Record from PROTA4U "Sida alba L."
https://www.prota4u.org/protav8.asp?h=M4&t=Sida,rhombifolia&p=Sida+alba#Synonyms

468.. Journal of Ethnobiology and Ethnomedicine20073:14
Biodiversity, traditional medicine and public health: where do they meet?
Rômulo RN Alves, Ierecê ML Rosa

469.. WORLD JOURNAL OF PHARMACY AND PHARMACEUTICAL SCIENCES Volume 5, Issue 4,
1505-1512
EXPERIMENTAL STUDY ON IMMUNOMODULATORY ACTIVITY OF NAGBALA (SIDA
HUMILIS CAV)
Dr. Shobha Khilari (Asso. Professor), Dr. Pallavi Anand Sathe* (MD Scholar)

470.. Asian Pac J Trop Biomed. 2014 Jan;4(1):18-24. doi: 10.1016/S2221-1691(14)60202-1.
Phytopharmacological evaluation of ethanol extract of Sidacordifolia L. roots.
Momin MA1, Bellah SF, Rahman SM, Rahman AA, Murshid GM, Emran TB.

471.. Modern Phytomorphology. 2014;6:91-91
Virginia mallow (Sida hermaphrodita (L.) Rusby) – properties and application
Anna Kasprzyk, Agata Leszczuk, Ewa Szczuka

472.. Polish Journal of Environmental Studies Vol. 12, No. 1 (2003), 119-122
Some Effects of Sida hermaphrodita R. Cultivation on Sewage Sludge
H Borkowska, K Wardzinska

473.. Polish J. of Environ. Stud. Vol. 18, No. 4 (2009), 563-568
Virginia Fanpetals (Sida hermaphrodita Rusby) Cultivated on Light Soil; Height of Yield and Biomass
Productivity
H. Borkowska1*, R. Molas2**, A. Kupczyk3

474.. Biomass and Bioenergy Volume 36, January 2012, Pages 234–240
Two extremely different crops, Salix and Sida, as sources of renewable bioenergy
Halina Borkowskaa, Roman Molasb, ,

475.. Journal of Applied Botany and Food Quality 87, 36 - 45 (2014)
Investigations on plant functional traits, epidermal structures and the ecophysiology of the novel bioenergy species Sida hermaphrodita Rusby and Silphium perfoliatum L.
J. Franzaring*, I. Schmid, L. Bäuerle, G. Gensheimer, A. Fangmeier

476.. Polish Journal of Chemical Technology, 14, 2, 9-15, 10.2478/v10026-012-0064-7
The effect of industrial wastes and municipal sewage sludge compost on the quality of virginia fanpetals (SIDA HERMAPHRODITA RUSBY) biomass. Part 1. Macroelements content and their upatke dynamics
Ewa Krzywy-Gawronska

477.. Annals of Warsaw University of Life Sciences – SGGW Forest and Wood Technology No 71, 2010: 83-86
Estimating the possibilities of applying Sida hermaphrodita Rusby to the production of low-density particleboards
RAFAà CZARNECKI, DOROTA DUKARSKA

478.. Int. Rev. Appl. Sci. Eng. 4 (2013) 2, 137–142
IMPROVEMENT OF GERMINATION CAPACITY OF SIDA HERMAPHRODITA (L.) RUSBY BY SEED PRIMING TECHNIQUES
E. KURUCZ 1a, M. G. FÁRI 1,2

479.. Annual Set The Environment Protection-Rocznik Ochrona Srodowiska Vol 15. 2013 Inline Plantation of Virginia Mallow (Sida hermaphrodita R.) as Biological Acoustic Screen
Joanna Szyszlak-Barglowicz, Tomasz Slowik,Grzegorz Zajac, Wieslaw Piekarski

480.. Applied Soil Ecology Volume 84, December 2014, Pages 12–15
Impact of land-use change towards perennial energy crops on earthworm population
C. Emmerling,

481.. Phytochemistry Volume 58, Issue 3, October 2001, Pages 451–454
Betaine distribution in the Malvaceae
Gerald Blundena, , Asmita V. Patela, Nigel J. Armstronga, John Gorhamb

482.. Acta univ. agric. et silvic. Mendel. Brun., 2004, LII, No. 1, pp. 113-120
The use of heavy metal accumulating plants for detoxication of chemically polluted soils.
Antonkiewicz, J., Jasiewicz, Cz., Ryant, P.

483.. Chem Nat Compd (1987) 23: 551
Study of the kinetics of the extraction of flavonoids from plant raw material I. Extraction of rutin fromSida hermaphrodita
Bandyukova, V.A. & Ligai, L.V.

484.. Chemia I Inzynieria Ekologiczna T.7, Nr 10, 2000
Chemical composition of Sida hermaphrodita Rusby Cultivated in Soil Contaminated with Heavy Metals
Czeslawa Jasiewicz, Jacek Antonkiewicz

485.. J Zhejiang University Sci 2006; B. 7: 713-718
Conservation of indigenous medicinal botanicals in Ekiti State, Nigeria.
Kayode J.

486.. Proceedings International Symposium on Biomedicines, Bogor, 18-19 September 2003; Lestari, Y et al. (eds)
Effect of sidaguri extract as an uric acid lowering agent on the activity of xanthine oxidase enzyme
Iswantini, D; Darusman, LK

487.. http://www.butterfliesandmoths.org/
Butterflies and Moths of North America website
BAMONA was one of 25 web sites to be recognized by MARS in 2011 as an outstanding site for reference information. MARS is the "MARS: Emerging Technologies in Reference" section of the Reference and User Services Association of the American Library Association.

488.. http://www.seedsplants.com/Fiche2.php?Lang=en&Ref=426&
Designation=Sida%20cordifolia
(Directions for the cultivation of Sida cordifolia)
Le Jardin Naturel is a botanical garden and a traditional nursery (sells cordifolia seed). Situated in
Reunion, a French tropical island in the Indian Ocean, near South Africa, Madagascar and Mauritius.

489.. Department of Atomic Energy, Bombay (India). Food and Agriculture Committee; p. 211-220; 1975;
Use of radiations and radioisotopes in studies of plant productivity, proceedings of a symposium held at
G.B. Pant University of Agriculture and Technology, Pantnagar, April 12-14, 1974
Effect of gamma rays on fibre of sida rhombifolia Linn
VR Dnyansagar, MM Mhaske

490.. Brazilian Journal of Medical and Biological Research (2016) 49(8)
Sida tuberculata (Malvaceae): a study based on development of extractive system and in silico and in vitro
properties
H.S. da Rosa, A.C.F. Salgueiro, A.Z.C. Colpo, F.R. Paula, A.S.L. Mendez, V Folmer

491.. Phytochemical Analysis Volume 12, Issue 2, pages 110–119, March/April 2001
Phytoecdysteroid profiles in seeds of Sida spp. (Malvaceae)
Laurence Dinan*, Pauline Bourne andPensri Whiting   xxx dup of 56, 263 also dup

492.. Rapid Communications in Mass Spectrometry Volume 22, Issue 16, pages 2413–2422, 30 August
2008
Structural characterization and identification of ecdysteroids from Sida rhombifolia L. in positive
electrospray ionization by tandem mass spectrometry
Yan-Hong Wang1, Bharathi Avula1, Atul N. Jadhav1, Troy J. Smillie1 andIkhlas A. Khan1,2,*

493.. Phytochemistry Volume 62, Issue 8, April 2003, Pages 1179–1184
Ecdysteroids and other constituents from Sida spinosa L.
Faten M.M Darwisha, Manfred G Reineckeb

494.. BMC Complementary and Alternative Medicine 2013, 13:276
Investigation on flavonoid composition and anti free radical potential of Sida cordata
Naseer Ali Shah1†, Muhammad Rashid Khan1*†, Bushra Ahmad1†, Farah Noureen1†, Umbreen
Rashid1†and Rahmat Ali Khan2†

495.. Journal of Gastroenterology and Hepatology (2002) 17, S370–S376
Herbal medicines for liver diseases in India
SP THYAGARAJAN, S JAYARAM, V GOPALAKRISHNAN, R HARI, P JEYAKUMAR AND
MS SRIPATHI

496.. BioMed Research International Volume 2014, Article ID 671294, 15 pages
Antidiabetic Effect of Sida cordata in Alloxan Induced Diabetic Rats
Naseer Ali Shah and Muhammad Rashid Khan

497.. Int.J.Curr.Microbiol.App.Sci (2013) 2(11): 247-255
Evaluation of Anthelmintic Activity of Different Leaf and Stem extract of Sida cordata burm.
F. A.R. Gulnaz1 and G. Savitha2*

498.. Journal of Evolution of Medical and Dental Sciences 2.15 (2013): 2514+
Phytochemical evaluation of leaf and stem extracts of Siddha medicinal plant: Sida Cordata
Gulnaz, A.R., and G. Savitha

499.. Annals of Clinical Microbiology and Antimicrobials 2013, 12:14
Anti-nociceptive properties in rodents and the possibility of using polyphenol-rich fractions from sida
urens L. (Malvaceae) against of dental caries bacteria
Kiessoun Konaté1*, Patrice Zerbo2, Maurice Ouédraogo3, Crépin I Dibala4, Hilou Adama5, Oksana
Sytar6, Marian Brestic7 and Nicolas Barro8

500.. Indian Journal of Pharmacology Volume: 40 Issue: Suppl 2 Pages: S112-S142 October 2008
Central nervous system depressant activity of Sida acuta root extract in mice
Bansod MS, Rajgure DT, Harle UN, Vyawahare NS, Yende SR

534

501.. International scholarly research notices 2014-10-30
Biochemical and Ultrastructural Changes in Sida cordifolia L. and Catharanthus roseus L. to Auto Pollution
Vijeta Verma, Neelam Chandra

502.. BMC Complementary and Alternative Medicine (2016) 16:276
In-Vitro dual inhibition of protein glycation, and oxidation by some Arabian plants
Maqsood A. Siddiqui1,3, Saima Rasheed2, Quaiser Saquib1,3, Abdulaziz A. Al-Khedhairy1, Mansour S. Al-Said5, Javed Musarrat4 and Muhammad Iqbal Choudhary2*

503.. Journal of Pharmacopuncture 2015;18[4]:012-019
Attenuation of Diabetic Conditions by Sida rhombifolia in Moderately Diabetic Rats and Inability to Produce Similar Effects in Severely Diabetic in Rats
Padmaja Chaturvedi, Tebogo Elvis Kwape

504.. Planta Daninha, Viçosa-MG, v. 32, n. 2, p. 311-317, 2014
Growth and Mineral Nutrition of Sida rhombifolia
BIANCO, S.2, CARVALHO, L.B.3 e BIANCO, M.S.2

505.. Rev. Ceres, Viçosa, v. 58, n.6, p. 749-754, nov/dez, 2011
Effects of seasonal variations on the emergence of Solanum viarum and Sida rhombifolia under different sowing depths
Marcelo Claro Souza1, Mariana Casari Parreira2, Carita Liberato do Amaral3, Pedro Luís da Costa Aguiar Alves4

506.. Pak. J. Bot., 38(2): 353-359, 2006.
HISTO-ARCHITECTURE OF THE PERICARP AND SEED LIBERATION IN THE SCHIZOCARPIC FRUIT OF SIDA RHOMBIFOLIA L. (MALVACEAE)
T. V. RAMANA RAO* AND YASH DAVE

507.. Indian Journal of Traditional Knowledge Vol. 5(3), July 2006, pp. 317-322
Ethnomedicinal studies of the Khamti tribe of Arunachal Pradesh
AK Das* & Hui Tag**

508.. Journal of Ethnobiology and Ethnomedicine20062:43
Medicinal plants used by traditional healers in Kancheepuram District of Tamil Nadu, India
Chellaiah Muthu, Muniappan Ayyanar, Nagappan Raja and Savarimuthu Ignacimuthu

509.. Rev. Ceres vol.61 no.2 Viçosa Mar./Apr. 2014
Leaf area and epicuticular wax content of Sida spp
Viviane Cristina da CunhaI; José Barbosa dos SantosII; Cintia Gonçalves GuimarãesI; Karina Guimarães RibeiroII; Roqueline Rodrigues Silva de MirandaIII; Daniel Valadão SilvaI; Germani ConcençoIV

510.. Planta Daninha, Viçosa-MG, v.21, n.1, p.181-189, 2003
Relationships Between Weed Seed Species Germination and Electrical Conductivity Use
VOLL, E.2 , BRIGHENTI, A.M.3, GAZZIERO, D.L.P.4 e ADEGAS, F.S.5

511.. Planta Daninha, v. 10, n. 1/2, 1992
LEVANTAMENTO E ANÁLISEFITOSSOCIOLÓGICA DAS PRINCIPAISESPÉCIES DE PLANTAS DANINHASDE PASTAGENS DA REGIÃO DE SELVÍRIA (MS)
S.L. CARVALHO1e, R.A. PITELLI2

512.. Planta Daninha, Viçosa-MG, v. 28, p. 1031-1039, 2010. Número Especial
Effect of Fertilization on Weeds and on the Period before Weed Interference in the Peanut Culture
YAMAUTI, M.S.2, ALVES, P.L.C.A.3, NEPOMUCENO, M.4 e MARTINS, J.V.F.5

513.. Planta Daninha, Viçosa-MG, v.21, n.2, p.219-227, 2003
Nutrient Contents of Coffee Plants Under Weed Interference
RONCHI, C.P.2, TERRA, A.A.4; SILVA. A.A.3 e FERREIRA, L.R.3

535

514..Bioresource Technology 98 (2007) 2723–2726   xxx dup of 430..
Cultivation of Pleurotus ostreatus on weed plants
Nirmalendu Das a, Mina Mukherjee b

515.. Planta April 1983, Volume 157, Issue 3, pp 224–232
Role of peroxidase in the development of water-impermeable seed coats in Sida spinosa L.
G. H. Egley, R. N. PaulJr., K. C. Vaughn, S. O. Duke

516.. Journal of Applied Entomology Volume 113, Issue 1-5, pages 202–208, January/December 1992
Toxicity of plant extracts to three storage beetles (Coleoptera)
B. Tierto Niber*, J. Helenius* andA.-L. Varis   xxx orig dup of 505..

517.. Weed Science Vol. 25, No. 2 (Mar., 1977), pp. 151-158
Competition of Spurred Anoda, Velvetleaf, Prickly Sida, and Venice Mallow in Cotton
J. M. Chandler

518.. Weed Research Volume 32, Issue 2, pages 103–109, April 1992
Arrowleaf sida (Sida rhombifolia) and prickly sida (Sida spinosa): germination and emergence
C. A. SMITH, D. R. SHAW andL. J. NEWSOM

519.. Planta Daninha, Viçosa-MG, v.22, n.1, p.11-17, 2004
Weed Emergence in Soil Covered with Sugarcane Harvest Straw Residue
CORREIA, N.M.2 e DURIGAN, J.C.3

520.. Int. J. Mol. Sci. 2011, 12(7), 4661-4677
Sida rhomboidea. Roxb Leaf Extract Down-Regulates Expression of PPAR?2 and Leptin Genes in High
Fat Diet Fed C57BL/6J Mice and Retards in Vitro 3T3L1 Pre-Adipocyte Differentiation
Menaka C. Thounaojam 1, Ravirajsinh N. Jadeja 1, Umed V. Ramani 2, Ranjitsinh V. Devkar 1,* and A.
V. Ramachandran 1

521.. Asian Journal of Traditional Medicines, 2009, 4 (4)
Plants-herbal wealth as a potential source of ayurvedic drugs
Ajay Kumar Meena *, Parveen Bansal, Sanjiv Kumar

522.. Int. J. Pharm. Sci. Rev. Res., 32(1), May – June 2015; Article No. 35, Pages: 209-216
An Overview on Therapeutic Potential and Phytochemistry of Sida rhombifolia Linn.
Goutam Ghosh*, Debajyoti Das

523.. Journal of Pure and Applied Microbiology 2(2):415-418 • August 2008
Comparative Studies on Antimicrobial Activity of Sida acuta (Malvaceae) Leaf Extracts
1 Kaladhar SVGK Dowluru, 2 Challa Surekha, D. Srinivas, I Bhaskar Reddy

524.. http://www.stuartxchange.org/Escobilla.html
Sida rhombifolia Linn. - A very common weed in the Philippines.
Dr. Godofredo Umali-Stuart,

525.. http://www.stuartxchange.com/Gulipas
Sida cordifolia
Dr. Godofredo Umali-Stuart,

526.. http://www.stuartxchange.com/Ualisualisan.html
Ualisualisan - Sida acuta Burm. f.
Dr. Godofredo Umali-Stuart

527.. http://www.stuartxchange.com/Ualisualisan.html
Ualis - Sida retusa Linn
Dr. Godofredo Umali-Stuart

528.. http://www.stuartxchange.com/Ualisualisan.html
Igat-igat - Sida javensis Cav.
Dr. Godofredo Umali-Stuart

529.. Japan J. Pharmcol. 21, 137 (1971)   xxx dup of 435
CENTRAL NERVOUS SYSTEM EFFECTS OF SIDA RETUSA ROOT
 Thangam JOSEPH* and G. SHANTHAKLMARI**

530.. American Journal of Drug Discovery and Development, 3: 194-199 2013.
Effects of Ethanol Extract of Sida acuta Leaves on Some Organ Function Parameters and Physiologically
Important Electrolytes in Normal Wistar Albino Rats.
V.H.A. Enemor, V.N. Okoye and U.L. Awoke

531.. Journal of Biology, Agriculture and Healthcare, Vol.3, No.10, 2013
The Electrolytic Effect of Sida Acuta Leaf Extract on the Kidney Electrolyte of Adult Wistar Rats
Kebe Obeten

532.. Int. J. of Pharm. & Life Sci. (IJPLS), Vol. 4, Issue 8: Aug: 2013,
Removal of fluoride from drinking water with the help of Sida acuta Burm f.
H. B.Trivedi and S. D.Vediya

533.. Web MD - http://www.webmd.com/vitamins-supplements/ingredientmono-837-
sida%20cordifolia.aspx?activeingredientid=837&activeingredientname=sida%20cordifolia
Sida cordifolia - Interactions

534.. Research Journal of Pharmacy and Technology 4(6):913-916 • June 2011
Comparative Cardiotonic Activity of Sida cordifolia Linn with Digoxin on Perfused Frog Heart.
Y. Dama Ganesh, P. Jori Mayuri, P. Joshi Prajakta, S. Bidkar Jayant

535.. Journal of Medicinal Plants Research Vol. 6(7), pp. 1106-1118, 23 February, 2012
Phytochemical and ethnobotanical study of some selected medicinal plants from Nigeria
Temitope Israel Borokini1* and Felix Oluwafemi Omotayo2

536.. Research Journal of Pharmaceutical, Biological and Chemical Sciences 3(2):488-493 • April 2012
Efficacy of Cardioprotective Effects in Ethanolic Extract of Sida Rhombifolia Linn. On Isoproterenol-
Induced Myocardial Infarction in Albino Rats
Ramadoss S*, KannanK,Balamurugan K, JeganathanNS,Manavalan R

537.. J. Chem. Pharm. Res., 2011, 3(6):136-142 (31)
Evaluation of Anti-inflammatory activities of Sida cordifolia Linn in Albino rats
Shailender Singh, Praveen Panchaksharimath* and Siddappa Devaru

538.. IJPBS, Volume 2, Issue 3, JULY-SEPT 2012, 303-309 (30)
PROXIMATE ANALYSIS OF SIDA RHOMBIFOLIA. L ROOT AND ITS EFFECT ON CADMIUM
CHLORIDE INDUCED ALTERATIONS IN BODY WEIGHT OF WISTAR RATS
Logeswari.P*,Dineshkumar.V ,Usha.P.T.A and PrathapKumar. S. M

539.. Medindia » Complementary Medicine http://www.medindia.net/alternativemedicine/bala.asp
Bala - Sida cordifolia
Dr. Sunil Shroff, MBBS, MS,FRCS(uk), D. UROL (Lond)

540.. International Journal of Research in Pharmacology & Pharmacotherapeutics, Vol 2, Issue 1, 2013
In vivo Antimalarial Activity of Aerial Part Extracts of Gardenia lutea and Sida rhombifolia
Baye Akele

541.. INTERNATIONAL JOURNAL OF RESEARCH IN PHARMACY AND CHEMISTRY 2011, 1(3)
FREE RADICAL SCAVENGING ACTIVITY OF THE ALCOHOLIC EXTRACT OF SIDA
RHOMBIFOLIA ROOTS IN ARTHRITIC RATS
Amarender Reddy Gangu*1, Prapulla P1, Anil Kumar CH1, Chamundeeswari D2 and Uma maheswara
Reddy C2

542.. Pharmacologyonline 3: 259-266 (2006)
Hepatoprotective Activity of Sida rhombifolia ssp. retusa Against Thioacetamide and Allyl Alcohol
Intoxication in Rats
Kamlesh Dhalwal*, Vaibhav Shinde, K.R. Mahadik and S.S. Kadam

543.. Hygeia.J.D.Med.vol.5 (1), April 2013 Page: 19-22
Phytochemical studies and pharmacological screening of Sida rhombifolia Linn.
R Sundaraganapathy1, V Niraimathi2, Ananda Thangadurai*1, M Jambulingam1, B Narasimhan3 and
Aakash Deep3

544.. Int. J. Pharm. Sci. Rev. Res., 20(2), May – Jun 2013 (21)
Anti-Tubercular Activity on Leaves and Roots of Sida rhombifolia L
N.Papitha*, N.Jayshree, S.Prabu Seenivasan, Vanaja Kumar

545.. Pharmacologyonline 2: 707-714 (2011)
ANALGESIC AND CYTOTOXIC ACTIVITIES OF SIDA RHOMBIFOLIA LINN
Md. Atiqur Rahman1*, Liton Chandra Paul1, Md. Solaiman1, A. A. Rahman1

546.. Ministry of Agriculture and Rural Development of Poland, Central Agricultural Library
Chemical composition of sida leaves in comparison with some plants used in rabbit feeding [1994]
Borkowska, H.

547.. Cardiovasc. Toxicol 2011, 11, 168–179.
In Vitro evidence for the protective role of Sida rhomboidea. Roxb extract against LDL oxidation and
oxidized LDL-induced apoptosis in human monocyte-derived macrophages.
Menaka C. ThounaojamRaviraysinh N. JadejaRanjisinh V. DevkarEmail authorA. V. Ramachandran

548.. Journal of Planar Chromatography Volume 18, Issue 105   xxx dup of 71
HPTLC method for chemical standardization of Sida species and estimation of the alkaloid ephedrine
Sayyada Khatoon, Manjoosha Srivastava, A. Rawat, Shanta Mehrotra

549.. Asian Pacific Journal of Tropical Medicine Volume 6, Issue 4, 13 April 2013, Pages 280-284
Protective effect of Sida cordata leaf extract against CCl4 induced acute liver toxicity in rats
Sunil Mistry a, KR Dutt b, J Jena

550.. Journal of Ethnopharmacology Volume 23, Issue 1, May–June 1988, Pages 27-37
Abortifacient properties of an extract from sida veronicaefolia
G.D. Lutterodt *

551.. Asian Pacific Journal of Tropical Biomedicine (2012)S947-S952
In vivo anti-inflamatory potential of various extracts of Sida tiagii Bhandari
Ramkumar Kumawat, Sunil Sharma, Neeru Vasudeva and Suresh Kumar*

552.. Acta Poloniae Pharmaceutica ñ Drug Research, Vol. 69 No. 6 pp. 1103ñ1109, 2012
EVALUATION OF ANALGESIC ACTIVITY OF VARIOUS EXTRACTS OF SIDA TIAGII
BHANDARI
RAM KUMAR KUMAWAT, SURESH KUMAR and SUNIL SHARMA*

553.. Acta Poloniae Pharmaceutica ñ Drug Research, Vol. 69 No. 4 pp. 69-706, 2012
ACUTE AND CHRONIC HYPOGLYCEMIC ACTIVITY OF SIDA TIAGII FRUITS IN N5-
STREPTOZOTOCIN DIABETIC RATS
ASHOK KUMAR DATUSALIA1, CHANDER PARKASH DORA and SUNIL SHARMA*

554.. Polish Journal of Environmental Studies Vol. 10, No. 5 (2001), 379-381
Suitability of Cultivation of Some Perennial Plant Species on Sewage Sludge
H. Borkowska*, I. Jackowska**, J. Piotrowski**, B. Styk*

555.. Taiwania 61(3): 243?252, 2016
A Synopsis of the genus Sida L. (Malvaceae) from Maharashtra, India
Gajanan M. TAMBDE*, Ramchandra D. GORE and Milind M. SARDESAI

556.. ActaBiochimicaPolonica Vol. 54 No. 4/2007, 727–732
The search for polyprenols in dendroflora of Vietnam
Andrzej Marczewski1, Ewa Ciepichal2, Le Xuan Canh3, Tran The Bach3,Ewa Swiezewska2 and Tadeusz
Chojnacki2

557.. India Journal of Natural Products and Resources, Vol 4(4), December 2013, pp. 339-347
Fibre-yielding plant resources of Odisha and traditional fibre preparation knowledge-An overview
SC Sahu, SK Pattnaik,SS Dash, NK Dhal

558.. Springer London - http://link.springer.com/referenceworkentry/10.1007/978-0-85729-323-7_2066
Lipids, Lipophilic Components and Essential Oils from Plant Sources pp 635-635
Shakhnoza S. Azimova, Anna I. Glushenkova

559.. Journal of the American Oil Chemists Society May 1973, Volume 50, Issue 5, pp 168–169
Studies on fixed oil of seeds of Sida acuta burm
Rao, R.E., Dixit, V.K. & Varma, K.C.

560.. Journal of Medicinal Plants Research Vol. 3(4), pp. 301-314, April, 2009
Ethnobotanical survey of plants used to treat diseases of the reproductive system and preliminary
phytochemical screening of some species of malvaceae in Ndop Central Sub-division, Cameroon
Focho D. A.1, Nkeng E. A. P.2, Lucha C. F.1*, Ndam W, T.1and Afegenui A.1

561.. Doctoral Thesis, Department of Botany, Faculty of Science,
The Maharaja Sayajirao University of Baroda
Studies on the Chemical Diversity and Biomarkers of the Plants Used as Bala and Bioprospecting of Their
Allied Species
Anamika Kumari

562.. Strickly Medicinal website
http://www.strictlymedicinalseeds.com/product.asp?specific=565
Bala (Sida cordifolia)

563.. SIDA, Contributions to Botany Vol. 11, No. 2 (DECEMBER 1985), pp. 215-225
OBSERVATIONS ON THE DISTRIBUTION AND ECOLOGY OF SIDA HERMAPHRODITA (L.)
RUSBY (MALVACEAE)
DAVID M. SPOONER, ALLISON W. CUSICK, GEORGE F. HALL and JERRY M. BASKIN

564.. International Review of Applied Sciences and Engineering Volume 4, Issue 2
Improvement of germination capacity of Sida hermaphrodita (L.) Rusby by seed priming techniques
manuskript
Erika Kurucz1* and Miklós Gábor Fári1,2

565.. Journal of the Chinese Chemical Society, 2007, 54, 41-45
Tocopherols and Triterpenoids from Sida acuta
Chiy-Rong Chen1,Li-Hui Chao3,Yun-Wen Liao2,Chi-I Chang2,Min-Hsiung Pan3

566.. J. Nat. Prod. Plant Resour., 2011, 1 (4):35-39
In-vitro antibacterial activity of Sida spinosa Linn
Pesaramelli, K., A.P. Kumar, and A.K. Harsha,
Could not find where this came from – not in Google scholar

567.. Fitoterapia 77 (2006) 19 – 27
Cardiovascular effects of Sida cordifolia leaves extract in rats
I.A. Medeiros *, M.R.V. Santos, N.M.S. Nascimento, J.C. Duarte

568.. A Textbook of Medicinal Plants from Nigeria
edited by Tolu Odugbemi, 2008
628 Pages.   UniLag Press

569.. Planta Med 1981; 43(12): 384-388
Alkaloid Constituents of Sida acuta, S. humilis, S. rhombifolia and S. spinosa*
A. Prakash, R. K. Varma, S. Ghosal

570.. Planta Med 1976; 30(6): 174-185
PHYTOCHEMICAL INVESTIGATION OF ABUTILON INDICUM
K. N. Gaind, K. S. Chopra

571.. Phytochemistry Letters Volume 1, Issue 4, 12 December 2008, Pages 179–182
Bioactive flavones of Sida cordifolia
Ranajit K. Sutradhara, , , A.K.M. Matior Rahmanb, , Mesbah U. Ahmadc, , Sitesh C. Bachard,

572.. IOSR Journal of Applied Physics (IOSR-JAP) Volume 4, Issue 1 (May. - Jun. 2013), PP 60-66
The evaluation of the effect of Sida acuta leaf extract on the microanatomy and some biochemical
parameters on the liver of Wistar rats
Kebe. E. Obeten1, Kelechi C. Uruakpa,2 Victoria Isaac3   xxx 256 dup

573.. Phytochemistry Volume 62, Issue 8, April 2003, Pages 1179–1184
Ecdysteroids and other constituents from Sida spinosa L.
Faten M.M Darwisha, Manfred G Reineckeb

574.. Chem Ind (London) 1985: 483-4.
Sida cordifolia seed oil: a rich source of hydrobromic acid-reactive fatty acids.
Farooqi JA, Ahmad M.

575.. J Am Chem Soc (1976) 53: 698.
Cyclopropenoid fatty acids in seed oils ofSida acuta andSida rhombifolia (malvaceae)
Ahmad, M.U., Husain, S.K., Ahmad, M. et al.

576.. Annals of Botany 88: 387-391, 2001
Herbivory and Calcium Concentrations A?ect Calcium Oxalate Crystal Formation in Leaves of Sida
(Malvaceae)
BRENDA MOLANO-FLORES*

577.. Ministry of Agriculture and Rural Development of Poland, Centralna Biblioteka Rolnicza/Central
Agricultural Library
Utilization of sida forage (Sida hermaphrodita Rusby) for silage [2003]
Tarkowski, A. (Akademia Rolnicza, Lublin (Poland). Inst. Zywienia Zwierzat)

578.. J Ethnopharmacol. 2012 Jul 13;142(2):422-31. doi: 10.1016/j.jep.2012.05.012. Epub 2012 May 21.
Anti-proliferative activities on HeLa cancer cell line of Thai medicinal plant recipes selected from
MANOSROI II database.
Manosroi J1, Boonpisuttinant K, Manosroi W, Manosroi A.

579.. Indo Global Journal of Pharmaceutical Sciences, 2012; 2(2): 98-102
Phytochemical Screening of a Vended Antimalarial - Malatreat
Terrumun A. Tor-Anyiin*, Kolapo A. Danisa

580.. J Ethnopharmacol. 2006 Jul 19;106(3):425-8. Epub 2006 Mar 27.
Analgesic activity of some Indian medicinal plants.
Malairajan P1, Geetha Gopalakrishnan, Narasimhan S, Jessi Kala Veni K.

581.. Pharmatutor website   xxx dup of 186
http://www.pharmatutor.org/articles/anti-inflammatory-analgesic-activity-methanolic-extract-whole-plant-
sida-acuta
ANTI-INFLAMMATORY AND ANALGESIC ACTIVITY OF METHANOLIC EXTRACT OF WHOLE
PLANT OF SIDA ACUTA (LINN.F.ND)
*Virendra Sharma, Pooja Sinoriya, Sunil Sharma

582.. Biochimie (2003), vol. 85, pp. 535-547.
Interactions of cryptolepine and neocryptolepine with unusual DNA structures
Lionel Guittat a,1 Patrizia Alberti a,1 Frédéric Rosu b,1 Sabine Van Miertc , Emilie Thetiot a , Luc Pieters
c , Valérie Gabelica d , Edwin De Pauw d , Alexandre Ottaviani a , Jean-François Riou e , Jean-Louis
Mergny a

583.. Planta Med 1981; 41(4): 392-396
Studies on Cryptolepine II: Inhibition of Carragenan Induced Oedema by Cryptolepine
S. O. A. Bamgbose, B. K. Noamesi

540

584.. Toxicology Letters 207 (2011) 322–325
Effects of the anti-malarial compound cryptolepine and its analogues in human lymphocytes and sperm in the Comet assay
Rajendran C. Gopalana, Esra Emerce b, Colin W. Wright a, Bensu Karahalil b, Ali E. Karakaya b, Diana Andersona,*

585.. Mahidol Univ J Pharm Sci 1982; 9 4: 88-91.
The antimicrobial activity of some Thai Medicinal Plants.
Pongpan A, Chumsri P and Taworasate T .

586.. Journal of Medicinal and Aromatic Plant Sciences 2004 26 1 34-38
Juvenoid activity in plant extracts against filarial mosquito Culex quinquefasciatus.
Neraliya, S.; Ratna Gaur

587.. Pakistan Journal of Biological Sciences   Year: 2003, Volume 6, Issue 1, Page No.: 73-75
Larvicidal Activity of a New Glycoside, Phenyl Ethyl ß-D Glucopyranoside from the Stem of the Plant Sida rhombifolia
Md. Ekramul Islam , Naznin Ara Khatune , M. I. I. Wahed , Md. Ekramul Haque and Md. Ashiik Mosaddik

588.. Research Gate, September 2011
Evaluation of the Anti-Hyperglycemic Activity of the Crude Leaf Extracts of Sida Acuta in Normal and Diabetic Rabbits
1 Chukwugozie Okwuosa, 2 Nc Azubike, 2 II NEBO

589-Cited in 471- III International Conference 'Plant - the source of research material' 16th – 18th October 2013, Lublin, Poland
MORPHOLOGICAL AND CHEMICAL CHANGES OF MYCOBACTERIUM SMEGMATIS CELLS AFTER EXPOSURE TO SIDA HERMAPHRODITA (MALVACEAE) EXTRACT
Lewtak K., Fiolka M., Szczuka E., Wydrych J., Keller R., Mendyk E., Rawski M., Skrzypiec K. (Poland)

590.. Materials Letters 170 (2016) 101–104
Synthesis of biofunctionalized AgNPs using medicinally important Sida cordifolia leaf extract for enhanced antioxidant and anticancer activities
B.Srinithya a , V. Vinod Kumar c , Vellingiri Vadivel b , Brindha Pemaiah b , Savarimuthu Philip Anthony c,n ,

591.. Int. J. Pharm. Sci. Rev. Res., 23(2), Nov – Dec 2013; n? 22, 126-132
Evaluation of Anticancer Activity of Sida cordifolia l. against Aflatoxin B1 induced Hepatocellular Carcinoma
Mallikarjuna G 1*, Jaya Sankar Reddy V1, Prabhakaran V11

592.. Int J Oncol. 2007 Oct;31(4):915-22.
The plant alkaloid cryptolepine induces p21WAF1/CIP1 and cell cycle arrest in a human osteosarcoma cell line.
Matsui TA1, Sowa Y, Murata H, Takagi K, Nakanishi R, Aoki S, Yoshikawa M, Kobayashi M, Sakabe T, Kubo T, Sakai T.

593.. Eur J Sci Res 44.4 (2010): 570-580.
Polyphenol contents, antioxidant and anti-inflammatory activities of six malvaceae species traditionally used to treat hepatitis B in Burkina Faso
Konaté, K., et al.

594.. Ethnobotanical Leaflets: Vol. 2005: Iss. 1, Article 5.
Available at: http://opensiuc.lib.siu.edu/ebl/vol2005/iss1/5
Ethnomedicinal Plant Resources of Southeastern Nigeria
Obute, Gordian C.

595.. Ethnobotanical Leaflets 13: 1353-61, 2009 opensiuc.lib.siu.edu
Ethnomedical Knowledge of Plants used by the Tribal people of Purandhar in Maharashtra, India
Bhosle S. V., Ghule V. P., Aundhe D. J.1 and Jagtap S. D.

541

596.. Ethnobotanical Leaflets 12: 851-65. 2008.
An Ethnobotanical Survey of Herbal Markets and Medicinal Plants in Lagos State of Nigeria
Olowokudejo J. D., Kadiri A. B*. and Travih V.A.

597.. Ethnobotanical Leaflets 13: 1-32. 2009.
Wound Healing Plants of Jalgaon District of Maharashtra State, India
1 M.Z. Chopda and 2R.T. Mahajan

598.. Conservation of Botanicals Used for Dental and Oral Healthcare in Ekitii State, Nigeria 11/13/08
Ethnobotanical Leaflets 12: 7-18. 2008. opensiuc.lib.siu.edu
Conservation of Botanicals Used for Dental and Oral Healthcare in Ekiti State, Nigeria
Kayode, Joshua and Omotoyinbo, Michael Ayorinde

599.. Ethnobotanical Leaflets 13: 1-32. 2009.
Wound Healing Plants of Jalgaon District of Maharashtra State, India
1M.Z. Chopda and 2R.T. Mahajan

600.. Ethnobotanical Leaflets 13: 379-87. 2009. opensiuc.lib.siu.edu
Ethnomedicinal practices of Kol tribes in Similipal Biosphere Reserve, Orissa, India
S.D Rout1 and H.N. Thatoi2

601.. Ethnobotanical Leaflets 13: 480 opensiuc.lib.siu.edu
Ethnobotanical Uses of Plants Among the Binis in the Treatment of Ophthalmic and ENT (Ear, Nose and
Throat) Ailments
Idu M., G.O. Obaruyi and J. O. Erhabor

602.. Ethnobotanical Leaflets 13: 548-63, 2009. opensiuc.lib.siu.edu
Ethnobotanical Plants Used for Oral Healthcare Among the Esan Tribe
of Edo State, Nigeria.
1Idu, M., 2Umweni, A. A., 1Odaro, T. and 1Ojelede L.

603.. Ethnobotanical Leaflets 13: 1113- 39, 2009. opensiuc.lib.siu.edu
Medicinal Plants of Sewa River Catchment Area in the Northwest Himalaya and its Implication for
Conservation
Mahroof Khan, Satish Kumar and Irshad Ahmed Hamal

604.. Cooperative Wildlife Research Laboratory, Final Reports 2003. Paper 16.
http://opensiuc.lib.siu.edu/cwrl_fr/16
HABITAT PREFERENCES OF MIGRATORY SHOREBIRDS AND WATERFOWL ON THE EAST
SHORELINE OF REND LAKE REFUGE
Woolf, Alan; Nawrot, Jack R.; Kirk, Laura; and Elliot-Smith, Elise,

605.. International Journal of Pharmacognosy, 29, 1991, 19-23.
Antimalarial activity of traditional plants against erythrocytic stages of Plasmodium berghei,
Mishra P, Pal NL, Guru PY, Katiyar JC, Tandon JS,

606.. Journal of Ethnopharmacology, 58, 1997, 75-83.
Antimicrobial screening of selected medicinal plants from India,
Valsaraj R, Pushpangadan P, Smitt UW, Adsersen A, Nyman U,

607.. Journal of Health Science, 55 (4) 641-648 (2009)
Antidepressant like potential of Sida tiagii Bhandari Fruite in Mice
Ashok Kumar Datusallia, Sunil Sharma, Pankaj Kalra, Manas Kumar Samal

608.. Philippine Journal of Veterinary Medicine Volume: 41 Issue: 1 Pages: 25-31 Published: 2004
Reproductive effects of gulipas (Sida cordifolia) on immature female Sprague-Dawley rats.
Presa J. D.; Valle-Paraso M. G. R.; Luis E. S.; et al.

609.. Journal of Ethnopharmacology Volume 176, 24 December 2015, Pages 135–176
The genus Sida L. – A traditional medicine: Its ethnopharmacological, phytochemical and pharmacological
data for commercial exploitation in herbal drugs industry

542

Biswanath Dindaa, , , Niranjan Dasb, Subhajit Dindac, Manikarna Dindad, Indrajit SilSarmaa

610.. Oxford and IBH Publishing, 1994.
Ayurvedic Drugs and Their Plant Sources
V. Sivarajan and I. Balachandran, cited by 496

611.. Am Oil Chem Soc (1984) 61: 1345.   dup of 352
Characteristics and composition of six malvaceae seeds and the oils
Rao, K.S. & Lakshminarayana, G. J

612.. Journal of Medicinal Plants Studies 2015; 3(4): 127-131
Micro-Morphological Study of 'BALA' Plant (Sida cordifolia L., Malvaceae) With Special Reference to
Its Propagation Technique
Debasmita Dutta Pramanick, GG Maiti, Amber Srivastava

613.. Food Chemistry Volume 182, 1 September 2015, Pages 193–199
Ecdysteroids in Sida tuberculata R.E. Fries (Malvaceae): Chemical composition by LC–ESI-MS and
selective anti-Candida krusei activity
Hemerson Silva da Rosaa, Vanessa Brum de Camargob, Graziela Camargoc, Cássia V. Garciad, Alexandre
M. Fuentefriac, d, Andreas S.L. Mendeza, d, ,

614.. Curr Drug Targets. 2011 October 1; 12(11): 1595–1653.
Identification of Novel Anti-inflammatory Agents from Ayurvedic Medicine for Prevention of Chronic
Diseases - "Reverse Pharmacology" and "Bedside to Bench" Approach
Bharat B. Aggarwal, Sahdeo Prasad, [...], and Bokyung Sung

615.. J. Nutr. Biochem. 14, 64-73 (2003)
Redox-sensitive mechanisms of phytochemical-mediated inhibition of cancer cell proliferation (Review).
Loo, G.

616.. Clin Infect Dis (2008) 46 (2): 155-164.
The Epidemic of Antibiotic-Resistant Infections: A Call to Action for the Medical Community from the
Infectious Diseases Society of America
Brad Spellberg Robert Guidos David Gilbert John Bradley Helen W. Boucher W. Michael Scheld John
G. Bartlett John Edwards, Jr the Infectious Diseases Society of America

617.. Clin Infect Dis (2013) 56 (12): 1685-1694.
10 × '20 Progress—Development of New Drugs Active Against Gram-Negative Bacilli: An Update From
the Infectious Diseases Society of America
Helen W. Boucher George H. Talbot Daniel K. Benjamin, Jr John Bradley Robert J. Guidos Ronald N.
Jones Barbara E. Murray Robert A. Bonomo David Gilbert for the Infectious Diseases Society of
America

618.. Center for Indectious Disease Research and Policy News, Jan 27, 2017
Studies show spread of MCR-1 gene in China
Chris Dall, News Reporter

619.. Pharm Biol. 2017 Dec;55(1):920-928. doi: 10.1080/13880209.2017.1285322.
Anti-inflammatory, anti-cholinergic and cytotoxic effects of Sida rhombifolia.
Mah SH1, Teh SS2, Ee GC3.

620.. Toxicon. 2017 Mar 15;128:1-4. doi: 10.1016/j.toxicon.2016.12.011. Epub 2017 Jan 16.
Swainsonine-induced lysosomal storage disease in goats caused by the ingestion of Sida rodrigoi Monteiro
in North-western Argentina.
Micheloud JF1, Marin R2, Colque-Caro LA3, Martínez OG4, Gardner D5, Gimeno EJ6.

621.. Vet Pathol. 2000 Mar;37(2):153-9.
Lysosomal storage disease caused by Sida carpinifolia poisoning in goats.
Driemeier D1, Colodel EM, Gimeno EJ, Barros SS.

622.. Molecules. 2017 Jan 6;22(1).
Alkaloids and Phenolic Compounds from Sida rhombifolia L. (Malvaceae) and Vasorelaxant Activity of Two Indoquinoline Alkaloids.
Chaves OS1, Teles YC2,3, Monteiro MM4, Mendes Junior LD5, Agra MF6, Braga VA7, Silva TM8, Souza MF9,10.

623.. Environ Sci Pollut Res Int. 2016 Dec 19. [Epub ahead of print]   630 a dup
The evaluation of growth and phytoextraction potential of Miscanthus x giganteus and Sida hermaphrodita on soil contaminated simultaneously with Cd, Cu, Ni, Pb, and Zn.
Kocon A1, Jurga B2.

624.. J Zoo Wildl Med. 2016 Sep;47(3):862-867.
POISONING BY THE SWAINSONINE-CONTAINING PLANT SIDA CARPINIFOLIA IN CAPTIVE SAMBAR DEER (CERVUS UNICOLOR).
Anjos BL, Peixoto PV, Caldas SA, Bhaltazar D, França TN, Armién AG.

625.. J Zoo Wildl Med. 2009 Sep;40(3):583-5.
Sida carpinifolia (Malvaceae) poisoning in fallow deer (Dama dama).
Pedroso PM1, Von Hohendorf R, de Oliveira LG, Schmitz M, da Cruz CE, Driemeier D.

626.. Equine Vet J. 2003 Jul;35(5):434-8.
Lysosomal storage disease in Sida carpinifolia toxicosis: an induced mannosidosis in horses.
Loretti AP1, Colodel EM, Gimeno EJ, Driemeier D.

627.. Vet Hum Toxicol. 2002 Jun;44(3):177-8.
Identification of swainsonine as a glycoside inhibitor responsible for Sida carpinifolia poisoning.
Colodel EM1, Gardner DR, Zlotowski P, Driemeier D.

628.. Toxicon. 2009 Apr;53(5):591-4.
Urinary oligosaccharides: a peripheral marker for Sida carpinifolia exposure or poisoning.
Bedin M1, Colodel EM, Giugliani R, Zlotwski P, Cruz CE, Driemeier D.

629.. Int J Phytoremediation. 2017 Apr 3;19(4):309-318. doi: 10.1080/15226514.2016.1225283.
Phytoextraction of heavy metals from municipal sewage sludge by Rosa multiflora and Sida hermaphrodita.
Antonkiewicz J1, Kolodziej B2, Bielinska EJ3.

630.. Environ Sci Pollut Res Int. 2016 Dec 19. [Epub ahead of print]   xxx dup of 623
The evaluation of growth and phytoextraction potential of Miscanthus x giganteus and Sida hermaphrodita on soil contaminated simultaneously with Cd, Cu, Ni, Pb, and Zn.
Kocon A1, Jurga B2.

631.. International Journal of Plant, Animal and Environmental Sciences, Vol. 2, Issue 1, March 2017
IN VITRO SEED GERMINATION STUDIES ON SIDA SCHIMPERIANA HOCHST. EX A.RICH. A RARE MEDICINAL PLANT
Prabhu.Va Ramar.Kb*and Dhinesh.Vc

632.. https://www.flowersofindia.net/catalog/slides/Schimper's%20Sida.html
Common name: Schimper's Sida
Botanical name: Sida schimperiana Hochst. ex A. Rich. Sida schimperiana Family: Malvaceae (Mallow family)

633.. International Journal of Chemical and Life sciences, 2012, 01 (02), 1039-1041
Antimicrobial Profile of the Selected Medicinal Plants
Nisar Ahmad1*, Amir MK1, Sultan Ayaz2, Shakeel ahmad3, Akber Jan1, Ashraf JS1 and Fatima Tu Zuhra1

634.. Journal of Medicinal Plants Studies 2017; 5(1): 91-95
Screening of edible plants in Sri Lanka for antioxidant activity
Chethana Galketiya, T Sampath Weerarathna, J Chamini Punchihewa, M Nirmali Wickramaratne and DBM Wickramaratne

544

635.. Oecologia Australis 14(1): 16-39, Março 2010
BEES AND MELITTOPHILOUS PLANTS OF SECONDARY ATLANTIC FOREST HABITATS AT
SANTA CATARINA ISLAND, SOUTHERN BRAZIL
Josefina Steiner 1, Anne Zillikens 2, Rafael Kamke 1, Eduardo Pickbrenner Feja 1 & Daniel de Barcellos
Falkenberg 3

636.. International Journal of Science and Research (IJSR) Volume 6 Issue 1, January 2017
Allelopathic Effect Abutilon indicum and Parthenium hysterophorus on Seed Germination and Seedling
Growth of Wheat
Dr. Rajendra Kumar

637.. Journal of Advanced Applied Scientific Research   JANUERY-2017
Kinetic, thermodynamic and isotherm studies on the removal of rhodamine b dye using acid
activated Abutilon Indicum
P. Pandian1 and A. Kasthuri2

638.. Cien. Inv. Agr. 43(3):464-475. 2016
Yield, yield features, phytochemical composition, antioxidant and antibacterial activities of Abutilon
indicum cultivated under different fertilizers
Gulsum Yaldiz1, Arzu Birinci Yildirim1, Yeliz Kasko Arici2,and MahmutCamlica1

639.. I J R B A T, Vol. V, Issue (1), Jan.- 2017
ANTIMICROBIAL POTENTIAL OF SOME MEDICINAL PLANTS AGAINST SELECTED HUMAN
PATHOGENS
Ravindrakumar Dhande

640.. Pharm Methods, 2017; 8(1): 209-212
A modified TLC bioautographic technique for the detection of antilithiatic potential of therapeutic plants
from Indigenous Ayurvedic System
Ankit Subhash Kale1, Anita Surendra Patil1*, Hariprasad Madhukarrao Paikrao2

641.. BMC Complement Altern Med. 2016 Aug 5;16:276. doi: 10.1186/s12906-016-1225-7.
In-Vitro dual inhibition of protein glycation, and oxidation by some Arabian plants.
Siddiqui MA1,2, Rasheed S3, Saquib Q1,2, Al-Khedhairy AA1, Al-Said MS4, Musarrat J5, Choudhary
MI6.

642.. Arabian Journal of Chemistry Volume 9, Supplement 1, September 2016, Pages S209–S224
Corrosion inhibition by leaves and stem extracts of Sida acuta for mild steel in 1 M H2SO4 solutions
investigated by chemical and spectroscopic techniques
S.A. Umoren, , U.M. Eduok, M.M. Solomon, A.P. Udoh

643.. J. Livestock Sci. 7: 1-12
Studies on the diversity of medicinal plant species utilized for goat reproduction in Abia State Nigeria
I.P. Ogbuewua,*, F.C. Ukaegbua, V.U. Odoemelama, F.O. Ugwuokeb,E.C. Echereobiac, I.C. Okolia,
M.U.Iloejea

644.. International Journal of Pharmacognosy and Phytochemical Research 2016; 8(4); 663-667
Phytochemical Screening and Free Radical Scavenging Activity of Chloroform Extract of Sida acuta
Burm. F.
Perumalsamy Muneeswari1, Subburaj Deepika1, Palanisamy Chella Perumal2, VelliyurKanniappan,
Gopalakrishnan1,2, Kannappan Poornima1*

645.. Int.J.Res.Ins.,Vol 3 (Issue2).,pp 191-201
PHYTOCHEMICAL ANALYSIS AND INVITRO ANTIBACTERIAL SCREENING OF SIDA ACUTA
EXTRACTS AGAINST EXTENED SPECTRUM BETA-LACTAMASE PRODUCING PATHOGENS
K. Prabhu

646.. International Conference of Science, Engineering & Environmental Technology (ICONSEET),
1(17): 121-127, 2016
Chemical Analysis of an Isolated Potentially Medicinal Active Ingredient of Sida Acuta Plant
Asimi Tajudeen1, LT. Z.U. Aghanti2, Kolawole Ajewole1, Lawal Isiaka Abife1, AsimiyuBabatunde
Olasupo3

647.. Der PharmaChemica, 2016, 8(19):396-402
In vitro and In vivo Evaluation of Sida Acuta burm.f. (Malvaceae) for its Anti-oxidant and Anti-Cancer Activity
Mahesh Thondawadaa*, Shashank Mulukutlab, Kalidhindi Rama Satyanarayana Rajub,Dhanabal S. Pc and Ashish Devidas Wadhwania

648.. Journal of Biology and Nature 5(4): 185-195, 2016
PHENOTYPIC PLASTICITY OF Euphorbia heterophylla L. AND Sida acuta Burm. F. IN RESPONSE TO SOIL FERTILITY, IRRIGATION INTERVAL AND PLANT DENSITY IN NORTHERN GUINEA SAVANNAH, NIGERIA
USMAN A. YUGUDA1*, WISDOM S. JAPHET1,2, BASHIR Y. ABUBAKAR2,SAIDU ABDULLAHI2 AND SULAIMAN DAUDA2

649.. Journal of Pharmacognosy and Phytochemistry 2016; 5(2): 275-279
Investigation of in-vitro Cytotoxicity and Thrombolytic activity of methanolic extract of Sida acuta (flower)
Md. Hossan sakib, Muhammad Sazzad Hossain, Sadequr Rahman, Ahsan Ullah, Mohammad Shahin Alam, Limon Kanti Shill, Md. Yasin Sarkar

650.. International Journal of Pharmacy and Pharmaceutical Sciences, 8 (5). pp. 122-126. (2016)
Evaluation of diuretic and antiurolithiatic properties of ethanolic extract of sida acuta burm F. in wistar albino rats
Mathew, Manu and Adiga, Shalini and Avin, S and Tripathy, Amruta

651.. J Exp Integr Med ? 2016 ? Volume 6 ? Issue 2
Effect of ethanol extract of Sida acuta Burm F. leaves on egg albumin-induced inflammation
Obioma Benedeth Eze1, Okwesili Fred Nwodo2, Victor Nwadiogo Ogugua2,Parker Elijah Joshua2

652.. J Invest Biochem ? 2016 ? Vol 5 ? Issue 2 37
Uterine Contractile Effect of Ethanol Extracts of Sida acuta Burm F. Leaves
Obioma Benedeth L. Eze1, Okwesili Fred C. Nwodo2,Victor Nwadiogo Ogugua2, Parker Elijah Joshua2

653.. Saudi Journal of Medical and Pharmaceutical Sciences 2016.2.8.5 198
Comparative In-vitro antioxidant activity on Melochia corchorifolia, Sida acuta and Saccharum officinarum leaf extracts and their Phenolic contents
M. N. Palaksha*, K. Ravishankar1 & V. Girija Sastry2

654.. PHYTOLOGIA BALCANICA 22(3): 363–376, Sofia, 2016 363
Pollination ecology of Sida acuta, S. cordata and S. cordifolia (Malvaceae)
A.J. Solomon Raju & D. Sandhya Rani

655.. J Exp Integr Med ? 2016 ? Volume 6 ? Issue 3
In-vitro stability and aggregatory effect of ethanol extract leaves of Sida acuta Burm F. on human erythrocyte
Obioma Benedeth Eze, Okwesili Fred Nwodo

657.. International Journal of Science, Environment and Technology, Vol. 5, No 1, 2016, 17 – 24
THE SURVIVAL OF FOUR TROPICAL PLANTS ON SOILS ARTIFICIALLY POLLUTED WITH TOXIC LEVELS OF ZINC
U.F. Umeoguaju*1, C.J. Ononamadu2, M.C. Okonkwo1 and O.C. Ezeigwe1

658.. Journal of Research in Forestry, Wildlife & Environment Vol. 8(3) September, 2016
POTENTIALS OF FLORA SPECIES ON THE YIELD OF HONEY IN DAKKA FOREST RESERVE, BALI LOCAL GOVERNMENT AREA OF TARABA STATE, NIGERIA
1Kwaga, B.T., 1Akosim, C., 1 Dishan, E. E. and 2Khobe, D.

659.. Int J Pharm Bio Sci 2015 Oct; 6(4): (B) 1005 - 1012
POLYPHENOL PROFILING IN THE LEAVES OF PLANTS FROM THE CATCHMENT AREA OF RIVER BEAS, INDIA
V. KUMAR, A. SHARMA, R. BHARDWAJ* AND ASHWANI KUMAR THUKRAL

660.. Entomol Ornithol Herpetol 2016, 5:2
Bee Fauna in and Around Kakum National Park
Rofela Combey* and Peter Kwapong

661.. Doctoral Thesis http://hdl.handle.net/10603/68059
Survey and screening of certain wild dicotyledonous plants of Sibsagar district western part Assam for
fungitoxic properties
Chandra Nath, Subhan

662.. Materials Letters 170 (2016) 101–104
Synthesis of biofunctionalized AgNPs using medicinally important Sida cordifolia leaf extract for
enhanced antioxidant and anticancer activities
B.Srinithya a, V. Vinod Kumar c, Vellingiri Vadivel b, Brindha Pemaiah b,Savarimuthu Philip Anthony
c,n, Meenakshi Sundaram Muthuraman a,nn

663.. Journal of Pharmacognosy and Phytochemistry 2016; 5(2): 30-34
Quantitative phytochemical analysis of some medicinal plant seed by using various organic solvents
V Sailaja, M Madhu, V Neeraja

664.. IJSR Volume 5 Issue 8, August 2016
Studies on the Phytochemistry, Spectroscopic Characterization and Antibacterial Efficacy of Sida
cordifolia (Linn)
Bibhu Prasad Sahu1, Panchanan Gouda2, Chakrapani Patnaik3

665.. International Journal of Scientific and Research Publications, Volume 6, Issue 1, January 2016
Effect of Temperature and Light on the seed germination of Sida cordifolia L.
Sangeeta Mishra

666.. Remarking Vol-II * Issue-VI* November - 2015
An Eco-Friendly Dyeing of Woollen Fabric by Sida Cordifolia Natural Dye
Lalit Jajpura

667.. Adv J Pharm Life sci Res, 2016 4;1:10-16
Comparative studies on Anti bacterial activity of Sida cordifolia Linn., and Sida spinosa Linn
S.Navaneetha , R.Vadivu*, R.Radha , S.C. Suruthi

668.. National Academy of Agricultural Science Vol. 34, No. 1, January-March 2016
Phytochemical Variations in Different Species of Sida Found in Kerala
C. Beena

669.. International Journal of Polymer Analysis and Characterization Volume 21, 2016 - Issue 2
Characterization of new cellulosic fiber from the stem of Sida rhombifolia
R. Gopinath, K. Ganesan, S. S. Saravanakumar & R. Poopathi

670.. Acta Physiol Plant (2016) 38:23
Identification of the medicinal plant species with the potential for remediation of hydrocarbons
contaminated soils
Refugio Rodri´guez-Va´zquez1 • Salvador Sa´nchez1 • Xenia Mena-Espino1 •Myriam A. Amezcua-
Allieri2

671.. http://www.shaman-australis.com.au/shop/sida_spp_cp_108.php
Shaman Australis Botanicals

 672.. J. Chem. Pharm. Res., 2016, 8(1):770-774
Pharmacological Evaluation Of Ethanol Extract Of Sida Rhombifolia L. Roots (Malvaceae)
Maria Tanumihardja et al

 673.. A Dissertation Submitted to the Graduate Faculty of the Louisiana State University and Agricultural
and Mechanical College, The School of Plant, Environmental, and Soil Sciences
PRICKLY SIDA (SIDA SPINOSA L.) - BIOLOGY AND IN-CROP AND POST-HARVEST
MANAGEMENT PROGRAMS

Josh T. Copes

674.. Colloids and Surfaces B: Biointerfaces 143 (2016) 499–510
Polyphenol stabilized colloidal gold nanoparticles from Abutilon indicum leaf extract induce apoptosis in HT-29 colon cancer cells
Rani Mata, Jayachandra Reddy Nakkala, Sudha Rani Sadras

675.. Mintage Journal of Pharmaceutical and Medical Sciences, Vol 2 Issue 4, Oct – Dec 2013
Effect of medicinal herb extracts treated on cotton denim fabric
M.Sumithra*1 and N.Vasugi Raaja2

676.. Int J Pharm Bio Sci 2013 Oct; 4(4): (P) 898 - 901
DETERMINATION OF THE BIOACTIVE COMPONENTS OF Abutilon indicum Linn.
KUMAR AMIT1 AND SAXENA GYANENDER2

677.. Journal of Biomedical and Pharmaceutical Research Volume 5, Issue 6: November-December; 2016, 68-74
Bioguided extraction and Evaluation of Antioxidant studies of Abutilon indicum fruits
Rajesh Bolleddu*1,3 , Sama Venkatesh1, Azmathunnisa Begum1, Ravi Alvala1, Rachamalla Shyamsunder2

678.. International Journal of Applied Research 2016; 2(2): 291-293
Phytochemical study of Abutilon indicum Linn. Medicinal plant
Neeta Mishra, SK Agnihotri

679.. International Journal of Basic & Clinical Pharmacology | May-June 2016 | Vol 5 | Issue 3
Nephroprotective effect of ethanolic extract of abutilon indicum root in gentamicin induced acute renal failure
Jacob Jesurun RS*, Lavakumar S.

680.. Asian Journal of Science and Technology Vol. 07, Issue, 05, pp.2980-2983, May, 2016
PHYTOCHEMICAL ANALYSIS AND IN VITRO ANTI-INFLAMMATORY ACTIVITY OF ABUTILON INDICUM
*Shanmugapriya, S. and Anuradha, R.

681.. I J A B E R, Vol. 14, No. 2 (2016): 1109-1125
THE EFFECT OF INDIAN MALLOW (ABUTILON INDICUM) HYDROETHANOLIC EXTRACT ON LEVELS OF REPRODUCTIVE HORMONES OF FEMALE ALBINO RATS
Kathleen Bersabal, Adorico M. Aya-ay, Chukwudum Kingsley

682.. Advances in Pharmacology and Toxicology; Jalgaon17.3 (Dec 2016): 19-24.
EVALUATION OF ANTI INFLAMMATORY ACTIVITY OF ABUTILON INDICUM LINN. AND TO COMPARE EFFECTIVENESS OF IT'S ROOTS AND SEEDS
Purnima Devi A*, Anand Pal T, Manasa S, Mounika M, Sindhura R and Lakshmi B

683.. Pharmacognosy Journal, Vol 8, Issue 2, Mar-Apr, 2016
In vitro Cytotoxicity Studies of Zn (Zinc) Nanoparticles Synthesized from Abutilon indicum L. against Human Cervical Cancer (HeLa) Cell Lines
Badarinath Druvarao Kulkarni1, Samim Sultana2, Mayuri Bora2, Ishita Dutta2, Padmaa Milaap Paarakh3,Vedamurthy Ankala Basappa1*

684.. RSC Adv., 2016, 6, 48336
Extraction and purification of phytol from Abutilon indicum - cytotoxic and apoptotic activity
Parth Thakor,a Japan B. Mehta,b Ravi R. Patel,a Disha D. Patel,a Ramalingam B. Subramaniana and Vasudev R. Thakkar*a

685.. Indian J.Sci.Res. 7(1) : 81-84, 2016
EVALUATION OF ANTICATARACT POTENTIAL OF Abutilon indicum - AN INVITRO STUDY
N. ROSHENI , K. NITHYA , S. BRINDHA , N. ELANGO , V. GOKILA , S. NISHMITHA AND S. KOKILA

686.. Cien. Inv. Agr. 43(3):464-475. 2016
Yield, yield features, phytochemical composition, antioxidant and antibacterial activities of Abutilon indicum cultivated under different fertilizers
Gulsum Yaldiz1, Arzu Birinci Yildirim1, Yeliz Kasko Arici2,and Mahmut Camlica1

687.. WORLD JOURNAL OF PHARMACY AND PHARMACEUTICAL SCIENCES Volume 5, Issue 5, 1182-1196
EVALUATION OF IN VITRO HEMOLYTIC ACTIVITY OF DIFFERENT PARTS OF ABUTILON INDICUM (LINN.)
S. Shobana1 and R. Vidhya1*

688.. IJPIB|Vol 1|Issue 1|07-13
SUPPLEMENTATION OF ETHANOLIC EXTRACT OF ABUTILON INDICUM (L) SWEET PREVENTS UROLITHIASIS IN EXPERIMENTAL RATS
Chitikela P Pullaiah1*, Narasimha Kumar. GV1, Vineela Ruth Madhuri P2, Dhanunjaya S1, Pushpa Kumari B1, Ranganayakulu.D1

689.. Pak. J. Weed Sci. Res. 22(4): 587-593. 2016.
Investigation of antimicrobial activity of some selected weed species.
Khan, W.M., S. Ali, M.S. Khan, N. Akhtar, K. Ali and H. Khan.

690.. Folia Biologica et Oecologica 11: 1–8 (2015)
Loliolide - the most ubiquitous lactone
MALGORZATA GRABARCZYK*, KATARZYNA WINSKA, WANDA MACZKA, BARTLOMIEJ POTANIEC & MIROSLAW ANIOL

691.. Asian Journal of Pharmaceutical Sciences Available online 25 November 2015
Determination of N-trans-feruloyltyramine content and nitric oxide inhibitory and antioxidant activities of Tinospora crispa
Attawadee SaeYoona, , Bhudsaban Sukkarna, Wichit Nosoongnoenb, Chutima Jantarata, Poonsit Hiransaic, Pajaree Sakdiseta, Jiraporn Chingunpitaka, Sunita Makchuchitd, Arunporn Itharatd

692.. http://www.illinoiswildflowers.info/weeds/plants/prickly_sida.htm
Prickly Sida   Sida spinosa
Dr. John Hilty, Illinois Wildflowers website

693.. Journal of Apiculture 31(4) : 379~387(2016)
A Checklist of Nectariferous and Polleniferous Plants of African Honeybees (Apis mellifera adansonii L.) in Awka, Nigeria
Akunne, C. E.1, Akpan, A. U.2 and Ononye, B. U.1

694.. Animal Research International (2007) 4(3): 750 – 752 750
PERFORMANCE OF WEANER RABBITS FED PANICUM MAXIMUM, CENTROSEMA PUBESCENS AND SIDA ACUTA SUPPLEMENTED WITH POULTRY GROWERS MASH
1UDEH Ifeanyichukwu, 2EKWE Okechukwu Okorie and 1AARON Evylene 1

695.. European Scientific Journal February 2017 edition vol.13, No.6 ISSN: 1857 – 7881
Importance Du Couplage De L'inventaire Des Plantes Mellifères Et De L'analyse Pollinique Des Miels De La Saison Des Pluies En Zone Ouest Soudanienne Au Nord-Bénin
Sfich T. B. Ahouandjinou, Monique G. Tossou, Hounnankpon Yédomonhan, Adéline Zanou, Aristide C. Adomou Akpovi Akoègninou

696.. The International Journal Of Engineering And Science (IJES) Volume 6, Issue 1, Pages 22-33, 2017
Modelling of Corrosion Inhibition of Mild Steel in Hydrochloric Acid by Crushed Leaves of Sida Acuta (Malvaceae)
Agha Inya Ndukwe1 and C. N. Anyakwo2

697... World Scientific News 61(2) (2017) 69-85
An approach for butterfly conservation through setting up a garden in an urban area, Kolkata, India
Debapriya Chakraborty Thakur1, Pinakiranjan Chakrabarti2 and Anuradha Chaudhuri1,*

698.. Data Sheet: Sida acuta (sida)
Centre for Agriculture and Biosciences International (CABI)
https://www.cabi.org/

699.. http://www.southernhabitats.com/sweet-tea-seed.asp
Information Sheet: Sweet Tea (Sida acuta)
Southern Habitats LLC, commercial sellers of Sweet Tea seed

700.. mBio 6(2):e00009-15. doi:10.1128/mBio.00009-15.
Sublethal Exposure to Commercial Formulations of the Herbicides Dicamba, 2,4-Dichlorophenoxyacetic
Acid, and Glyphosate Cause Changes in Antibiotic Susceptibility in Escherichia coli and Salmonella
enterica serovar Typhimurium
Brigitta Kurenbach,a Delphine Marjoshi,a Carlos F. Amábile-Cuevas,b Gayle C. Ferguson,c William
Godsoe,d Paddy Gibson,a Jack A. Heinemann

701.. AgBioForum, The Journal of Agrobiotechnology Managment and Economics Vol 2, Number 3&4,
Article 3
Book Chapter in Ethical Issues in Biotechnology, Rowman & Littlefield Publishers (October 9, 2002)
Ten Reasons Why Biotechnology Will Not Ensure Food Security, Protect The Environment, And Reduce
Poverty In The Developing World
Miguel A. Altieri and Peter Rosset

702.. https://www.worldseedsupply.com/product/sida-cordifolia-bala-seeds/
Seed listing: Sida cordifolia
World Seed Supply website

703.. http://davesgarden.com/guides/pf/go/74728/#b
Listing for cultivation of Sida cordifolia
Dave's Garden site

704.. Pharmaceutical Biology, 46:10-11, 673-676 92 (2008)
Biological Activity of Extracts in Relationship to Structure of Pure Isolates of Abutilon indicum
Sammia Yasmin, Muhammad Akram Kashmiri, Iftikhar Ahmad, Ahmad Adnan & Mushtaq Ahmad

705.. Fitoterapia 56, 3, 169--171; also in: Indian Drugs 22, 1984, 69--72
Preliminary pharmacological screening of Abutilon indicum. II. Analgesic activity [1985]
Bagi, M.K. Kalyani, G.A. Dennis, T.J. Akshaya Kumar, K. Kakrani, H.K.

706.. Global Journal of Pharmacology 2 (2): 23-30, 2008
Investigation into the Mechanism of Action of Abutilon indicum in the Treatment of Bronchial Asthma
Archana N. Paranjape and Anita A. Mehta

707.. Colloids and surfaces B: Biointerfaces • February 2015
Biogenic silver nanoparticles from Abutilon indicum: Their antioxidant, antibacterial and cytotoxic effects
in vitro.
Rani Mata, Jayachandra Reddy Nakkala, Sadras Sudha Rani

708.. Journal of Chemical and Pharmaceutical Research, 2012, 4(8):3959-3965
Chemical investigation and biological activity of phytoconstituents from methanol extract of Abutilon
indicum leaves
Ambarsing, P. Rajput1* and Milind, K. Patel2

709.. American Journal of BioScience Vol. 3, No. 2-1, 2015, pp. 5-11 Special Issue: Pharmacological and
Phytochemicals Investigation.
Pharmacologicals and Phytochemicals Potential of Abutilon indicum - A Comprehensive Review
Md. Reyad-ul-ferdous, Mehedi Rahman, Md. Kawsar Mahamud, Sharmi Sultana Ayshi, Md.
Didaruzzaman Sohel.

710.. Asian Journal of Pharmacy & Life Science, Vol. 1 (2), March-June, 2011
Comprehensive review - Abutilon indicum Linn
Akash Jain*1, Gaurav Saini1 U.B.Moon2, D. Kumar2

711.. Research Journal of Pharmaceutical, Biological and Chemical Sciences 2010 Vol.1 No.4 pp.718-729
A Review on Some Important Medicinal Plants of Abutilon spp.
Khadabadi SS 1 and Bhajipale NS2*

712.. Journal of Pharmacognosy and Phytochemistry 2015; 3(5): 66-72
Ethnomedicinal uses and phytochemistry of Abutilon indicum (Linn.) Sweet - an overview
A. Saini, D. K. Gahlawat, C. Chauhan, S. K. Gulia, S. A. Ganie, Archita and S. S. Yadav

713.. International Journal of Pharmacognosy and Phytochemical Research 2010; 2(1);1-4
Cytotoxic and Antimicrobial Activity of the Crude Extract of Abutilon Indicum
Muhit Md. Abdul *, Apu Apurba Sarker, Islam Md. Saiful, Ahmed Muniruddin

714.. Indian Journal of Natural Products 2000 Vol.16 No.2 pp.25-27 ref.11
Hepatoprotective activity of leaves of Abutilon indicum.
Dash, G. K.; Samanta, A.; Kanungo, S. K.; Sahu, S. K.; Suresh, P.; Ganapaty, S.

715.. Journal of Pharmacy Research 2009 Vol.2 No.4 pp.644-645 ref.7
In-vitro anti-arthritic activity of Abutilon indicum (Linn.) sweet.
Vallabh Deshpande; Jadhav, V. M.; Kadam, V. J.

716.. Pharmaceutical Biology, 48:3, 282-289, (2010)
Antioxidant potential and radical scavenging effects of various extracts from Abutilon indicum and
Abutilon muticum
Sammia Yasmin, Muhammad Akram Kashmiri, Muhammad Nadeem Asghar, Mushtaq Ahmad & Ayesha
Mohy-ud-Din

717.. Article in Medicinal Plants - International Journal of Phytomedicines and Related Industries 2(3):215
• September 2010
Antifungal activity of a new steroid isolated from Abutilon indicum (L.) Sw.
S.K. Prabhuji, Deepak Kumar Singh1, Atul Kumar Srivastava2 and Rahul Sinha1

718.. Ancient Science of Life Vol : XXVI (1&2) July, August, September, October, November, December
2006
ANTIBACTERIAL ACTIVITY OF LEAF EXTRACT OF Abutilon indicum
M. POONKOTHAI

719.. International Journal of PharmTech Research   Vol.1, No.4, pp 1314-1316, Oct-Dec 2009
ANTIOXIDANT ACTIVITY OF ABUTILON INDICUM LEAVES
Guno Sindhu Chakraborthy

720.. http://www.itis.gov/servlet/SingleRpt/SingleRpt?search_topic=TSN&search_value=21725
ITIS website, Taxonomy and Nomenclature, "Sida L."
The ITIS is the result of a partnership of federal agencies formed to satisfy their mutual needs for
scientifically credible taxonomic information. The original ITIS partners include: Department of
Commerce,National Oceanic and Atmospheric Administration (NOAA), Department of Interior (DOI),
Geological Survey (USGS), Environmental Protection Agency (EPA), Department of Agriculture
(USDA), Agriculture Research Service (ARS), Natural Resources Conservation Service (NRCS),
Smithsonian Institution, National Museum of Natural History (NMNH)

721.. Herbal Antiobiotics: Natural Alternatives for Treating Drug-Resistant Bacteria (book),
Storey Books, Second edition, 2012
Stephen Harrod Buhner

722.. The Ayurveda Way: 108 practices from the World's Oldest Healthing System fo Better Sleep, Less
Stress, Optimal Digestions, and More (book)
Storey Publishing, 2017
Anata Ripa Ajmera

723.. The Washington Post, May 27, 2016
https://www.washingtonpost.com/news/to-your-health/wp/2016/05/26/the-superbug-that-doctors-have-
been-dreading-just-reached-the-u-s/?utm_term=.b58183429816
The superbug that doctors have been dreading just reached the U.S.

Lena H. Sun and Brady Dennis

724.. https://plants.usda.gov/java/
Plants database
US Department of Agriculture, Natural Resources Conservation Service

725.. http://eol.org/pages/595806/overview
Encyclopedia of Life listing for "Sida rhombifolia/Sidratusa"
EOL is an international consortium of national agencies combing their expertise

726.. Dave's Garden website
 "About abutilons" March 2, 2015
Audrey Stallsmith

727.. Ayurtimes website (ayurtimes.com)
Abutilon Indicum (Indian Mallow – Atibala)
Dr. Jagdev Singh is a founder of Ayur Times. He is an Ayurvedic Physician and Herbalist.
Education: Bachelor of Ayurvedic Medicine and Surgery, M.Sc. in Medicinal Plants,
Board of Ayurvedic and Unani Medicine, Chandigarh – 2009 to present

728.. Handbook of Ethnopharmacology, 2008: 393-420 ISBN: 978-81-308-0213-8 Editor: Mohamed Eddouks
Chapter 12: Ayurveda, drug discovery and immunomodulation: Review and case study of Withania somnifera
Bhushan Patwardhan 1*, Manish Gautam 1, Sarang Bani 2, Qazi G.N 2 and Ashok DB Vaidya 3

729.. http://www.stuartxchange.com/Malbas.html
Malbas - Abutilon indicum (Linn.) Sweet - CHINESE BELL FLOWER
Dr. Godofredo Umali-Stuart

730.. Ayurhelp website
 http://www.ayurhelp.com/articles/ayurveda-medicinal-properties-bala-sida-cordifolia#.V8zzMFQrKvs
Ayurveda Medicinal properties of Bala (Sida Cordifolia):
An ayurveda site dedicated to propagate ayurveda. Symptomatic treatment is NOT the complete cure.
Treat the root cause. Treat it through Ayurveda

731.. Medinform Publishers (U.K.) 2010
Gut and Psychology Syndrome (book)
Dr. Natasha Campbell-McBride MD,

732.. Cardiovasc Drug Rev. 2001 Fall;19(3):234-44.
Cardiovascular actions of berberine.
Lau CW1, Yao XQ, Chen ZY, Ko WH, Huang Y.

733.. Scientific Reports | 7:44040 | DOI: 10.1038/srep44040
Identification of berberine as a direct thrombin inhibitor from traditional Chinese medicine through structural, functional and binding studies
XingWang1,*, Yuxin Zhang2,*, YingYang3, XiaWu1, Hantian Fan1 & YanjiangQiao2

734.. http://www.medicinenet.com/script/main/art.asp?articlekey=4168
MedicineNet website topic: Lipids

735.. IJRPC 2013, 3(1)
ABUTILONS INDICUM LINN - A PHYTOPHARMACOLOGICAL REVIEW
Vadnere Gautam P1*, Pathan Aslam R1, Kulkarni Bharti U1and Abhay Kumar Singhai2

736.. Drug Invention Today 2009, 1(2),137-139
Antimycotic activity of the componenets of Abutilon indicum (Malvaceae)
 Rajalakshmi Padma Vairavasundaram,1*.and Kalaiselvi Senthil2

737.. Indian J. Pharm. Sci., 2012, 74 (2): 163-167
Relationship between Antioxidant Properties and Chemical Composition of Abutilon Indicum Linn

552

A. R. SRIVIDYA*, S. P. DHANABAL, S. JEEVITHA, V. J. VISHNU VARTHAN AND R. RAJESH KUMAR

738.. Google dictionary

739.. Drug Design, Development and Therapy 2015:9 5737–5747
Mechanism and pharmacological rescue of berberine-induced hERG channel deficiency
Meng Yan1 Kaiping Zhang1 Yanhui Shi1 Lifang Feng1 Lin Lv1 Baoxin Li 1,2

740.. Int. J. Pharm. Sci. Rev. Res., 20(1), May – Jun 2013; n? 20, 120-127
Phytochemical and Pharmacological Profile of Abutilon Indicum L. Sweet : A Review
Archna Sharma1, R.A. Sharma2, andHemlata Singh2*

741.. PLoS Med 14(7): e1002344. Published: July 7, 2017
http://journals.plos.org/plosmedicine/article?id=10.1371/journal.pmed.1002344
Copyright: © 2017 World Health Organization. Licensee Public Library of Science.
Antimicrobial resistance in Neisseria gonorrhoeae: Global surveillance and a call for international collaborative action.
Wi T, Lahra MM, Ndowa F, Bala M, Dillon J-AR, Ramon-Pardo P, et al. (2017)

742.. Thomson Reuters Foundation   Thursday, 6 July 2017 23:01 GMT
WHO warns of imminent spread of untreatable superbug gonorrhoea
Kate Kelland, Reuters Health and Science Correspondent

 743.. Weed Research Volume 32, Issue 2, April 1992, Pages 103–109
Arrowleaf sida (Sida rhombifolia) and prickly sida (Sida spinosa): germination and emergence
C. A. SMITH, D. R. SHAW, L. J. NEWSOM

744.. J. Clin. Microbiol. December 2013 vol. 51 no. 12 3937-3943
Scopulariopsis, a Poorly Known Opportunistic Fungus: Spectrum of Species in Clinical Samples and In Vitro Responses to Antifungal Drugs
Marcelo Sandoval-Denisa, Deanna A. Suttonb, Annette W. Fothergillb, Josep Cano-Liraa, Josepa Genéa, C. A. Decockc, G. S. de Hoogd and Josep Guarroa

745.. National Institute of Sida
http://nischennai.org/siddhamedicine.html
The National Institute of Siddha (NIS), located in Chennai, is a center of excellence with research and higher education in Siddha System of Medicine as its mission.

746.. Hawaiian Native Plant Propagation Database
http://www2.hawaii.edu/~eherring/hawnprop/sid-fall.htm
College of Tropical Agriculture and Human Resources, University of Hawaii at Manoa

747.. Flora of China http://foc.eflora.cn/
Flora of China contains 31,362 species of vascular plants in 3,328 genera and 312 families in 25 volumes of books.

748.. International Environmental Weed Foundation (IEWF)
http://www.iewf.org
A registered non-profit based in Sydney Australia.

749.. India Biodiversity Portal
http://indiabiodiversity.org/species/show/263548
Sida rhomboidea Roxb. ex Fleming (Synonym of Sida spinosa L.)
Dr. N Sasidharan, Kerala Forest Research Institute, Peechi

750.. Flora of Zimbabwe website
http://www.zimbabweflora.co.zw/speciesdata/species.php?species_id=139150
A private website run by three individuals.
Partners: Kew Royal Botanic Gardens and Botanic Garden Meise (An internationally important Botanic Garden, situated just north of Brussels, in the centre of Belgium)

553

751.. Virginia Tech Weed Identification Guide
Sida spinosa
M. Flessner

752.. Folia Biologica et Oecologica 11: 1–8 (2015)
Loliolide - the most ubiquitous lactone
MALGORZATA GRABARCZYK*, KATARZYNA WINSKA, WANDA MACZKA,
BARTLOMIEJ POTANIEC & MIROSLAW ANIOL

753.. Planta Med 2013; 79(06): 437-446
The Effects of Berberine on Blood Lipids: A Systemic Review and Meta-Analysis of Randomized
Controlled Trials
Hui Dong1, *, Yan Zhao2, Li Zhao1, *, Fuer Lu1

754.. Planta Med. 1981 Dec;43(4):384-8.
Alkaloid constituents of Sida acuta, S. humilis, S. rhombifolia and S. spinosa.
Prakash A1, Varma RK, Ghosal S.

755..European Bioinformatics Institute (EMBL-EBI)
http://www.ebi.ac.uk
part of the European Molecular Biology Laboratory

756.. PubChem, open chemistry database
https://pubchem.ncbi.nlm.nih.gov
National Center for Biotechnology Information,
U.S. National Library of Medicine, Bethesda, MD

757.. Self Hacked website   https://selfhacked.com
Science based site led by PhD level researchers in altnerative health. SelfHacked's aim is to help you
understand exactly why your body isn't functioning optimally, and what to do about it.

758.. Biol Pharm Bull. 2007 Oct;30(10):1972-4.
N-trans-feruloyltyramine as a melanin biosynthesis inhibitor.
Efdi M1, Ohguchi K, Akao Y, Nozawa Y, Koketsu M, Ishihara H.

759.. Doctor Mercola's website http://www.mercola.com/
The World's #1 Natural Health Website
Doctor Joseph Mercola
DO, State of Illinois Licensed Physician and Surgeon, Chairman, Department of Family Practice at St.
Alexius Medical CenterNew York Times bestselling author

760.. International Journal for Research in Applied Science & Enginerring Technology (IJRASET)
Vol. 3, Isss 6, June 2015
Comparative Study of DPPH, ABTS and FRAP Assays for Determination of Antioxidant Activity
Pooja Shah, H.A. Modi

761.. Planta Med 1980; 39(5): 66-72
Studies on Medicinal Plants of Sri Lanka III: Pharmacologically Important Alkaloids of some Sida Species
A. A. Leslie Gunatilaka1 , S. Sotheeswaran1 , S. Balasubramaniam2 , A. Indumathie Chandrasekara1 , H.
T. Badra Sriyani1

762.. Fitoterapia 1989, 60, 163–164.
Neutral constituents of the aerial parts of Sida rhombifolia var. rhomboidea.
Goyal, MM; Rani, KK.

763.. Journal of Acute Disease Volume 2, Issue 4, 2013, Pages 304-309
Syringic acid, a novel natural phenolic acid, normalizes hyperglycemia with special reference to
glycoprotein components in experimental diabetic rats
JayachandranMuthukumaran b, SubramaniSrinivasan a, Rantham SubramaniyamVenkatesan b,
VinayagamRamachandranaUdaiyarMuruganathan a

764.. Hokkaido University Collection of Scholarly and Academic Papers 2014
Isolation of antitrypanosomal compounds from Myanmar medicinal plants
KHINE SWE NYUNT

765.. ChemFaces website (China) www.chemfaces.com
high-quality natural product library for drug research and development

766.. Planta Med 2006; 72(4): 351-357
New Cytotoxic Tetrahydrofuran- and Dihydrofuran-Type Lignans from the Stem of Beilschmiedia tsangii
Jih-Jung Chen1 , En-Tzu Chou1 , Chang-Yih Duh2 , Sheng-Zehn Yang3 , Ih-Sheng Chen4

767.. Genet Resour Crop Evol (2008) 55:1239–1256
Traditional leafy vegetables and their use in the Benin Republic
A. Dansi Æ A. Adjatin Æ H. Adoukonou-Sagbadja ÆV. Falade´ Æ H. Yedomonhan Æ D. Odou Æ B.
Dossou

768.. Volume 8 of the series Parasitology Research Monographs pp 99-153 Date: 15 January 2016
Chapter - Nanoparticles in the Fight Against Parasites
Green Synthesized Silver Nanoparticles: A Potential New Insecticide for Mosquito Control
Marimuthu Govindarajan

769.. The Journal of Antibiotics Vol. 38 (1985) No. 7 P 936-940
STUDIES OF AN IMMUNOMODULATOR, SWAINSONINE II. EFFECT OF SWAINSONINE ON
MOUSE IMMUNODEFICIENT SYSTEM AND EXPERIMENTAL MURINE TUMOR
TOHRU KINO1), NORIAKI INAMURA1), KUNIO NAKAHARA1), SUMIO KIYOTO1), TOSHIO
GOTO1), HIROSHI TERANO1), MASANOBU KOHSAKA1), HATSUO AOKI1), HIROSHI
IMANAKA1)

770.. Cancer Research March 1988 Volume 48, Issue 6
Augmentation of Murine Natural Killer Cell Activity by Swainsonine, a New Antimetastatic
Immunomodulator
Martin J. Humphries, Kazue Matsumoto, Sandra L. White, Russell J. Molyneux and Kenneth Olden

771.. Pharmacology & Therapeutics Volume 50, Issue 3, 1991, Pages 285-290
The potential importance of swainsonine in therapy for cancers and immunology
KennethOlden*PascalBreton*KrzysztofGrzegorzewski*YoshiakiYasuda*Barry L.Gause†Oladipo
A.Oredipe*Sheila A.Newton*Sandra L.White‡

772.. Phytomedicine Volume 14, Issue 5, 21 May 2007, Pages 353-359
Inhibition of the growth of human gastric carcinoma in vivo and in vitro by swainsonine
Author links open overlay panelJ.-Y.SunaM.-Z.ZhubS.-W.WangaS.MiaoaY.-H.XieaJ.-B.Wanga

773.. JNCI: Journal of the National Cancer Institute, Volume 81, Issue 13, 5 July 1989, Pages 1028–1033,
Inhibition of Human HT29 Colon Carcinoma Growth In Vitro and In Vivo by Swainsonine and Human
Interferon-a2
James W. Dennis Kay Koch David Beckner

774.. British Journal of Cancer (1999) 80(1/2), 87–95
Swainsonine protects both murine and human haematopoietic systems from chemotherapeutic toxicity
J-LD Klein1,*, JD Roberts1, MD George1, J Kurtzberg2, P Breton3, J-C Chermann4 and K Olden1

775.. JNCI: Journal of the National Cancer Institute, Volume 81, Issue 13, 5 July 1989, Pages 1024–1028
Swainsonine Inhibition of Spontaneous Metastasis
Sheila A. Newton Sandra L. White Martin J. Humphries Kenneth Olden

776.. Asian-Australasian Journal of Animal Sciences 1997 Vol.10 No.1 pp.28-34
Variability in ash, crude protein, detergent fiber and mineral content of some minor plant species collected
from pastures grazed by goats.
Serra, A. B.; Serra, S. D.; Orden, E. A.; Cruz, L. C.; Nakamura, K.; Fujihara, T.

777.. Systematic Botany (2003), 28(2): pp. 352–364
Phylogenetic Relationships and Classification of the Sida Generic Alliance (Malvaceae) Based on nrDNA ITS Evidence
JAVIER FUERTES AGUILAR1, PAUL A. FRYXELL, and ROBERT K. JANSEN2

778.. SIDA, Contributions to Botany Vol. 11, No. 1, JUNE 1985, pp. 62-91
SIDUS SIDARUM — V. THE NORTH AND CENTRAL AMERICAN SPECIES OF SIDA
PAUL A. FRYXELL

779.. Journal of Equine Veterinary Science September 2006
Poisoning of Horses by Bamboo, Bambusa vulgaris
José Diomedes Barbosa,a Carlos Magno C. de Oliveira,a Marcos Dutra Duarte,a Gabriela Riet-Correa,a Paulo Vargas Peixoto,b and Carlos Hubinger Tokarniab

780.. Tropical Grasslands (2002) Volume 36, 123–125
Manure production by goats grazing native pasture in Nigeria
C.U. OSUHOR1, J.P. ALAWA2 and G.N. AKPA2

781.. J. Livestock Sci. 7: 1-12
Studies on the diversity of medicinal plant species utilized for goat reproduction in Abia State Nigeria
I.P. Ogbuewua,*, F.C. Ukaegbua, V.U. Odoemelama, F.O. Ugwuokeb,E.C. Echereobiac, I.C. Okolia, M.U.Iloejea

782.. Small Ruminant Research 107 (2012) 49– 64
Goat grazing, its interactions with other herbivores and biodiversity conservation issues
R. Rosa García*, R. Celaya, U. García, K. Osoro

783.. Journal of Ethnobiology and Ethnomedicine 2015, 11:12
Local knowledge about fodder plants in the semi-arid region of Northeastern Brazil
Alissandra Trajano Nunes1, Reinaldo Farias Paiva de Lucena2, Mércia Virgínia Ferreira dos Santos3 and Ulysses Paulino Albuquerque1*

784.. Faculty of Agriculture, The University of the West Indies, St. Augustine, Trinidad
Goat Production in Jamaica (1970)
C. DEVENDRA

785.. Annals of Applied Biology Volume 170, Issue 2, March 2017, Pages 204–218
The ever increasing diversity of begomoviruses infecting non-cultivated hosts: new species from Sida spp. and Leonurus sibiricus, plus two New World alphasatellites
C.G. Ferro1, J.P. Silva1, C.A.D. Xavier1, M.T. Godinho1, A.T.M. Lima1,3, T.B. Mar1, D. Lau2 & F.M. Zerbini1

786.. http://www.sciencedirect.com/topics/agricultural-and-biological-sciences/daucosterol
Chemical Ecology, in Comprehensive Natural Products II, 2010
Falko P. Drijfhout, E. David Morgan,

787.. NeoStrata Company, Inc., Princeton, NJ, USA
Maltobionic Acid, a Powerful yet Gentle Skincare Ingredient with Multiple Benefits to Protect Skin and Reverse the Visible Signs of Aging
Irina Brouda, MA, Brenda L. Edison, BA, Ronni L. Weinkauf, PhD, Barbara A. Green, RPh, MS

788.. Plant Physiol. (1968) 43, 1466-1470
Tests Whether a Head to Head Condensation Mechanism Occurs in the Biosynthesis of n-Hentriacontane, the Paraffin of Spinach and Pea Leaves
P. E. Kolattukudy

789.. Archives of Insect Biochemistry and Physiology 18:71-79 (1991)
Makisterone C: A 29-Carbon Ecdysteroid From Developing Embroyos of the Cotton Stianer Bug, Dysdercus fasciatus
Mark Feldlauger, Gunter Weirich, William Lusby, James Svoboda

556

790.. Phytotherapy Research. 3. 201 - 206. (1989).
Immunomodulatory and CNS effects of sitoindosides IX and X, two new glycowithanolides from Withania somnifera.
Ghosal, Shibnath & Lal, Jawahar & Srivastava, Radheyshyam & K. Bhattacharya, Salil & N. Upadhyay, Sachidananda & Jaiswal, Arun & Chattopadhyay, Utpala.

791.. The Lancet   www.thelancet.com Vol 385 April 11, 2015
http://www.thelancet.com/pdfs/journals/lancet/PIIS0140-6736%2815%2960696-1.pdf
Offl ine: What is medicine's 5 sigma?
Richard Horton

792.. Indian Journal of Traditional Knowledge Vol 7(1)- October 2007- pp 678-686
Herbs used in Siddha medicine for arthritis – A review
Eugene Wilson*1, GV Rajamanickam1, Neera Vyas2, A Agarwal3 & GP Dubey3

793.. https://keyserver.lucidcentral.org/weeds/data/media/Html/sida_cordifolia.htm
Sida cordifolia fact sheet, Similar Species
Queensland Government, Weeds of Australia, Biosecurity Queensland Edition

794.. The Washington Post, To Your Health May 27, 2016
The superbug that doctors have been dreading just reached the U.S.
By Lena H. Sun and Brady Dennis

795.. JSS University PhD Thesis   http://hdl.handle.net/10603/30854 MARCH, 2013
Investigation of the antiviral properties of select medicinal plants from the genus sida
Wadhwani, Ashish Devidas

796.. Database of Indian Plants - Efloraofindia (2007 onwards).
Developed by the members of Efloraofindia Google group.
Accessed at https://sites.google.com/site/efloraofindia/
on [10 November 2017]."

797.. Connecticut Center for Health website on July 25, 2017
Magnesium: Health Benefits, Facts, Research
Megan Ware RDN LD

798.. Pest Management Science   Volume 67, Issue 8 August 2011 Pages 1015–1022
Soyasapogenol B and trans-22-dehydrocam- pesterol from common vetch (Vicia sativa L.) root exudates stimulate broomrape seed germination
Antonio Evidente, Alessio Cimmino, Mónica Fernández-Aparicio, Diego Rubiales, Anna Andolfi, Dominique Melck

799.. Reference.MD website: encyclopedia of medical concepts
http://www.reference.md/files/C087/mC087806.html
acanthoside B

800.. The LibreTexts libraries (website) are based upon work supported by the National Science Foundation
https://chem.libretexts.org/Core/Analytical_Chemistry/Electrochemistry/Redox_Chemistry/Oxidizing_and_Reducing_Agents
"Oxidizing and Reducing Agents", Last updatedJul 28, 2015
Diana Pearson, Connie Xu, Luvleen Brar (UCD)

801.. Linus Pauling Institute, Micronutrient Information Center
Choline
Jane Higdon, Ph.D., Steven H. Zeisel, M.D., Ph.D

802.. Science Direct www.sciencedirect.com/topics/neuroscience/coumarins
Medicinal Plant Research in Africa - Pharmacology and Chemistry
(Book) Edited by Victor Kuete, Pages 261-300,
"Coumarins and Related Compounds from the Medicinal Plants of Africa"
Hervé Martial Poumale Poumale, Rebecca Hamm, Yanqing Zang, Yoshihito Shiono, Victor Kuete

557

Coumarins (1-benzopyran-2-one) are chemical compounds in the benzopyrone class of organic compounds found in many plants. Coumarins possess a variety of biological properties, including antimicrobial, antiviral, antiinflammatory, antidiabetic, antioxidant, and enzyme inhibitory activity.

803.. National Center for Biotechnology Information. PubChem Compound Database; CID=5793,
https://pubchem.ncbi.nlm.nih.gov/compound/5793 (accessed Jan. 8, 2018).
Pub Chem Open Chemistry Database - D-Glucose

804.. Encyclopedia.com. - www.encyclopedia.com
"pheophytin." A Dictionary of Biology. Accessed 8 Jan. 2018,
sources like Oxford University Press and Columbia Encyclopedia

805.. Res Pharm Sci. 2016 Jan-Feb; 11(1): 1–14.
Quinazolinone and quinazoline derivatives: recent structures with potent antimicrobial and cytotoxic activities
Elham Jafari,1,2 Marzieh Rahmani Khajouei,2,3 Farshid Hassanzadeh,1,2 Gholam Hossein Hakimelahi,4 and Ghadam Ali Khodarahmi1,2,*

806.. Journal of Ethnopharmacology Volume 23, Issues 2–3, July–August 1988, Pages 313-322
Responses of gastrointestinal smooth muscle preparations to a muscarinic principle present in Sida veronicaefolia
George D.Lutterodt

807.. Planet Ayurveda website, http://www.planetayurveda.com/library/nagabala-sida-veroni-caefolia
"Sida Veronicaefolia"
Dr. Vikram Chauhan MD (Ayurvedic medicine, Herbal Pharacology and Pharacognosy,
Dr. Meenakshi Chauhand MD (Altharnative medicine), BAMS Gold Medalist from Panjab University

808.. PlastiPure Company - Solutions for Safer Products
http://www.plastipure.com/%20safer-products/what-is-estrogenic-activity/
"What is Estrogenic Activity?"

809.. https://www.nature.com/articles/srep27258.pdf
Scientific Reports: Antimicrobial activity, improved cell selectivity and mode of action of short PMAP-36-derived peptides
against bacteria and Candida
Yinfeng Lyu, YangYang, Xiting Lyu, Na Dong & Anshan Shan

....

Use of natural products for curing wide variety of human and domestic animal diseases has a long history that goes to human civilization. These products have been used as good sources of many modern drugs for treatment of several human diseases such as cardiovascular, cancer, malaria, mental diseases, etc. Most of these modern drugs have been obtained or discovered from medicinal plants. Such drugs have been discovered after observing the medicinal use of a particular plant or its parts (leaves, roots, barks, fruits or seed or whole plant) by herbalists, and subsequent isolation of bioactive compounds from the plant or part of the plant that was traditionally used for treatment of different human illnesses. [278]

Conclusion: The antibacterial flavonoids from S. acuta could be used in developing novel antibacterial drugs. [271]

558

About the Author

I have been a plant person most of my adult life. My wife and I started **Bountiful Gardens Seeds** in 1982, which is part of **Ecology Action of the Midpeninsula**, an organization that has been desperately trying to save the world's soil for the last 45 years, while refining a farming method (biointensive) that actually creates soil while being very productive.

We started **Bountiful Gardens** because heirloom, open-pollinated seeds were hard to come by in the 1980s, and disappearing. At the time it was not certain that theser heirloom seeds would continue to be available to the general public. We offered a considerable number of varieties that otherwise would not have been available. Back then we also had a "Healing Herbs Garden Club" that really educated me in medicinals of all sorts. BG has always carried a strong section of medicinal plant seed.

For years I selected many of the varieties we carried in our catalog, which was not unlike being an Indiana Jones of the plant world. All of this has given me good experience with discovering everything about a plant. It also helps to be married to a biologist who fills in any blanks. I retired as the third longest-tenured employee ever at Ecology Action after our founders.

I consider myself a personal herbalist. I do not have the intimate, extensive knowledge of hundreds of herbs that a professional herbalist would know, but rather I know very well the few plants that I need, seeking only my health, and the health of my family. Medicinal herbs and preventative medicine have been at the core of my family's health for at least 50 years. I know the plants I use very well, and when I discover a new one that is as good as Sida is, I am completely on board right away, and want to know everything about it. The next step is a thorough and intensive research into its known benefits. So for over a year I intensely scoured the internet for peer-review research on Sida, and in particular studies on Sida acuta, the species that I use. The results have exceeded my wildest expectations.

Former Lives

Walked away from two degrees at Cal Berkeley. Spent time in the Haight-Ashbury. Spent some time on the margins of society - until I became a father. That changed everything. Both my son and step-daughter eventually graduated from Stanford University.

For better or worse, I am one of the people who brought personal computers into being. I am a "76er" – anyone involved before 1976 was a genuine pioneer. I worked for the People's Computer Company of digital legend, as well as running database marketing for the very first Computer Faires. Once it stopped being a crusade and became industry I became a gardener of sorts, but having a computer background was very helpful when starting a seed company in the 1980s.

Around 1990 I created a poster, **The Vegetable Gardener's Guide** (in its third printing), that has been a perennial favorite of master gardeners – they are grateful to have all the essential questions beginners ask right there on the wall.

In 2004 I decided to put my enthusiasm for the French bidet into a book. As often happens with me, this book turned out to be the first book on the topic, ever! Could not find anything in print. There was nothing in the Library of Congress at the time except a note by President Thomas Jefferson on the bidet as a result of his visit to Paris in the 1700s. What a treat to write the first book on anything in 2004! Depite this I discovered everything known at the time, and went beyond by adding information from other knowledge bases, resulting in a book whose information is still very complete and current today.

Unpublished authors in 2004 had few options for publication. I ended up physically making every book and selling them on Amazon on consignment. Create Space publishing did not exist. So I printed pages through a cheap home printer, punched the spiral binding and bound the book.

The Bidet immediately became the reference on the subject. It was also commonly known in the business as the "bidet bible", because it included every thing known about the bidet, and more.

I soon grew tired of physically producing books for small margins and stopped publication. Nevertheless used copies (when available) are selling for $30. It is intereting how many thousand times it has been pirated on the web over those years! People really wanted this little book! My reference books are complete beyond anyone's expectations. I hope to replicate this thoroughness with this "Sida bible".

The Bidet (book)

The Bidet Everything There Is To Know From The First And Only Book On The Bidet An Elegant Solution For Comfort Health Happiness Ecology And About The Device That Can Save Your Health
ISBN 0-9748799-0-8   LCCN 2004096271
2004 $7.95

Praise for The Bidet (book)

Library of Online Book Shopping
http://1lg09.hostfree.pw/
Ronald G. Rubin   4.9 out of 5 stars.

"First, it's important to say this is not only a great little book, but it is a primer for our culture to shift into the 21st century... This book received significant support from the bidet industry while it was being written, but is an independent work that surveys the industry as a whole. This book presents and documents the medical literature that largely supports the many health benefits that bidet users claim."

Librabook website   http://librarbook.com/
Rating: 4.6/5 from 1158 votes.

Australian Bidet - the largest supplier of Bidets, Electronic Bidet Seats, Integrated Toilet Bidets, Non-Electric Bidet Seats, Bidet Attachments and Personal Hygiene products for Australia, New Zealand and South-east Asia.

"Known in the bidet industry as 'The Bidet Bible', this book will save you many times its price while improving your health and personal comfort. The Bidet contains everything known about the bidet."

Library Thing Review - A community of 2,100,000 book lovers.
Toby Marotta, May 12, 2011

"This unprecedented American introduction to bidet use is a self-published paperback composed and periodically updated by Bill Bruneau."

English dictionary englishdictionary.education/en/bidet
The English Dictionary project is a powerful English dictionary online with many examples of use: definitions, synonyms, translations, related news and books.

"This is the only complete and impartial source of bidet information. This book has interesting history, drama, suspense, some real eye-opening facts, and is pretty good reading for a reference book."

The Sunday Times Sri Lanka
http://www.sundaytimes.lk/080706/Mirror/mirror0010.html
In defense of the hand-held hygiene gun!
By Rukshani Weerasooriya

"An obviously bored and very creative man. William Bruneau actually took the time to write The Bidet Book which is a 90 page guide on everything you ever wanted to know about your bidet. This book is often referred to as the Bible of the bidet industry. As fascinating a fact that this may be, I have spent many lonely moments of my day wondering how in the world a person could write 90 whole pages on the bidet."

562

Disclaimer   (continued from inside title page)

The content of this book is for general information purposes only. The content should not be construed as medical advice or a professional medical opinion on any facts or circumstances. Information in this book is not guaranteed to be accurate or complete, and you should not rely on it to make any medical or other decisions.

I am not a doctor and I am not qualified to give you direct medical advice. I report research on all aspects of the genus Sida, including medical research. The sources are peer-review research, and other expert sources. I do not warrant that any claims here are true or accurate - the reader is obliged to look up the sources of the information in this book, or to contact the authors of this information, to ascertain the quality of the information.

No health benefits in this book have been evaluated or approved by the FDA. They should not be used in place of personal judgment or medical treatment when needed, nor is anything in this book intended to diagnose, treat, cure or prevent any disease. Only your doctor can diagnose and treat disease.

None of the information in this book is intended to be taken as direct medical advice. Always consult with your medical practitioner before trying any knowledge you have learned from this book. Readers should not act upon any information provided in this book without seeking advice from a licensed physician.

I expressly disclaim all liability with respect to actions taken or not taken based on any of the contents of this book. If I provide any specific examples of medical outcomes here, please be advised that I personally do not recommend them. This book is compilation of peer-review research and expert commentary. It is for informational purposes only and not meant to be medical advice.

The information in this book is intended only for scientific exchange. It has not been approved by the United States Food and Drug Administration for publication nor does it have any official status. Information herein is from the public domain. Any copyrighted or privately owned material inadvertently included will be removed as soon as possible.

For information or concerns about the toxicity of plants, contact the local Poison Control Center in your area. A directory of these is available from The American Association of Poison Control Centers (http://www.aapcc.org/)

www.ingramcontent.com/pod-product-compliance
Lightning Source LLC
Chambersburg PA
CBHW051946270326
41929CB00015B/2545